ANTICANCER DRUG DEVELOPMENT GUIDE

CANCER DRUG DISCOVERY AND DEVELOPMENT

Beverly A. Teicher, Series Editor

Proteasome Inhibitors in Cancer Therapy, edited by *Julian Adams, 2004*

Nucleic Acid Therapeutics in Cancer, edited by *Alan M. Gewirtz, 2004*

Cancer Chemoprevention, Volume 1: *Promising Cancer Chemopreventive Agents,* edited by *Gary J. Kelloff, Ernest T. Hawk, and Caroline C. Sigman, 2004*

DNA Repair in Cancer Therapy, edited by *Lawrence C. Panasci and Moulay A. Alaoui-Jamali, 2004*

Hematopoietic Growth Factors in Oncology: *Basic Science and Clinical Therapeutics,* edited by *George Morstyn, MaryAnn Foote, and Graham J. Lieschke, 2004*

Handbook of Anticancer Pharmacokinetics and Pharmacodynamics, edited by *William D. Figg and Howard L. McLeod, 2004*

Anticancer Drug Development Guide: *Preclinical Screening, Clinical Trials, and Approval, Second Edition,* edited by *Beverly A. Teicher and Paul A. Andrews, 2004*

Handbook of Cancer Vaccines, edited by *Michael A. Morse, Timothy M. Clay, and Kim H. Lyerly, 2004*

Drug Delivery Systems in Cancer Therapy, edited by *Dennis M. Brown, 2003*

Oncogene-Directed Therapies, edited by *Janusz Rak, 2003*

Cell Cycle Inhibitors in Cancer Therapy: *Current Strategies,* edited by *Antonio Giordano and Kenneth J. Soprano, 2003*

Chemoradiation in Cancer Therapy, edited by *Hak Choy, 2003*

Fluoropyrimidines in Cancer Therapy, edited by *Youcef M. Rustum, 2003*

Targets for Cancer Chemotherapy: *Transcription Factors and Other Nuclear Proteins,* edited by *Nicholas B. La Thangue and Lan R. Bandara, 2002*

Tumor Targeting in Cancer Therapy, edited by *Michel Pagé, 2002*

Hormone Therapy in Breast and Prostate Cancer, edited by *V. Craig Jordan and Barrington J. A. Furr, 2002*

Tumor Models in Cancer Research, edited by *Beverly A. Teicher, 2002*

Tumor Suppressor Genes in Human Cancer, edited by *David E. Fisher, 2001*

Matrix Metalloproteinase Inhibitors in Cancer Therapy, edited by *Neil J. Clendeninn and Krzysztof Appelt, 2001*

Farnesyltransferase Inhibitors in Cancer, edited by *Saïd M. Sebti and Andrew D. Hamilton, 2001*

Platinum-Based Drugs in Cancer Therapy, edited by *Lloyd R. Kelland and Nicholas P. Farrell, 2000*

Apoptosis and Cancer Chemotherapy, edited by *John A. Hickman and Caroline Dive, 1999*

Signaling Networks and Cell Cycle Control: *The Molecular Basis of Cancer and Other Diseases,* edited by *J. Silvio Gutkind, 1999*

Antifolate Drugs in Cancer Therapy, edited by *Ann L. Jackman, 1999*

Antiangiogenic Agents in Cancer Therapy, edited by *Beverly A. Teicher, 1999*

Anticancer Drug Development Guide: *Preclinical Screening, Clinical Trials, and Approval,* edited by *Beverly A. Teicher, 1997*

Cancer Therapeutics: *Experimental and Clinical Agents,* edited by *Beverly A. Teicher, 1997*

Anticancer Drug Development Guide

Preclinical Screening, Clinical Trials, and Approval

Second Edition

Edited by

Beverly A. Teicher, PhD

*Vice President and
Director of Oncology Portfolio
Genzyme Corporation
Framingham, MA*

Paul A. Andrews, PhD

*Senior Director, Preclinical Sciences
Aton Pharma Inc.
Tarrytown, NY*

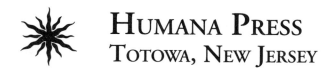

Humana Press
Totowa, New Jersey

© 2004 Humana Press Inc.
999 Riverview Drive, Suite 208
Totowa, New Jersey 07512

www.humanapress.com

Cover design by Patricia F. Cleary.

Cover illustration: from Fig. 1 in Chapter 14, "Discovery of TNP-470 and Other Angiogenesis Inhibitors," by Donald E. Ingber, in *Cancer Therapeutics: Experimental and Clinical Agents*, edited by Beverly A. Teicher, Humana Press, 1997.

This publication is printed on acid-free paper. ∞

ANSI Z39.48-1984 (American National Standards Institute)Permanence of Paper for Printed Library Materials

For additional copies, pricing for bulk purchases, and/or information about other Humana titles, contact Humana at the above address or at any of the following numbers: Tel.:973-256-1699; Fax: 973-256-8341; Email: humana@humanapr.com; or visit our Website: http://humanapress.com

Printed in the United States of America.   10 9 8 7 6 5 4 3 2 1

E-ISBN 1-59259-739-4

Library of Congress Cataloging-in-Publication Data

Anticancer drug development guide : preclinical screening, clinical trials, and approval / edited by Beverly A. Teicher, Paul A. Andrews.—2nd ed.
      p. ; cm. — (Cancer drug discovery and development)
Includes bibliographical references and index.
      ISBN 1-58829-228-2 (alk. paper)
  1. Antineoplastic agents—Development.
      [DNLM: 1. Antineoplastic Agents—standards. 2. Clinical Trials. 3. Drug Approval. 4. Drug Design. 5. Drug Evaluation, Preclinical. QV269 A62953 2004] I. Teicher, Beverly A., 1952-   . II. Andrews, Paul A. III. Series.
      RC271.C5A6722 2004
      616.99'4061—dc22
                                                                                        2003024925

For the beautiful ones

Emily and Joseph

Katie and Matt

PREFACE

This unique volume traces the critically important pathway by which a "molecule" becomes an "anticancer agent." The recognition following World War I that the administration of toxic chemicals such as nitrogen mustards in a controlled manner could shrink malignant tumor masses for relatively substantial periods of time gave great impetus to the search for molecules that would be lethal to specific cancer cells. We are still actively engaged in that search today. The question is how to discover these "anticancer" molecules. *Anticancer Drug Development Guide: Preclinical Screening, Clinical Trials, and Approval, Second Edition* describes the evolution to the present of preclinical screening methods. The National Cancer Institute's high-throughput, in vitro disease-specific screen with 60 or more human tumor cell lines is used to search for molecules with novel mechanisms of action or activity against specific phenotypes. The Human Tumor Colony-Forming Assay (HTCA) uses fresh tumor biopsies as sources of cells that more nearly resemble the human disease.

There is no doubt that the greatest successes of traditional chemotherapy have been in the leukemias and lymphomas. Since the earliest widely used in vivo drug screening models were the murine L1210 and P388 leukemias, the community came to assume that these murine tumor models were appropriate to the discovery of "antileukemia" agents, but that other tumor models would be needed to discover drugs active against solid tumors. Several solid tumor models were developed in mice that are still widely used today and have the advantage of growing a tumor in a syngeneic host. In the meantime, a cohort of immunodeficient mice was developed, including nude, beige, and SCID mice, allowing the growth of human tumor cell lines and human tumor biopsies as xenografts in the mice. Through the great advances in our knowledge of intracellular communication by secreted growth factors, cytokines, chemokines, and small molecules, the importance of the normal cellular environment, both stromal and organal, to the growth of malignant tumors has come to the fore. Now preclinical tumors in which malignant cells are implanted into the organ of origin, that is, in the orthotopic site, add this additional level of sophistication to drug discovery. In addition, new endpoints for preclinical testing, such as quantified tumor cell killing and detection of tumor cells in sanctuary sites, have been developed.

Of the hundreds of thousands of molecules passing through the in vitro screens, few reach clinical testing. In the United States, the FDA must grant permission to enter new investigational agents into human testing, whether the clinical testing is sponsored by an academic investigator, the NCI, or the pharmaceutical industry. Patient safety is the foremost concern. Nonclinical safety testing programs need to be carefully designed to allow identification of potential hazards so that they can be appropriately monitored and so that safe starting doses can be selected. The ongoing costs and timelines for toxicology studies need to be realistically factored into overall development plans so that clinical testing is not unnecessarily delayed. The phase I clinical trial allows the initial study of a candidate therapeutic's pharmacokinetics, pharmacodynamics, toxicity profile, and tolerated dose. In phase II clinical trials, the goal becomes demonstration of disease-specific activity. In phase III clinical trials, statistically significant clinical benefit in well-designed and adequate clinical trials is required for success and FDA marketing approval. Phase III trial designs and statistical plans need to be appropriate relative to the current standard therapy for the intended indication. Poorly conceived and poorly executed clinical development can sabotage promising agents with recognizable activity. Much of the world's community of physicians and investigators now participate in clinical trials of potential new anticancer agents; however, the century-old goal of discovering molecules that control the growth and spread of malignancies as well as being viable as therapeutics in humans remains elusive.

The systems for finding molecules to manage malignancy are in place worldwide and our knowledge of cell growth and regulation is increasing daily; thus, one must remain optimistic of success in cancer drug discovery. This volume provides a guide for navigating the treacherous path from molecule discovery to a commercial therapy. This development path is mined with ample opportunity for failure. For anticancer drug development programs to succeed, promising compounds need to be expeditiously and intelligently selected; toxicology programs need to be thorough, relevant, timely, and informative; clinical development needs to be focused and executed with the highest scientific and administrative integrity; and FDA regulations and guidance have to be understood and followed. It is our hope that *Anticancer Drug Development Guide: Preclinical Screening, Clinical Trials, and Approval, Second Edition* will help all those engaged in developing new treatments for this dread disease to avoid the pitfalls that await. Our friends, colleagues, and family members who are burdened with a diagnosis of cancer await your successes.

Beverly A. Teicher, PhD
Paul A. Andrews, PhD

CONTENTS

Preface vii
Contributors xi
Value-Added eBook/PDA xiv

Part I: In Vitro Methods

1   High-Volume Screening 3
    Michel Pagé

2   High-Throughput Screening in Industry 23
    Michael D. Boisclair, David A. Egan, Kety Huberman,
      and Ralph Infantino

3   The NCI Human Tumor Cell Line (60-Cell) Screen:
    Concept, Implementation, and Applications 41
    Michael R. Boyd

4   Human Tumor Screening 63
    Axel-R. Hanauske, Susan G. Hilsenbeck, and Daniel D. Von Hoff

Part II: In Vivo Methods

5   Murine L1210 and P388 Leukemias 79
    William R. Waud

6   In Vivo Methods for Screening and Preclinical Testing:
    Use of Rodent Solid Tumors for Drug Discovery 99
    Thomas Corbett, Lisa Polin, Patricia LoRusso, Fred Valeriote,
      Chiab Panchapor, Susan Pugh, Kathryn White, Juiwanna Knight,
      Lisa Demchik, Julie Jones, Lynne Jones, and Loretta Lisow

7   Human Tumor Xenograft Models in NCI Drug Development 125
    Michael C. Alley, Melinda G. Hollingshead, Donald J. Dykes,
      and William R. Waud

8   NCI Specialized Procedures in Preclinical Drug Evaluations 153
    Melinda G. Hollingshead, Michael C. Alley, Gurmeet Kaur,
      Christine M. Pacula-Cox, and Sherman F. Stinson

9   Patient-Like Orthotopic Metastatic Models of Human Cancer 183
    Robert M. Hoffman

10 Preclinical Models for Combination Therapy 213
    Beverly A. Teicher

11 Models for Biomarkers and Minimal Residual Tumor 243
    Beverly A. Teicher

12   Spontaneously Occurring Tumors in Companion Animals As Models
     for Drug Development 259
     David M. Vail and Douglas H. Thamm

Part III: Nonclinical Testing to Support Human Trials

13   Nonclinical Testing: *From Theory to Practice*...287
     Denis Roy and Paul A. Andrews

14   Nonclinical Testing for Oncology Drug Products 313
     Paul A. Andrews and Denis Roy

15   Nonclinical Testing for Oncology Biologic Products 325
     Carolyn M. Laurençot, Denis Roy, and Paul A. Andrews

Part IV: Clinical Testing

16   Working With the National Cancer Institute 339
     Paul Thambi and Edward A. Sausville

17   Phase I Trial Design and Methodology for Anticancer Drugs 351
     Patrick V. Acevedo, Deborah L. Toppmeyer, and Eric H. Rubin

18   Phase II Trials: *Conventional Design and Novel Strategies
     in the Era of Targeted Therapies*..363
     Keith T. Flaherty and Peter J. O'Dwyer

19   Drug Development in Europe: *The Academic Perspective* 381
     Chris Twelves, Mike Bibby, Denis Lacombe, and Sally Burtles

20   The Phase III Clinical Cancer Trial 401
     Ramzi N. Dagher and Richard Pazdur

21   Assessing Tumor-Related Symptoms and Health-Related Quality of Life
     in Cancer Clinical Trials: *A Regulatory Perspective* 411
     Judy H. Chiao, Grant Williams, and Donna Griebel

22   The Role of the Oncology Drug Advisory Committee
     in the FDA Review Process for Oncologic Products 421
     Leslie A. Vaccari

23   FDA Role in Cancer Drug Development and Requirements
     for Approval 429
     Susan Flamm Honig

     Index 443

CONTRIBUTORS

PATRICK V. ACEVEDO, MD • *The Cancer Institute of New Jersey, UMDNJ-Robert Wood Johnson Medical School, New Brunswick, NJ*

MICHAEL C. ALLEY, PhD • *Biological Testing Branch, Developmental Therapeutics Program, Division of Cancer Treatment and Diagnosis, National Cancer Institute, Frederick, MD*

PAUL A. ANDREWS, PhD • *Aton Pharma Inc., Tarrytown, NY*

MIKE BIBBY, PhD, DSc, CBiol, FIBiol • *Tom Connors Cancer Research Centre, University of Bradford, West Yorkshire, UK*

MICHAEL D. BOISCLAIR, PhD • *OSI Pharmaceuticals Inc., Farmingdale, NY*

MICHAEL R. BOYD, MD, PhD • *Cancer Research Institute, University of South Alabama, Mobile, AL*

SALLY BURTLES, BSc, PhD • *Division of Drug Development, Cancer Research UK, London, UK*

JUDY H. CHIAO, MD • *Oncology Clinical Research and Development, Aton Pharma Inc., Tarrytown, NY*

THOMAS CORBETT, PhD • *Division of Hematology and Oncology, Barbara Ann Karmanos Cancer Institute, Wayne State University School of Medicine, Detroit, MI*

RAMZI N. DAGHER, MD • *Division of Oncology Drug Products, Food and Drug Administration, Rockville, MD*

LISA DEMCHIK, BS • *Division of Hematology and Oncology, Wayne State University School of Medicine, Detroit, MI*

DONALD J. DYKES, BS • *Cancer Therapeutics, Southern Research Institute, Birmingham, AL*

DAVID A. EGAN, PhD • *OSI Pharmaceuticals Inc., Farmingdale, NY*

KEITH T. FLAHERTY, MD • *Developmental Therapeutics Program, Abramson Cancer Center, University of Pennsylvania, Philadelphia, PA*

DONNA GRIEBEL, MD • *Division of Oncology Drug Products, Food and Drug Administration, Rockville, MD*

AXEL-R. HANAUSKE, MD, PhD • *Section of Medical Oncology, AK St. George, Hamburg, Germany*

SUSAN G. HILSENBECK, PhD • *Section of Biostatistics, Division of Medical Oncology, Department of Medicine, University of Texas Health Science Center, San Antonio, TX*

ROBERT M. HOFFMAN, PhD • *AntiCancer Inc., San Diego, CA; Department of Surgery, University of California at San Diego, La Jolla, CA*

MELINDA G. HOLLINGSHEAD, DVM, PhD • *Biological Testing Branch, Developmental Therapeutics Program, Division of Cancer Treatment and Diagnosis, National Cancer Institute, Frederick, MD*

SUSAN FLAMM HONIG, MD • *Division of Oncology Drug Products, Food and Drug Administration, Rockville, MD*

KETY HUBERMAN, MS • *OSI Pharmaceuticals Inc., Farmingdale, NY*

RALPH INFANTINO, BS • *OSI Pharmaceuticals Inc., Farmingdale, NY*

JULIE JONES, BS • *Division of Hematology and Oncology, Wayne State University School of Medicine, Detroit, MI*

LYNNE JONES, BS • *Division of Hematology and Oncology, Wayne State University School of Medicine, Detroit, MI*

GURMEET KAUR, MS • *Biological Testing Branch, Developmental Therapeutics Program, Division of Cancer Treatment and Diagnosis, National Cancer Institute, Frederick, MD*

JUIWANNA KNIGHT, BA • *Division of Hematology and Oncology, Wayne State University School of Medicine, Detroit, MI*

DENIS LACOMBE, MD, MSc • *New Drug Development Program, European Organization for Research and Treatment of Cancer, Brussels, Belgium*

CAROLYN M. LAURENÇOT, PhD • *Cato Research Ltd., Rockville, MD*

LORETTA LISOW, BA • *Division of Hematology and Oncology, Wayne State University School of Medicine, Detroit, MI*

PATRICIA LORUSSO, DO • *Division of Hematology and Oncology, Wayne State University School of Medicine, Detroit, MI*

PETER J. O'DWYER, MD • *Developmental Therapeutics Program, Abramson Cancer Center, University of Pennsylvania, Philadelphia, PA*

CHRISTINE M. PACULA-COX, MS • *Biological Testing Branch, Developmental Therapeutics Program, Division of Cancer Treatment and Diagnosis, National Cancer Institute, Frederick, MD*

MICHEL PAGÉ, PhD • *Department of Medical Biology, Faculty of Medicine, Université Laval, Sainte-Foy, Québec, Canada*

CHIAB PANCHAPOR, BS • *Division of Hematology and Oncology, Wayne State University School of Medicine, Detroit, MI*

RICHARD PAZDUR, MD • *Division of Oncology Drug Products, Food and Drug Administration, Rockville, MD*

LISA POLIN, PhD • *Division of Hematology and Oncology, Wayne State University School of Medicine, Detroit, MI*

SUSAN PUGH, BS • *Division of Hematology and Oncology, Wayne State University School of Medicine, Detroit, MI*

DENIS ROY, PhD • *Cato Research Ltd., San Diego, CA*

ERIC H. RUBIN, MD • *The Cancer Institute of New Jersey, UMDNJ-Robert Wood Johnson Medical School, New Brunswick, NJ*

EDWARD A. SAUSVILLE, MD, PhD • *Developmental Therapeutics Program, Division of Cancer Treatment and Diagnosis, National Cancer Institute, Rockville, MD*

SHERMAN F. STINSON, PhD • *Biological Testing Branch, Developmental Therapeutics Program, Division of Cancer Treatment and Diagnosis, National Cancer Institute, Frederick, MD*

BEVERLY A. TEICHER, PhD • *Oncology Discovery and Research, Genzyme Corporation, Framingham, MA*

PAUL THAMBI, MD • *Medical Oncology Research Unit, National Cancer Institute, National Institutes of Health, Bethesda, MD*

DOUGLAS H. THAMM, VMD • *Department of Medical Sciences, School of Veterinary Medicine; Comprehensive Cancer Center, University of Wisconsin, Madison, WI*

DEBORAH L. TOPPMEYER, MD • *The Cancer Institute of New Jersey, UMDNJ-Robert Wood Johnson Medical School, New Brunswick, NJ*

CHRIS TWELVES, BMedSci, MB ChB, MD, FRCP (London & Glasgow) • *New Drug Development Program, European Organization for Research and Treatment of Cancer, Brussels, Belgium; and Tom Connors Cancer Research Center, University of Bradford, Bradford, West Yorkshire, UK*

LESLIE A. VACCARI, BSN, RAC • *Cato Research Ltd., Rockville, MD*

DAVID M. VAIL, DVM • *Department of Medical Sciences, School of Veterinary Medicine, Comprehensive Cancer Center, University of Wisconsin, Madison, WI*

FRED VALERIOTE, PhD • *Division of Hematology and Oncology, Wayne State University School of Medicine, Detroit, MI*

DANIEL D. VON HOFF, MD • *Departments of Medicine, Pathology and Molecular and Cellular Biology, Arizona Cancer Center, University of Arizona, Tucson, AZ*

WILLIAM R. WAUD, PhD • *Cancer Therapeutics, Southern Research Institute, Birmingham, AL*

KATHRYN WHITE, BS • *Division of Hematology and Oncology, Wayne State University School of Medicine, Detroit, MI*

GRANT WILLIAMS, MD • *Division of Oncology Drug Products, Food and Drug Administration, Rockville, MD*

Value-Added eBook/PDA

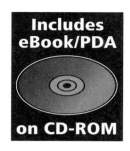

This book is accompanied by a value-added CD-ROM that contains an Adobe eBook version of the volume you have just purchased. This eBook can be viewed on your computer, and you can synchronize it to your PDA for viewing on your handheld device. The eBook enables you to view this volume on only one computer and PDA. Once the eBook is installed on your computer, you cannot download, install, or e-mail it to another computer; it resides solely with the computer to which it is installed. The license provided is for only one computer. The eBook can only be read using Adobe® Reader® 6.0 software, which is available free from Adobe Systems Incorporated at www.Adobe.com. You may also view the eBook on your PDA using the Adobe® PDA Reader® software that is also available free from Adobe.com.

You must follow a simple procedure when you install the eBook/PDA that will require you to connect to the Humana Press website in order to receive your license. Please read and follow the instructions below:

1. Download and install Adobe® Reader® 6.0 software

   You can obtain a free copy of Adobe® Reader® 6.0 software at www.adobe.com

   *Note: If you already have Adobe® Reader® 6.0 software, you do not need to reinstall it.

2. Launch Adobe® Reader® 6.0 software

3. Install eBook: Insert your eBook CD into your CD-ROM drive

   PC: Click on the "Start" button, then click on "Run"

   At the prompt, type "d:\ebookinstall.pdf" and click "OK"

   *Note: If your CD-ROM drive letter is something other than d: change the above command accordingly.

   MAC: Double click on the "eBook CD" that you will see mounted on your desktop.

   Double click "ebookinstall.pdf"

4. Adobe® Reader® 6.0 software will open and you will receive the message

   "This document is protected by Adobe DRM" Click "OK"

   *Note: If you have not already activated Adobe® Reader® 6.0 software, you will be prompted to do so. Simply follow the directions to activate and continue installation.

   Your web browser will open and you will be taken to the Humana Press eBook registration page. Follow the instructions on that page to complete installation. You will need the serial number located on the sticker sealing the envelope containing the CD-ROM.

If you require assistance during the installation, or you would like more information regarding your eBook and PDA installation, please refer to the eBookManual.pdf located on your cd. If you need further assistance, contact Humana Press eBook Support by e-mail at ebooksupport@humanapr.com or by phone at 973-256-1699.

*Adobe and Reader are either registered trademarks or trademarks of Adobe Systems Incorporated in the United States and/or other countries.

I

IN VITRO METHODS

1

High-Volume Screening

Michel Pagé, PhD

CONTENTS

INTRODUCTION
HISTORY
TECHNIQUE DEVELOPMENT
REPORTING TOXICITY

1. INTRODUCTION

The evaluation of compounds such as cancer cytotoxic agents necessitates screening of a great number of chemicals. Animal models have always played an important role in drug evaluation, but with the development of a large number of cytotoxic drugs, animal models are too costly and the delay is too long for these models to be used for large-scale screening.

Up to 1985, when the National Cancer Institute (NCI) started a large program for improving drug discovery (1), screening was performed mostly in vivo, with murine P388 tumors followed by various murine tumor models and three human tumor models xenografted in nude mice.

Compounds that had a minimal activity on P388 leukemia tumors were usually rejected unless they had some special characteristics using other biological or biochemical test models. An evaluation panel for compounds selected from 1975 to 1985 concluded that this approach had a low predictive value and that this screening protocol had only defined a few new anticancer drugs *(2–4)*.

Since the first step in drug screening was performed on P388 leukemia model, this technique could have been selective for drugs that were effective against leukemia and lymphoma, thus limiting the potential for different types of compounds that would be active against solid tumors. The new approach for large-scale screening was favored also for financial considerations, since in vitro testing had considerable economic advantages over the in vivo models.

Animal models were limited by metabolic differences between humans and rodents. There was also some pressure for using fewer animals for experimentation. Thus, it was concluded that, although costly, animal models will not give more information than in vitro screening using a large panel of human tumor cell lines.

From: *Cancer Drug Discovery and Development:*
Anticancer Drug Development Guide: Preclinical Screening, Clinical Trials, and Approval, 2nd Ed.
Edited by: B. A. Teicher and P. A. Andrews © Humana Press Inc., Totowa, NJ

Major efforts were dedicated to the development of in vitro assays based on a large panel of human cell lines representing various tumor types. The requirement using this in vitro system was first that the assay gives reproducible dose-response curves over a concentration range that includes the probable in vivo exposure doses, and second, these dose-response curves obtained in vitro should predict the in vivo effect of the drug. This in vitro prescreening should lead to in vivo testing with suitable tumor models either in the mouse or in human tumors xenografted in nude mice (5).

2. HISTORY

The use of in vitro screening of cytotoxic drugs started with the development of nitrogen mustard derivatives in 1946. The historical development of this technique was reviewed by Dendy (6). The first test for measuring the cytotoxic effect was mainly qualitative with explants of tumor biopsies growing in undefined media, which made the evaluation very difficult. The development of chemically defined media in the 1950s, and of techniques for growing cells as a monolayer on glass or in plastic Petri dishes made this assay easier. Using this technique and protein dyes, the dose-response relationship between the number of colonies and a drug concentration could be determined (7). At the same period, Puck reported the conditions for cell growth in Petri dishes and better defined media were developed by Ham in 1963 (8).

Although useful, monolayer cultures were difficult to use for drug screening, since tumor cells from explants were often contaminated with fibroblasts or other cell types. The successfull development of the in vitro agar plate assay for antibiotic screening led to the interest in the development of a similar approach for cytotoxic drugs, thus eliminating normal cells that could not grow in soft agar. This technique was applied experimentally by Wright et al. (9) using explants of human tumor tissues. This first report was followed by many investigators who correlated the in vitro sensitivity to drugs in the soft agar assay with clinical results.

The correlation that was obtained between in vitro and in vivo results (10,11) provided some arguments for its use in drug screening. This method was, however, time-consuming and difficult to automate, and it was not acceptable for large-scale screening.

Although some of the following techniques are limited in terms of applications for large-scale screening, they are important steps in the development of techniques that lead to large-scale methods used nowadays. The properties of the techniques that will be described may bring some ideas for further development of approaches that will be as close as possible to the clinical situation.

3. TECHNIQUE DEVELOPMENT

3.1. Organ Culture

Organ culture offers many advantages, since tissue integrity is maintained as well as cell-cell relationship, thus giving closer analogy to the in vivo situation. This technique is, however, limited by the difficulty for measuring drug effect as well as variations related to specimen differences. The method had been used in the 1950s for drug screening, but it is difficult to believe that this approach may be used for large-scale screening.

3.2. Spheroids

This technique results from the spontaneous aggregation of cells into small spherical masses that grow and differentiate. The structure of spheroids is closer to the in vivo system than monolayer growth, and the use of these small masses for measuring cytotoxicity is a better model, since it takes into account the three-dimensional structure and mimics the diffusion of drugs into tissues. Spheroids allow the determination of drug penetration into nonvascularised tissues, the effect of the pO_2, pCO_2, and of the diffusion of nutrients into these tissues.

Most of the studies performed with spheroids are performed with cell lines, and they require about 2 wk before drug sensitivity testing. They are, therefore, not suitable for large-scale screening.

3.3. Suspension Culture

Suspension cultures are more suitable for studying drug sensitivity on cells growing in suspension, such as the ones isolated from small-cell carcinoma of the lung, which grow like small floating islets or leukemia or lymphoma, which normally grow in liquid media. Also, some cells are modified in such a way that they grow in suspension in culture; this is going further away from natural growth, and this may result in bias in drug evaluation.

3.4. Monolayer Culture

Growing cells in monolayers has been most frequently applied to cytotoxicity testing, because it is easily adapted to automation. It may be difficult to use with primary cultures using human biopsy material, since this material is often contaminated with normal cells that may overgrow tumor cells. Some modifications may be applied to media, mostly to defined media to prevent growth of nontumor cells, but in general, these tests are performed with cell lines. This technique, however, may be performed using outgrowths from tumor biopsy explants.

This method offers great flexibility for possible drug exposure and recovery, and for drug effect measurement. Among the various methods described, monolayer culture may be automated more easily, and it is adaptable to microscale methodology.

3.5. Clonogenic Growth and Soft Agar

Clonogenic assays have the advantage of selecting tumor cells in a mixed population, since only the latter have the capacity to grow in suspension in soft agar. Cloning efficiencies, however, using such techniques are very low, often less than 1% with single-cell suspensions, and the measurement of inhibition of colony formation is performed after about six generations. This means that the measurement of the number of colonies and their diameter is often performed on a small number, and colonies of small diameters cannot be measured. The number of technical problems in culture, however, and the difficulty in performing this assay prevent its use in large-volume screening.

Also, the determination of the number of colonies is somewhat subjective, and very recently, we have reported a colony amplification method that is described later (12). Various modifications of the clonogenic assay have been proposed, but the major problem remains that it is a time-consuming technology that is difficult to adapt to large-volume screening *(13–17)*.

3.6. Large-Scale Screening

With the development of a myriad of cytotoxic compounds, it became urgent to develop methods that could be automated. The criteria for the development of methods for large-scale screening are the following:

- The method should be economical. The stress applied to drug companies and government agencies for reducing the production cost requires that screening of new compounds should be economical. Techniques should be predictive enough so that in vivo testing in nude mice xenografted with human tumors be used only in the second phase of drug screening.
- Methods that require too much technician time or expensive reagents should be avoided. The need for large-scale screening required automation. The development of 96-well plates for this purpose is now widely accepted and used in various laboratories around the world. Instruments for reading these plates, either in fluorescence or in the visible spectrum, are also available. Data acquisition is also simple, since all these instruments are connected to microcomputers or to central facilities.
- The method should be reproducible with a low interassay coefficient of variation.
- Cells needed for cytotoxicity should not be a limiting factor; large-scale screening should be performed with various cell lines, rather than primary cells.
- The choice of cell lines should represent as close as possible the clinical situation; cell lines should be chosen to be representative of the various tumors, including resistance to various cytotoxic agents.
- The assay should be sensitive so that one may detect the influence of very low concentrations of the test compounds on cell viability.
- The relationship should be as linear as possible, so that interpretation and data treatment could be more easily performed using simple regression.
- The range of drug concentrations used should be comparable to what could be expected for in vivo treatment.
- Substrate or dyes used for the assay should be as stable as possible so that large quantities may be prepared in advance to reduce variation; chemicals used for the assay should not then be toxic.

The development of a practical in vitro test to evaluate the efficacies of various drugs for cancer treatment has been the goal of many investigators, and many tests have been developed that give good sensitivity, but their use for large-scale screening is very limited.

In the 1950s, Puck reported inhibition of colony formation using either primary cells or cell lines. This method could not be used for large-scale screening, because it was tedious and very costly in terms of labor. The automatic determination of colony size and the number of colonies as reported by Emond et al. in 1982 made this approach more accurate, but still very far from an application for large-scale screening. Colony counting, however, does not always reflect cell growth because of the large variation in colony diameter to overcome this difficulty, a semiautomated method in which the surface occupied by the colony was integrated has already reported *(18)*.

The soft agar cloning assay developed by Salmon et al. *(19,20)* gives a very good predictive value, but it has many technical disadvantages, thus limiting its application in preclinical drug screening.

Very recently, we have reported an optimization of the soft agar technique using tetrazolium salt to detect very small colonies *(21)*. Although very sensitive, this method cannot be applied to the large scale, because it has the same limitation as the other soft agar techniques.

Dye exclusion techniques are widely used for cells growing in suspension, but for low cell numbers, the method is not applicable *(22)*. Assays using uptake of radioactive precursors are not practical and, because of potential hazards, cannot be used in large-scale routine cytotoxicity measurements.

The ability of fibroblasts to exclude a variety of dyes in the presence of the physiological saline solutions has been used extensively for cell death measurement *(23–27)*. Already in 1978, Durkin et al. *(23)* had reported a very good correlation between in vitro dye exclusion and the results obtained on seven patients with Hodgkin's lymphoma receiving chemotherapy. This was usually performed by counting preparations of cells with a hemocytometer in the presence of such agents as trypan blue, eosin, or erythrocin B.

The uptake of dye over long periods may not be representative of viable cells. Also, it is sometimes difficult to distinguish between viable tumor cells and viable nontumor cells present in the preparation.

Moreover, the acute toxicity of chemotherapeutic agents on the membrane integrity as a criteria may not reflect cell viability for long-time exposure.

In 1983, Weisenthal et al. *(22)* reported a dye exclusion method for in vitro chemosensitivity testing in human tumors. In this method, dissociated cancer cells are exposed to antineoplasic drugs and cultured for 4–6 d in liquid medium. After this period, cells are stained with fast green, sedimented on two slides, and counterstained with hematoxylin eosin.

Living cells are stained with fast green, and all cells are stained with hematoxylin eosin. The assay could be performed on about 50% of human cancer specimens obtained. The assay demonstrated a very good correlation between the in vitro chemosensitivity of different types of tumors and the clinical response. However, it is aimed at determining the prognosis of chemotherapy treatment of specific cancer patients rather than large-sale drug screening.

In 1983, Tseng and Safa reported an in vitro screening test for anticancer agents using monodispersed tumor cells derived from rat mammary tumors in rat *(28)*. Monolayer cell cultures in multiwell plates were maintained in medium supplementated with hormones and fetal calf serum. Using a randomnized table, drugs like tamoxifen, adriamycin, thiotepa, and methotrexate were administrated to cultures singly or in combination. They found that adriamycin consistently exhibited a greater cytotoxic effect for a given concentration as expected.

Combination of these drugs was also studied. Using this procedure, they tested human tumor biopsies. Although useful, this method is also designed for individual patients.

In 1989, the National Cancer Institute has initiated a panel of human tumor cell lines for primary anticancer drugs screening for discovery of compounds with potential antitumor activity and possibly disease-oriented specificity. This method was initiated for the screening of up to 10,000 new substances/yr. The screening panel consisted of 60 human cell lines representing various tumor sites, such as lung, colon, melanoma, kidney, ovary, leukemia, and lymphoma. The cell inoculum was performed in 96-well tissue-culture plates, and the cells were incubated for 24 h. Then test agents were added in 5- to 10-fold dilutions from the highest soluble concentration and incubated for 48 h. For each cell line, a dose-response curve was generated, and the activity of a new compound was compared to known compounds, such as adriamycin and tamoxifen.

The cell growth and viability were measured using a protein stain sulforhodamine (SRB). This dye binds to basic amino acids of cellular macromolecules. This assay was found valid for attached cells. The bound dye was solubilized and measured spectrophotometrically on the plate reader interfaced with a microcomputer. This was the first attempt of the NCI for large-scale screening of new drugs.

This assay is valid only for attached cells, since the determination of the dose-response relationship is based on the intensity of the color generated by cells that remain attached on the micro wells.

This is also limited by the effect that certain drugs may have on cell function on long-term viability. The determination of this factor is thus limited, since this assay measures only the cells that after treatment become detached from the plastic support compared to controls (29).

As mentioned earlier, cell viability may be determined using vital stains, such as the most common trypan blue. In 1990, Cavanaugh et al. reported the use of neutral red as a vital stain that accumulates in the lysosomal compartment following uptake via non-ionic diffusion. This viability dye has already been reported by Nemez et al. (30), and Allison and Young (31). Its use to evaluate cell number was reported earlier by Fintner (32), as a vital stain for assaying viral cytopathogenecity and its application have been demonstrated in the interferon assay.

The use of neutral red as a vital stain for the determination of toxicity was already reported by Borenfreund and Puerner (33), to determine the toxicity of various compounds in vitro. The advantages of this compound is that it may be used in the semiautomatic mode and incorporated into various cell lines for large-scale screening of compounds as indicated by Cavanaugh et al. (34).

In this assay, neutral red is used for the rapid screening of potential anticancer agents using solid tumor cell lines. The assay is performed in microwells, and cells are incubated for short periods of 2 h followed by the measurement of cell number by neutral red absorbance following four cell doubling times.

The cell number correlated very well with the absorbance at 540 nm. However, it is important to determine the optimal dye concentration and staining times, which vary between cell Unes. •

This assay provided a reproducible and technically simple method for measuring cell number. The response was relatively linear over a wide range of cell concentrations. The method is not dependent on the metabolism, which is the case for MTT, XTT, or alamar blue, which will be described later. It allows the direct measurement of cell number following various treatments.

The method is semiautomatic, as is data treatment. This allowed the analysis of the steepness of the concentration-response curve, thus discriminating potentially active compounds. This assay, however, is not sensitive enough at about 1000 cells/well. The method requires little technician time, and it is applicable for large-scale screening.

The method suggests the use of only two cell lines, and it would be interesting to verify its application with a variety of cell lines, such as the one used by the NCI screening program. The assay may be used for suspension cultures by the addition of centrifugation steps, but this renders the procedure long and tedious.

The reduction of soluble tetrazolium salts to insoluble color formazans has been applied for many years in zymograms for the determination of isoenzyme activities *(35,36)*. In one of the earliest efforts to develop practical in vitro drug screening, Mosmann in 1983 described a rapid colorimetric assay for the measurement of cell growth. Ideally, the colorometric assay should transform a colorless substrate and modify it into a colored product by any living cell, but not by dead cells. The tetrazolium salts, which are used for measuring various dehydrogenases, were applied for this purpose. In this assay, the tetrazolium ring is modified in active mitochondria, which makes it selective for living cells. Mosmann has developed a new tetrazolium salt MTT [3-(4.5-dimethylthiazol-2-yl)-2,5-difenyl tetrazolium bromide] that measures only leaving cells and can be read by the ELISA reader *(37)*.

Tetrazolium salts had already been used by Schaeffer and Friend *(38)* for identification of viable colonies of tetrazolium salts in soft agar and for measuring the sensitivity of tumor cells in primary cultures by Alley and Lieber *(39)*. In this assay, cells are treated with various concentration of drugs for different periods, MTT solution is added to each well, and the plate is incubated at 37°C for 4 h. The insoluble tetrazolium salt is then solubilized in acid propanol, and after a few minutes, all crystals are dissolved, and the plates are then read at 570 nm.

The first demonstration of this assay was performed to measure the activity of interleukin-2 in vitro. The use of MTT has several advantages for assaying cell survival and proliferation. The substrate is cleaved by all living and metabolically active cells, but not by dead cells or erthrocytes.

The amount of formazan generated is proportional to the metabolically active cell number over a wide range of drug concentrations. The advantages of the colorimetric assay are the ease and speed with which samples can be processed. The substrate does not interfere with the measurement of the product, and absorbance may be measured directly after a few minutes of solubilization. The color generated is stable for a few hours at room temperature. The MTT assay was compared with thymidine incorporation, and a good correlation was found between the thymidine incorporation and the visual examination of the cell density. However, the incorporation of thymidine may differ in terms of quality from the MTT assay, because these assays do not measure exactly the same parameters. Thymidine incorporation is proportional to cells in the S phase, whereas the MTT assay measures viable cells or metabolically active cells. The reduction of MTT varies from one cell type to another. Standard curves show differences in the metabolic activity between cell lines. Therefore, a standard curve must be run for each cell line.

Several modifications of the Mosmann MTT assay have been reported for the measurement of cell growth *(40–42)*. We have already reported the optimization of the tetrazolium-based colorimetric assay for the measurement of cell toxicity in large-scale screening *(43)*.

In this paper, we reported some modifications of MTT assay for the measurement of anchorage-dependent and independent cells. The various factors affecting color production, such as the concentration of tetrazolium, incubation period, and solvent volume, were optimized. Using cyanide and daunorubicin, the influence of dead cells on the measurement was also studied. The assay was tested in both anchorage-independent mouse leukemia P388 cells, H69 small-cell carcinoma growing as small islets, and anchorage-dependent adenocarcinoma cells. Centrifugation of the microtitration plate was

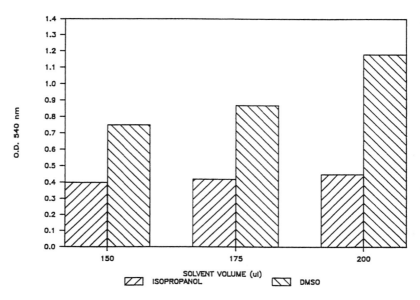

Fig. 1. Optimization of the extraction of reduced MTT using various volumes of either DMSO or isopropanol.

eliminated by the use of a supernatant collection system. Although the use of the MTT assay was rapid and precise, we found that care had to be taken when using this assay for short-term cytotoxicity testing, since nonviable cells could also metabolize tetrazolium salts.

Many variables were tested to achieve the optimal assay conditions when suspension cultures were used; we found that the supernatant could be removed easily with a Scatron supernatant collection system (Emendale Scientific Workwood Ontario, Canada), since the crystals set at the bottom of the plate. Acid isopropanol was replaced by dimethyl sulfoxide *(42)* to increase solubilization. On a routine basis, all plates should be read after 60 min to reduce variations in color development.

Results shown on the next figure show the efficiency of DMSO as compared to acid isopropanol (Fig. 1).

Also, increasing the volume of DMSO yielded a higher optical density. For practical reasons and because of the limited volume of the wells, 200 µL of DMSO were used to solubilize reduced formaran in routine assays.

A typical standard curve for leukemia P388 cells is shown in Fig. 2. We observed a linear relationship between the optical density and the incubation period from 0–3 h. For routine assays, a 4-h incubation period was chosen as described by Mosman. No benefit could be obtained from longer solubilization periods.

The centrifugation step used by many authors before extraction of the reduced tetrazolium salt was avoided by the use of a supernatant collection system. This device efficiently separated insoluble crystals from the supernatant.

Since reduced MTT is a product of functional mitochondria, nonviable cells could also reduce MTT and thus influence cell measurement. To test this hypothesis, cells were heat-killed in a hot growth medium before being assayed, treated with high doses of

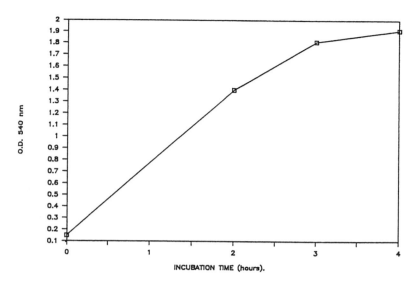

Fig. 2. Determination of the optimal incubation time for P388 cells in the presence of 20 µL MTT solution (5 mg/mL).

daunorobucin, or cells were incubated for 45 min in complete medium supplemented with $10^{-2}M$ potassium cyanide. At various periods, aliquots were taken for MTT measurement.

It is well known that oxidation reactions occur in active mitochondria. Thus, measurement of cells using the MTT should be related to the oxidation potential of each cell. I could not find any report where the influence of dead cells was studied on color development using the MTT method. Since active mitochondria could be isolated, it is then possible that nonviable cells could interfere and give a positive MTT reaction. We found that the killing of cells by heat or by cyanide treatment did not cause color development or interfere with the assay. These factors, also, inhibited the oxidation process in mitochondria.

However, antimitotic drugs, such as daunorobucin, are cytotoxic mainly because they intercalate into the DNA and cause cell death over longer periods while living functional mitochondria. Figure 3 shows that when P388 cells were treated with a very high concentration of daunorobucin, color development after 24 h was still 50% of the control, although these cell could be considered nonviable by the trypan blue exclusion method. The presence of dead cell was no longer interfering after 4 d, which is the time required to test cytotoxic drugs in vitro. Although the assay was found valid and that the influence of dead cells was negligible after 4 d, one must take into account this factor when using the MTT assay for short-term cytotoxocity testing.

The same applies to other assays using mitochondrial dehydrogenases, since most of the drugs tested are not targeted toward mitochondrial activity.

Although the MTT assay is valid, the amount of reduced MTT must be dissolved in DMSO. This may be a safety hazard for laboratory personnel, and it has a deleterious effect on laboratory plasticware. Also, the use of a solvent increases the inherent error in the assay.

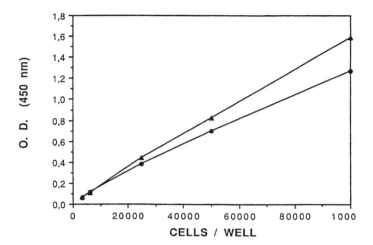

Fig. 3. Standard curves for (▲) LoVo (incubation 4 h, 5 µL PMS 10 m*M*, XTT 1.5 mg/mL) and (●) H-69 (incubation 16 h, 5 µL PMS 5 m*M*, XTT 1.0 mg/mL). Various concentrations of cells were seeded in microtitration plates, and the XTT assay was performed immediately.

In 1988, the National Cancer Institute developed a new tetrazolium derivative of which the reduced form (XTT) is soluble in cell culture *(44,45)*. We have optimized the assay with XTT and reported results that were comparable to the MTT assay in terms of color development, but it could be performed safely and more easily *(46)*.

The next figure shows that the maximum absorbance of reduced XTT at 465 nm with a minimum absorption at 400 nm. Measurement could be performed on the normal ELISA reader (Fig. 3).

After optimization of the XTT assay, we found that this substrate was not reduced as easily as MTT by mitochondrial enzymes and some electron couplers, such as PMS (phenazinemethosulfate), had to be used for the rapid electron transfer to XTT. We also found that optical density decreased by increasing the XTT concentration over 75 µg/ well. This was probably owing to an inhibition of the enzymatic reaction related to the toxicity of the product at high concentrations. The assay could be performed in 4 h using XTT at 75 µg/well containing 5 µL of 10 m*M* PMS/well. The influence of dead cells for short incubation periods was comparable to MTT.

Figure 4 shows the linear relationship obtained between the optical density (450 nm) and cell concentration using two cell lines, adenocarcinoma Lovo cells, and small-cell carcinoma of the lung H69. The lower limit of detection for these cell lines varies between 1500 and 3000 cells/well.

The growth of anchorage-dependent and independent cells was followed by the XTT assay. Figure 5 shows these growth curves. The cytotoxicity of daunorobucin was measured with the XTT assay, and results were found comparable to the ones obtained with MTT.

Based on the various parameters tested for the optimization of the XTT method. The assay could be performed as follows: 50 µL of a solution containing 5 µL of 10 m*M* PMS/ well and XTT (1.5 mg/mL). The incubation period could be varied from one cell line to another depending on the level of metabolism of these cells, but for each analysis with many cell Unes, a fixed period of 4 h was compatible with the metabolism of most of the cell lines.

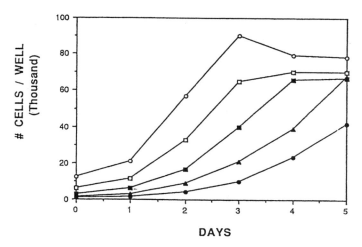

Fig. 4. Growth curves for LoVo cells (incubation 4 h, 5 μL PMS 10 m*M*, XTT 1.5 mg/mL) (●) 1000, (▲) 2000, (■) 4000, (□) 8000, (○) 16,000 cells/well. Cells were seeded at different concentrations, and cell growth was determined every day by XTT assay.

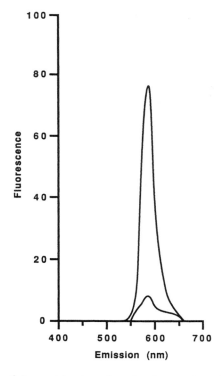

Fig. 5. Fluorescence spectra of alamar blue in reduced and nonreduced forms. Alamar was reduced by addition of sodium borohydride.

There are some advantages for using the XTT method of compared to the MTT, since the former is soluble both in reduced and oxidized forms; it allows a direct optical density reading, therefore eliminating the solubilization step. This method could be used efficiently for measuring cell growth of either anchorage-dependent or independent cells.

The assay offers the same advantages as the widely used MTT assay, but it offers the added advantage of being more reproducible. It also could be automated, and it avoids the use of toxic solvents.

MTT and XTT solutions are, however, unstable, and these must be prepared shortly before being used; these products are also cytotoxic. Very recently, a new reagent, alamar blue, was developed by Alamar Bioscience. This nonfluorescent substrate yields after reduction in living cells a very strong fluorescent product. We have used this new substrate to replace MTT or XTT. On reduction alamar blue yields a fluorescent pink product. Using the automated fluorescent plate reader Cytofluor (Millipore Corporation), we have evaluated the various parameters, such as substrate concentration, time of incubation temperature of incubation with respect to linearity, and lower limit of detection.

Alamar blue was obtained from Alamar Bioscience Inc. (Sacramento, CA). This product is supplied as a ready-to-use solution that may be stored in the dark at 4°C for long periods. For comparison, XTT was used as a reference method as described above (47), The fluorescence spectra of oxidized and reduced alamar blue are shown in Fig. 5.

As shown in Fig. 5, the fluorescence of reduced alamar blue is extremely high at 590 nm. The assay is similar to the XTT assay. Briefly, cells are inoculated into 96-well flat-bottom microplates in 200 µL of culture medium; various volumes of alamar blue were added and the cells were incubated at 37° in the presence of 5% CO_2 for fluorescence development by living cells. After various periods, fluorescence was measured with an excitation at 530 nm and an emission at 590 nm. The Cytofluor systems software was used for data management. The development of fluorescence was followed with time and at various alamar blue concentrations. For standard curves, exponentially growing cells were seeded into 100 µL of complete culture medium. Ten micro-liters of Alamar Blue were added per well, and the microplate was inoculated for 2 h at 37°C before fluorescence measurement. When the optimized assay was used for cytotoxicity measurement, human ovarian carcinoma cells SKOV3 were plated at 2500 cells/well in the presence of various concentrations of daunorubicin. Cells were incubated for 4 d at 37°C, and alamar blue assay was performed.

When the development was followed over various periods of incubation, we observed an almost linear relationship between fluorescence and incubation time. It was only when 1 µL of alamar blue was used/well that we found a reduced fluorescence. We found no significant difference in fluorescence development for volumes varying from 5–15 µL/well.

As already noted for MTT or XTT assays, a standard curve must be run for each cell line because of the inherent difference in the metabolism between one cell line to the other. In Fig. 6, we found a lower detection limit of 200 cells/well for most of the cell Unes tested. This assay gives a good relationship between the number of cells and the fluorescence obtained over a wide range of concentrations. For low cell numbers from 200–3000 cells, the assay was nearly linear. When alamar blue assay was compared to the XTT for testing the cytotoxicity of daunorubicin, we obtained the following (Figs. 7 and 8).

This new fluorogenic indicator for cell measurement has many advantages, since it yields a soluble product in culture medium with a low background for the oxidized form of alamar blue. We found no interference with culture medium, except that high serum concentrations may cause some quenching. The method may be used for anchorage-dependent or independent cells, since no solubilization or centrifugation is needed. The

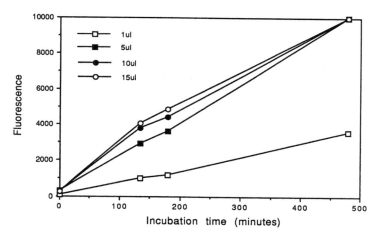

Fig. 6. Time-course for reduction of alamar blue (fluorescence development) by SKOV3 cells (12,500 cells/well), for different concentrations of alamar blue; 1 (□), 5 (■), 10 (●), and 15 μL (○) were added to the medium.

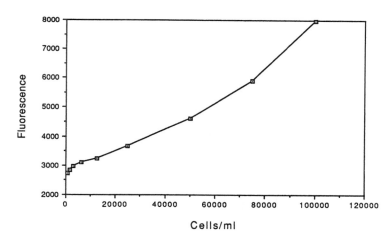

Fig. 7. Standard curves for SKVLB; incubation time was 2 h with 10 μL/well of alamar blue. Various concentrations of cells (serially diluted) were seeded in 96-well plates, and alamar blue was added immediately.

lower limit of detection obtained was about 200 cells for the cell lines tested. This is markedly lower than most of the previous assays. The assay was used recently for measuring the activity of interleukin-2 (48).

The assay is sensitive and highly reproducible, but it is limited since automated fluorescence plate readers are not found frequently in laboratories. In 1995, we have reported the conditions for using alamar blue as a substrate in a colorimetric cytotoxic assay. When alamar blue is reduced in the presence of mitochondrial dehydrogenases in living cells, the production of a fluorescent product is accompanied by a change in color, which may be used for cytotoxicity measurement. The absorption spectra of alamar blue in reduced and oxidized forms are shown in Fig. 9.

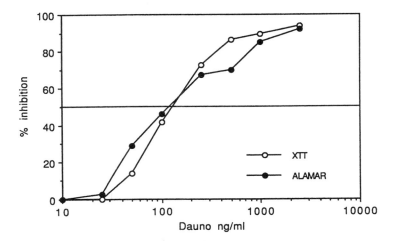

Fig. 8. Cytotoxicity of daunorubicin on SKOV3 cells (12,000 cells/well). Cells were treated with various daunorubicin concentrations. On day 4 of treatment, the living cell population was measured by XTT or by the addition of 10 µL/well of alamar blue. Fluorescence was measured after an incubation of 2 h.

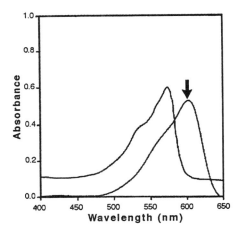

Fig. 9. Absorption spectra of alamar blue in reduced and oxidized (arrow) forms. Alamar was reduced by the addition of sodium borohydride.

The assay was optimized, and the optical density was read at 600 nm with the ELISA plate reader. The colormetric assay was compared to the fluorescence assay or to the XTT for cytotoxicity measurement of daunorobucin in vitro. For this assay, human ovarian teratocarcinoma cells were plated at 2500 cells/well in the presence of various concentrations of daunorubicin in complete culture medium. Cells were incubated for 4 d at 37°C, alamar blue was added and optical density was measured at 600 nm. We noticed again differences in the metabolism of alamar blue by various cell Unes. The decrease in optical density at 600 nm as a function of cell number is given in Fig. 10.

For the colorimetric assay, 20 µL of alamar blue had to be used/well as compared to 10 µL for the fluorometric assay. We found for this colorimetric assay a lower limit of

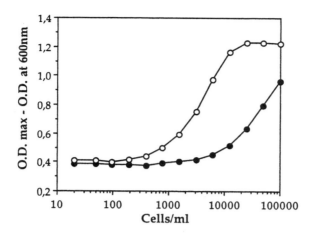

Fig. 10. Standard curves for (**A**) CRL 1572, (**B**) CEM/vbl 100, and (**C**) SKOV 3; incubation time 4 (●) and 24 (○) for (**C**) only. Cells were seeded in 200 µL of culture medium, and 20 µL of alamar blue were added.

detection of 2000 cells/well for most of the cell lines tested. If one increases the incubation period to 24 h, a lower limit of detection of 200 cells/well was found, and this is comparable to the one obtained with the fluorescence assay. In Fig. 10, we compared the cytotoxicity of daunorubicin in vitro with three assays. We found no significant difference among the three assays and the IC_{50} was 2.1 ng/mL for the fluorescence alamar blue assay, 1.6 ng for the XTT assay, and 2.1 ng for the colorimetric alamar blue assay.

This colorimetric assay may be less sensitive, but it could be performed with a common ELISA plate reader. It is economical, and it could replace many of the formazan salts discussed earlier or other cytotoxicity measurement techniques, thus avoiding potentially hazardous chemicals. Alamar blue is nontoxic, and viable cells may be recovered for further experimental procedures.

One of the main problems encountered in cancer chemotherapy is multiple drug resistance (MDR), where cell populations treated in vivo with a single agent subsequently exhibited a broad crossresistance to other chemicals unrelated chemically or to which the cells have never been exposed. This phenomenon has been extensively studied recently (49–54). This crossresistance is related to a membrane glycoprotein, which is used as a membrane efflux pump. There are also many other mechanisms of resistance that are not related to the MDR-like alteration in the topoisomerase, which influences the toxicity of VP16 or VP26 resistance to methotrexate, which is related to DHFR amplification. Owing to the importance of drug resistance in cancer chemotherapy, resistant cell lines were included in the NCI panel for large-scale screening of new drugs, such as the one reported in 1992 by Wu et al. at the National Cancer Institute (55). The cell panels manifested a broad range of sensitivities to drugs associated with MDR as well as other types of resistance.

Wu et al. found a strong correlation between drugs, which share the same intracellular mechanism of action as expected, and for seven MDR drugs, the coefficient was larger than 0.8. Such correlations between relative cellular sensitivities and intracellular mechanisms of action were recently used as a basis for the selection of other drugs, such as tubulin binding compounds.

Wu et al. showed very clearly the importance of using the cytotoxicity assay for the measurement of resistance and also for screening potential cytotoxic agents that could be used to overcome MDR.

This panel or a disease-oriented panel is used for large-scale screening of new anti-cancer drugs. With proper data management, this panel may also be used for getting information related to the mechanism of drug action. The NCI is presently using this panel for screening of about 20,000 new drugs/y (56).

4. REPORTING TOXICITY

When reporting toxicity of a drug, the IC_{50} represents the dose that is needed to inhibit 50% cell growth. In other words, this is the concentration of the drug in wells that contain one-half of the cells that are present in the control wells. Since most of the drugs have an action on dividing cells, one may assume that the cell population is dividing rapidly. The amount of drug needed to obtain 50% growth in these rapidly dividing cells will be lower than the amount of drug needed to inhibit slow-growing cells. Since the IC_{50} does not take into account the growth rate, the former may vary with various cell growth rates. The aim of these screenings is to predict if a certain drug may be used at a certain concentration to slow down cancer without being toxic for a patient or to determine if the cells tested are resistant to the drug. However, in a clinical situation, the aim is not only to slow down cancer growth rate, but to reduce the tumor mass to zero. This may be represented in the following equation:

$$IC_{50} = (T_5 \times 100/NT_5) \tag{1}$$

IC_{50} is the dose that inhibits 50% of the cells present in the control wells. GI50 is the dose that inhibits 50% of cell growth.

$$GI_{50} = (T_1 - T_5 \times 100 / T_1 - NT_5) \tag{2}$$

T_5 is the number of cells in treated wells on day 5, NT_5 is the number of cells in non-treated wells on day 5. T_1 is the number of cells in wells (treated or nontreated) on day 1. Figure 11 gives a representation of these data (Tremblay ML, personal communication).

Since the GI_{50} takes into account cell growth in the treated wells compared with the nontreated wells, one would expect that the GI_{50} would not vary with growth rate. If one varies the growth rate of 3T3 cells with various concentrations of calf serum and measures the GI_{50} and the IC_{50} at these various growth rates, very important differences are observed in the IC_{50} without much variation in the GI_{50} (Table 1).

The same is true for human colon adenocarcinoma Lovo cells when they are cultured in 1% compared with 10% calf serum. We found no significant difference in the GI_{50}, whereas the IC_{50} was 55 ng/mL for 1% serum and 40 ng/mL for 10% calf serum. This method was applied to various cell lines, and we found that the GI_{50} did not vary significantly whatever the growth rate of the cells. We also observed that the faster the cell growth rate, the lower the IC_{50}.

These results show the importance of reporting the data, so that one may predict the usefulness of a certain drug as a potential cancer treatment. The results show that the GI_{50} should be added to the information when reporting cytotoxicity, since it allows one to predict that not only could a drug be cytostatic, but also it could have a potential in terms of tumor reduction.

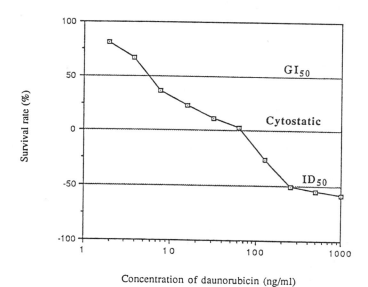

y-axis: Survival rate (%)
x-axis: Concentration of daunorubicin (ng/ml)

Fig. 11. Cytotoxicity of daunorubicin for cancer cells.

Table 1
Comparison Between GI50 and ID50
for the Measurement of Daunorubicin Cytotoxicity, MTT Method, in Swiss 3T3
and LOVO Cells Cultured in Different Concentrations of Calf Serum (1, 5,10, and 20%)

Type of cells	Measure	GI50 ng/mL	ID50 mg/mL
3T3	Slow growth 1 % serum	40.0	40.0
3T3	Slow growth 5% serum	5.0	20.0
3T3	Normal growth 10% serum	5.0	6.0
3T3	Rapid growth 20% serum	6.0	5.0
Lovo	Slow growth 1 % serum	7.5	55.0
Lovo	Normal growth 10% serum	8.0	40.0

The description of the various methods used for drug screening shows that it is now possible at an acceptable cost to obtain information on a new drug in terms of its potential use as an anticancer agent with a panel consisting of cells from various target organs and different types of resistance. It is now possible not only to predict toxicity and resistance, but also their mechanism of action.

REFERENCES

1. Shoemaker RH, McLemore TL, Abbott BJ, Fine DL, Gorelik E, Mayo JG, Fodstad O, Boyd MR. Human tumour xenograft models for use with an *in vitro*-based disease-oriented anti-tumour drug screening program. In: Winograd B, Peckham MJ, Pinedo, HM, eds., *Human Tumour Xenografts in Anticancer Drug Development*. Berlin and Heidelberg: Springer-Verlag. 1988:115–120.
2. Staquet MJ, Byar DP, Green SB, Rozencweig M. Clinical predictivity of transplantable tumor systems in the selection of new drugs for solid tumors: rationale for a three-stage strategy. *Cancer Treat Rep* 1983; 67:753–765.

3. Venditti JM. The National Cancer Institute antitumor drug discovery program, current and future perspectives: a commentary. *Cancer Treat Rep* 1983; 67:767–772.

4. Atassi G, Staquet M. The clinical predictive value of the mouse screening methods. In: Hilgard P, Hellmann K, eds. *Anticancer Drug Development*. Barcelona: JR Prous Publishers. 1983:27–34.

5. Pinedo HM. Development of new anti-cancer drugs. *Med Oncol Tumor Pharmacother* 1986; 3:63–69.

6. Dendy PP, Hill BT, eds. *Human Tumour Drug Sensitivity Testing in Vitro: Techniques and Clinical Applications*. Academic. 1983.

7. Eagle H, Fooley GE. *Am J Med* 1956; 21:739.

8. Ham RG. *Science* 1963; 140:802.

9. Wright JC, Cobb JP, Gumport SL, Golomb FM, Safadi D. *New Engl J Med* 1957; 257:1207.

10. Wilson AP, Neal FE. *Br J Cancer* 1981; 44:189.

11. Silvestrini R, Sanfilippo O, Daidone MG. In: Dendy PP, Hill BT, eds., *Human Tumour Drug Sensitivity Testing In Vitro*. Academic, 1983:281

12. Lemieux P, Michaud M, Pagé M. A new formazan amplified clonogenic assay for cytotoxicity testing. *Biotechnol Techniques* 1993; 7:597–602.

13. Agrez MW, Kovach JS, Lieber MM. *Br J Cancer* 1982; 46:88.

14. Bertoncello I, et al. *Br J Cancer* 1982; 45:803.

15. Rupniak HT, Hill BT. *Cell Biol M Rep* 1980; 4:479.

16. Hamburger AW, Salmon SE, Kim MB, Trent JM, Soehnlen B, Alberts DS, Schmidt HJ. *Cancer Res* 1978; 38:3438.

17. Salmon SE, ed. *Cloning of Human Tumour Stem Cells. Progress in Clinical and Biological Research*, vol. 48. New York: Alan R. Liss, 1980.

18. Emond JP, Pagé M. A semi-automatic *in vitro* method for the measurement of the pharmacological activity of drug-antibody conjugates used in drug targeting. European Association of Cancer Research, Tumor Progression and Markers. 1981:467–470.

19. Salmon SE, Alberts DS, Durie BGM, Meyskens PL, Soehnlen , Chen H-S G, Moon T. Clinical correlations of drug sensitivity in the human tumor stem cell assay. *Recent Results Cancer Res* 1980; 74: 300–305.

20. Salmon SE, Hamburger AW, Soehnlen BJ, Durie BGM, Alberts DS, Moon TC. Quantitation of differential sensitivities of human tumor stem cells to anticancer drugs. *N Engl J Med* 1978; 298: 1321–1327.

21. Lemieux P, Michaud M, Pagé M. A new formazan amplified clonogenic assay for cytotoxicity testing. *Biotechnol Techniques* 1993; 7:597–602.

22. Weisenthal LM, Marsden JA, Dill PL, Macaluso CK. A novel dye exclusion method for testing in vitro chemosensitivity of human tumors. *Cancer Res* 1983; 43:749–757.

23. Durkin WJ, Chanta VK, Balch CM, Davis DW, Hiramoto RN. A methodological approach to the prediction of anticancer drug effect in humans. *Cancer Res* 1978; 39:402–407.

24. Grinnell F, Milan M, Srere PA. Studies on cell adhesion. II. Adhesion of cells to surfaces of diverse chemical composition and inhibition of adhesion by sulfhydryl binding reagents. *Arch Biochem Biophys* 1972; 153:193–198.

25. Hansen HH, Bender RA, Shelton BJ. The cytocentrifuge and cerebrospinal fluid cytology. *Acta Cytol* 1974; 18:259–262.

26. Holmes HL, Litle JM. Tissue culture microtest for predicting response of human cancer to chemotherapy. *Lancet* 1974; 2:985–987.

27. Kaltenbach JP, Kaltenbach MH, Lyons WB. Nigrosin as a dye for differentiating live and dead ascites cells. *Exp Cell Res* 1958; 15:112–117.

28. Tseng and Safa. *Cancer Detect Prev* 1983; 6:371.

29. Monks A, Scudiero D, Skehan P, Boyd M. Implementation of a pilot-scale, high flux anticancer drug screen utilizing disease-oriented panels of human tumor cells lines in culture. AACR, 1988.

30. Nemes Z, Dietz R, Luth JB, Gomba S, Hackenthal F, Gross F. The pharmacological relevance of vital staining with neutral red. *Experientia* 1979; 35:1475–1476.

31. Allison AC, Young MR. Vital staining in fluorescence microscopy of lysosomes. In: Dingle JT, Fell HB, eds. *Lysosomes in Biology and Pathology* Vol. 2, New York: American Elsevier Publishing. 1969: 600–626.

32. Fintner NB. Dye uptake methods for assessing viral cytopathogenicity and their application to interferon assays. *J Gen Virol* 1969; 5:419–427.

33. Borenfreund E, Puerner JA. Toxicity determined in vitro by morphological alterations and neutral red absorption. *Toxicol Lett* 1985; 24:199–124.

34. Cavanaugh PF, Moskwa PS, Donish WH, Pera PJ, Richardson D, Andrese AP. A semi-automated neutral red based chemosensitivity assay for drug screening. *Invest New Drugs* 1990; 8: 347–354.

35. Pearse AGE. Principles of oxidoreductase histochemistry. In: *Histochemistry, Theoretical and Applied*. Edinburgh: Churchill Livingston, 1972.

36. Altman FP. Tetrazolium salts and formazans. *Prog Histochem Cytochem* 1977; 9:1–56.

37. Mosmann T. Rapid colorimetric assay for cellular growth and survival: application to proliferation and cytotoxicity assays. *J Immunol Methods* 1983; 65:55–63.

38. Schaeffer WI, Friend K. Efficient detection of soft-agar grown colonies using a tetrazolium salt. *Cancer Lett* 1976; 1:275–279.

39. Alley MC, Lieber MM. Improved optical detection of colony enlargement and drug cytotoxicity in primary soft agar cultures of human solid tumour cells. *Br J Cancer* 1984; 49:225–233.

40. Pagé M, Bejaoui N, Cinq-Mars B, Lemieux P. Optimization of the tetrazolium-based colorimetric assay for the measurement of cell number and cytotoxicity. *Int J Immunopharmacol* 1988; 10:785–793.

41. Green LM, Reade JL, Ware CF. Rapid colorimetric assay for cell viability: application to the quantitation of cytotoxic and growth inhibitor lymphokines. *J Immunol Meth* 1984; 70:257–268.

42. Denizot F, Lang R. Rapid colorimetric assay for cell growth and survival. Modifications to this tetrazolium dye procedure giving improved sensitivity and reliability. *J Immunol Meth* 1986; 89:271–277.

43. Carmichael J, DeGraff WG, Gazdar AF, Minna ID, Mitchell JB. Evaluation of a tetrazolium-based semiautomated colorimetric assay: assessment of chemosensitivity testing. *Cancer Res* 1987; 47: 936–942.

44. Scudiero DA, Shoemaker RH, Paull KD et al. Evaluation of a soluble tetrazolium/formazan assay for cell growth and drug sensitivity in culture. *Cancer Res* 1988; 48:4827–4833.

45. Parsons JL, Risbood PA, Barbera WA, Sharman MN. The synthesis of XTT: a new tetrazolium reagent that is bioreducible to a water soluble formazan. *J Heterocyclic Chem* 1988; 25:911–914.

46. Lamontagne P, Maion G, Pagé M. Cytotoxicity testing using a soluble tetrazolium formazan derivative. *Cell Pharmacol* 1994; 1:171–174.

47. Pagé B, Pagé M. Sensitive colorimetric cytotoxicity measurement using alamar blue. *Oncol Rep* 1995; 2:59–61,

48. Harvey M, Pagé M. Determination of Interleukin 2 activity by a new fluorometric method. *Biotechnol Techniques* 1995; 9:69–73.

49. Moscow JA, Cowan KH. Multidrug resistance. *J Natl Cancer Inst* 1983; 80:14–20.

50. Roninson IB, Patel MC, Lee I, Noonan KE, Chen CJ, Choi K, Chin JE, Kaplan R, Tsuruo T. Molecular mechanism and diagnosis of multidrug resistance in human tumor cells. *Cancer Cells* 1989; 7:81–86.

51. Juranka PF, Zastawny RL, Lingn V. P-glycoprotein: multidrug-resistance and a superfamily of membrane-associated transport proteins. *FASEB J* 1989; 3:2583–2592.

52. Fuqua SA, Merkel DE, McGuire WL. Laboratory aspects of multidrug resistance. *Cancer Treat Res* 1989; 42:45–59.

53. Kane SE, Pastan I, Gottesman MM. Genetic basis of multidrug resistance of tumor cells. *J Bioenerg Biomembr* 1990; 22:493–618.

54. Nooter K, Herweijer H. Multidrug resistance (MDR) genes in human cancer. *Br J Cancer* 1991; 63: 663–669.

55. Wu L, Smvthe AM, Stinson SF, Mullendore LA, Monks A, Scudiero DA, Paull KD, Koutsoukos AD, Rubinstein LV, Boyd MR, Shoemaker RH. Multidrug-resistant phenotype of disease-oriented panels of human tumor cell lines used for anticancer drug screening. *Cancer Res* 1992; 52:3029–3034.

56. Monks A, Scudiero D, Skehan P, Shoemaker R, Paull K, Vistica D, Hose C, Langley J, Cronise P, Vaigro-Wolff A, Gray-Goodrich M, Campbell H, Mayo J, Boyd M. Feasibility of high-flux anticancer drug screening using a diverse panel of cultured human tumor cell lines. *J Natl Cancer Inst* 1991; 83:757–766.

2

High-Throughput Screening in Industry

Michael D. Boisclair, PhD, David A. Egan, PhD, Kety Huberman, MS, and Ralph Infantino, BA

CONTENTS

INTRODUCTION
HIGH-THROUGHPUT ASSAY METHODOLOGIES
AUTOMATION FOR HIGH-THROUGHPUT SCREENING
SCREEN MINIATURIZATION
COMPOUND LIBRARY MANAGEMENT
HIGH-THROUGHPUT ADME-TOX ASSAYS
DATA MANAGEMENT FOR HIGH-THROUGHPUT SCREENING
CONCLUSIONS

INTRODUCTION

1.1. Anticancer Drug Discovery Today

Drug discovery operations have been transformed over the past 20 yr by a series of technological innovations and scientific advances that the pharmaceutical industry has been quick to exploit. The trend has been to embrace automation and high-throughput techniques and to integrate research functions into a consolidated framework for drug discovery.

Truly automated high-throughput screening (HTS) dates from the late 1980s and was one of the earliest of the current new wave of technological innovations to be adopted for drug discovery. HTS involves testing collections ("libraries") of hundreds of thousands of natural products or synthetic compounds against a biological target using a quantitative bioassay. Its purpose is to identify screening "hits" that modulate the activity of the biological target and that form the starting point for a collaborative discovery effort between medicinal chemists and biologists. In essence, HTS is an effective way of reducing a prohibitively large number of diverse chemical starting points to a few promising structures that can be explored in more depth. Initially, the goal of the collaborative effort is to identify "lead" compounds from among the hits. Ultimately, the goal of drug discov-

From: *Cancer Drug Discovery and Development:*
Anticancer Drug Development Guide: Preclinical Screening, Clinical Trials, and Approval, 2nd Ed.
Edited by: B. A. Teicher and P. A. Andrews © Humana Press Inc., Totowa, NJ

ery is to transform lead compounds into drug candidates for clinical development. The strategic importance of HTS is that it requires no prior knowledge of the types of structures that will modulate the target molecule.

Bioinformatics and functional genomics have expanded the number of biological targets available for drug discovery. Furthermore, high-throughput screens for ADME-Tox (absorption, distribution, metabolism, excretion, and toxicity) have improved the chances of identifying better quality, more drug-like lead compounds. The new approaches to drug discovery, when combined with more traditional research methods, are starting to bear fruit, and we are now witnessing the emergence of a new generation of molecularly targeted anticancer drugs.

In this chapter we review the use of HTS for anticancer drug discovery and provide a general overview of an industrial screening operation. In particular, we focus on novel technologies and approaches that are helping to shrink screening timelines. Given that the bottlenecks in drug discovery have moved downstream of HTS in the screening pathway, we review new screening approaches that are being used to improve the drug-like quality of leads entering preclinical testing.

1.2. Mechanism-Based Anticancer Drug Discovery

Historically, drugs for the treatment of cancer were discovered through testing the cytotoxic effects of compounds on whole cells, organs, and even complete organisms. Subsequent work was required to elucidate the mechanism of action of the cytotoxic drugs. In contrast, modern anticancer drug discovery typically starts with the identification of a molecular target: either a protein or its RNA or DNA precursors. The strategic shift has been made possible by a dramatic improvement in our understanding of the molecular mechanisms underlying the pathogenesis of cancer.

The pharmaceutical industry's current strategy for controlling tumor growth selectively is to develop drugs that interfere with targets important in tumor angiogenesis, tumor invasion, tumor metastasis, cell cycle control, and apoptosis. Selection of individual targets for drug discovery is usually based on information obtainable from the academic literature or unpublished original research to which the pharmaceutical company has direct access. Once sequence information is known for a molecular target, bioinformatics can be employed to search for structurally related targets. Bioinformatics can uncover previously unknown proteins and thereby expand the number of potential targets that may require HTS for leads discovery.

The viability of a molecular target for drug discovery is based on a number of criteria that differ somewhat from one organization to another. In essence, for a target to be considered viable, some experimental validation is needed to show that interfering with its function will produce the desired effect in vivo. A number of strategies are generally employed to validate a target for drug discovery. The validation strategies include the use of gene knockouts, ribozymes, antisense technology, and RNA interference (RNAi). Gene knockouts in mice are particularly valuable since they will demonstrate the effect, in an in vivo setting, of abolishing the normal function of a gene product (1,2). However, gene knockouts also have several disadvantages for target validation; experimental timelines are long, costs are high, and the findings may relate more to developmental function than to adult function. As a consequence, the results of gene knockout experiments are sometimes difficult to interpret. Alternatively, antisense oligonucleotides or ribozymes (RNA enzymes that cleave messenger RNA) can be used to study the effect of abrogating specific gene transcripts (3–5). RNAi is a new technology that uses gene silencing to manipulate gene expression in a number of cellular systems, including mammalian cells (6). RNAi can be employed in a high-throughput fashion to explore the function of a large number of putative molecular targets for anticancer drug discovery.

One caveat with the biological methods of validating a target, as described above, is that they do not always represent the effect that a small molecule has on a target. Moreover, it may not be worthwhile committing the time or resources into validating certain targets before proceeding to leads discovery. In some instances a pharmaceutical company may make the strategic decision to proceed with HTS against a nonvalidated target and to use the lead compounds themselves to demonstrate the effect of interfering with the target's function.

A research organization uses the approaches described above to create a list of potential targets for drug discovery. Further practical considerations are used to prioritize the targets for further consideration. The latter considerations include (1) the freedom to operate without infringing on intellectual property owned by another organization, (2) the feasibility of establishing a screening assay for discovering hit compounds and (3) the overall balance within the target portfolio of novelty (novel targets incur less competition from other pharmaceutical companies) versus validation (established pharmaceutical targets have undergone more experimental and clinical validation than novel targets and therefore present less risk of a negative outcome from drug discovery). An organization will often concentrate on certain classes of targets. For example, protein tyrosine kinases and G protein-coupled receptors (GPCRs) have received (and continue to receive) considerable attention as drug targets. Further efficiencies can be realized by employing the same assay technology for families of targets; this approach simplifies assay development and expedites HTS.

Table 1 outlines the cascade of screening steps that are taken in anticancer drug discovery for an enzyme target. The screening pathway begins with a high-throughput biochemical "primary" screen and the testing of a compound library of hundreds of thousands of compounds. The more advanced screening laboratories can easily achieve throughputs of 100,000 compounds or more per week. In general, it is usually possible to complete an HTS campaign, including the confirmation testing of hits, in less than 2 mo. Some simple measures are taken to remove nuisance or uninteresting compounds from the list of hits. A common first step is for an experienced chemist to review the structures and remove compounds that do not constitute good starting points for medicinal chemistry.

The compounds in a library are stored for HTS as solutions in dimethyl sulfoxide (DMSO); some compounds degrade during long-term storage. Purity testing is performed to address the possibility that a compound that was active in a screen was not the original structure. Liquid chromatography (LC) is employed, coupled with analysis by mass spectrometry (MS), to determine the structure or structures in the sample on the basis of compound mass. LC-MS can be performed in high throughput, which permits an entire set of a few hundred screening hits to be analyzed in less than a week.

Once the original hits have been selected, they are tested for potency in the primary high-throughput screen and ranked by their IC_{50} or EC_{50} values (concentrations that produce 50% inhibition or effective stimulation, respectively). The most potent com-

Table 1
Anticancer Screening Pathway (Enzyme Target)

1. In vitro screening
    1.1. HTS (inhibition of target in primary biochemical assay)
    1.2. Inhibition of target in cellular assay
    1.3. Inhibition of cell proliferation
    1.4. Selectivity assays
2. In vitro ADME-Tox profiling
    2.1. Metabolic stability
    2.2. Cytochrome P450 inhibition
    2.3. Solubility
    2.4. Protein binding
    2.5. Cell permeability
3. In vivo screening
    3.1. Rapid PK
    3.2. Full PK on selected compounds
    3.3. In vivo pharmacodynamic assay
    3.4. Tumor growth inhibition

ABBREVIATIONS: ADME-Tox, absorption, distribution, metabolism, excretion, and toxicity; HTS, high-throughput; PK, pharmacokinetics.

pounds are assayed to determine whether they also inhibit the enzyme in a whole cell screen. At this juncture, the data are reviewed to decide whether there is a basis for allocating medicinal chemistry resources and continuing drug discovery.

If HTS has been successful in identifying potent hit compounds, a collaborative effort is initiated in which various chemical strategies are employed to synthesize compounds with improved inhibitory activity. Medicinal chemistry usually incorporates combinatorial approaches capable of generating large numbers of structurally related compounds; HTS is capable of delivering the throughput required for a timely analysis of the combinatorial libraries. The synthetic compounds are screened in the biochemical assay and the mechanistic cellular assay. Active compounds are also tested for their ability to inhibit proliferation of a tumor cell line in a functional screen. The selectivity of certain compounds for the target molecule may be explored using a panel of enzyme assays, which usually includes enzymes from the same family as the target molecule and may include unrelated enzymes.

Historically, the classical strategy taken for drug discovery was to focus initially on synthesizing compounds with maximal potency for the target molecule and to postpone testing of pharmacokinetic (PK) properties until efficacy testing in animal models was already under way. As a consequence, a high percentage of compounds with good potency for the target molecule turned out to show little efficacy in vivo because of poor PK properties, thus wasting many months or even years of research. It has also been argued that HTS strategies are biased toward the discovery of lipophilic compounds with inappropriate PK properties, especially when biochemical screening is employed (7). However, a paradigm shift toward optimizing PK properties has occurred in the last 5 yr. The modern approach is to eliminate compounds with poor PK properties early in the drug discovery cycle and thereby improve the likelihood that lead compounds will be successful during in vivo testing. A panel of in vitro screens is used to profile the molecular properties of lead compounds and predict which compounds will have appropriate PK properties. The latter screens are usually run in parallel and include assays for metabolic stability, P450 inhibition, solubility, protein binding, and cell permeability. Computational approaches are also employed to predict which compounds possess properties in common with developmental drugs by calculating molecular properties such as molecular weight, numbers of hydrogen bond donors and acceptors, number of rotatable bonds, cLogP (calculated octanol-water partition coefficient; a predictor of lipophilicity), and polar surface area (PSA; a predictor of absorption) *(7–9)*.

Compounds that demonstrate the most appropriate properties in the in vitro assays and computational models are advanced to the in vivo phase of testing. A favored approach is to test compounds initially in a high-throughput PK assay using a single dose in mice; only a small quantity of each compound is required. A caveat of the low-dose testing procedure is that it does not properly represent the PK that can be expected when the drug is given in higher doses or when it is formulated as a tablet. Higher throughputs can be achieved using cassette dosing techniques, in which each animal is dosed with several compounds or, preferably, pooling strategies in which plasma samples from several animals are combined before analysis *(10)*. Only those compounds that achieve sufficiently high plasma concentrations and are cleared slowly will be advanced further down the discovery pathway. More extensive PK testing is carried out on compounds that achieve the selection criteria set for high-throughput PK testing. Two types of in vivo assay are commonly used for testing the anticancer activity of lead compounds. Pharmacodynamic assays are used to measure the efficacy of a compound in inhibiting the target enzyme in tumors, whereas a tumor growth inhibition (TGI) assay measures the efficacy of a compound in inhibiting tumor growth. Compounds that show excellent efficacy in preventing disease progression in the animal model will be considered for nomination as clinical candidates.

1.3. Leads Discovery

HTS is best considered as one of several approaches that can be employed to find lead compounds for drug discovery. One alternative approach to HTS is structure-based drug design, which employs computer modeling to design compounds that bind to regions of the target molecule known to be important for its normal function *(11)*. A three-dimensional structure of the target molecule is a prerequisite for structure-based design. The molecular coordinates of the target structure can be obtained either by X-ray crystallography or by homology modeling. In the latter approach, the primary sequence of a novel protein is compared with the sequence of a protein whose structure is already known using software that is able to predict the novel structure. A caveat of homology modeling, however, is that it fails to consider the flexibility of protein conformations; therefore, the homology models may not always be accurate.

A second alternative approach to HTS is to initiate a drug discovery project based on a compound with published activity against the target. If freedom to operate on the published structure is restricted by intellectual property, a pharmaceutical company will sometimes adopt medicinal chemistry approaches to discover similar compounds that have activity against the target, yet are not covered by any patent.

In practice, most organizations use a flexible research strategy for discovering lead compounds. Whenever feasible, HTS is supplemented with structure-based drug design and/or medicinal chemistry approaches based on published structures to increase the likelihood of finding successful lead compounds.

An emerging innovation for leads discovery is to make strategic use of advances in high-performance computing platforms. *Virtual screening* is used to expand the screening of structures beyond those compounds existing in an organization's physical inventory *(11–13)*. A virtual library is created containing compounds in vendors' compound collections, compounds in the screening library, and even compounds created computationally that are not available from any known source. By expanding structure-based drug design to virtual libraries of compounds held in huge databases, millions of virtual compounds can be "docked" computationally against the target molecule in just a few days. Computational scoring methods are used to identify those compounds that bind tightly to the target. The virtual hits are subsequently purchased from vendors or synthesized in-house if no commercial source can be found. Virtual screening is also used to identify those compounds in the screening library that are most likely to be hits. When used tactically in this way, virtual screening can accelerate lead identification and reduce costs. As a consequence, some companies have installed industrial-scale "cherry-picking" systems that allow focused collections of a few thousand compounds, identified as potential hits by virtual screening, to be selected quickly from the library and compiled into plates for subsequent in vitro screening.

2. HIGH-THROUGHPUT ASSAY METHODOLOGIES

Knowledge of the molecular target and expertise in assay design are important prerequisites for developing a high-throughput screen. HTS assays can be run using either cells or purified molecular targets. Cell types can be mammalian, yeast, or bacterial. Cells are engineered to overexpress a target protein or are transfected with a reporter gene. The criteria used in deciding which assay technology to use for HTS include sensitivity, speed, ease of automation, reliability, safety, and cost.

Early high-throughput screens relied on measurements of absorbance and radioisotopes. Luminescent assay techniques were subsequently exploited, most notably for reporter gene assays *(14)*. More recently, fluorescence detection has gained prominence for HTS because of its high sensitivity, versatility, and compatibility with assay miniaturization *(15)*. Fluorescence-based screening techniques include prompt fluorescence intensity, time-resolved fluorescence (TRF), fluorescence resonance energy transfer (FRET), and fluorescence polarization (FP).

2.1. Homogeneous and Heterogeneous Assay Technologies

The assay design will impact both the timeline required to develop a screen and the screening throughput. A simple screen with few operational steps can be optimized quickly and is very amenable to automation. Homogeneous assays (e.g., FRET and FP) have become increasingly popular for HTS: they use "mix-and-measure" methods that avoid separation steps and provide excellent precision. Heterogeneous assays (e.g., enzyme-linked immunosorbent assays [ELISAs]) require separation steps that go beyond simple fluid additions, incubations, and readings to include manipulations such as washing steps, filtration steps, or plate-to-plate transfers. Despite the operational limitations

Table 2

Protein Kinase Assay Methodologies Commonly Used for HTS

Assay Methodology	Assay type	Assay readout	Source
DELFIA®	Heterogeneous	Time-resolved fluorescence	Perkin Elmer Life Sciences (Boston, MA)
ELISA	Heterogeneous	Absorbance	Multiple
ALPHAScreen™	Homogeneous	Fluorescence	Perkin Elmer Life Sciences
FlashPlate®	Homogeneous	Scintillation (radiometric)	Perkin Elmer Life Sciences
FP	Homogeneous	Prompt fluorescence	Multiple
FRET	Homogeneous	Prompt or time-resolved fluorescence	Multiple
SPA	Homogeneous	Scintillation (radiometric)	Amersham Biosciences (Piscataway, NJ)

ABBREVIATIONS: DELFIA®, dissociation-enhanced lanthanide fluoroimmunoassay; ELISA, enzyme-linked immunosorbent assay; ALPHAScreen™, amplified luminescent proximity homogeneous assay; FP, fluorescence polarization; FRET, fluorescence resonance energy transfer; SPA, scintillation proximity assay.

of heterogeneous assays for HTS, they do offer some advantages. One advantage of heterogeneous assays is that compounds are not present when the signal is measured, which obviates the possibility that compounds will interfere with the assay readout. A second advantage of heterogeneous assays is that they typically generate a higher signal-to-background ratio.

HTS methodologies have evolved enormously over the past decade. For example, when HTS was in its infancy, tyrosine kinases were commonly screened by measuring the incorporation of ^{32}P into substrate from radiolabeled ATP or by using ELISAs employing anti-phosphotyrosine antibodies. An adaptation of ELISA methodology—DELFIA® (dissociation-enhanced lanthanide fluoroimmunoassay)—which employs a TRF readout, has also been used (16). The above screening methods require a separation step before measuring the assay signal. More recently, homogeneous assay technologies such as SPA (scintillation proximity assay), FP, FRET, ALPHAScreen™ (amplified luminescent proximity homogeneous assay), and scintillating microplates (FlashPlate®) have all become available for HTS (15–20). Table 2 lists the assay methods that are commonly used to screen for inhibitors of protein kinases. Many of the more novel assay technologies have been commercialized for HTS and are easy to use; in some cases the vendors offer kits for HTS. Consequently, assay development for kinases and certain other target classes can be reduced down to a simple set of guidelines, which enables new screens to be developed and transferred to HTS in a rapid and streamlined process. Stocks of generic screening reagents can sometimes be used for multiple screens, which can further accelerate assay development and screening.

2.2. Cell-Based and Biochemical Screens

Screening for inhibitors of novel biological targets is often performed using a well-characterized biochemical assay established with purified components. The biochemical assays typically examine a single biochemical event such as an enzymatic reaction or a binding interaction. With enzyme targets, most of which are intracellular, a biochemical assay is usually preferred for HTS. Cell-based HTS is sometimes preferred for targets expressed within the cell membrane and for screening against several targets in a pathway simultaneously. The complexity of cell-based screens, compared with most biochemical screens, usually results in less reproducible screening data. For a biochemical screen, large stocks of reagents can be prepared and frozen down for the entire screening campaign, which simplifies the screening operation. However, for some targets, it may be impractical to produce and isolate large quantities of specialized reagents (such as a membrane-bound receptor), and a cell-based screen becomes more attractive for HTS than a biochemical assay. For example, yeast-based reporter gene assays offer a cheap and straightforward alternative to biochemical methods for screening against GPCRs (21). Since cell-based and biochemical assays each offer advantages for certain targets, it is usually advisable for HTS laboratories to use both approaches for leads discovery.

2.3. Advanced Fluorescence Assay Technologies

Advances in imaging and assay technologies have led to the emergence of high-content screening (HCS), which yields far more information on cells than single-measurement screens (22). Through HCS, changes in cell shape and size, changes in the distribution of intracellular proteins, and multiple cellular targets can be assayed simultaneously through judicious selection of fluorescent probes (23). An example of the use of HCS is for measuring apoptosis, in which changes in nuclear morphology, cytoskeleton organization, and mitochondrial physiology are measured in a multiparameter fashion (24). A caveat with HCS is that it can generate huge quantities of data, presenting a data analysis challenge that has tended to limit its application to screens downstream of HTS in the drug discovery pathway.

Another advanced fluorescence assay technology involves the use of confocal laser techniques to measure the fluorescence properties of single molecules as they move through tiny volumes as small as 1 fl (25). The best known example of a single-molecule detection (SMD) assay is fluorescence correlation spectroscopy (FCS). Because the detection volume for SMD assays is so small, they are ideally suited to miniaturization and have found application in the densest plate formats, including 1536-well plates.

3. AUTOMATION FOR HIGH-THROUGHPUT SCREENING

There has been tremendous growth in the number and variety of robotic instruments specifically designed for automated drug discovery. A research organization now has a variety of options for equipping the HTS laboratory according to the prevailing types of assays, the required throughput, and the available budget (Table 3).

The early history of HTS was characterized by the use of fully integrated robotic screening systems that incorporated a method of moving assay plates from station to station, generally a robotic arm located centrally or on a linear rail. A drawback of integrated robotic systems is that many months are required to design, build, and test the systems. Deployment of integrated robotic systems is quite slow compared with workstations, which can be installed quickly in the laboratory and which require less testing before becoming operational.

Table 3
Equipment Platforms for HTS

Parameter	Manual devices	Workstations	Laboratory robotics	Industrial robotics
Cost	Low	Medium	High	Very high
Throughput capability (tests/d)	5000	50,000	75,000	250,000
Advantages	Cheap	High throughput, flexible, quick to deploy	Suited to heterogeneous assays, unattended operation	Capable of uHTS, component of drug discovery factory
Disadvantages	Low throughput, subject to human error	Requires human intervention, low throughput for heterogeneous assays	Expensive, slow to deploy, difficult error recovery	Very expensive and complex, dedicated facility

HTS, high-throughput; uHTS, ultra-high-throughput.

Two of the most important recent advances for HTS have been the development of homogeneous assay formats and an increase in the use of workstations for screening. The use of homogeneous fluorescence assay technologies has resulted in assays that require fewer steps and thus less plate manipulation. Liquid-handling workstations, with the capability of moving large numbers of plates on tracks, can be very productive when applied to homogeneous assays (an example is the MiniTrak™ from Perkin Elmer Life Sciences, Boston, MA). Plates can be transferred manually from the liquid-handling workstation to an incubator or reader by using removable plate stackers.

Integrated robotic systems still have a role to play in screening, especially when complex assays involving multiple steps are involved (e.g., ELISAs or cell-based assays). Moreover, robotic systems can run for long periods unattended and are capable of achieving high throughputs by functioning during periods when laboratory personnel are not normally in attendance. It is therefore easy to understand why traditional robotic systems are still commonplace in most HTS facilities.

A more recent trend, which has found most resonance with the largest pharmaceutical companies, is toward industrial-scale automation that is compatible with the vision of a drug discovery factory (26). When applied to HTS, the approach is to build very large robotic systems capable of achieving throughputs well in excess of 100,000 tests per day; this is the realm of ultra high-throughput screening (uHTS).

In the case of the traditional robotic systems, the robotic arm tends to be in constant demand while many of the individual equipment modules stand idle, awaiting delivery of plates. In short, the robotic arm can become a bottleneck in the system, preventing higher levels of productivity from being attained. Industrial-scale robotic systems (such

Table 4
Impact of Assay Miniaturization on Reagent Costs and Screening Throughput

Plate density (wells/plate)	Assay volume (μL)	Throughput (tests/d)	Reagent costs/well ($)
96	50–200	10,000	0.50
384	20–50	40,000	0.20
1536	2.5–10	60,000	0.05

as those supplied by The Automation Partnership [Royston, UK] and RTS Thurnall [Manchester, UK]) have solved the productivity problem by managing to keep all components of the robotic system working continuously. Plates progress along tracks at a constant pace, instead of being moved individually by robotic arms. When there is potential for one step of an assay to hold up the progress of plates along the system (e.g., when a plate needs to be subjected to three cycles of washing) an engineering solution is found to minimize the impact on overall productivity (e.g., using three washers, one for each washing cycle). The factory-style approach to HTS is enabling large pharmaceutical companies to keep pace with the numbers of targets that have been unleashed by functional genomics.

4. SCREEN MINIATURIZATION

There has been a trend in the industry over the last 5 yr toward high-density plate formats and low-volume assays. Miniaturization has been driven by a desire to reduce reagent costs, to conserve compound libraries, and to allow for uHTS by enhancing throughput (27). The benefits of screen miniaturization are illustrated in Table 4. The greatest increase in throughput comes when switching from 96-well to 384-well plates. Screens that would take weeks or months to complete in 96-well plates can be carried out in weeks or days in 384-well plates.

The equipment required to perform 384-well HTS is well proven and is available at reasonable cost from many different manufacturers. In fact, the introduction of the 384-well format has been so successful that more than half of all HTS was performed in 384-well plates in 2001 (28). Specialized equipment is required to perform HTS in volumes below 5 μL. Miniaturizing a screen to run in a 1536-well plate can greatly reduce costs, but custom-designed liquid handling becomes a necessity. The technological challenges posed by 1536-well HTS probably explain why less than 4% of all HTS was performed in 1536-well plates in 2001 (28).

Low-volume dispensing technologies can be divided into two classes: noncontact dispensing and contact dispensing. Cartesian Technologies (Irvine, CA) has long been a leader in noncontact dispensing; its SynQuad™ technology can accurately dispense volumes as low as 50 nL very rapidly. Equipment introduced more recently (e.g., the Spot-On™ technology from Allegro Technologies, Dublin, Ireland) promises improved accuracy at even lower volumes. Contact dispensing involves the use of pin tools that were originally developed for generating DNA microarrays; volumes as low as 5 nL can be handled in this way. Contact dispensing has proved to be very useful for transferring compound libraries to high-density plates.

5. COMPOUND LIBRARY MANAGEMENT

It is axiomatic that the hits generated from an HTS campaign will only be as good as the compound library that was screened. Over the past few years a number of changes have taken place to enhance the quality of screening collections. Many discovery organizations have retreated from screening natural products because of the costs and timelines involved in isolating and identifying active compounds from natural mixtures.

When it comes to synthesized compound libraries, the emphasis is now more on quality than quantity. Companies are increasingly using computational methods to select compounds for their collections, either to increase diversity or to generate sublibraries for specific target classes. The increasing reliance on more focused compound collections has obviated the need to screen huge compound libraries against every target.

Compound handling has also benefited from innovations in robotics. Companies such as RTS Thurnall, The Automation Partnership, and REMP (Oberdiessbach, Switzerland) can supply fully automated compound stores. The stores can hold millions of compounds in a variety of formats including standard vials, plates, and minitubes. The storage units are incorporated into environmental enclosures with temperature and humidity control. Integrated liquid-handling stations generate compound plates preformatted for HTS. An innovation that has greatly aided focused screening efforts is the development of 96-well minitubes that can be tracked individually. Compounds in minitubes are managed robotically within automated stores; thousands of compounds can be cherry-picked and transferred into screening plates within a 24-h period.

6. HIGH-THROUGHPUT ADME-TOX ASSAYS

Discovery teams are now tasked with generating information on the ADME-Tox properties of promising compounds. This has led to a requirement for higher throughput ADME-Tox assays that can be automated for testing compounds early in the discovery pathway *(29)*.

6.1. High-Throughput ADME Screens

The solubility of a compound is critical to its bioavailability. A number of automated assays have been developed to measure compound solubility, but the method most amenable to high-throughput applications is probably the laser nephelometry method that can be performed in 96-well plates *(30)*. Laser nephelometry involves passing a polarized laser beam through a compound solution to measure light scattering caused by precipitated compound.

Orally available drugs have to be able to get into the bloodstream through the gut epithelium. Small rodent animal models can be used for testing compound absorption, but are not suitable for high-throughput applications. In vitro methods have been developed that utilize both cultured cell monolayers and artificial membranes. The cell-based absorption assays most commonly use Caco-2 cells *(28)*, but Madin-Darby canine kidney (MDCK) cells are also used. The cells are grown in a monolayer on a membrane built into an insert in a 24-well plate. The cells form tight junctions; compound added to the apical compartment can only get to the basolateral compartment through the cells. The amount of compound in the basolateral medium, as measured by LC-MS, can be used to calculate an apparent permeability coefficient (P_{app}) using Artursson's equation *(31)*. Artificial membrane assays are run in a similar manner to the cell-based absorption assays but use an immobilized artificial membrane in place of the cell layer. One example is the parallel artificial membrane permeability assay (PAMPA) that can be carried out in the 96-well format (32).

Drug stability can be assayed using cultured human hepatocytes, human microsomes, or animal hepatocytes (29). Tissue from human sources is expensive and can create safety concerns, but the use of animal hepatocytes may not provide a good reflection of the rate of drug metabolism in humans. Drug metabolism in metabolic stability assays is generally monitored by LC-MS (10).

Screens for cytochrome P450 (CYP) inhibition are widely used in drug discovery to eliminate compounds that might cause drug-drug interactions. Commercially available assays for CYP inhibition exist that are easily automated (33).

6.2. High-Throughput Toxicity Screens

The simplest measure of a compound's toxicity is to test its effect on the viability of cultured cells. Since most in vivo toxicity is a reflection of hepatotoxicity, human hepatocyte cell lines are frequently used. Cell viability can be measured using an assay that measures the color change when 3-(4,5-dimethylthiazol-2-yl)-2,5-diphenyl tetrazolium bromide (MTT) is metabolized by the mitochondria of living cells. An alternative cell viability assay measures cellular ATP content. Both the MTT assay and the ATP assay are easily automated (34).

Genotoxicity tests use specifically engineered strains of *Salmonella typhimurium* that can be used to screen for mutagenic compounds (35). The assay detects a change in pH; a spectrophotometer measures the color change indicated by a pH-sensitive dye in the culture medium. The advent of DNA microarrays and other genomics technologies has allowed the simultaneous monitoring of transcripts from thousands of genes known to be involved in responses to toxic insult (36). The latter genes include heat shock genes, cytochrome P450s, and glutathione-*S*-transferase (GST). Transcription profiling enables discovery groups to build a detailed genotoxic profile on compounds of interest.

Mutations in the hERG gene, which encodes a cardiac potassium channel, can cause long Q-T syndrome (LQTS), which can lead to sudden death induced by cardiac arrythmia (37). Pharmacological blockade of the hERG channel can result in a similar cardiac effect; consequently there is much interest in screening for hERG channel effects. The traditional electrophysiological hERG channel assays such as patch clamping do not have sufficient throughput, so a number of higher throughput assays have been developed for drug discovery (38). Two assays use fluorescent voltage-sensitive dyes; they measure a change in membrane potential when cells transfected with the hERG channel are treated with hERG channel blockers. A third assay uses atomic absorption spectrometry to measure the efflux of rubidium ions from hERG-transfected cells.

7. DATA MANAGEMENT FOR HIGH-THROUGHPUT SCREENING

Since so much information is generated during a drug discovery program, a good data management system is indispensable to the pharmaceutical organization. The data management system is used for capturing and storing data that are generated at different stages of the discovery pathway and for making the data available to the multidisciplinary discovery teams. Research groups use the data management system to make informed

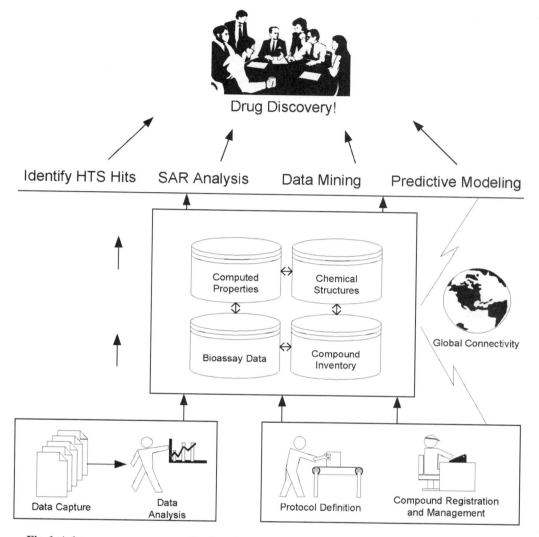

Fig. 1. A data management system for drug discovery. The discovery data are held in a series of interfaced Oracle® databases. Mechanisms exist to streamline the entry of data into the databases and to control data quality. A variety of software tools are used to derive knowledge from the data for drug discovery. HTS, high-throughput screening; SAR, structure-activity relationship.

decisions about which series of compounds to synthesize and which compounds to advance down the discovery pathway. It is quite common for some research organizations to be distributed across different countries and different time zones. A company's data management system can therefore play a vital role in coordinating the activities of geographically distributed groups. The data management system acts as a central resource that collects and collates data in real time and organizes the information for dissemination to researchers across the organization.

A typical data management system for drug discovery is illustrated in Fig. 1. A database or series of interconnected databases lies at the heart of the system. Most systems utilize the Oracle® database (Redwood Shores, CA), which facilitates system integration and data exchange between different products and employs technologies that enable deployment through client-server and web-based technologies. The compound inventory system records the corporate identifier, location, and other critical information (e.g., batch details) about each compound. Structural information is usually maintained in a commercial chemical database (e.g., MDL® ISIS/Host from MDL®, San Leandro, CA) that permits compound searches based on chemical substructures. Many companies have built their own databases to store bioassay and compound inventory information, but commercial options also exist. The modern data management system includes a large database for storing multiple physiochemical properties that are computed for each compound held in the inventory.

The data management system includes mechanisms to assist the flow of data into the databases, to regulate quality, and to enforce the business rules of the organization. Database protocols (metadata) describe the assays and are established for each screen. A compound registration system is used to enter structural and other critical information about each compound that is received into the inventory. Researchers submit compound requests using an application that accesses the compound inventory database to report the availability of individual compounds and to control access to restricted samples (not shown in Fig. 1). A data capture application is necessary to process large volumes of data rapidly and to streamline their entry into the database. Software applications are used to analyze the assay data and to detect aberrant results as part of standard quality control (QC) procedures.

Data stored in the database do not directly translate into knowledge that can be used by the drug discovery teams. A variety of software applications are used to query the database and to report results that are important to the decision-making process for drug discovery. In an environment of rapid change, expansion, and merger, it is considered best practice to build data management systems that facilitate multisite access and good performance at remote locations. A combination of client-server and web-based technologies for querying the database will generally achieve the correct balance between application functionality and ease of deployment.

The archived data form the basis for future reporting by scientists throughout the company. Data may also be collected and reorganized into a data warehouse to improve query and reporting efficiency (not shown in Fig. 1). An obvious example of a database query is one used to identify hits from HTS. Further down the discovery cascade, structure-activity relationships (SAR) are built by querying the database. SAR analyses combine biological and chemical information and are used to identify the structural features of compounds that are important for biological activity against the target molecule. SAR analyses are also used to determine the chemical features that produce undesirable pharmaceutical effects. Data mining is a strategy for analyzing large quantities of data held in databases to reveal trends and relationships that would otherwise remain hidden. Data mining software is frequently employed to look for trends in HTS data: to identify hits that would be overlooked by conventional data analysis and to perform sophisticated QC analyses. Modeling techniques, using data acquired from a limited screening "training set," can be used to predict other compounds in the screening library that are likely to be hits. Predictive modeling, when combined with industrial cherry-picking capabilities and a sequential approach to screening, can be used to identify useful hits without needing to screen the entire compound library (39).

8. CONCLUSIONS

The alternative approaches to drug discovery notwithstanding, most biopharmaceutical companies have adopted HTS as a cornerstone of their leads discovery operation. Indeed, it is fair to say that HTS has established itself over recent years as an essential component of drug discovery. However, the role of HTS laboratories is changing. At the start of the HTS revolution, screening against a drug target to find hits required many months or even years of concentrated effort. As the field has progressed, advances in assay methodologies, miniaturization, high-density plate formats, and screening automation have resulted in a dramatic reduction in the cycle time for HTS, which is now completed in a matter of a few weeks. Consequently, in most pharmaceutical companies, the primary screen is no longer seen as the bottleneck in drug discovery.

At the current time, business imperatives in the pharmaceutical industry are driving program managers to shorten research timelines and discover increasing numbers of clinical candidates. Research efforts are focusing on how to identify high-quality lead compounds that are less likely to fail in preclinical testing and HTS laboratories are ideally placed to assist in this regard. Much of the infrastructure that has been established for running a primary screen at high throughput (notably laboratory automation, assay methodologies, and data management systems) is being applied to downstream needs in drug discovery. Many HTS departments are shouldering the responsibility for running preliminary ADME-Tox screens, and the trend toward automating assays that have traditionally been run in low throughput is likely to continue. Some companies are even taking the automation of drug discovery to the extreme, with the establishment of factory-like facilities.

Many companies cannot afford to screen their entire compound library against all the targets proposed for HTS. It is a measure of how far screening laboratories have progressed that logistical concerns no longer dominate decisions over how many primary targets to investigate by HTS. Miniaturization has reduced the cost of individual screening campaigns, but the flood of new targets produced by genomics approaches (for which HTS is often the only viable option for leads discovery) has driven running costs even higher. It is partly as a consequence of the financial considerations that, in the future, we are likely to witness a symbiotic relationship forming between HTS (in vitro screening) and virtual (*in silico*) screening. HTS and virtual screening are complementary approaches for leads discovery: they can be employed independently of each other or in combination, both methodologies play the "numbers game," and both ultimately require large sets of compounds to be screened in vitro. In the anticancer field, HTS (both of random libraries and focused compound collections) will continue to play a pivotal role in mechanistic discovery as high-throughput approaches are increasingly applied to accelerate the identification of new clinical drug candidates.

REFERENCES

1. Bast RC, Kufe DW, Pollock RE, Weichselbaum RR, Holland JF, Frei E, eds. *Cancer Medicine*, 5th ed. Toronto: BC Decker, 2000.
2. Harris S. Transgenic knockouts as part of high-throughput, evidence-based target selection and validation strategies. *Drug Discov Today* 2002; 6:628–636.
3. Dean NM. Functional genomics and target validation approaches using antisense oligonucleotide technology. *Curr Opin Biotechnol* 2001; 12:622–625.
4. Goodchild J. Hammerhead ribozymes for target validation. *Expert Opin Ther Targets* 2002; 6:235–247.
5. Goodchild J. Hammerhead ribozymes: biochemical and chemical considerations. *Curr Opin Mol Ther* 2000; 2:272–281.

6. Hannon GJ. RNA interference. *Nature* 2002; 418:244–251.
7. Lipinski CA, Lombardo F, Dominy BE, Feeney PJ. Experimental and computational approaches to estimate solubility and permeability in drug discovery and development settings. *Adv Drug Deliv Rev* 1997; 23:3–25.
8. Spalding DJM, Harker AJ, Bayliss MK. Combining high-throughput pharmacokinetic screens at the hits-to-leads stage of drug discovery. *Drug Discov Today* 2000; 5(suppl):S70–76.
9. Clark DE, Pickett SD. Computational methods for the prediction of 'drug-likeness.' *Drug Discov Today* 2000; 5:49–58.
10. Watt AP, Morrison D, Evans DC. Approaches to higher-throughput pharmacokinetics (HTPK) in drug discovery. *Drug Discov Today* 2000; 5:17–24.
11. Rowland RS. Using X-ray crystallography in drug discovery. *Curr Opin Drug Discov Devel* 2002; 5:613–619.
12. Leach AR, Hann MM. The in silico world of virtual libraries. *Drug Discov Today* 2000; 5:326–336.
13. Bajorath J. Integration of virtual and high-throughput screening. *Nat Rev Drug Discov* 2002; 1:882–894.
14. Dhundale A, Goddard C. Reporter gene assays in the high throughput laboratory: a rapid and robust first look? *J Biomol Screen* 1996; 1:115–118.
15. Pope AJ, Haupts UM, Moore KJ. Homogeneous fluorescence readouts for miniaturized high-throughput screening: theory and practice. *Drug Discov Today* 1999; 4:350–362.
16. Hemmilä I, Webb S. Time-resolved fluorometry: an overview of the labels and core technologies for drug screening applications. *Drug Discov Today* 1997; 2:373–381.
17. Cook ND Scintillation proximity assay—a versatile high throughput screening technology. *Drug Discov Today* 1996; 1:287–294.
18. Glickman JF, Wu X, Mercuri R, et al. A comparison of ALPHAScreen, TR-FRET and TRF as assay methods for FXR nuclear receptors. *J Biomol Screen* 2002; 7:3–10
19. Kolb AJ, Kaplita PV, Hayes DJ, et al. Tyrosine kinase assays adapted to homogeneous time-resolved fluorescence. *Drug Discov Today* 1998; 3:333–342
20. Earnshaw DL, Pope AJ. FlashPlate scintillation proximity assays for characterization and screening of DNA polymerase, primase, and helicase activities. *J Biomol Screen* 2001; 6:39–46.
21. Berg M, Undisz K, Thiericke R, Moore T, Posten C. Miniaturization of a functional transcription assay in yeast (human progesterone receptor) in the 384- and 1536-well plate format. *J Biomol Screen* 2000; 5:71–76.
22. Ramm P. Imaging systems in assay screening. *Drug Discov Today* 1999; 4:401–410.
23. Kain SR. Green fluorescent protein (GFP): applications in cell-based assays for drug discovery. *Drug Discov Today* 1999; 4:304–312.
24. Liptrop C. High content screening—from cells to data to knowledge. Drug Discov Today 2001;6:832–834.
25. Moore KJ, Turcone S, Ashman S, et al. Single molecule detection techniques in miniaturized high-throughput screening: fluorescence correlation spectroscopy. *J Biomol Screen* 1999; 4:335–353.
26. Archer R. Faculty or factory? Why industrializing drug discovery is inevitable. *J Biomol Screen* 1999; 5:235–237.
27. Wolcke J, Ullmann D. Miniaturized HTS technologies—uHTS. *Drug Discov Today* 2001; 6:637–646.
28. Fox S, Wang H, Sopchack L, et al. *High-Throughput Screening 2002: New Strategies and Technologies.* Moranga, CA: HighTech Business Decisions. 2002.
29. Li AP. Screening for human ADME/Tox drug properties in drug discovery. *Drug Discov Today* 2001; 6:357–366.
30. Valkó K. Measurements and predictions of physicochemical properties. In: Darvas F, Dormán G, eds., *High Throughput ADMETox Estimation*: In Vitro and In Silico *Approaches*. Westborough, MA: Eaton. 2002:1–24.
31. Artursson P, Karlsson J. Correlation between oral drug absorption in humans and apparent drug permeability in human epithelial (Caco-2) cells. *Biochem Biophys Res Commun* 1991; 175:880–885.
32. Kansy M, Senner F, Gubernator K. Physicochemical high throughput screening: parallel artificial membrane permeation assay in the description of passive absorption. *J Med Chem* 1998; 41:1007–1010.
33. Crespi CL, Miller VP, Penman BW. High throughput screening for inhibition of cytochrome P450 metabolism. *Med Chem Res* 1998; 8:457–471.
34. Slater K. Cytotoxicity tests for high throughput drug discovery. *Curr Opin Biotechnol* 2001; 12:70–74.
35. Ames BN, McCann J, Yamasaki E. Methods for detecting carcinogens and mutagens with the salmonella/mammalian microsome mutagenicity test. *Mutat Res* 1975; 31:347–367.

36. Krajcsi P, Dravas F. High-throughput in vitro toxicology. In: Darvas F, Dormán G, eds., *High Throughput ADMETox Estimation*: In vitro and In Silico *Approaches*. Westborough, MA: Eaton. 2002:75–81.
37. Netzer R, Ebneth A, Bischoff U, Pongs O. Screening lead compounds for QT interval prolongation. *Drug Discov Today* 2001; 6:78–84.
38. Tang W, Kang J, Wu X, et al. Development and evaluation of high throughput functional assay methods for hERG potassium channel. *J Biomol Screen* 2001; 6:325–331.
39. Engels MFM, Venkatarangan P. Smart screening: approaches to efficient HTS. *Curr Opin Drug Discov Dev* 2001; 4:275–283.

3

The NCI Human Tumor Cell Line (60-Cell) Screen

Concept, Implementation, and Applications

Michael R. Boyd, MD, PhD

CONTENTS

INTRODUCTION
IMPLEMENTATION
OPERATION
CONCLUSIONS

1. INTRODUCTION

This chapter is not intended to provide a comprehensive review of applications of the National Cancer Institute (NCI) 60-cell screen to anticancer drug discovery and development. The literature is now replete with such examples, given the NCI operation and provision of the screen to researchers worldwide for well over a decade. Selected examples are used here to illuminate the kind of output that has been routinely available from the screen and to show how some of the simplest applications of this output have been and perhaps remain of substantial utility to researchers engaged in the challenging and uncertain field of anticancer drug discovery and development. Readers may also wish to examine and consider the current operational details, as well as the wealth of related information and research tools based on the 60-cell screen, now provided by the NCI Developmental Therapeutics Program (DTP) at its internet website (http://dtp.nci.nih.gov). What follows here is intended as an historical and personal perspective on how the 60-cell screen came to be and the value and legitimacy of the screen as a research tool. I attempt to convey a sense of the breadth and depth of the diverse participants and their contributions to the screen's conceptual development, implementation, and oversight, and I offer one participant's view of obstacles encountered, choices and compromises made, and other issues that may have contributed to the utility as well as limitations of the current screen.

From: *Cancer Drug Discovery and Development:*
Anticancer Drug Development Guide: Preclinical Screening, Clinical Trials, and Approval, 2nd Ed.
Edited by: B. A. Teicher and P. A. Andrews © Humana Press Inc., Totowa, NJ

1.1. Background

Since 1955, the U.S. NCI has provided screening support to cancer researchers worldwide. Until 1985, the NCI screening program and the selection of compounds for further preclinical and clinical development under NCI auspices had relied predominantly on the in vivo L1210 and P388 murine leukemias and certain other transplantable tumor models *(1)*. From 1975 to 1985, the in vivo P388 mouse leukemia model was used almost exclusively as the initial or primary screen. With few exceptions, agents that showed minimal or no activity in the P388 system were not selected by the NCI for further evaluation in other tumor models or alternative screens.

1.2. The Concept

In June of 1984, the author presented to the Board of Scientific Counselors (BSC) of the NCI Division of Cancer Treatment (DCT) a preliminary concept of a so-called disease-oriented in vitro primary anticancer drug screen as a potential replacement to the P388 in vivo primary screen. Although the new concept was greeted initially with limited enthusiasm, the presenter nonetheless was encouraged to return to the subsequent fall meeting of the DCT-BSC with a more fully developed concept for further review and discussion. The new screening model proposed to the Board at the October 1984 meeting *(2,3)* comprised the essence of the operational screen that was formally launched *(4–11)* in 1990 and that is embodied in the present-day (2002) screen *(12,13)*.

1.3. Debate and Decision

Following the October, 1984 presentation of the new screen concept to the DCT-BSC, the Board expressed sufficient interest to name a BSC subcommittee to meet separately with the leadership and staff of the DTP to consider the concept in further detail. Subsequently we, and the subcommittee under the chairmanship of Dr. Mortimer M. Elkind, joined in the planning and organization of a workshop entitled "Disease-Oriented Antitumor Drug Discovery and Development." That workshop, held in Bethesda, Maryland on January 9–10, 1985, provided a forum for extensive discussion and debate concerning the justification, or otherwise, of such a proposed radical departure from the existing NCI drug screening paradigms. Participants in the workshop, in addition to NCI staff, represented a wide cross-section of experts from academia and industry, from both the United States and abroad *(see* Appendix A, p. 60). The debate, well documented by a verbatim transcript *(14)*, was vigorous but did not reveal any clear unanimity of opinion either as to the shortcomings of existing screens or as to alternative screening models or strategies. Nevertheless, there was a consensus that new screening and discovery strategies in general merited consideration, particularly given the prevailing dearth of effective therapeutic agents for most human cancers. Following the workshop, the author again presented the new screen concept to the DCT-BSC at the February 1985 meeting *(4)* for final review, further debate, and vote. The Board voted affirmatively, recommending an initial 2-yr exploratory effort, to be pursued in parallel with a continuing, albeit substantially downsized, P388 in vivo screen *(4)*. The Board additionally approved the author's proposed concurrent DTP-NCI implementation of a comprehensive new natural products collection, extraction, and repository program *(4)*.

In mid-1985, we began the phase-down, and eventual termination, of the in vivo P388 primary screen, the human tumor colony-forming assay (HTCFA) screen *(15)*, and the "tumor-panel" secondary screens *(1)*. Simultaneously, we launched the pilot program to explore the feasibility of the proposed new in vitro primary screening model. The screen would employ a diverse panel of human tumor cell lines organized into subpanels representing major tumor types. Compounds would be tested over a wide range of concentrations for cytotoxic or growth-inhibitory effects against each cell line comprising the panel. A secondary stage of screening on selected compounds would be performed in vivo in xenograft models using a subset of the cell lines found to be sensitive in the in vitro screen.

Although simple in concept, the development and implementation of the new in vitro NCI primary screen presented unprecedented challenges. Nevertheless, the feasibility of the pilot screen was firmly established by mid-1989, and, in April 1990 the screen was established in fully operational status. Samples were screened initially at a rate of about 20,000 per year, with the input shared between pure compounds submitted to the NCI and extracts or fractions thereof originating primarily from the NCI natural products repository. In its operational configuration, the cell line panel consisted of a total of 60 human tumor cell lines arranged in multiple subpanels representing diverse histologies including leukemias, melanomas, and tumors of the lung, colon, kidney, ovary, breast, prostate, and brain.

2. IMPLEMENTATION

2.1. Overview and Oversight

Efforts to establish the feasibility of the proposed new in vitro primary screen were focused initially on three main fronts: investigation of various alternative assays of in vitro drug sensitivity *(16–23)*; development of the cell line panel *(23–25)*; and information technology *(6,26,27)*. The technical challenges to implementation of such a screen, requiring on the order of 10–20 million individual culture well assays a year to achieve the scope of operations envisaged, were daunting. Also, many critical choices had to be made with respect to the design principles of the screening model, which would in turn have a profound impact on screening operational logistics as well as the nature of the data output and its potential utility. To assist us in making such critical decisions, as well as to provide in-depth, regular oversight of implementation of the new program, we organized an international, external Ad Hoc Review Committee for the NCI *In Vitro/In Vivo* Disease-Oriented Screening Project under the chairmanship of Professor Kenneth R. Harrap. The participants (non-NCI) in one or more meetings of that key committee (the Harrap Committee) during its 1985–1990 existence are given in Appendix B. The Harrap-committee, or a subcommittee thereof, met at least once annually with NCI staff for detailed discussions, debate, and critique of the new program. The 1987 meeting of the Harrap Committee was combined with a second workshop entitled "Selection, Characterization, and Quality Control of Human Tumor Cell-Lines for the NCI's New Drug Screening Program," which we jointly organized and held in Bethesda, Maryland on May 27–28, 1987. Participants in that meeting are given in Appendix C. Verbatim transcripts of all these meetings *(14,28–32)* provide interesting documentation of the progress, as well as the challenging technical problems encountered, during the 1985–1990 period. In addition to the Harrap Committee reviews, the development of the new screen was also reviewed periodically during regular meetings of the full membership of the DCT-BSC and likewise by the National Cancer Advisory Board (NCAB).

2.2. In Vitro Microculture Assays of Cell Growth and Viability

Three alternative assays for cellular growth and viability for possible use in the new primary screen were extensively investigated (16–23). Two were metabolic assays (16,18); the cellular reduction of a colorless tetrazolium salt, 3-(4,5-dimethylthiazol-2-yl)-2,5-diphenyl tetrazolium bromide (MTT), or 2,3-bis(2-methoxy-4-nitro-5-sulfophenyl)-5-([penylamino]-carbonyl)-2H tetrazolium hydroxide (XTT), yielded a colored formazan in proportion to viable cell number. The formazans could be measured conveniently in an automated colorimeter.

Development of the XTT tetrazolium assay (18) was stimulated by the desire to simplify further the MTT procedure by eliminating an aspiration/solubilization step; the reduction of MTT yielded an insoluble formazan that had to be dissolved in dimethylsulfoxide prior to colorimetry. In contrast, the XTT reagent (17) was metabolized by viable cells directly to a water-soluble formazan, allowing the immediate reading of optical density in the culture wells without further processing. Although simple and convenient, the XTT procedure gave relatively high background readings (low signal-to-noise ratio). XTT also shared with MTT the feature of an unstable (i.e., time-critical) endpoint, compromising the potential use of either of the tetrazolium assays in a high-flux antitumor screen employing a large panel of cell lines.

Although the XTT tetrazolium assay ultimately was not adopted for the anticancer screen, it did prove to have an immensely valuable application in the DTP-NCI high-flux anti-HIV drug discovery screen. The concept and development of the anti-HIV screen was first proposed by the author in November 1986, subsequently presented to and formally approved by the DCT-BSC in February 1987, and pursued thereafter by the DTP in parallel with the anticancer screen (33,34). We also organized a separate external Ad Hoc Advisory Committee, initially under the chairmanship of Dr. Dani P. Bolognasi and later under Dr. William M. Mitchell, to provide critique and oversight of development of the anti-HIV screen. Verbatim transcripts of the three major meetings of that committee during 1987–1990 were similarly recorded (35–37); the names of the committee members are available in the transcripts. This committee met concurrently with the Harrap Committee at its 1989 meeting.

For the anticancer screen application, two especially troublesome problems encountered with the tetrazolium assays eventually prompted the development of a third alternative microculture assay method. For either MTT or XTT, tetrazolium reduction was dependent on the cellular generation of NADH and NADPH. This raised concern about the influence of glucose concentration on the formation of the colored tetrazolium formazan, which was measured colorimetrically as an estimate of cellular growth or viability. Studies with MTT indicated that a progressive reduction in MTT-specific activity (MTT formazan formed/μg cell protein), which was observed during the course of a typical 7-d assay, was paralleled by a progressively decreasing glucose concentration (19). For XTT, there was a further problem owing to the additional requirement of an electron transfer reagent, phenazine methylsulfate (PMS), to promote adequate cellular reduction of the tetrazolium. With XTT/PMS, variations in pH of the standard growth medium (RPMI-1640), typically caused by temporary removal of culture plates from the relatively high 5% CO_2 incubator environment, resulted in occasional formation of a crystalline material causing erratic optical density measurements. Crystal formation occurred in the pH range of 7.0–9.0 and could be attributed to the reaction of PMS with glutathione (19).

In an attempt to eliminate the pH instability problem, a new culture medium was developed by the NCI Program Development Research Group (PDRG)(20). The medium had a stable physiological pH of 7.4 at normal atmospheric levels of CO_2 and derived its buffering capacity primarily from β-glycerophosphate. The new medium was optimized to facilitate growth in atmospheric CO_2 by inclusion of biotin, L-asparagine, pyruvate, and oxaloacetate for metabolic stimulation of intracellular CO_2 production. With either the MTT assay or a non-tetrazolium assay (described below), similar dose-response curves were obtained for various standard anticancer drugs against cell cultures maintained either in the new medium (PDRG-basal growth medium) under ambient CO_2 or in RPMI-1640 under a 5% CO_2 environment. However, a decision was subsequently made, consistent with a specific recommendation of the Harrap committee, not to incorporate the PDRG medium into the new screen, but rather to consider an alternative endpoint assay that was not as dependent on the particular CO_2 environment.

In an attempt to identify a suitable, non-tetrazolium assay for use in the in vitro primary drug screen, a series of protein and biomass stains were investigated (21). These included anionic dyes that bound to the basic amino acid residues of proteins, as well as cationic dyes that bound to the negative, fixed charges of biological macromolecules. Of all the reagents tested, sulforhodamine B (SRB) gave the best combination of stain intensity, signal-to-noise ratio, and linearity with cell number. SRB is a bright pink anionic dye that, in dilute acetic acid, binds electrostatically to the basic amino acids of trichloroacetic acid (TCA)-fixed cells.

2.3. Selection of Assay Parameters and Methodology

Under in vitro assay conditions, exposure to an antitumor agent may decrease the number of viable tumor cells by direct cell killing or by simply decreasing the rate of cellular proliferation. Many in vitro assays of drug sensitivity typically employ relatively low initial cell inoculation densities (e.g., a few hundred cells/well) followed by relatively long continuous drug exposure times (e.g., 6–7 d or considerably longer than the doubling times of many tumor lines). Such a selection of assay parameters, although favoring the detection of antiproliferative effects (i.e., growth inhibition), might, however, obscure otherwise potentially interesting patterns of differential cytotoxicity (e.g., net cell killing). Moreover, with an antiproliferative or growth inhibition endpoint, cell lines with very short doubling times (e.g., leukemias) might appear hypersensitive in comparison with more slowly growing tumor lines (e.g., from solid tumors). Additionally, potential problems of nutrient deprivation, as well as practical limitations on the use of pulsed drug exposures, might, in the course of an assay, necessitate removal and replacement of medium. On the other hand, a longer assay duration might facilitate the detection of activity of relatively insoluble compounds or active trace constituents in mixtures or extracts. Furthermore, the longer assay format might be essential for detection of agents that required several cell cycles for expression of lethal drug effects.

An alternative selection of assay parameters was considered in order to enhance the screen's ability to discern interesting differences in net cell killing (i.e., actual reduction of biomass) among the sensitive panel lines. This required the use of a relatively large initial cell inoculum (e.g., 20,000 cells/well) and a relatively short drug exposure/incubation time (e.g., 1–2 d). Optimal exploitation of this format required a high level of sensitivity and reproducibility of the assay methodology, as well as the capability to measure reliably the initial viable cell densities (t_0 values) just prior to drug introduction.

There were reasonable arguments for or against selection of either of these two alternative sets of assay parameters, or some compromise in between. Indeed, we extensively investigated the impact of these parameters on the screen's performance and, not surprisingly, found that certain kinds of compounds yielded results that contrasted greatly, depending on the particular choice of assay parameters. However, for purposes of further studies with the pilot-scale screen, as well as for initiation of the full-scale screen, the high-cell- inoculum/short-assay protocol was selected for routine use. This selection was based principally on the desire to minimize the effects of variable doubling times of the diverse cell lines in the panel, to optimize the chances of detection of cell line-specific or subpanel-specific cytotoxins, and to minimize the chances of obscuring such activities by nonspecific antiproliferative effects. This choice of assay parameters was also emphatically endorsed by the Harrap Committee, after much discussion, debate, and extensive review of the relevant available experimental data.

Given the above decisions concerning assay parameters, the optimal choice of a tetrazolium assay (e.g., MTT or XTT) versus the SRB assay had to be determined for the desired application to a large-scale screening operation employing many diverse tumor lines simultaneously. Pilot screening studies (22,23) were performed on a common set of compounds using both MTT and SRB with the selected assay parameters. Under the experimental conditions employed, and within the limits of the data analyses applied, the assays gave quite comparable results. However, the SRB assay had important practical advantages for large- scale screening. Although the SRB procedure was more labor-intensive (e.g., required multiple washing steps), it had the distinct advantage of a stable endpoint (i.e., not time-critical, in contrast to either of the tetrazolium assays). Screening capacity, reproducibility, and quality control all appeared to be markedly enhanced by adoption of SRB for the primary screen (23). Therefore, the SRB assay was used subsequently for all routine screening operations.

2.4. Cell Line Panel

The initial panel incorporated a total of 60 different human tumor cell lines derived from seven cancer types including lung, colon, melanoma, renal, ovarian, brain, and leukemia. Selection of lines for inclusion in the panel required that they adequately met minimal quality assurance criteria (testing for mycoplasma, mitogen-activated protein [MAP], human isoenzyme, karyology, in vivo tumorigenicity), that they were adaptable to a single growth medium, and that they showed reproducible profiles for growth and drug sensitivity. Mass stocks of each of the lines were prepared and cryopreserved; these stocks provided the reservoir for replacement of the corresponding lines used for drug screening after no more than 20 passages in the screening laboratory (6,23,24).

Although many of the lines were well known and had been widely used in research, the clinical histories and/or original tumor pathologies of many of the lines were incomplete or unavailable. All cell lines in the interim panel were nevertheless subjected to detailed, specialized characterizations (e.g., histopathology, ultrastructure, immunocytochemistry) to verify or determine tissue and tumor type (25). Moreover, parallel projects were launched for the acquisition of better and more diverse candidate cell lines and for the development of new lines directly from surgical specimens or from nude mouse xenografts for which the corresponding clinical backgrounds were more complete. Special focus was placed on major cancer types (e.g., breast and prostate) that were not represented in the initial panel because of unavailability of suitable lines.

2.5. Pilot Screening Operations: Standardization and Reproducibility

A pilot screening operation *(6,23)* was initiated in which the panel lines were inoculated onto a series of standard 96-well microtiter plates on d 0, in most cases at 20,000 cells/well and then preincubated in absence of drug for 24 h. Test agents were then added in five 10-fold dilutions starting from the highest soluble concentration, and the lines were incubated for a further 48 h. The cells were then fixed *in situ*, washed, and dried. SRB was added, followed by further washing and drying of the stained, adherent cell mass. The bound stain was solubilized and measured spectrophotometrically on automated plate readers interfaced with personal computers, which in turn were interfaced with a central computer.

A series of approx 170 known compounds, comprising commercially marketed (New Drug Application [NDA]-approved) anticancer agents, investigational (Investigational New Drug Application [INDA]-approved) anticancer agents, and other candidate antitumor agents (compounds previously approved by the NCI Decision Network Committee for preclinical development based on activities in prior screens) was selected for pilot screening studies *(6)*. The repetitive screening of these prototype "standard agents" was aimed at providing a suitable database from which a variety of novel approaches to data display and analysis could be explored. The "standard agent database" was also the basis for calibration and standardization of the screen, for the assessment of reproducibility of the screening data, and for the development of procedures for quality control monitoring *(6,27)*.

2.6. Information Technology

Facilitating the above analyses were the development of the COMPARE pattern-recognition methodology, and the mean-graph display, which supported both visual and automated analyses of the differential activity profiles of agents tested against the 60-cell panel *(6,12,13,26,27)*. The mean-graph profiles of standard agents were highly reproducible over time; for example, the characteristic mean-graph profile of a given standard agent could be shown by COMPARE to be highly correlated among separate screening runs of the same compound over many months *(6,27)*.

2.7. Review and Recommendation to Operational Status

In November of 1989, a pivotal review meeting *(5,32)* was held at the NCI-Frederick Cancer Research and Development Center in Frederick, Maryland, the site of the newly constructed screening facilities. The full current memberships of the Harrap Committee, the Natural Products Program Advisory Subcommittee, the DCT-BSC, the NCAB, and the President's Cancer Panel, were invited to review jointly in detail the progress of implementation of the in vitro screen and to provide recommendations as to further directions. The resulting consensus recommendation was that the feasibility, reproducibility, and calibration of the screen was sufficiently established that full-scale operation should be formally initiated as soon as possible *(5)*. DTP staff responded accordingly, and full operational status of the screen was established shortly thereafter. Table 1 summarizes the assay protocol and parameters for the operational screen as launched in 1990. Table 2 summarizes some of the pertinent screening laboratory operations and logistics. The annual operational costs of the new in vitro primary screen were budgeted at approx $3–4 million/yr, or approx one-third the operational costs of the P388 in vivo primary screen that it replaced.

Table 1
Assay Protocol and Parameters for the NCI In Vitro Antitumor Screen as Initiated in 1990[a]

Cell line panel
Sixty lines total
Seven subpanels initially (lung, colon, renal, ovary, melanoma, brain, leukemia)
Lines used at ≤ 20 passages from master stock
Culture medium
RPMI-1640
5% serum
Cell inoculation density
5000–40,000 cells per well (96-well microtiter plate)
Preincubation
24 h (no drug)
Sample dilutions
Routinely 10^{-4}, 10^{-5}, 10^{-6}, 10^{-7}, and 10^{-8} M or as specified
Duplicates performed at all concentrations
T_0 and "no-drug" controls included
Drug incubation
48 h
Endpoint assay
Sulforhodamine B protein stain

[a]Further details are available in refs. 6, 21, 23, and 25.

3. OPERATION

3.1. Service Screening Operations

Initially, for routine screening, each sample was tested in the 2-d, continuous drug exposure protocol using five $\log_{10}$-spaced concentrations starting at an upper limit of $10^{-4} M$ (or 100 μg/mL for natural product extracts or fractions thereof) against all the 60 cell lines comprising the panel. Most crude extracts were initially "prescreened" using only a single concentration (100 μg/mL) against the entire 60-cell line panel; extracts that produced 50% or more net cell killing of three or more of the panel lines were routinely selected for testing in the full screen. A 3-d prescreen was subsequently also introduced for pure compounds. Current details of the 60-cell screening operations are available at the DTP website (http://dtp.nci.nih.gov).

Details of the particular cell lines comprising the original panel and the individual inoculation densities and other assay features used initially in routine screening operations were as published (23,25). After December 1, 1992, a modified panel, in which 10 of the original cell lines were replaced by a selection of breast and prostate cancer lines, was employed. Details of the replacement cell lines, inoculation densities, and other aspects of the revised routine screening operations were as published (13).

The testing of a sample in the full 60-cell line screen generates a corresponding set of 60 dose-response curves. Figure 1 illustrates four contrasting sets of composite dose-response curves. In Fig. 1A, the particular test compound had essentially no effect on the growth or viability of any of the 60 cell lines. Figure 1B shows the effect of a test

Table 2
Primary Screening Laboratory Operations and Logistics as Initiated in 1990[a]

Laboratory
  Total space, 8051 ft^2
  Two floors
  Four general support modules
  Screening modules, 20
  Laminar-flow hoods, 50

Staffing
  Technicians, 44
  Senior supervisors (PhD), 2

Cell inoculations/drug additions
  Lines assigned per technician, 6
  Three lines/2 compounds per 96-well plate

Colorimetric endpoint determinations
  Ten plates/compound
  Plates/week, 4000
  Automated plate readers, 12

Quality control
  Manual
  Automated

Computer support
  In-lab PCs networked to central computer, 20

Calibration/standardization of screen
  Daily standards
  Monthly standards
  Standard agent database

[a]Further details are available in refs. *6, 23,* and *27.*

compound that was cytotoxic, albeit with essentially equivalent potency to all the panel lines. Neither of these screening results are particularly useful. In contrast, Fig. 1C illustrates results from a compound showing pronounced cytotoxicity, albeit with considerably divergent potencies among the individual cell lines. Screening profiles, such as exemplified by Fig. 1C, that manifest "differential" growth inhibition and/or cytotoxicity have been of particular interest as the basis for research applications of the screen, as well as for the selection and prioritization of compounds for in vivo evaluation.

Figure 1D shows the characteristic dose-response composite profile from a highly potent natural product, dolastatin 10 (Fig. 2; *see* also refs. *38* and *39*); there appears to be a marked degree of differential growth inhibition and/or cytotoxicity among the various panel lines; however, for any given line the inhibitory effect of the compound, within the tested concentration range, is not concentration-dependent. A more detailed analysis and explanation of the basis for this type of profile has been provided elsewhere *(13).* Critical to any research application of the screen is the remarkably high degree of reproducibility of the screening profile of a given compound tested repetitively over time in the NCI screen *(6,13,27).*

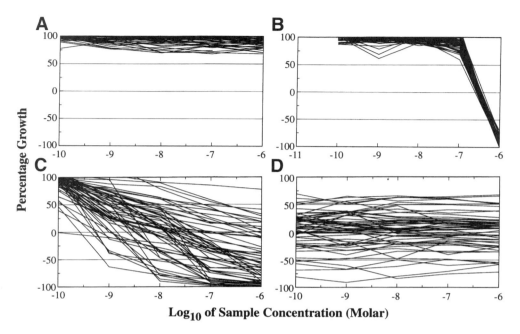

Fig. 1. Examples of composite 60-cell dose-response profiles of various compounds tested in the NCI in vitro screen. Composite **A** is from the screening of a compound that produced little or no growth inhibition or cytotoxicity in any of the cell lines. Composite **B** is from the screening of a compound showing general ("nondifferential") cytotoxicity at the highest tested concentration. Composite **C** shows results of screening of a compound that produced markedly "differential" cytotoxicity among the panel cell lines. Composite **D** illustrates another type of differential activity profile, in which there is no apparent dose dependence of the effects within the tested concentration range of the particular compound.

3.2. Research Applications

NCI staff, collaborators, and others have explored diverse data analysis strategies and methods with data generated by the in vitro screen. Examples, reviews and other publications describing such studies are available *(6,12,13,40–44,48).* As discussed elsewhere *(13),* the appealingly simple mean-graph and COMPARE analysis methodologies have provided useful support for a number of research applications. Such applications have encompassed the discovery of new members of known mechanistic classes. For example, the mean-graph screening profiles (not shown) of halichondrin B *(45,46)* and spongistatin 1 *(47)* (Fig. 2) were revealed by COMPARE to resemble closely the mean-graph profile (not shown) of dolastatin 10 *(38,39)* (Fig. 2) and other known members (e.g., vinca alkaloids, taxol, rhizoxin, maytansine) of the general class comprising tubulin-interactive antimitotics *(48).* Follow-up biochemical studies *(49,50)* confirmed the general antimitotic mechanism anticipated from the initial evaluation of halichondrin B and spongistatin 1 in the 60-cell screen.

The counterpoint to discovery of new members of known mechanistic classes is the discovery of new antitumor mechanistic classes and new members therein. Such application of the 60-cell screen is exemplified by studies of 9-methoxy-N^2-methyl-ellipticinium acetate (MMEA) and related ellipticinium derivatives. MMEA produced an

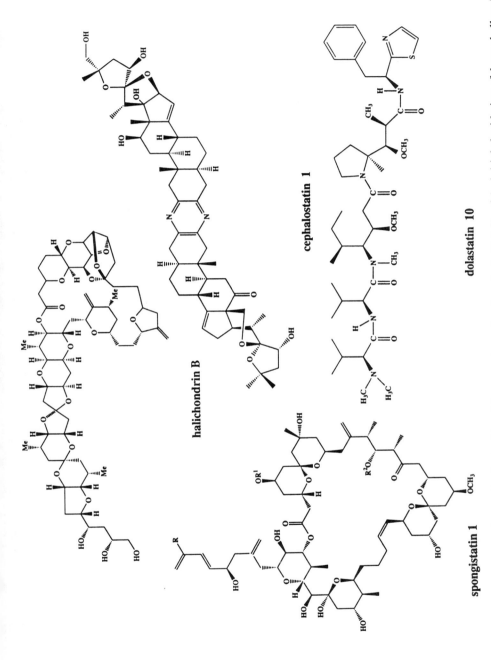

cephalostatin 1

dolastatin 10

halichondrin B

spongistatin 1

Fig. 2. Structures of some novel antitumor leads elucidated from marine natural products. Details of the initial elucidation of these challenging structures by the original investigators can be found in refs. *38*, *45–47*, and *54*. Samples of the compounds were provided by Professor George R. Pettit for study in the NCI screen. Figure 1D is the composite dose-response profile obtained from testing of dolastatin 10. The composite screening profiles of spongistatin 1 and halichondrin B (not shown) closely resembled that of dolastatin 10 (Fig. 1D). Figure 1C is the composite dose-response profile from testing of cephalostatin 1 in the in vitro screen.

unprecedented screening profile, in which the brain tumor cell line subpanel showed consistently higher sensitivity to MMEA cytotoxicity than did other lines comprising the panel (6,51). Subsequent studies revealed a high correlation between uptake and accumulation of MMEA, and/or metabolite(s) thereof, and MMEA cytotoxicity in the sensitive brain tumor cell lines (52). Both uptake and cytotoxicity of MMEA were blocked by reserpine. Other experiments further suggested a resemblance of the MMEA transporter in the brain tumor lines to a constitutive biogenic amine transport process characteristic of certain glial elements of normal brain (52). In vivo studies of the 9-chloro analog of MMEA showed evidence of in vivo antitumor activity against an intracranially implanted brain tumor cell line (53).

Another novel lead that showed an unprecedented profile in the 60-cell line screen is cephalostatin 1 (54,55) (Fig. 3). Figure 1C is from the screening of this compound. Figure 3 shows the median growth inhibition (GI_{50}), the total growth inhibition (TGI) and the median lethal concentration (LC_{50}) mean-graphs, constructed from the data of Fig. 1C, as defined in detail elsewhere (13). COMPARE analyses were performed, using described procedures (13), with the mean graph profiles of cephalostatin 1 as the "seed" against the entire available screening database from approx 40,000 pure compounds tested to date. When the profiles were ranked in order of degree of similarity to the seed, the top-ranking 13 profiles were all found to be derived from prior tests of cephalostatin 1 or other closely related members of the cephalostatin series (55). On the other hand, the characteristic screening profile of the cephalostatins did not show comparable correlations to any member(s) of the standard agent database, suggesting that the differential cytotoxicity of this lead derives from an unprecedented, but as yet undefined, mechanism of action.

Another important research application emerged from studies of structure-activity relationships (SARs) and chemical analog synthesis. In these applications the NCI in vitro screen has provided an opportunity for lead optimization based on the feedback of both quantitative and qualitative biological data. For example, members of a chemically related series can be compared not only with respect to relative potencies, but also with respect to the degree to which they do or do not retain the desired cell line specificity or subpanel activity of the lead compound. Research applications of this nature are illustrated by studies (51) with the aforementioned ellipticinium series and also by SAR investigations related to the novel cytotoxin halomon (56,57).

The 60-cell screen has also been used for the selection and bioassay-guided fractionation of natural product extracts from the NCI repository. The screen can be used either to select or, alternatively, to eliminate from further consideration extracts having screening profiles either similar to or distinctly different from any known standard agent or mechanistic class. Bioassay support for fractionation has typically employed one or a few individual cell lines selected on the basis of the 60-cell screening profile. A recent example of use of the 60-cell screen in natural products research is the discovery of a novel antitumor benzolactone enamide class (Fig. 4) that selectively inhibits mammalian vacuolar-type (H^+)-ATPases (V-ATPases) (58). This class comprises the marine natural products salicylihalamides (59) and lobatomides (60,61) and microbial metabolites including the apicularens (62,63), oximidines (64), and others (65) (Fig. 5). Although they are structurally unrelated to the classical V-ATPase inhibitors bafilomycin A and concanamycin A (Fig. 6), the benzolactone enamides show 60-cell mean-graph profiles

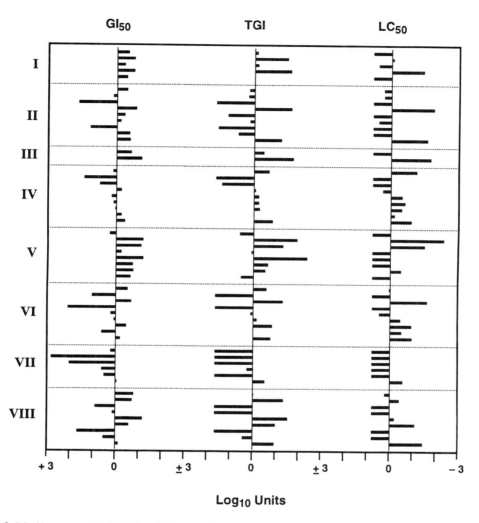

Fig. 3. Median growth inhibition (GI_{50}), total growth inhibition (TGI) and mean lethal concentration (LC_{50}) mean graphs for cephalostatin 1 constructed from the data illustrated in Fig. 1C. Response parameter definitions, methods of construction, and interpretation of mean graphs have been reviewed recently in detail elsewhere (*see* ref. 13). The tumor cell line subpanels are identified as follows: I, leukemia; II, lung, nonsmall cell; III, lung, small cell; IV, colon; V, brain; VI, melanoma; VII, ovary; VIII, kidney. These mean graph "fingerprints" can be shown by pattern-recognition analyses (e.g., *see* methods of COMPARE analyses also reviewed recently in refs. *13* and *44*) to be highly correlated with those of other cephalostatins; in contrast, they were not similarly correlated with any of the "standard agents" *(6,13)*.

essentially indistinguishable from the classical inhibitors (Fig. 7). However, further analyses of these various compounds in specific V-ATPase assays revealed that the benzolactone enamide class has unprecedented specificity for mammalian V-ATPase isoforms. It is anticipated that the elucidation and availability of these new compounds will facilitate further exploration of the validity of V-ATPase as a molecular target for cancer therapeutics.

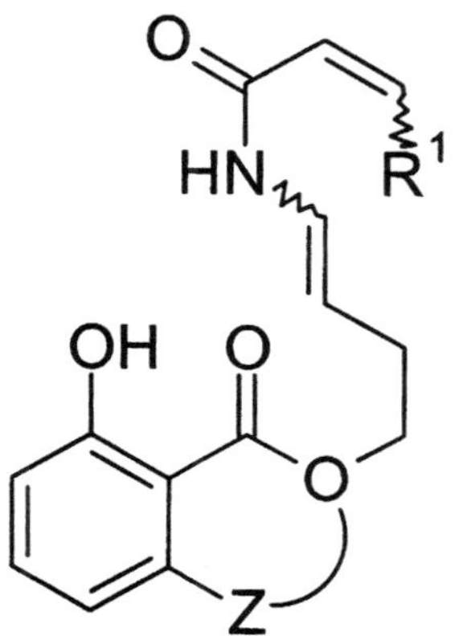

Fig. 4. Generic structure of the new benzolactone enamide V-ATPase inhibitor class, wherein Z represents a linker of variable length, composition, and stereochemistry, R^1 is a substituent of variable composition and geometric orientation, and geometric isomers are possible at the enamide linkage.

There have been other research applications of the NCI in vitro screen aimed at exploiting advances in knowledge of tumor biology and the molecular genetics of cancer. For example, experimental measurements of the differential expression in the panel cell lines of potential cell growth regulatory and/or drug sensitivity or resistance determinants have been used to construct hypothetical mean-graph profiles that were then used to search the available databases for compounds that produced actual screening profiles similar to the desired hypothetical one(s). For instance, a hypothetical mean-graph fingerprint constructed from quantitative expression values for the *mdr*-1/P-glycoprotein in each of the panel cell lines was used as the seed for COMPARE analyses *(66)*. A series of compounds was thereby identified having screening profiles highly correlated with the constructed probe. Subsequent biochemical analyses confirmed that the selected compounds were indeed substrates for the P-glycoprotein. In a related study *(67)*, comparably high correlations were found for the same compounds with respect to a probe constructed of rhodamine efflux values, which are functional assay counterparts of *mdr*-1 expression. NCI staff and collaborators have continued to explore similar research strategies with numerous other potential sensitivity or resistance determinants, such as oncogene or tumor suppressor gene products, growth factor receptors, transporters, and the like.

4. CONCLUSIONS

It is approaching two decades since the concept for the NCI 60-cell screen was first proposed. The initial 5 yr, 1985–1990, were consumed with developing key elements of the screening model and physical facilities to accommodate the screening operations, recruiting and training staff, implementing and evaluating a pilot-scale screen and data management operations, and calibration and standardization of the screen. During the subsequent years of operation of the screen, hundreds of thousands of materials, including pure compounds as well as natural product extracts, have been tested either in the prescreen and/or the full-screen assay against the 60- cell panel. The accrued databases have provided a rich source of information having considerable utility in certain research

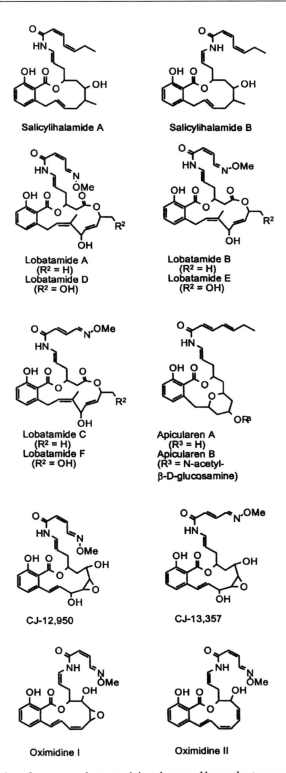

Fig. 5. Specific examples of compounds comprising the novel benzolactone enamide structural class.

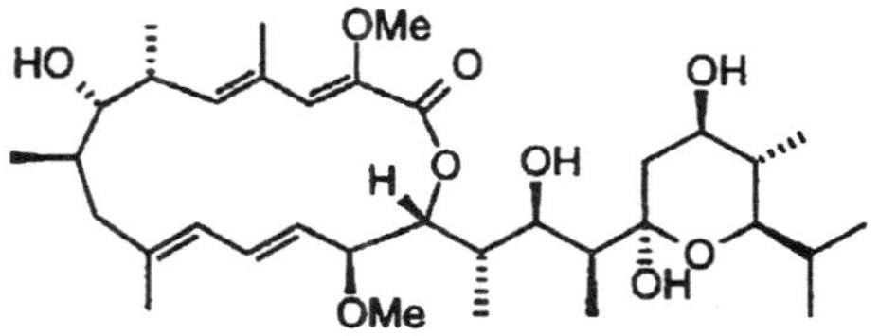

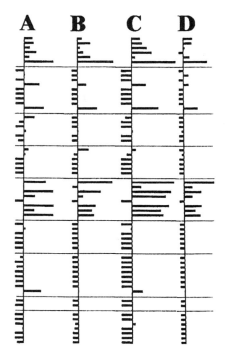

Bafilomycin A₁

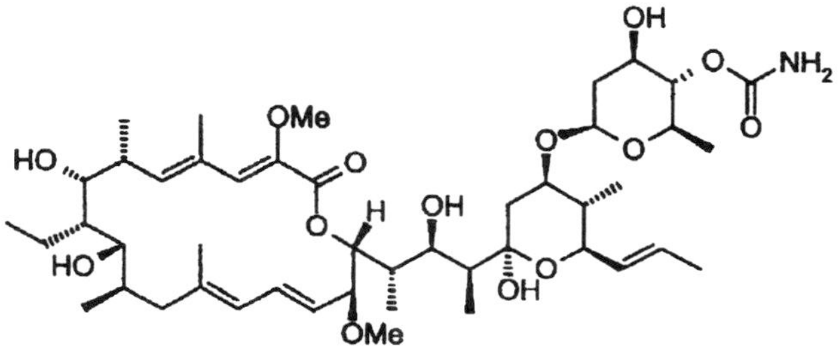

Fig. 6. Specific examples of compounds of the bafilomycin/concanamycin macrocyclic lactone class.

A   B   C   D

Fig. 7. Total growth inhibition (TGI)-based mean-graph profiles derived from testing of bafiloymcin A₁ (**A**), salicylihalamide A (**B**), lobatamide A (**C**), and oximidine II (**D**) in the NCI 60-cell screen. Each horizontal bar represents the sensitivity of an individual cell line relative to the average sensitivity (represented by the central vertical line) of the full 60-cell panel. Bars projecting to the right represent relatively more sensitive cell lines and those to the left the less sensitive lines. The horizontal lines delineate the nine cell line subpanels, as follows, from top to bottom: leukemia, nonsmall cell, lung, colon, brain, melanoma, ovary, kidney, prostate, and breast. Individual cell line identifiers have been omitted for clarity. Cell line identities and specific response values for each line from a typical testing of salicylihalamide A can be found in ref. *59*.

applications. To add new potential dimensions of utility, the NCI Developmental Therapeutics Program has continued to pursue the "molecular characterization" of the cell lines of the NCI screen with respect to selected genes, gene products, and other possible "molecular targets" contributing to maintenance or reversion of the malignant phenotype (*see* the DTP website at http://dtp.nci.nih.gov). It is hoped that such information will facilitate further use of the 60-cell screen and/or the accrued screening databases to discover novel molecular target-directed leads.

REFERENCES

1. Driscoll JS. The preclinical new drug research program of the National Cancer Institute. *Cancer Treat Rep* 1984; 68:63–76.
2. Boyd JD, ed. National Cancer Institute planning to switch drug development emphasis from compound to human cancer-oriented strategy. *Cancer Lett* 1984; 10:1–2.
3. Boyd MR. National Cancer Institute drug discovery and development. In: Frei E II, Freireich E, eds., *Accomplishments in Oncology*. Philadelphia: Lippincott. 1986:68–76.
4. Boyd JD, ed. Division of Cancer Treatment Board approves new screening program, natural products concepts. *Cancer Lett* 1985; 11:4–5.
5. Boyd JD, ed. Reviewers report progress in new drug prescreen system development. *Cancer Lett* 1989; 15:1–5.
6. Boyd MR. Status of the NCI preclinical antitumor drug discovery screen. In: DeVita VT Jr, Hellman S, Rosenberg SA, eds., *Cancer: Principles and Practice of Oncology Updates*, vol. 3, no. 10. Philadelphia: Lippincott. 1989:1–12.
7. Friend T. Plants, sea could yield new drugs. *USA Today* 1989; September 5:D1.
8. Kolberg RJ. Casting a wider net to catch cancer cures. *J NIH Res* 1990; 2:82–84.
9. Ansley D. Cancer Institute turns to cell line screening. *Scientist* 1990; 4:3–9.
10. Stehlin D. Harvesting drugs from plants. *FDA Consumer* 1990; October:20–24.
11. Thompson D. Giving up on the mice. Time 1990; September 17:79.
12. Boyd MR. The future of new drug development. In: Niederhuber JE, ed., *Current Therapy in Oncology*. Philadelphia: BC Decker. 1993:11–22.
13. Boyd MR, Paull KD. Some practical considerations and applications of the National Cancer Institute *in vitro* anticancer drug discovery screen. *Drug Dev Res* 1995; 34:91–109.
14. Developmental Therapeutics Program, Division of Cancer Treatment, National Cancer Institute. Proceedings, Workshop on Disease-Oriented Antitumor Drug Discovery and Development, Bethesda, MD, January 9–10. 1985:1–273.
15. Shoemaker RH, Wolpert-DeFilippes M, Kern D, et al. Application of a human tumor colony forming assay to new drug screening. *Cancer Res* 1985; 45:2145–2153.
16. Alley MC, Scudiero DA, Monks A, et al. Feasibility of drug screening with panels of human tumor cell lines using a microculture tetrazolium assay. *Cancer Res* 1988;48:589–601.
17. Paull KD, Shoemaker RH, Boyd MR, et al. The synthesis of XTT: a new tetrazolium reagent that is bioreducible to a water-soluble formazan. *J Heterocyclic Chem* 1988; 25:911–914.
18. Scudiero DA, Shoemaker RH, Paull KD, et al. Evaluation of a soluble tetrazolium/formazan assay for cell growth and drug sensitivity in culture using human and other tumor cell lines. *Cancer Res* 1988; 48:4827–4833.
19. Vistica DT, Skehan P, Scudiero D, Monks A, Pittman A, Boyd MR. Tetrazolium-based assays for cellular viability: a critical examination of selected parameters affecting formazan production. *Cancer Res* 1991; 51:2515–2520.
20. Vistica DT, Scudiero D, Skehan P, Monks A, Boyd MR. New carbon dioxide-independent basal growth medium for culture of diverse tumor and nontumor cells of human and nonhuman origin. *J Natl Cancer Inst* 1990; 82:1055–1061.
21. Skehan P, Storeng R, Scudiero D, et al. New colorimetric cytotoxicity assay for anticancer-drug screening. *J Natl Cancer Inst* 1990; 82:1107–1112.
22. Rubinstein LV, Shoemaker RH, Paull KD, et al. Comparison of *in vitro* anticancer-drug-screening data generated with a tetrazolium assay versus a protein assay against a diverse panel of human tumor cell lines. *J Natl Cancer Inst* 1990; 82:1113–1118.

23. Monks A, Scudiero D, Skehan P, et al. Feasibility of a high-flux anticancer drug screen utilizing a diverse panel of human tumor cell lines in culture. *J Natl Cancer Inst* 1991; 83:757–766.

24. Shoemaker RH, Monks A, Alley MC, et al. Development of human tumor cell line panels for use in disease-oriented drug screening. In: Hall T, ed., *Prediction of Response to Cancer Chemotherapy*. New York: Alan R. Liss. 1988:265–286.

25. Stinson SF, Alley MC, Fiebig H, et al. Morphologic and immunocytochemical characteristics of human tumor cell lines for use in an anticancer drug screen. *Anticancer Res* 1992; 12:1035–1054.

26. Paull KD, Shoemaker RH, Hodes L, et al. Display and analysis of patterns of differential activity of drugs against human tumor cell lines: development of the mean graph and COMPARE algorithm. *J Natl Cancer Inst* 1989; 81:1088–1092.

27. Boyd MR, Paull KD, Rubinstein LR. Data display and analysis strategies for the NCI disease-oriented *in vitro* antitumor drug screen. In: Valeriote FA, Corbett T, Baker L, eds., *Cytotoxic Anticancer Drugs: Models and Concepts for Drug Discovery and Development*. Amsterdam: Kluwer Academic Publishers. 1992:11–34.

28. Developmental Therapeutics Program, Division of Cancer Treatment, National Cancer Institute. Proceedings of the Ad Hoc Review Committee for the NCI *In Vitro/In Vivo* Disease-Oriented Screening Project, Bethesda, MD, September 23–24. 1985:1–243.

29. Developmental Therapeutics Program, Division of Cancer Treatment, National Cancer Institute. Proceedings of the Ad Hoc Review Committee for the NCI *In Vitro/In Vivo* Disease-Oriented Screening Project, Bethesda, MD, December 8–9. 1986:1–173.

30. Developmental Therapeutics Program, Division of Cancer Treatment, National Cancer Institute. Proceedings of Workshop on Selection, Characterization and Quality Control of Human Tumor Cell Lines for the NCI's New Drug Screening Program, Bethesda, MD, May 27–28, 1987:1–160.

31. Developmental Therapeutics Program, Division of Cancer Treatment, National Cancer Institute. Proceedings of the Ad Hoc Review Committee for the NCI *In Vitro/In Vivo* Disease-Oriented Screening Project, Bethesda, MD, May 19–20. 1988:1–218.

32. Developmental Therapeutics Program, Division of Cancer Treatment, National Cancer Institute. Proceedings of the Ad Hoc Review Committee for the NCI *In Vitro/In Vivo* Disease-Oriented Screening Project, Bethesda, MD, November 13–15. 1989:1–245.

33. Boyd MR. Strategies for the identification of new agents for the treatment of AIDS: a national program to facilitate the discovery and preclinical development of new drug candidates for clinical evaluation. In: DeVita VT, Hellman S, Rosenberg SA, eds., *AIDS, Etiology, Diagnosis, Treatment and Prevention*. Philadelphia: Lippincott. 1988:305–319.

34. Weislow, OS, Kiser R, Fine DL, Bader J, Shoemaker RH, Boyd MR. New soluble-formazan assay for HIV-1 cytopathic effects: application to high-flux screening of synthetic and natural products for AIDS-antiviral activity. *J Natl Cancer Inst* 1989; 81:577–586.

35. Developmental Therapeutics Program, Division of Cancer Treatment, National Cancer Institute. Proceedings of Workshop on Issues for Implementation of a National Anti-HIV Preclinical Drug Evaluation Program; Critical Parameters for an *In Vitro*, Human Host-Cell Based, Primary Screen, Bethesda, MD, April 8–9. 1987:1–136.

36. Developmental Therapeutics Program, Division of Cancer Treatment, National Cancer Institute. Proceedings of the Ad Hoc Advisory Committee for the Anti-HIV Drug Screening Program, Bethesda, MD, April 7–8. 1988:1–113.

37. Developmental Therapeutics Program, Division of Cancer Treatment, National Cancer Institute. Proceedings of the Ad Hoc Expert Advisory Committee for the Anti-HIV Drug Screening Program, Bethesda, MD, November 13–15. 1989:1–226.

38. Pettit GR, Kamano Y, Herald CL, et al. The isolation and structure of a remarkable marine animal constituent: dolastatin 10. J Am Chem Soc 1987; 109:6883–6885.

39. Bai R, Pettit, GR, Hamel E. Dolastatin 10, a powerful cytotoxic peptide derived from a marine animal; inhibition of tubulin polymerization mediated through the vinca alkaloid binding domain. *Biochem Pharmacol* 1990; 39:1941–1949.

40. Hodes L, Paull K, Koutsoukos A, Rubinstein L. Exploratory data analytic techniques to evaluate anticancer agents screened in a cell culture panel. *J Biopharmaceut Stat* 1992; 2;31–48.

41. Weinstein JN, Kohn KW, Grever MR, et al. Neural computing in cancer drug development: predicting mechanism of action. *Science* 1992; 258:447–451.

42. van Osdol WW, Myers TG, Paull KD, Kohn KW, Weinstein JN. Use of the Kohonen self-organizing map to study the mechanisms of action of chemotherapeutic agents. *J Natl Cancer Inst* 1994; 86: 1853–1859.
43. Weinstein JN, Myers T, Buolamwini J, et al. Predictive statistics and artificial intelligence in the U.S. National Cancer Institute's drug discovery program for cancer and AIDS. *Stem Cells* 1994; 12:13–22.
44. Paull KP, Hamel E, Malspeis L. Prediction of biochemical mechanism of action from the in vitro antitumor screen of the National Cancer Institute. In: Foye O, ed., *Cancer Chemotherapeutic Agents*. Washington DC: American Chemical Society Books. 1995:9–45.
45. Hirata Y, Uemura D. Halichondrins-antitumor polyether macrolides from a marine sponge. *Pure Appl Chem* 1986; 58:701–710.
46. Pettit GR, Herald CL, Boyd MR, et al. Isolation and structure of the cell growth inhibitory constituents from the pacific marine sponge *Axinella* sp. *J Med Chem* 1991; 34:3339–3340.
47. Pettit GR, Cichacz ZA, Gao F, et al. Isolation and structure of spongistatin 1. *J Org Chem* 1993; 58: 1302–1304.
48. Paull KD, Lin CM, Malspeis L, Hamel E. Identification of novel antimitotic agents acting at the tubulin level by computer-assisted evaluation of differential cytotoxicity data. *Cancer Res* 1992; 52: 3892–3900.
49. Bai R, Paull KD, Herald CL, Malspeis L, Pettit GR, Hamel E. Halichondrin B and homohalichondrin B, marine natural products binding in the vinca domain of tubulin; discovery of tubulin-based mechanism of action by analysis of differential cytotoxicity data. *J Biol Chem* 1991; 24:15,882–15,889.
50. Bai R, Chiacz ZA, Herald CL, Pettit GR, Hamel E. Spongistatin 1, a highly cytotoxic, sponge-derived, marine natural product that inhibits mitosis, microtubule assembly, and the binding of vinblastine to tubulin. *Mol Pharmacol* 1993; 44:757–766.
51. Acton EM, Narayanan VL, Risbood P, Shoemaker RH, Vistica DT, Boyd MR. Anticancer specificity of some ellipticinium salts against human brain tumors *in vitro*. *J Med Chem* 1994; 37:2185–2189.
52. Vistica DT, Kenney S, Hursey ML, Boyd MR. Cellular uptake as a determinant of cytotoxicity of quaternized ellipticines to human brain tumor cells. *Biochem Biophys Res Commun* 1994; 200: 1762–1768.
53. Shoemaker RH, Balaschak MS, Alexander MR, Boyd MR. Antitumor activity of 9-Cl-2-methylellipticinium acetate against human brain tumor xenografts. *Oncol Rep* 1995;2:663–667.
54. Pettit GR, Inoue M, Kamano Y, et al. Isolation and structure of the powerful cell growth inhibitor cephalostatin 1. *J Am Chem Soc* 1988; 110:2006–2007.
55. Pettit GR, Kamano Y, Inoue M, et al. Antineoplastic agents 214. Isolation and structure of cephalostatins 7-9. *J Org Chem* 1992; 57:429–431,
56. Fuller RW, Cardellina JH II, Kato Y, et al. A pentahalogenated monoterpene from the red alga, *Portieria hornemannii*, produces a novel cytotoxicity profile against a diverse panel of human tumor cell lines. *J Med Chem* 1992; 35:3007–3011.
57. Fuller RW, Cardellina JH II, Jurek J, et al. Isolation and structure/activity features of halomon-related antitumor monoterpenes from the red alga, *Portieria hornemanii*. *J Med Chem* 1994; 37:4407–4411.
58. Boyd MR, Farina C, Belfiore P, et al. Discovery of a novel antitumor benzolactone enamide class that selectively inhibits mammalian vacuolar-type (H+)-ATPases. *J Pharmacol Exp Ther* 2001; 297: 114–120.
59. Erickson KL, Beutler JA, Cardellina JH II, Boyd MR. Salicylhalamides A and B, novel cytotoxic macrolides from the marine sponge *Haliclona* sp. *J Org Chem* 1997; 62:8188–8192.
60. Galinis DL, McKee TC, Pannell L, Cardellina JH II, Boyd MR. Lobatamides A and B, novel cytotoxic macrolides from the tunicate *Aplidium lobatum*. *J Org Chem* 1997; 62:8968–8969.
61. McKee TC, Galinis DL, Pannell LK, et al. The lobatamides, novel cytotoxic macrolides from the tunicate *Aplidium lobatum*. *J Org Chem* 1998; 63:7805–7810.
62. Kunze B, Jansen R, Sasse R, Hofle G, Reichenbach H. Apicularens A and B, new cytostatic macrolides from *Chondromyces* species (myxobacteria): production, physico-chemical and biological properties. *J Antibiot* 1998; 51:1075–1080.
63. Jansen R, Kunze B, Reichenbach H, Hofle G. Antibiotics from gliding bacteria LXXXVI. Apicularens A and B, cytotoxic 10-membered lactones with a novel mechanism of action from *Chondromyces* species (myxobacteria): isolation, structure elucidatin, and biosynthesis. *Eur J Org Chem* 2000; 913–919.

64. Kim JW, Shinya K, Furihata K, Hayakawa Y, Seto H. Oximidines I and II: novel antitumor macrolides from *Pseudomonas* sp. *J Org Chem* 1999: 64:153–155.
65. Dekker KA, Aiello R, Hirai H, et al. Novel lactone compounds from *Mortierella verticillata* that induce the human low density lipoprotein receptor gene: fermentation, isolation, structural elucidation and biological activities. *J Antibiot* 1998; 51:14–20.
66. Alvarez M, Paull K, Monks A, et al. Generation of a drug resistance profile by quantitation of *mdr*-1/ P-glycoprotein expression in the cell lines of the NCI anticancer drug screen. *J Clin Invest* 1995; 95:2205–2214.
67. Lee J-S, Paull KP, Hose C, et al. Rhodamine efflux patterns predict PGP substrates in the NCI drug screen. *Mol Pharm* 1994; 46:627–638.

APPENDIX A

Participants (Non-NCI) in the NCI Workshop on Disease-Oriented Antitumor Drug Discovery and Development, January 9–10, 1985, Bethesda, MD

Dr. Michael Alley
Dr. Ghanem Atassi
Dr. Bruce Baguley
Dr. Laurence Baker
Dr. Ralph Bernacki
Dr. Bijoy Bhuyan
Dr. Arthur Bogden
Mr. Jerry Boyd
Dr. William Brodner
Dr. Martin Brown
Dr. James Catino
Dr. Thomas Corbett
Dr. Daniel Dexter
Dr. Benjamin Drewinko
Dr. Gertrude Elion
Dr. Mortimer Elkind
Dr. Edward Elslager
Dr. David Ettinger
Dr. Oystein Fodstad
Dr. Martin Forbes
Dr. Henry Friedman
Dr. David Gillespie

Dr. David Goldman
Dr. Robert Goodman
Dr. Michael Grever
Dr. Daniel Griswold
Dr. Ladislav Hanka
Dr. Kenneth Harrap
Dr. David Hesson
Dr. David Houchens
Dr. Peter Houghton
Dr. Susan Horwitz
Dr. Robert Jackson
Dr. Randall Johnson
Dr. John Johnston
Dr. Michael Johnston
Dr. John Kovach
Dr. Victor Levin
Dr. Daniel Martin
Dr. Patrick McGovern
Dr. Christopher Mirabelli
Dr. John Montgomery
Dr. Franco Muggia
Dr. Ronald Natale

Dr. Robert Newman
Dr. Kent Osborne
Dr. George Pettit
Dr. Theodore Phillips
Dr. Alexander Pihl
Dr. Mark Rosenblum
Dr. Alan Rosenthal
Dr. Marcel Rozencweig
Dr. Youcef Rustum

Dr. Dale Stringfellow
Dr. Robert Sutherland
Dr. Raymond Taetle
Dr. Ken Tew
Dr. Richard Tuttle
Dr. David Van Echo
Dr. Daniel Von Hoff
Dr. George Weber
Dr. Larry Weisenthal

Dr. Clifford Schold
Dr. John Schurig
Mr. Alan Shefner

Dr. Thomas Wiliams
Dr. Benjamin Winogard
Dr. Charles Young

APPENDIX B

Members of the Ad Hoc Review Committee for NCI In Vitro/In Vivo Disease-Oriented Screening Project[a]

Dr. Bruce Baguley
Dr. Ralph Bernacki
Dr. Arthur Bogden
Dr. Michael Buas
Dr. Thomas Carey
Dr. Thomas Connors
Dr. Thomas Corbett
Dr. Mortimer Elkind
Dr. John Faulkner
Dr. Isaiah Fidler
Dr. Heinz-Herbert Fiebig
Dr. Oystein Fodstad
Dr. James Goldie

Dr. David Goldman
Dr. Daniel Griswold
Dr. Kenneth Harrap[b]
Dr. Sydney Hecht
Dr. Susan Horwitz
Dr. Peter Houghton
Dr. George Pettit
Dr. Alexander Pihl
Dr. Alan Rosenthal
Dr. Sydney Salmon
Dr. Phillip Skehan
Dr. Larry Weisenthal
Dr. Robert Whitehead

[a]Each named member participated in at least one or more regular meetings of the Committee during 1985–1989.

[b]Committee Chair

APPENDIX C

Participants (Non-NCI) in the NCI Workshop on Selection, Characterization and Quality Control of Human Tumor Cell-Lines for the NCI's New Drug Screening Program, May 27–28, 1987, Bethesda, MD

Dr. Bruce Baguley
Dr. Ralph Bernacki
Dr. June Biedler
Dr. Arthur Bogden
Dr. Michael Brattain
Dr. Thomas Carey
Dr. Desmond Carney
Dr. Thomas Corbett
Dr. Joseph Eggleston
Dr. Eileen Friedman
Dr. David Goldman
Dr. Daniel Griswold
Dr. Kenneth Harrap

Ms. Janine Einspahr
Dr. Howard Fingert
Dr. Oystein Fodstad
Dr. Ian Freshney
Dr. Susan Friedman
Dr. Robert Hay
Dr. Steven Jacobs
Dr. Edward Keenan
Dr. James Kozlowski
Dr. Chung Lee
Col. Al Liebovitz
Dr. John Masters
Dr. Stanley Mikulski

Dr. Mary Pat Moyer
Dr. Charles Plopper
Dr. Mark Rosenblum
Dr. Phillip Skehan
Dr. Robert Sutherland
Dr. Raymond Taetle
Dr. Peter Twentyman
Dr. John Wallen
Dr. Michael Wiemann
Dr. Larry Weisenthal
Dr. James Willson
Dr. Bernd Winterhalter

4 Human Tumor Screening

Axel-R. Hanauske, MD, PhD,
Susan G. Hilsenbeck, PhD,
and Daniel D. Von Hoff, MD

CONTENTS

INTRODUCTION
CONCEPTUAL CONSIDERATIONS WITH IN VITRO DRUG SCREENING
CLONOGENIC VS NONCLONOGENIC TESTS
CHEMOSENSITIVITY ASSAYS VS CHEMORESISTANCE ASSAYS
METHODOLOGY
SUMMARY

1. INTRODUCTION

In 2003, an estimated 1.33 million patients will be diagnosed with cancer in the United States, and the number of predicted cancer deaths will be in excess of 550,000 *(1)*. Similar incidences and death rates for the most important cancers are reported from other industrialized Western countries. Most patients diagnosed with cancer will receive one or more chemotherapy regimens during the course of their disease. Retrospective and prospective clinical trials have improved the likelihood of response in individual patients and have been pivotal in the development of curative regimens for patients with a variety of malignancies. These major advances include patients with childhood tumors, testicular cancer, and some types of leukemias and malignant lymphomas. The empiric clinical approach has also led to the development of successful adjuvant therapies for patients with breast cancer, osteogenic sarcomas, and colorectal cancer.

Despite this progress, treatment options are still marginal for patients with the majority of cancer types. For this reason, many attempts have been made to develop new therapeutic compounds with improved antitumor activity or decreased clinical toxicity while preserving activity. The development of methodologies that allow for the prediction of a clinical tumor response with acceptable accuracy is of pivotal importance in order to focus the available resources on the pursuit of promising agents. Of course, it is necessary to demonstrate that these assays also can predict clinical tumor response to agents that are already established in clinical practice.

From: *Cancer Drug Discovery and Development:*
Anticancer Drug Development Guide: Preclinical Screening, Clinical Trials, and Approval, 2nd Ed.
Edited by: B. A. Teicher and P. A. Andrews © Humana Press Inc., Totowa, NJ

Table 1
Principles of In Vitro Tumor Screening

Goals
  Identify tumor types with particular sensitivity to developmental agents as a rationale for
    subsequent clinical Phase II trials
  Provide experimental support for choice of optimal clinical administration schedule
  Determine shape of concentration-response relationship

Conceptual issues
  Adequate choice of drug concentration
  Intratumoral heterogeneity
  Intertumoral heterogeneity
  Interference with physiological tumor cell microenvironment
  Selection pressure might lead to selection of clinically insignificant clones
  Optimal time for clinical treatment with in vitro active agents
  Limited value of in vitro assays to study agents requiring metabolic activation

2. CONCEPTUAL CONSIDERATIONS WITH IN VITRO DRUG SCREENING

Several conceptual problems have been identified with in vitro or in vivo predictive assays. First, the choice of a drug concentration relevant for the clinical situation is largely arbitrary. Second, the problem of biological intratumoral and intertumor heterogeneity (different metastases in the same patient) has not been overcome. Third, experimental systems will inevitably create a tumor microenvironment that is vastly different from the physiologic microenvironment in the patient. Fourth, all experimental systems exert a selection pressure on tumor cells that may arbitrarily produce an advantage for clinically insignificant tumor subpopulations (Table 1). These considerations not only apply for the prediction of an individual cancer patient's response to chemotherapy, but also to the prediction of whether a new chemical compound will be active against certain tumor types in the clinical setting.

In patients with curable malignancies receiving standard first-line chemotherapy regimens, chemosensitivity assays would only be helpful if they had such excellent positive and negative predictivity to allow identification of the rare patient with intrinsic tumor resistance. At present, none of the available chemosensitivity assays has convincingly demonstrated such a predictivity. However, in patients with refractory tumors or in diseases with low response rates, chemosensitivity assays may be helpful to avoid excessive and unwarranted toxic side effects, and may therefore help to preserve quality of life. Although there is not yet evidence for improved disease-free or overall survival by assay-guided chemotherapy, recent evidence suggests that clinical response rates may be superior if chemotherapy regimens are selected using predictive in vitro assays *(2)*. There is also evidence that certain in vitro assays may be helpful in the choice of tumors to be studied in a clinical Phase II setting with new antineoplastic agents *(see below) (3)*.

3. CLONOGENIC VS NONCLONOGENIC TESTS

Table 2 summarizes in vitro and in vivo techniques that have attracted attention because of their potential for clinical predictivity. For most systems, an extensive prospective validation of their predictive value has not been performed.

Table 2
In Vitro and In Vivo Techniques That Have Been Utilized
to Predict Tumor Response in Individual Patients

In vitro systems
 Clonogenic
  Human tumor cloning assay
  Cellular adhesive matrix
Nonclonogenic
 Dye exclusion
 Explant (organoid) cultures
 Precursur incorporation
 Fluorescence
 Intracellular ATP concentration
 Intracellular drug concentrations
 Specific molecular markers (e.g., alteration of drug transport, alteration of enzyme
  activities, gene amplification)
In vivo systems
 Subrenal capsule
 Nude mouse xenograft

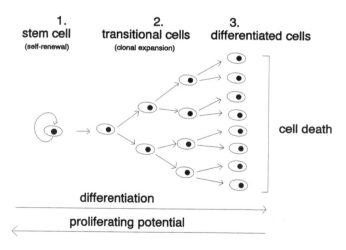

Fig. 1. The stem cell model for human tumors and normal tissues. The stem cell is defined by micro-environmental factors and has the potential of unlimited self-renewal. It generates a population of cells with limited growth capacity and increasing differentiation (clonogenic cells). Finally, growth and differentiation have either reached a balance (normal tissue) or are left at various stages in the chaotic growth of a tumor.

Clonogenic assay systems rest on the concept that tumor stem cells are the ultimate driving force of tumor growth in vitro and in vivo *(4)* (Fig. 1). This concept has been derived from normal human tissues and forms the basis for all clonogenic test systems *(5–7)*. The main representative of this type of assay is the human tumor cloning assay (HTCA) with several technical variations of the original technique having been reported over time *(4,8–11)*. Thus, the HTCA is used to determine the effects of clinically used or investigational antineoplastic agents on actively growing tumor cells *(12)*.

Nonclonogenic assay systems rest on the concept that total tumor cell kill rather than clonogenic tumor cell kill is the most important variable for in vitro chemosensitivity tests. Supporters of this concept have argued that true stem cells have not yet been identified in solid human tumors and that recruitment of resting tumor cells into the clonogenic pool may occur after this pool has been depleted by chemotherapy.

4. CHEMOSENSITIVITY ASSAYS VS CHEMORESISTANCE ASSAYS

Although the ultimate goal clearly is to identify the individual patient or the specific type of tumor sensitive to a given agent or combination of antineoplastic agents, there is indisputable evidence that all available in vitro assays predict drug resistance much more reliably than drug sensitivity. Published reports on the most widely used assay, the HTCA, demonstrate that sensitivity and positive predictive value compare well with other clinically used diagnostic procedures (e.g., antibiograms, and estrogen and progesterone receptor determination in breast cancer patients). However, in light of limited evaluability rates, many investigators believe that this is not sufficient to warrant the use of in vitro chemosensitivity assay as part of the clinical routine.

For these reasons, several investigators have attempted to focus the negative predictive value of in vitro assay systems (13). However, it has to be kept in mind that rather than knowing where an agent is inactive, clinicians and researcher involved in drug development need to know where an agent is active. This need clearly points to the limitations of exclusive resistance testing.

5. METHODOLOGY

5.1. HTCA

Of all in vitro systems studied to date, none has been investigated as thoroughly as the HTCA. The inhibition of cellular proliferation of clonogenic cells is the experimental endpoint (4,8,9,14). The assay has been widely used for work with cell lines and has also been used to assess the effects of radiotherapy. It has attracted particular interest when used with freshly explanted human tumor tissue. Biopsies from solid tumors or pleural/ascitic effusions are processed into single-cell suspensions and are exposed to anticancer agents. For cell-cycle-dependent agents, like cytosinarabinoside, a long-term exposure for the whole incubation period is required, whereas other agents are removed by washings after a 1-h exposure. The cells are then seeded into a semisolid medium (agar, agarose, or methylcellulose) to prevent growth of nonmalignant bystander cells in the specimen. Traditionally, Petri dishes are used for this assay, but soft agar cloning of freshly explanted tumor specimens in glass capillaries has also been reported, and appears to have some technical and conceptual advantages (11,15,16). After 14–28 d, clonogenic cells will have divided several times and have produced tumor cell colonies that are subsequently quantified. In addition to negative controls with untreated cells, each experiment must include controls treated with an agent to identify cell clumps that might give spuriously high colony counts (17).

The HTCA is useful for the conduct of several types of studies. First, it has been extensively used to investigate the biologic behavior of clonogenic cells from freshly explanted human tumors. Second, it has been used to determine whether an individual patient's tumor response to chemotherapy can be accurately predicted. Third, the HTCA has been demonstrated to be a valuable tool in the arena of anticancer drug development.

5.2. Statistical Considerations

There are a number of statistical issues that must be addressed in the analysis and interpretation of results from the HTCA, including definition of an evaluable assay; estimation of tumor specific outcome; analysis of concentration-response; analysis of patterns of cross resistance; and prediction of patient sensitivity to cytotoxic drugs. Tumor growth in the assay is extremely heterogenous, with some tumors producing hundreds of colonies under control conditions, whereas others produce very few colonies. Even under optimal experimental conditions, a substantial percentage of tumors show no growth at all. As a result, drug and concentration effects have to be interpreted relative to control colony formation in the same tumor. The following criteria to determine sample evaluability have been established: In Petri dishes, replicate negative (solvent-only) control plates ($N = 3$–6) without cytostatic agents must average more than 20 colonies. In capillaries, the average number of colonies in controls must be more than 3. Growth under positive (toxic) control conditions must average < 30% of negative controls. Replication is important because it allows one to compute within-sample standard deviations and coefficients of variation (CTs). Outliers or "bad" plates can be detected and discarded.

Individual tumor-specific results of the HTCA are most often reported as the ratio of treated to control colony counts and are expressed as a percentage. Survival fractions near 100% suggest a lack of cytotoxic effect, whereas values that are substantially < 100% suggest that the drug reduces colony formation. Important issues are the determination of biologically relevant and clinically predictive reductions of colony growth as well as the reproducibility of these results. In computing the percent survival, both the numerator and denominator are derived from sample data that are subject to random variation. Exact calculation of the sample standard deviation of percent survival is problematic, but an approximation computed based on a Taylor series expansion of the ratio gives the following:

$$SD = [(CV^2_D / N_D) + (CV^2_C / N_C)]^{1/2} \times \text{percent survival} \qquad (1)$$

where CV_D and CV_C are the coefficients of variation (i.e., $CV_D = \text{standard deviation}_D / \text{mean}_D * 100\%$) for drug-treated and control replicate samples, respectively, and N_D and N_C are the number of plates in each sample. Table 3 illustrates this calculation for a hypothetical set of data. An approx 95% confidence interval could be calculated as % survival $\pm 2 \times SD = 56 \pm 18\%$. Since this interval does not include 100%, it would be reasonable to suggest that the drug treatment has had a cytotoxic effect. This assumes that under null conditions of no effect, colony formation is similar in both treated and control plates. In actual practice, growth tends to be slightly lower in treated plates, and a safer approach would be to require the 95% confidence interval to be below 85 or 90% survival. Alternatively, investigators often choose a particular cutoff value for % survival (i.e., 50%) in order to classify tumors as sensitive or resistant. We have reviewed results from 924 evaluable assays in which the drug effect was expected to be negligible. Treatments were limited to drugs known to be noncytotoxic, or in the case of cytotoxic drugs, to doses at least two orders of magnitude below the equivalent clinically achievable plasma concentrations. The median survival was 85%, and only 5% of assays had survivals below 48%. The analysis provides empirical support for the use of the 50% cutoff as a statistically reasonable approximation to a 5% level test of whether % survival is less than would be expected if the drug has no effect.

Table 3
Hypothetical Results of the HTCA

Treatment regimen	Colony counts				Survival	SD^c
	No. plates	Mean	SD^a	CV^b		
Control	4	50	10	10%	100	
Drug	4	27	7	25%	56%	9%

[a]Standard deviation.
[b]Coefficient of variation.
[c]See text for computational formula.

Rather than reporting individual outcomes, a panel of tumors might be tested against a range of concentrations of an investigational drug in an effort to detect possible efficacy, especially in specific tumor types. Clinically achievable plasma concentrations may not be known, and it is therefore highly desirable to demonstrate a concentration-response in the HTCA. Analysis can be based on counts of sensitive (% survival < 50%) and resistant tumors using contingency tables. Alternatively, more powerful methods, such as analysis of variance, can be used to analyze counts of raw or transformed percent survivals. Regardless of the method, it is essential to recognize that data arising from testing the same tumor at different concentrations are not independent. For example, if a particular tumor is sensitive to a drug at one concentration, it is invariably sensitive at all higher concentrations. This lack of independence must be accounted for in the analysis. Appropriate methods include McNemar's test for 2 × 2 tables or analysis of variance with repeated measures. The analysis can be further complicated if some tumors are not tested at all concentrations.

As a tool in the development of new drugs, the HTCA can be used to identify possible crossresistance with clinically established drugs. For example, a panel of tumors could each be tested against a standard drug and selected concentrations of the investigational drug. The tumors, cross-classified as sensitive or resistant to each drug, can be analyzed with a test for independence such as Fisher's Exact Test. Survivals or counts for each drug can be analyzed using linear regression to determine the extent to which knowledge of the outcome for one drug alters predictions for the outcome on the other drug.

5.3. Clinical Applications

Clinical correlative trials using variations of the HTCA have been performed retrospectively and prospectively in large patient populations using established compounds. Table 4 summarizes the results of clinical correlation studies for different types of tumors. Most investigators have included patients with a broad variety of different tumors in their analyses. Although this approach allows for an overall estimate of predictive accuracy, the value of the HTCA for specific tumor types requires separate analysis, and only a few tumor-specific correlative trials have been reported. For several tumor types, the available information is difficult to interpret because of a small sample size. The analysis of published data on clinical correlations also has to take into account the fact that investigators have used different cutoff points and different definitions of in vitro evaluability. Also, the impact of prior chemotherapy on the predictive performance of the

Table 4
Summary of Clinical Correlative Trials With the HTCA

Tumor type	Trial design	No. of published studies	No. of patients	No. of correlations	In vitro/in vivo correlations[a]				Sensitivity (95% CI[b])	Specificity (95% CI[b])	Positive predictive value (95% CI[b])	Negative predictive value (95% CI[b])
					S/S	S/R	R/S	R/R				
Miscellaneous	RS	14	797	959	209	84	40	616	0.84 (0.79–0.88)	0.87 (0.84–0.89)	0.69 (0.64–0.74)	0.94 (0.92–0.96)
	PS	7	378	380	60	35	38	247	0.61 (0.50–0.71)	0.88 (0.84–0.91)	0.63 (0.53–0.73)	0.87 (0.83–0.91)
Bladder	RS	1	13	15	3	2	1	9	0.75 (0.19–0.99)	0.82 (0.48–0.98)	0.60 (0.15–0.95)	0.90 (0.56–1.00)
Brain	PS	1	10	10	3	1	0	6	1.00	0.86 (0.35–0.97)	0.75 (0.19–0.99)	1.00
Breast	RS	3	57	57	14	4	6	33	0.70 (0.50–0.90)	0.89 (0.79–0.99)	0.78 (0.59–0.97)	0.85 (0.73–0.96)
	PS	2	49	49	16	13	6	13	0.70 (0.51–0.88)	0.50 (0.31–0.69)	0.55 (0.37–0.73)	0.65 (0.44–0.86)
Cervix	RS	1	13	13	3	3	0	7	1.00	0.79 (0.35–0.93)	0.50 (0.12–0.89)	1.00
Colorectal	PS	2	21	23	12	2	0	9	1.00	0.82 (0.48–0.98)	0.86 (0.57–0.98)	1.00
Kidney	PS	1	7	7	2	2	0	3	1.00	0.60 (0.15–0.95)	0.50 (0.07–0.93)	1.00
Lung	RS	1	33	33	4	3	4	22	0.50 (0.16–0.84)	0.88 (0.69–0.98)	0.57 (0.18–0.90)	0.85 (0.65–0.96)
Melanoma	RS	1	39	49	10	1	0	38	1.00	0.97 (0.87–1.00)	0.91 (0.59–1.00)	1.00
	PS	4	106	124	20	26	5	73	0.80 (0.59–0.93)	0.74 (0.65–0.83)	0.44 (0.29–0.59)	0.94 (0.89–0.99)
Myeloma	RS	2	49	73	21	8	4	40	0.84 (0.70–0.98)	0.83 (0.72–0.84)	0.72 (0.56–0.88)	0.91 (0.82–0.99)
	PS	1	14	28	21	3	0	4	1.00	0.57 (0.18–0.90)	0.88 (0.69–0.98)	1.00
Ovary	RS	4	58	97	23	7	1	66	0.96 (0.88–1.00)	0.90 (0.83–0.97)	0.77 (0.62–0.92)	0.99 (0.97–1.00)
	PS	2	59	114	22	9	1	82	0.96 (0.88–1.00)	0.90 (0.84–0.96)	0.71 (0.55–0.87)	0.99 (0.97–1.00)
Unknown primary	RS	1	10	10	1	5	1	3	0.50 (0.00–0.98)	0.38 (0.09–0.76)	0.17 (0.00–0.64)	0.75 (0.01–0.81)

[a]S, Sensitive; R, Resistant; RS, retrospective; PS, prospective.
[b]95% Confidence interval.
Adapted from ref. 43.

HTCA has not been studied. A cumulative analysis of all published correlative trials indicates that the probability of a partial or better response is 69% if the patient's tumor specimen is sensitive in vitro. On the other hand, if a tumor is resistant in vitro, there will only be a 9% chance for tumor response *(18)*. Keeping all criticisms and limitations in mind, it is still important to acknowledge that the overall predictive performance of the HTCA is comparable to other clinically accepted tests, e.g., the determination of steroid hormone receptors on breast cancer cells for the prediction of tumor response, exercise ECG for the detection of ischemic heart disease, or the use of tumor markers for the detection of cancer or prediction of disease recurrence *(19)*.

Despite encouraging evidence from retrospective studies, only a few prospective clinical correlative trials have been performed using established anticancer compounds. In a trial with 133 patients with advanced malignancies, treatment groups were stratified according to performance status, tumor type, and prior chemotherapy followed by randomization either to receive single-agent chemotherapy as determined by a medical oncologist or to be treated with single-agent chemotherapy according to in vitro sensitivity data obtained in a capillary cloning system *(2)*. For a variety of reasons, only 36 of the 65 patients assigned to the clinician's choice group actually received treatment as compared to 19 of 68 patients assigned to the assay-guided group. In the clinician's choice group, one patient achieved a partial response (3%), and in the assay-guided group, four patients had partial responses (21%, $p = 0.04$). In addition, 26% of patients receiving the assay-guided treatment had stable disease as compared to 8% receiving empirical treatment. No difference in the survival was observed. In a Southwest Oncology Group trial in 211 patients with ovarian cancer, the response rate was significantly higher (28%) in patients receiving HTCA-guided chemotherapy compared to patients treated empirically (11%, $p = 0.03$). However, in contrast to earlier reports *(see below)* there was no survival difference between the two groups (6.25 vs 7 mo) *(20)*. Although these studies provide encouraging leads for future trials, they also point to several technical limitations of the HTCA that still need to be resolved *(21)*. These include lack of growth in 30–50% of all specimens and an incubation time of 2–4 wk. A modified assay combining precursor incorporation (^{3}H-thymidine or ^{3}H-uridine) and soft agar colony formation has been reported to increase the number of evaluable specimens to 80–90% and decrease the incubation time to several days *(10)*. However, this modification no longer allows for the direct determination of inhibition of clonal proliferation. Instead, the amount of trichloroacetic acid precipitable radioactivity is taken as representative of cell growth. The relationship between the number of colonies and radioactive precursor incorporation is nonlinear and can only be described by elaborate mathematical algorithms *(13,22)*. No randomized prospective correlative trials have been performed with this system.

5.4. The HTCA and Drug Development

In the field of anticancer drug development, the HTCA is used for in vitro Phase II studies to identify sensitive tumor types and to estimate the probability for response *(23,24)*. It is also used to show a concentration-response effect at concentrations that are clinically achievable *(25–32)*. It has been employed to compare the activity of developmental compounds with clinically used agents and to address questions of crossresistance or cross-sensitivity *(33)*. An important issue is the choice of biologically meaningful, i.e.,

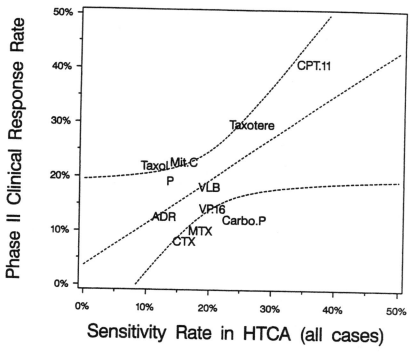

Fig. 2. Correlation of in vitro sensitivity rates and published clinical response rates for clinically established and experimental therapeutics in nonsmall-cell lung cancer *(3)*. Tumor specimens were considered sensitive if colony survival was 0.5 × control. Drug concentrations for in vitro testing corresponded to 10% of clinically achievable peak plasma concentrations. Drugs include: ADR, doxorubicin; Carbo. P, carboplatin; CTX, cyclophosphamide; CPT. 11, irinotecan; MTX, metho-trexate; Mito. C, mitomycin C; P, cisplatin; VLB, vinblastine; VP. 16, etoposide; Taxol and Topotecan. Linear regression and 95% confidence regions are shown.

clinically relevant, concentrations. Lack of clinical predictivity may result from selection of unrealistically high or low drug concentrations for in vitro testing. Ideally, in order to define definitively its utility for the selection of drugs and tumor types for future development, the HTCA should be studied in a setting where patients enrolled in clinical trials have their tumors tested against the same investigational agent that is administered clinically. Clinical response and in vitro sensitivity to various concentrations could then be analyzed. However, this type of study is not likely to be performed, because it will be very difficult to accrue a sufficient number of patients. In addition, since only small cohorts of patients are enrolled in early clinical trials, the statistical power may not be large enough for meaningful correlations. Attempts have been made to correlate clinical Phase II data with in vitro results *(34,35)*. In recent analyses of data from our laboratory we have found that the correlation of in vitro response rates and published clinical single-agent activity depends on the type of tumor tested. As shown in Fig. 2, a reasonable correlation was observed for nonsmall-cell lung cancer *(3)*. However, in vitro response and clinical response correlated less well in ovarian cancer and breast cancer.

On the opposite end of the drug development spectrum, the HTCA has been used to investigate the biological effects of cytokines or polypeptide growth factors, with tumor growth stimulation being used as an additional endpoint *(36–40)*. Finally, the assay could be suitable to study potential synergisms between treatment components.

In summary, at the present time, in vitro Phase II studies cannot replace clinical Phase II testing, since the correlation of in vitro response to clinical response is still poorly understood. Activity of a new compound in the HTCA, however, may support the clinician's decision to investigate further its clinical value in a particular type of tumor in patients.

5.5. Comparison With Other In Vitro and In Vivo Chemosensitivity Tests

As summarized in Table 5, a number of chemosensitivity assays have been developed during the past decade. Most of these assays use surrogate endpoints for cell kill or inhibition of proliferation. Some of the newer assays are based on the hypothesis that total cell kill is more important than selective cell kill of clonogenic cells and are thus not selective for colony-forming units or other features of clonogenic cells. However, none of these assays has undergone clinical testing as thoroughly as the HTCA. In particular, the predictive value of most of these assays has not been investigated in prospective or randomized studies. For the ATP cell viability assay, a multicenter prospective correlative clinical trial has been recently initiated by the Swiss Cancer Research Group. No results are yet available from this study.

Yanagawa and coworkers have studied 71 tumor specimens using a nude mouse isotope assay, the subrenal capsule assay, the ATP cell viability assay, and the HTCA. Except for the HTCA, evaluability rates were above 90%. In this study, only 42.9% of specimens were evaluable for the human tumor cloning assay. However, the prediction of clinical response was reported to be 100% accurate and was clearly superior to the two in vivo tests examined *(41)*. The same group of investigators recommended in a clinical correlative study with 391 patients using these four chemosensitivity assay that separate assays should be used to predict for clinical sensitivity or resistance to certain cytostatic agents *(42)*. This study points to the limitations of each assay system and suggests that multiple assay endpoints are needed for an accurate clinical predictive value. However, there are no independent prospective trials available that validate this complicated approach.

6. SUMMARY

Of all predictive tests, soft agar cloning of freshly explanted human tumors has been the most extensively studied. Although technically difficult, this experimental approach has been demonstrated to be of value for clinical and preclinical research. It is employed for cell biologic studies as well as for early drug development. In the clinical setting, it may help identify active agents and may spare undue toxicity in carefully selected patients. It is important that prospective randomized studies be performed to obtain definitive data on the impact of human tumor cloning assay-guided therapy on patient survival.

Table 5

Comparision of HTCA with Other Commonly Used Chemosensitivity Tests[a]

Assay	Endpoint	Time to achieve results	% Supplies that can be studied	Correlative studies available			Impact on			Comment
				Retrospective	Prospective	Randomized	Response rate	Relapse-free survival	Survival	
Human Tumor Cloning Assay (12)	Growth inhibition of clonogenic tumor cells	14–28 d	Average of 50%–70% variations between different tumor types	Many	Few	?	Yes	Unknown	No	Detection of sensitivity and resistance
Radiolabelled Precursor uptake (44)	Incorporation of [³H]-thymidene or [³H]-uridine into DNA	Short-term Assay: 1 d	Approx 80%	Few	None	None	?	?	?	Detection of resistance only
Radiolabelled Precursor uptake (10)	Incorporation of [³H]-thymidene or [³H]-uridine into DNA	Combination with HTCA: 7 d	Approx 80%	Few	None	None	?	?	?	Detects sensitivity and resistance
Fluorescent Copyright (45)	Hydrolysis of fluorescine-acetate	5–10 d	?	Few	None	None	?	?	?	Standardization difficult
Differential Staining Cytotoxicity Assay (46)	Dye exclusion	6 d	70–80%	Few	None	None	?	?	?	Mostly used in hematological neoplasias; less well studied in solid tumors
ATP-Cell Viability Assay (47)	Depletion of intracellular ATP	6–7 d	Approx 90%	Few	None	None	?	?	?	
MTT Assay (48)	Mitochondrial reduction of tetrazolium dye	3–5 d	80%–90%	Few	None	None	?	?	?	Mostly used with cell lines; feasibility with fresh tumors questionable; High costs, labor-intensive;
Subrenal Capsule Assay (49)	In vivo tumor size reduction	4–11 d	60%–80%	Few	None	None	?	?	?	
Nude Mouse Xenograft (50)	In vivo tumor size reduction	>4 wk	≤40%	None	None	None	?	?	?	High cost, labor-intensive;

[a]Evidence for a predictive value with regard to tumor response has been largely derived from retrospective correlations. Data from prospective or randomized studies, as well as data concerning the potential impact on patient survival, are preliminary and will need further verification in carefully designed clinical studies.

REFERENCES

1. Jemal A, Murray T, Samuels A, Ghafoor A, Ward E, Thun MJ. *CA Cancer J Clin* 2003; 53:5–26.
2. Von Hoff DD, Sandbach JF, Clark GM, Turner JN, Forseth BF, Piccart MJ, Colombo N, Muggia FM. Selection of cancer chemotherapy for a patient by an in vitro assay versus a clinician. *J Natl Cancer Inst* 1990; 82:110–116.
3. Perez E, Eckardt J, Hilsenbeck S, Rothenberg M, Degen D, Von Hoff DD. Activity of cytotoxic agents against non-small cell lung cancer specimens using a human tumor cloning assay. *Proc Am Assoc Cancer Res* 1994; 35:203.
4. Hamburger AW, Salmon SE. Primary bioassay of human tumor stem cells. *Science* 1977; 197:461–463.
5. Buick RN, Pollack MN. Perspectives on clonogenic tumor cells, stem cells, and oncogenes. *Cancer Res* 1984; 44:4909–4918.
6. Mackillop WJ, Ciampi A, Till JE, Buick RN. A stem cell model of human tumor growth: implications for tumor cell clonogenic assays. *J Natl Cancer Inst* 1983; 70:9–16.
7. Potten CS, Schofield R, Lajtha LG. A comparison of cell replacement in bone marrow, testis and three regions of surface epithelium. *Biochim Biophys Acta* 1979; 560:281–299.
8. Hamburger AW, Salmon SE. Primary bioassay of human myeloma stem cells. *J Clin Invest* 1977; 60:846–854.
9. Salmon SF, Hamburger AW, Soehnlen B, Durie BGM, Alberts DS, Moon TE. Quantitation if differential sensitivity of human tumor stem cells to anticancer drugs. *N Engl J Med* 1978; 298:1321–1327.
10. Tanigawa N, Kern DH, Hikasa Y, Morton DL. Rapid assay for evaluating the chemosensitivity of human tumors in soft agar culture. *Cancer Res* 1982; 42:2159–2164.
11. Von Hoff DD, Forseth BJ, Huong M, Buchok JB, Lathan B. Improved plating efficiencies for human tumors cloned in capillary tubes versus Petri dishes. *Cancer Res* 1986; 46:4012–4017.
12. Hanauske A-R, Hanauske U, Von Hoff DD. The human tumor cloning assay in cancer research and therapy. *Curr Probl Cancer* 1985; 9:1–50.
13. Kern DH, Weisenthal LM. Highly specific prediction of antineoplastic drug resistance with an in vitro assay using suprapharmacologic drug exposures. *J Natl Cancer Inst* 1990; 82:582–588.
14. Courtenay D, Selby PJ, Smith IE, Mills J, Peckham MJ. Growth of human tumour cell colonies from biopsies using two soft-agar techniques. *Br J Cancer* 1978; 38:77–81.
15. Maurer HR, Ali-Osman F. Tumor stem cell cloning in agar-containing capillaries. *Naturwissen Schaften* 1981; 68:381–383.
16. Lathan B, Kerkhoff K, Scheithauer W, Von Hoff DD, Diehl V. Homogeneous growth of tumor cell colonies in agar containing glass capillaries. *Anticancer Res* 1989; 9:1897–1902.
17. Hanauske U, Hanauske A-R, Marshall MH, Muggia VA, Von Hoff DD. Biphasic effects of vanadium salts on in vitro tumor colony growth. *Int J Cell Cloning* 1987; 5:170–178.
18. Von Hoff DD. He's not going to talk about in vitro predictive assays again, is he? *J Natl Cancer Inst* 1990; 82:96–101.
19. Osborne CK, Yochmowitz MG, Knight WA. The value of estrogen and progesterone receptors in the treatment of breast cancer. *Cancer* 1980; 46:2884–2888.
20. Von Hoff DD, Kronmal R, Salmon SE, Turner J, Green JB, Bonorris JS, Moorhead EL, Hynes HE, Pugh RE, Belt RJ, Alberts DS. A Southwest Oncology Group study on the use of a human tumor cloning assay for predicting response in patients with ovarian cancer. *Cancer* 1991; 67:20–27.
21. Von Hoff DD. In vitro predictive testing: the sulfonamide era. *Int J Cell Cloning* 1987; 5:179–190.
22. Weisenthal LM, Dill PL, Kurnick NB, Lippmann ME. Comparison of dye exclusion assays with a clonogenic assay in the determination of drug-induced cytotoxicity. *Cancer Res* 1983; 43:258–264.
23. Von Hoff DD. Human tumor cloning assays: applications in clinical oncology and new antineo-plastic agent development. *Cancer Metastasis Rev* 1988; 7:357–371.
24. Salmon SE, Meyskens PL Jr, Alberts DS, Soehnlen B, Young L. New drugs in ovarian cancer and malignant melanoma: in vitro phase II screening with the human tumor stem cell assay. *Cancer Treatment Rep* 1981; 65:1–12.
25. Neumann HA, Herrmann DB, Boerner D. Inhibition of human tumor colony formation by the new alkyl lysophospholipid ilmofosine. *J Natl Cancer Inst* 1987; 78:1087–1093.
26. Von Hoff DD, Clark GM, Weiss OR, Marshall MH, Buchok JB, Knight WA III, LeMaistre CF. Use of in vitro dose response effects to select antineoplastics for high-dose or regional administration regimens. *J Clin Oncol* 1986; 4:1827–1834.

27. Arteaga CL, Kisner DL, Goodman A, Von Hoff DD. Elliptinium, a DNA intercalating agent with broad antitumor activity in a human tumor cloning system. *Eur J Cancer Clin Oncol* 1987; 11:1621–1626.
28. Hanauske A-R, Degen D, Marshall MH, Hilsenbeck SG, McPhillips JJ, Von Hoff DD. Pre-clinical activity of ilmofosine against human tumor colony forming units in vitro. *Anti-Cancer Drugs* 1992; 3:43–46.
29. Hanauske A-R, Degen D, Marshall MM, Hilsenbeck SG, Grindey GB, Von Hoff DD. Activity of 2' ,2 '-difluorodeoxycytidine (Gemcitabine) against human tumor colony forming units. *Anti-Cancer Drugs* 1992; 3:143–146.
30. Hanauske A-R, Degen D, Hilsenbeck SG, Bissery MC, Von Hoff DD. Effects of taxotere and taxol on in vitro colony formation of freshly explanted human tumor cells. *Anti-Cancer Drugs* 1992; 3:121–124.
31. Hanauske A-R, Ross M, Degen D, Hilsenbeck SG, Von Hoff DD. In vitro activity of the benzotriazene dioxide SR 4233 against human tumour colony-forming units. *Eur J Cancer* 1993; 29A:423–425.
32. Marshall MV, Marshall MH, Degen DR, Roodman GD, Kuhn JG, Ross ME, Von Hoff DD. In vitro cytotoxicity of Hepsulfam against human tumor cell lines and primary human tumor colony forming units. *Stem Cells* 1993; 11:62–69.
33. Vogel M, Hilsenbeck SG, Depenbrock H, Danhauser-Riedl S, Block T, Nekarda H, Fellbaum C, Aapro MS, Bissery MC, Rastetter J, Hanauske A-R. Preclinical activity of Taxotere (RP56976, NSC 628503) against freshly explanted clonogenic human tumour cells: Comparison with Taxol and conventional antineoplastic agents. *Eur J Cancer* 1993; 29A:2009–2014.
34. Lathan B, Von Hoff DD, Clark GM. Comparison of in vitro prediction and clinical outcome for two anthracene derivatives: mitoxantrone and bisantrene. In: Salmon SE, Trent JM, eds. *Human Tumor Cloning.* New York: Gruñe & Stratton. 1984:607–619.
35. Lathan B, Von Hoff DD, Melink TJ, Kisner DL. Screening of Phase I drugs to pinpoint areas of emphasis in Phase II studies. In: Salmon SE, Trent JM, eds. *Human Tumor Cloning.* New York: Gruñe & Stratton. 1984:669.
36. Hamburger AW, Lurie KA, Condon ME. Stimulation of anchorage-independent growth of human tumor cells by interleukin 1. *Cancer Res* 1987; 47:5612–5615.
37. Joraschkewitz M, Depenbrock H, Freund M, Erdmann G, Meyer H-J, DeRiese W, Neukam DF, Hanauske U, Krumwieh M, Poliwoda H, Hanauske A-R. Effects of cytokines on in vitro colony formation of primary human tumour specimens. *Eur J Cancer* 1990; 26:1070–1074.
38. Hanauske A-R, Degen D, Marshall MH, Hilsenbeck SG, Banks P, Stuckey J, Leahy M, Von Hoff DD. Effects of recombinant human interleukin-la on clonogenic growth of primary human tumors in vitro. *J Immunother* 1992; 11:155–158.
39. Hanauske A-R, DeRiese W, Joraschekewitz M, Freund M, Poliwoda H. Effects of cytokines on clonogenic growth of primary renal cancer cells: An in vitro Phase II study. *Onkologie* 1992; 15:147–150.
40. Bauer E, Danhauser-Riedl S, DeRiese W, Raab H-R, Sandner S, Meyer H-J, Neukam D, Hanauske U, Freund M, Poliwoda H, Rastetter J, Hanauske A-R. Effects of recombinant human erythropoietin on clonogenic growth of primary human tumour specimens in vitro. *Eur J Cancer* 1992; 28A:1769.
41. Yanagawa E, Nishiyama M, Saeki T, Kim R, Jinushi K, Kirihara Y, Takagami S, Niimoto M, Hattori T. Chemosensitivity tests in colorectal cancer patients. *Jpn J Surg* 1989; 19:432–438.
42. Nishiyama M, Takagami S, Kirihara Y, Saeki T, Niimi K, Nosoh Y, Hirabayashi N, Niimoto M, Hattori T. The indications of chemosensitivity tests against various anticancer agents. *Jpn J Surg* 1988; 18:647–652.
43. Von Hoff DD. In vitro predictive testing: the sulfonamide era. *Int J Cell Cloning* 1987; 5:179–190.
44. Sanfilippo O, Silvestrini R, Zaffaroni N, Piva L, Pizzocaro G. Application of an in vitro anti-metabolic assay to human germ cell testicular tumors for the preclinical evaluation of drug sensitivity. *Cancer* 1986; 58:1441–1447.
45. Leone LA, Meitner PA, Myers TJ, Grace WR, Gajewski WH, Fingert HJ, Rotman B. Predictive value of the fluorescent cytoprint assay (FCA): A retrospective correlation study of in vitro chemosensitivity and individual responses to chemotherapy. *Cell Immunol* 1991; 8:1–13.
46. Weisenthal LM, Marsden JA, Dill PL, Macaluso CK. A novel dye exclusion method for testing in vitro chemosensitivity of human tumors. *Cancer Res* 1983; 43:749–757.
47. Koechli OR, Avner BP, Sevin B-U, Avner B, Perras JP, Robinson DS, Averette HE. Application of the adenosine triphosphate-cell viability assay in human breast cancer chemosensitivity testing: A report on the first results. *J Surg Oncol* 1993; 54:119–125.

48. Furukawa T, Kubota T, Suto A, Takahara T, Yamaguchi H, Takeuchi T, Kase S, Kodaira S, Ishibiki K, Kitajima M. Clinical usefulness of chemosensitivity testing using the MTT assay. *J Surg Oncol* 1991; 48:188–193.

49. Bodgen AE, Cobb WR, Lepage DJ, Haskell PM, Guitón TA, Ward A, Kelton DE, Esber HJ. Chemotherapy responsiveness of human tumors as first transplant generation xenografts in the normal mouse: Six-day subrenal capsule assay. *Cancer* 1981; 48:10–20.

50. Bellet RE, Danna V, Mastrangelo MJ, Berd D. Evaluation of a "nude" mouse-human tumor panel as a predictive secondary screen for cancer chemotherapy. *J Natl Cancer Inst* 1976; 63:1185–1188.

II   IN VIVO METHODS

5

Murine L1210 and P388 Leukemias

William R. Waud, PhD

CONTENTS

INTRODUCTION
ROLE IN DRUG SCREENING
CHARACTERISTICS
SENSITIVITY TO CLINICAL AGENTS
PREDICTIVE VALUE
DRUG-RESISTANT LEUKEMIAS
CONCLUSIONS

1. INTRODUCTION

L1210 and P388 leukemias were developed in 1948 *(1)* and 1955 *(2)*, respectively. Each leukemia played an important role in both screening and detailed evaluations of candidate anticancer agents. Fifty years later, these in vivo models are still used to evaluate anticancer activity, although at a greatly reduced level. This chapter reviews their past and present role in the evaluation of anticancer drugs. Data on the sensitivity to clinically useful drugs of these two leukemias and the drug-resistant P388 sublines are reported.

2. ROLE IN DRUG SCREENING

The use of murine leukemias in drug screening had its beginning in the 19th century *(3)*. It was at this time that studies of rodent tumors were being conducted that would pave the way for large-scale drug screening programs. Although spontaneous tumors in animals were used as models, it was the ability to transplant tumors that made possible the development of tumor systems that could be used both for large-scale screening and detailed evaluations of candidate anticancer agents. Furthermore, the development in the 1920s of inbred strains of mice allowed the successful transplantation of numerous tumor systems *(4)*.

By the 1940s, it was recognized that systemic cancer would respond to drug treatment. As a result, drug discovery programs were begun at several institutions in the United States and abroad. Soon anticancer drug screening programs were initiated, one of which

From: *Cancer Drug Discovery and Development:*
Anticancer Drug Development Guide: Preclinical Screening, Clinical Trials, and Approval, 2nd Ed.
Edited by: B. A. Teicher and P. A. Andrews © Humana Press Inc., Totowa, NJ

was the Memorial Sloan-Kettering program that used the mouse sarcoma 180 (SA-180) as its screening model. Since additional drugs exhibited some anticancer activity and the supply of new candidate agents exceeded the screening capacity, the need for a national drug development program became apparent. In 1954, Congress directed the National Cancer Institute (NCI) to start such a program, and in 1955, the Cancer Chemotherapy National Service Center (CCNSC) was created.

The initial CCNSC screen consisted of three mouse tumors: L1210 leukemia, SA-180, and mammary adenocarcinoma 755 (5). Over the years, the primary screen changed from the original three tumors to L1210 plus two arbitrarily selected tumors to L1210 plus Walker 256 carcinosarcoma to L1210 plus the P388 leukemia to L1210 plus P388 plus B16 melanoma or Lewis lung tumor (6). Secondary evaluations of the most promising agents were conducted in a variety of other tumor models.

In 1976, a major change occurred in the NCI primary screen. The new screen consisted of a panel of colon, breast, and lung tumor models (murine and human); however, drugs were initially screened in P388 leukemia (7).

The low number of drugs with marked activity against human solid tumors led to a radical change in the screening program that had used murine leukemia models. In the mid-1980s, the NCI developed a new screen based on the use of established human tumor cell lines in vitro (8). The two screening systems were to be conducted in parallel so as to permit a comparison; however, in early 1987, budget cuts forced an end to large-scale P388 screening (9).

3. CHARACTERISTICS

L1210 and P388 leukemias were both chemically induced in a DBA/2 mouse by painting the skin with methylcholanthrene (1,2). The leukemias are propagated in DBA/2 mice by implanting ip 0.1 mL of a diluted ascitic fluid containing either 10^5 (L1210) or 10^6 (P388) cells. Testing is conducted in a hybrid of DBA/2 (e.g., $CD2F_1$ or $B6D2F_1$). Implant sites that are frequently used are ip, iv, or ic. For L1210 leukemia (10^5 cells), the median days of death and the tumor doubling times for these implant sites are 8.8, 9.9, 6.4, and 7.0 and 0.34, 0.46, 0.45, and 0.37 d, respectively. For P388 leukemia (10^6 cells), the median days of death and the tumor doubling times for these implant sites are 10.3, 13.0, 8.0, and 8.0 and 0.44, 0.52, 0.68, and 0.63 d, respectively.

Studies on the rate of distribution and proliferation of L1210 leukemia cells were conducted at Southern Research by Skipper and coworkers (10) using bioassays of untreated mice after ip, iv, and ic inoculation. After ip inoculation, most of the L1210 cells were found in the ascites fluid of the peritoneal cavity. On the median day of death from the leukemia, the most infiltrated tissues were the bone marrow, liver, and spleen. After iv inoculation, most of the L1210 cells were filtered out in the bone marrow. On the median day of death from the leukemia, the most infiltrated tissues were also the bone marrow, liver, and spleen. After ic inoculation, most of the L1210 cells remained in the brain (for 3–5 d). On the median day of death from the leukemia, the spleen was heavily infiltrated. (The extent of the leukemia in other tissues was not reported.)

At Southern Research, antitumor activity is assessed on the basis of percent median increase in life span (% ILS), net $\log_{10}$ cell kill, and long-term survivors. Calculations of net $\log_{10}$ cell kill are made from the tumor doubling time, which is determined from an internal tumor titration consisting of implants from serial 10-fold dilutions *(11)*. Long-term survivors are excluded from calculations of % ILS and tumor cell kill. To assess tumor cell kill at the end of treatment, the survival time difference between treated and control groups is adjusted to account for regrowth of tumor cell populations that may occur between individual treatments *(12)*. The net $\log_{10}$ cell kill is calculated as follows:

$$\text{Net } \log_{10} \text{ cell kill} = [(T - C) - (\text{duration of treatment in days})]/3.32 \times T_d$$

where $(T - C)$ is the difference in the median day of death between the treated (T) and the control (C) groups, 3.32 is the number of doublings required for a population to increase 1 $\log_{10}$ unit, and T_d is the mean tumor doubling time (in days) calculated from a log-linear least-squares fit of the implant sizes and the median days of death of the titration groups.

4. SENSITIVITY TO CLINICAL AGENTS

The sensitivities of L1210 and P388 leukemias to most of the clinically useful agents are shown in Figs. 1 and 2 and Figs. 3 and 4, respectively. Overall, P388 leukemia is more sensitive than is L1210 leukemia. For alkylating agents, the sensitivities are similar. Notable exceptions are chlorambucil, mitomycin C, and carboplatin, for which P388 is markedly more sensitive. For antimetabolites, the sensitivities are also similar. Exceptions are floxuridine (P388 being markedly more sensitive) and hydroxyurea (L1210 being markedly more sensitive). For DNA-binding agents, P388 leukemia is clearly more sensitive (e.g., actinomycin D, mithramycin, daunorubicin, teniposide, doxorubicin, and amsacrine). For tubulin-binding agents, P388 leukemia is again clearly more sensitive. The vinca alkaloids are active against P388 leukemia but ineffective against L1210 leukemia.

Although most of the sensitivity data are for ip implanted leukemia and ip administered drugs, valuable information can be obtained from separating the implant site and the route of administration. Table 1 shows the activity of melphalan, administered ip, against both L1210 and P388 leukemias implanted ip, iv, and ic. The use of ip melphalan is highly effective against both ip implanted leukemias. The activity is reduced to less than one-half when the implant site is changed to iv. The activity is further reduced when the implant site is changed to ic; however, melphalan can cross the blood-brain barrier to some extent. This principle is illustrated more fully with the data in Figs. 5 (L1210) and 6 (P388) for the leukemias implanted ic and various clinically useful agents administered ip. Thiotepa, CCNU, BCNU, and 1-β-D-arabinofuranosylcytosine (ara-C)/palmO-ara-C, administered ip, exhibit comparable activity against either ip or ic implanted leukemias. Cisplatin, cyclophosphamide, ifosfamide, and 6-mercaptopurine (L1210), in addition to melphalan, have reduced activity when the implant site is changed to ic. Several agents become inactive when the implant site is changed to ic (e.g., methotrexate [P388], 5-fluorouracil, floxuridine, actinomycin D, vincristine, doxorubicin, and etoposide).

Some comparisons using different treatment schedules can be misleading. Even though all values have been expressed as net cell kill (i.e., corrected for the treatment schedule), one schedule can be optimal, whereas another schedule is suboptimal. For nitrogen mustard, no conclusion can be drawn from the data about its ability to cross the blood-brain barrier. The agent is active against the ip implanted leukemia using a single ip

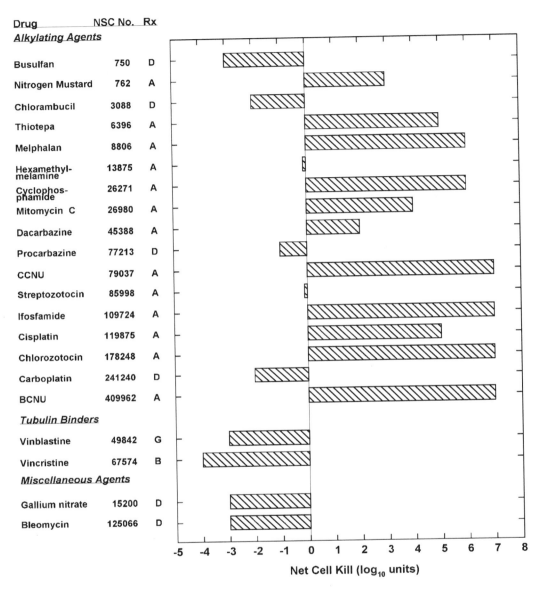

Fig. 1. Sensitivity of ip implanted L1210 leukemia to clinically useful alkylating agents, tubulin binders, and other miscellaneous agents. L1210 leukemia (10^5 cells except for hexamethylmelamine, which used 10^6 cells) was implanted ip on d 0. Beginning on d 1, the agents were administered ip using the indicated schedules. Treatment schedule (R_x): A, d 1; B, d 1, 5, 9; C, d 1–5; D, d 1–9; E, d 1, 4, 7, 10; F, q3h x 8, d 1, 5, 9; G, d 1–15.

injection (optimal) and is inactive against the ic implanted leukemia using 15 daily ip injections (suboptimal). This is further illustrated by chlorambucil, which is active against ic implanted L1210 (using a single ip injection) and inactive against ip implanted L1210 (using nine daily ip injections).

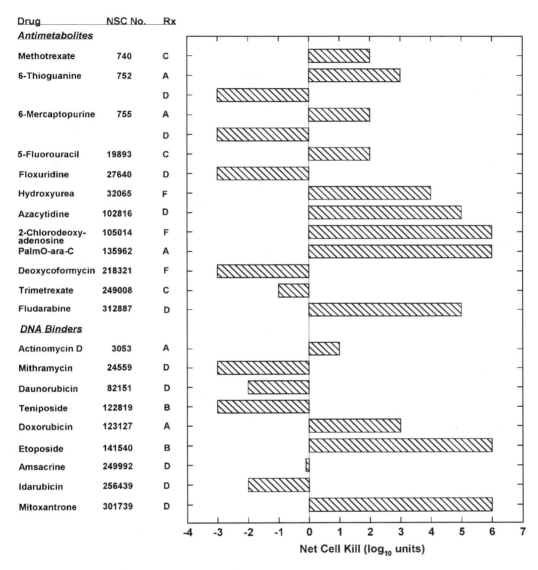

Drug	NSC No.	Rx
Antimetabolites		
Methotrexate	740	C
6-Thioguanine	752	A
		D
6-Mercaptopurine	755	A
		D
5-Fluorouracil	19893	C
Floxuridine	27640	D
Hydroxyurea	32065	F
Azacytidine	102816	D
2-Chlorodeoxy-adenosine	105014	F
PalmO-ara-C	135962	A
Deoxycoformycin	218321	F
Trimetrexate	249008	C
Fludarabine	312887	D
DNA Binders		
Actinomycin D	3053	A
Mithramycin	24559	D
Daunorubicin	82151	D
Teniposide	122819	B
Doxorubicin	123127	A
Etoposide	141540	B
Amsacrine	249992	D
Idarubicin	256439	D
Mitoxantrone	301739	D

Net Cell Kill ($\log_{10}$ units)

Fig. 2. Sensitivity of ip implanted L1210 leukemia to clinically useful antimetabolites and DNA binders. L1210 leukemia (10^5 cells, except for hydroxyurea, which used 10^4 cells and 6-thioguanine [d 1 only treatment] and daunorubicin, which used 10^6 cells) was implanted ip on d 0. Beginning on d 1 (d 2 for daunorubicin), the agents were administered ip using the indicated schedules. Treatment schedule (R_x): *see* legend for Fig. 1.

Studies with these screening models revealed that drug sensitivity was, in some cases, heavily dependent on drug concentration and exposure time, which in turn was impacted by the in vivo treatment schedule. As an example, studies conducted with ara-C pointed out the need for concentration and time of exposure studies. With L1210 leukemia in mice, it was shown that the optimal dosage and schedule for ara-C was 15–20 mg/kg/dose, given every 3 h for eight doses, and then repeated three times at 4-d intervals *(13)*.

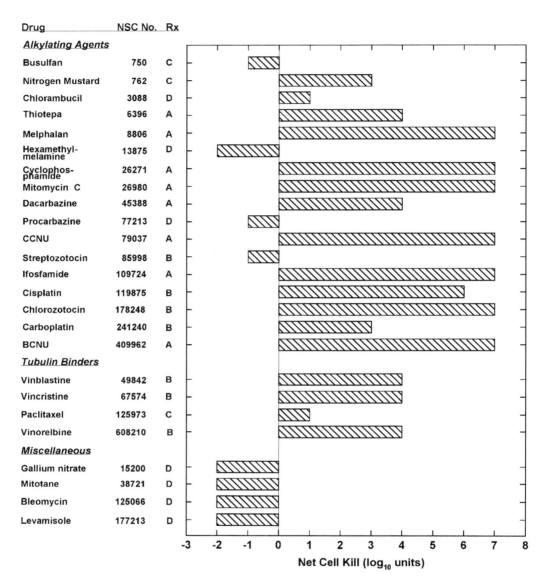

Fig. 3. Sensitivity of ip implanted P388 leukemia to clinically useful alkylating agents, tubulin binders, and other miscellaneous agents. P388 leukemia (10^6 cells except for CCNU, which used 10^7 cells) was implanted ip on d 0. Beginning on d 1 (d 2 for CCNU, streptozotocin, and chlorozotocin), the agents were administered ip using the indicated schedules. Treatment schedule (R_x): *see* legend for Fig. 1.

This regimen was curative. The single lethal dose for 10% of test subjects (LD_{10}) for mice was between 2500 and 3000 mg/kg, and using a single dose within that range would effect a 3-log_{10}-unit reduction in L1210 cells but was not curative. Although these in vivo results might give the appearance of a concentration-dependent effect, in vitro studies have clearly shown that cell kill of L1210 in culture was time-dependent at the higher concentration levels employed. The apparent concentration dependence observed in vivo

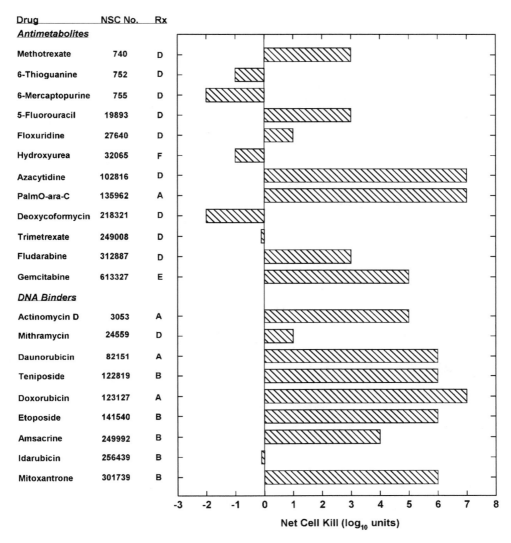

Fig. 4. Sensitivity of ip implanted P388 leukemia to clinically useful antimetabolites and DNA binders. P388 leukemia (10^6 cells) was implanted ip on d 0. Beginning on d 1, the agents were administered ip using the indicated schedules. Treatment schedule (R_x): *see* legend for Fig. 1.

Table 1
Activity of Melphalan Administered As a Single ip Injection
Against L1210 and P388 Leukemias Implanted ip, iv, and ic

		Net cell kill (log_{10} units)	
Site	*Inoculum size*	*L1210*	*P388*
ip	10^6	4.7	>6.5
iv	10^6	2.0	2.9
ic	10^4	1.2	2.4

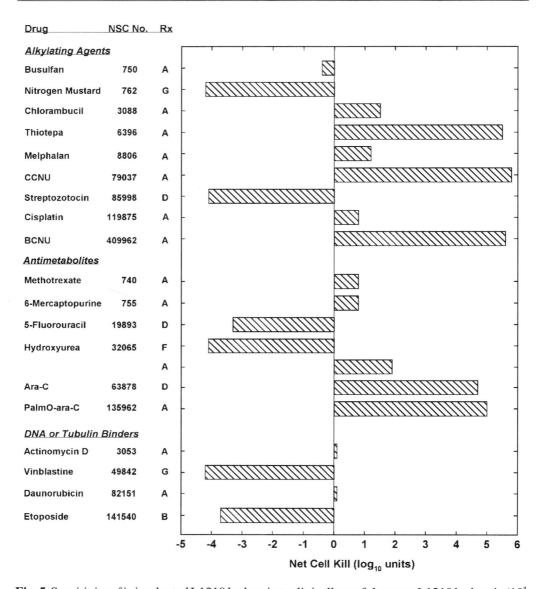

Fig. 5. Sensitivity of ic implanted L1210 leukemia to clinically useful agents. L1210 leukemia (10^4 cells except for CCNU, which used 10^5 cells) was implanted ic on d 0. Beginning on d 1 (d 2 for busulfan, chlorambucil, thiotepa, melphalan, hydroxyurea [single injection], cisplatin, BCNU, and daunorubicin), the agents were administered ip using the indicated schedules. Treatment schedule (R_x): *see* legend for Fig. 1.

over a range of single doses resulted from the extended time of exposure of those extremely high dosage levels.

5. PREDICTIVE VALUE

An argument has been made for years against the use of experimental leukemias as primary screening models. Since L1210 or P388 leukemia was used for many years as the

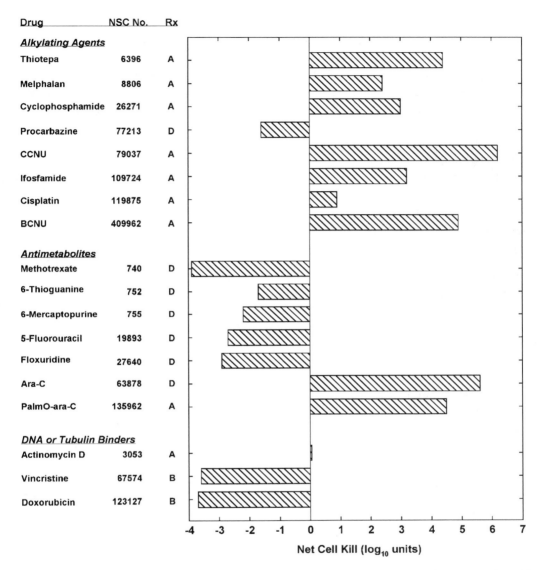

Fig. 6. Sensitivity of ic implanted P388 leukemia to clinically useful agents. P388 leukemia (10^4 cells except for ifosfamide, methotrexate, 6-thioguanine, 6-mercaptopurine, 5-fluorouracil, and floxuridine, which used 10^3 cells and CCNU and ara-C, which used 10^5 cells) was implanted ic on d 0. Beginning on d 1 (d 2 for ifosfamide), the agents were administered ip using the indicated schedules. Treatment schedule (R_x): *see* legend for Fig. 1.

initial screening model, it has been argued that no further evaluation of compounds emerging from the screen, even using solid tumor models, would detect anything but an antileukemic drug *(14)*. It would appear reasonable that in order to obtain agents that are active against specific tumor types or solid tumors in general, then the primary screen should consist of specific tumor types or solid tumors. However reasonable, such an approach depends on the hope that agents exist or can be developed that will selectively kill specific cancer histotypes.

A point often made is that many drugs are active against L1210 or P388 leukemia but inactive against experimental solid tumors. Of 1493 agents that were active against P388 leukemia, only 1.7% were active against murine Lewis lung carcinoma. Of 1507 agents that were active against P388 leukemia, only 2% were active against murine colon 38 adenocarcinoma. Finally, of 1133 agents that were active against P388 leukemia, only 2% were active against human CX-1 (HT29) colon tumor. Interestingly, of 1564 agents that were active against P388 leukemia, only 15% were active against L1210 leukemia (15).

Another point often made is that certain drugs are active against experimental solid tumors but inactive against P388 leukemia. Of 84 agents that were inactive against P388 leukemia, 15% were active against at least one of eight solid tumors tested (15). Flavone acetic acid has been cited as an example (14). The agent was inactive in the initial P388 screen; however, it exhibited activity against the leukemia when the appropriate treatment schedule was used (16). This example points out a weakness of large-scale screening—an appropriate treatment schedule may not be used.

Finally, the point is also made that certain experimental solid tumors (e.g., murine pancreatic 02 ductal adenocarcinoma) are not responsive in vivo to any clinically used agents, including many P388-active agents (14). However, pancreatic 02 adenocarcinoma is sensitive to numerous clinical agents in vitro after a 24-h exposure (17), suggesting that the in vivo insensitivity of this tumor is not owing to cellular characteristics but instead may be caused by some characteristic(s) of the tumor in the animal.

Recently, Southern Research evaluated a spectrum of compounds in the ip implanted P388 model in order to evaluate this model as a predictor for the response of human tumor xenografts to new candidate antitumor agents (unpublished results). The P388 data collected were compared with the data for various sc implanted human tumor xenografts, which were selected on the basis of the results of the NCI in vitro screen. In general, compounds that were active against P388 leukemia were active to a lesser degree in one or more of the xenografts in the in vivo tumor panel. However, there were isolated examples of a P388-active agent being inactive in the human tumor xenograft models tested and vice versa. There was no indication that the P388 model could predict compound efficacy for specific tumor xenografts.

Is P388 leukemia (or L1210) a poor predictor for solid tumor-active drugs? The question will be answered only when drugs without P388 activity but of proven value in the treatment of human solid tumors become available.

6. DRUG-RESISTANT LEUKEMIAS

At Southern Research, series of in vivo drug-resistant murine L1210 and P388 leukemias have been developed for use in the evaluation of crossresistance and collateral sensitivity. These in vivo models have been used for the evaluation of new drugs of potential clinical interest. Schabel and coworkers (18) have published the most extensive summary of in vivo drug resistance and crossresistance data available. Their initial report included results of in vivo crossresistance studies on 79 antitumor drugs in 7 drug-resistant L1210 leukemias and 74 antitumor drugs in 12 drug-resistant P388 leukemias. Previously, we expanded this crossresistance database for the drug-resistant P388 leukemias to include two new drug-resistant leukemias and more clinically useful drugs, and we updated the database to include new candidate antitumor agents entering clinical trials (19). Recently, three additional drug-resistant P388 leukemias were added to this database *(20)*. In this section, we report on this crossresistance database for 16 drug-resistant P388 leukemias and many of the clinically useful agents.

6.1. Resistance to Alkylating Agents

The crossresistance profile of cyclophosphamide-resistant P388 leukemia (P388/CPA) to 14 different clinical agents is shown in Table 2. The P388/CPA line was crossresistant[1] to one (mitomycin C) of the five alkylating agents, no antimetabolites, no DNA-binding agents, and no tubulin-binding agents. Crossresistance of P388/CPA has also been observed for two other alkylating agents (chlorambucil and ifosfamide) *(20)*. Interestingly, there are differences among these three agents. Chlorambucil and ifosfamide, like cyclophosphamide, each have two chloroethylating moieties, whereas mitomycin C is from a different chemical class. Ifosfamide, cyclophosphamide, and mitomycin C require metabolic activation, and chlorambucil does not. Although P388/CPA is crossresistant to two chloroethylating agents, the line is not crossresistant to other chloroethylating agents (melphalan and BCNU). Therefore, P388/CPA appears to be crossresistant only to a select group of alkylating agents with differing characteristics. P388/CPA appears to be collaterally sensitive to fludarabine.

The effect of 15 different clinical agents on melphalan-resistant P388 leukemia (P388/L-PAM) is shown in Table 2. The P388/L-PAM line was crossresistant to approx one-half of the agents—two of four alkylating agents, one of four antimetabolites, three of five DNA-binding agents, and one of two tubulin-binding agents. The alkylating agents involved in crossresistance represent different chemical classes. Similarly, the DNA-interacting agents involved in crossresistance include agents with different mechanisms of action—inhibitors of DNA topoisomerase II (amsacrine and mitoxantrone) and a DNA-binding agent (actinomycin D). However, the melphalan-resistant line did not exhibit crossresistance to other inhibitors of DNA topoisomerase II (e.g., doxorubicin and etoposide) or another DNA-binding agent (e.g., doxorubicin).

The sensitivity of cisplatin-resistant P388 leukemia (P388/DDPt) to 17 different clinical agents is shown in Table 2. The P388/DDPt line was not crossresistant to any of these agents. Interestingly, the cisplatin-resistant line was collaterally sensitive to three agents (fludarabine, amsacrine, and mitoxantrone). Of these three agents, the latter two have been reported to interact with DNA topoisomerase II *(21,22)*.

The crossresistance data for N,N'-*bis*(2-chloroethyl)-*N*-nitrosourea-resistant P388 leukemia (P388/BCNU) have been limited to the evaluation of alkylating agents. The crossresistance profile of P388/BCNU to four different clinical agents is shown in Table 2. The BCNU-resistant line was not crossresistant to melphalan, cyclophosphamide, mitomycin C, or cisplatin.

The crossresistance profile of mitomycin C-resistant P388 leukemia (P388/MMC) to 13 different clinical agents is shown in Table 2 *(23)*. The P388/MMC line was crossresistant to approx one-half of the agents—one of three alkylating agents, none of

---

[1]Crossresistance is defined as decreased sensitivity (by >2-$\log_{10}$ units of cell kill) of a drug-resistant P388 leukemia to a drug compared with that observed concurrently in P388/0 leukemia. Similarly, marginal crossresistance is defined as a decrease in sensitivity of approx 2-$\log_{10}$ units. Collateral sensitivity is defined as increased sensitivity (by >2-$\log_{10}$ units of cell kill) of a drug-resistant P388 leukemia to a drug over that observed concurrently in P388/0 leukemia.

Table 2
Crossresistance of P388 Sublines Resistant to Various Alkylating Agents and Antimetabolites to Clinically Useful Agents[a]

Drug	NSC no.	Rx[b]	CPA	L-PAM	DDPt	BCNU	MMC[c]	MTX	5-FU	ARA-C
Alkylating agents										
Melphalan	8806	A	–	+	–	–				±
Cyclophosphamide	26271	A	+	–	–	–	–			+
Mitomycin C	26980	A	±	+	–	–	+	–		+
Procarbazine	77213	D	–			–				
Cisplatin	119875	B	–	+	+	–	±[d]	–		+
BCNU	409962	A	–	–	–	+	–	–		–
Antimetabolites										
Methotrexate	740	D			–		–[e]	+	+	+
6-Thioguanine	752	A					–[e]	–		
6-Mercaptopurine	755	D						–		
5-Fluorouracil	19893	D	–		–		–[e]	–	+	=
PalmO-ara-C	135962	A	–	–	–		–[e]	–	–	+
Trimetrexate	249008	D	–	±	–			–		–
Fludarabine	312887	D	=	=	=			–	=	+
Gemcitabine	613327	E	–	–	–			–		+

DNA binders

	NSC	R_x				
Actinomycin D	3053	A	±	–	±	–
Doxorubicin	123127	A	+	–	–	–
Etoposide	141540	B	+[d]	–	–	–
Amsacrine	249992	B	–[d]	=	+	–
Mitoxantrone	301739	B		=	+	–
Tubulin binders						
Vinblastine	49842	A	+		+	–
Vincristine	67574	B	+[d]	+	+	+
Paclitaxel	125973	C		–	–	–

ABBREVIATIONS: ARA-C, 1-β-D-arabinofuranosylcytosine; BCNU, N,N'-*bis*(2-chloroethyl)-*N*-nitrosourea; CPA, cyclophosphamide; DDPt, cisplatin; 5-FU, 5-fluorouracil; L-PAM, melphalan; MMC, mitomycin C; MTX, methotrexate; NSC, National Service Center.

[a]$CD2F_1$ mice were implanted ip with 10^6 P388/0 or drug-resistant P388 cells on d 0. Data presented are for ip drug treatment at an optimal (≤LD_{10}) dosage. Symbols: resistance/crossresistance, +; marginal crossresistance, ±; no crossresistance, –; and collateral sensitivity, =.

[b]Treatment schedule (R_x): A, d 1; B, d 1, 5, 9; C, d 1–5; D, d 1–9; E, d 1, 4, 7, 10.

[c]Data from ref. 23.

[d]Treatment schedule was d 1.

[e]Treatment schedule was d 1 and 5.

four antimetabolites, three of four DNA-binding agents, and two of two tubulin-binding agents. The pattern was similar to that observed for P388/L-PAM.

6.2. Resistance to Antimetabolites

The effect of 14 different clinical agents on methotrexate-resistant P388 leukemia (P388/MTX) is shown in Table 2. The P388/MTX line was not crossresistant to any of these agents.

The crossresistance data for 5-fluorouracil-resistant P388 leukemia (P388/5-FU) have been limited to antimetabolites. The sensitivity of the P388/5-FU line to three different agents is shown in Table 2. The P388/5-FU line was not crossresistant to palmO-ara-C (a slow-releasing form of ara-C) or fludarabine (possible collateral sensitivity). Crossresistance was observed for methotrexate.

The crossresistance profile of ara-C-resistant P388 leukemia (P388/ARA-C) to 16 different clinical agents is shown in Table 2. The P388/ARA-C line was crossresistant to members of several functionally different classes of antitumor agents—four of five alkylating agents, three of five antimetabolites, none of four DNA-binding agents, and one of two tubulin-binding agents. Interestingly, the line was collaterally sensitive to 5-fluorouracil.

6.3. Resistance to DNA- and Tubulin-Binding Agents

The effect of 17 different clinical agents on actinomycin D-resistant P388 leukemia (P388/ACT-D) is shown in Table 3. P388/ACT-D was not crossresistant to any alkylating agents or antimetabolites. It was, however, crossresistant to all the drugs tested that are involved in multidrug resistance, except for amsacrine.

The crossresistance profile of doxorubicin-resistant P388 leukemia (P388/ADR) to 21 different clinical agents is shown in Table 3. The P388/ADR line was not crossresistant to any of the antimetabolites and was marginally crossresistant to only one alkylating agent (mitomycin C). Resistance was observed for all the drugs tested that are reported to be involved in multidrug resistance (actinomycin D, doxorubicin, etoposide, amsacrine, mitoxantrone, vinblastine, vincristine, and paclitaxel). P388/ADR was collaterally sensitive to fludarabine.

The sensitivity of amsacrine-resistant P388 leukemia (P388/AMSA) to 14 different clinical agents is shown in Table 3. P388/AMSA was not crossresistant to any of the alkylating agents and was marginally crossresistant to only one antimetabolite. Crossresistance was observed for all the drugs tested that are involved in multidrug resistance.

The crossresistance data for mitoxantrone-resistant P388 leukemia (P388/DIOHA) have been limited mainly to agents involved in multidrug resistance. The sensitivity of P388/DIOHA to seven different clinical agents is shown in Table 3. The P388/DIOHA line exhibited mixed multidrug resistance—crossresistance to amsacrine and vincristine but no crossresistance to actinomycin D, doxorubicin, etoposide, or paclitaxel.

The crossresistance profile of etoposide-resistant P388 leukemia (P388/VP-16) to 13 different clinical agents is shown in Table 3. The P388/VP-16 line was not crossresistant to any of the alkylating agents or antimetabolites; however, it was crossresistant to all the drugs tested that are reported to be involved in multidrug resistance.

The sensitivity of camptothecin-resistant P388 leukemia (P388/CPT) to seven different clinical agents is shown in Table 3 *(24)*. P388/CPT was not crossresistant to any of these agents.

The effect of 21 different clinical agents on vincristine-resistant P388 leukemia (P388/VCR) is shown in Table 3. The P388/VCR line was crossresistant to three of the agents—mitomycin C, cisplatin (marginal), and vinblastine. Unexpectedly, P388/VCR was not crossresistant to many of the drugs tested that are involved in multidrug resistance (e.g., actinomycin D, doxorubicin, etoposide, amsacrine, mitoxantrone, and paclitaxel).

The crossresistance data for paclitaxel-resistant P388 leukemia (P388/PTX) have been limited to agents involved in multidrug resistance. The sensitivity of P388/PTX to three different clinical agents is shown in Table 3. The P388/PTX line was crossresistant to drugs that are involved in multidrug resistance (doxorubicin, etoposide, and vincristine).

7. CONCLUSIONS

L1210 and P388 leukemia models have been extensively used over the last 50 yr. The models are rapid, reproducible, and relatively inexpensive (in comparison with human tumor xenograft models). However, as with any experimental animal tumor model, there are limitations. Neither leukemia is a satisfactory model for either human cancer in general or human leukemia in particular. (Of course this could be said of any animal tumor model.) P388, the more sensitive of the two leukemias, overpredicts the activity in both preclinical human tumor xenograft models and in the clinic. However, the question of whether P388 leukemia (or L1210) is a poor predictor for solid tumor-active drugs has yet to be sufficiently answered.

Despite the limitations of the murine leukemia models, these models have been useful in making progress in anticancer drug development, in the development of a number of therapeutic principles, and in understanding the biological behavior of tumor and host. These models are still useful today for conducting detailed evaluations of new candidate anticancer drugs (e.g., schedule dependency, route of administration dependency, formulation comparison, analog comparison, and combination chemotherapy).

The greatest utility of the murine leukemias today is derived from evaluations of the drug-resistant sublines for crossresistance and collateral sensitivity. Analysis of the crossresistance data generated at Southern Research for clinical agents has revealed possible non-crossresistant drug combinations. P388 leukemia lines selected for resistance to alkylating agents (e.g., P388/CPA, P388/L-PAM, P388/DDPt, P388/BCNU, and P388/MMC) differed in their crossresistance profiles, with respect to both alkylating agents and other functional classes. Similarly, P388 leukemia lines selected for resistance to antimetabolites (e.g., P388/MTX, P388/5-FU, and P388/ARA-C) differed in their crossresistance profiles, with respect to both antimetabolites and other functional classes. Clearly, the spectrum of crossresistance of an alkylating agent or an antimetabolite will depend on the individual agent. P388 leukemia lines selected for resistance to large polycyclic anticancer drugs (e.g., P388/ACT-D, P388/ADR, P388/AMSA, P388/DIOHA, P388/VP-16, P388/CPT, P388/VCR, and P388/PTX) were not generally crossresistant to alkylating agents or antimetabolites. However, the crossresistance profiles to DNA- and tubulin-binding agents were variable.

Table 3
Crossresistance of P388 Sublines Resistant to Various DNA and Tubulin Binders to Clinically Useful Agents[a]

Drug	NSC no.	R_x[b]	ACT-D	ADR	AMSA	DIOHA	VP-16	CPT[c]	VCR	PTX
Alkylating agents										
Melphalan	8806	A	–	–	–		–		–	
Cyclophosphamide	26271	A	–	–	–	–	–		–	
Mitomycin C	26980	A	±	±	–			–[f]	+	
Procarbazine	77213	D	–	–					–	
Cisplatin	119875	C	–	–	–[d]		–[d]	–[f]	±[f]	
BCNU	409962	A	–	–			–		–	
Antimetabolites										
Methotrexate	740	D	–	–	±				–	
6-Thioguanine	752	D	–	–					–	
6-Mercaptopurine	755	D	–	–[e]					–	
5-Fluorouracil	19893	D	–	–[e]	–[e]		–[d]		–	
PalmO-ara-C	135962	A	–	–	–				–	
Trimetrexate	249008	D		–					–	
Fludarabine	312887	D		=					–	
Gemcitabine	613327	E		–			–		–	

DNA binders

	NSC	R_x							
Actinomycin D	3053	A	+	+	−	+	−[f]	+	−
Doxorubicin	123127	A	±	+	−	+	−[f]	+	−
Etoposide	141540	B	+	+	−	+	−[f]	+	−
Amsacrine	249992	B	−	+	+	+	−[f]	+	−
Mitoxantrone	301739	B	+	+	+	+	−[f]	+	−
Tubulin binders									
Vinblastine	49842	B	+	+		+		+	+
Vincristine	67574	B	+	+	+	+	−[f]	+	+
Paclitaxel	125973	C	±	±	−		−[f]		+

ABBREVIATIONS: ACT-D, actinomycin D; ADR, doxorubicin; AMSA, amsacrine; CPT, camptothecin; DIOHA, mitoxantrone; NSC, National Service Center; PTX, paclitaxel; VCR, vincristine; VP-16, etoposide.

[a] $CD2F_1$ mice were implanted ip with 10^6 P388/0 or drug-resistant P388 cells on d 0. Data presented are for ip drug treatment at an optimal ($\leq LD_{10}$) dosage. Symbols: resistance/crossresistance, +; marginal crossresistance, ±; no crossresistance, −; and collateral sensitivity, =.

[b] Treatment schedule (R_x): A, d 1; B, d 1, 5, 9; C, d 1–5; D, d 1–9; E, d 1, 4, 7, 10.

[c] Data from ref. 24.

[d] Treatment schedule was d 1, 5, 9.

[e] Treatment schedule was d 1–5.

[f] Treatment schedule was d 1 and 5.

Five of the 16 drug-resistant leukemias exhibited collateral sensitivity to one or more drugs. These observations of collateral sensitivity suggest that a combination of one of the five drugs plus one of the corresponding agents for which collateral sensitivity was observed might exhibit therapeutic synergism.

Crossresistance data, coupled with knowledge of the mechanisms of resistance operative in the drug-resistant leukemias, may yield insights into the mechanisms of action of the agents being tested. Similarly, crossresistance data, coupled with the mechanisms of action of various agents, may yield insights into the mechanisms of resistance operative in the drug-resistant leukemias (19). Furthermore, crossresistance data may identify potentially useful guides for patient selection for clinical trials of new antitumor drugs (19).

In conclusion, the role of L1210 and P388 leukemias in the evaluation of anticancer agents has diminished considerably. However, the models are still appropriate for answering certain questions, and the drug-resistant sublines can provide valuable information concerning crossresistance and collateral sensitivity.

ACKNOWLEDGMENTS

Most of this work was supported by contracts with the Developmental Therapeutics Program, Division of Cancer Treatment and Diagnosis, NCI. The studies of gemcitabine and P388/VP-16 leukemia were supported by Eli Lilly and Company and by Burroughs Wellcome Company, respectively. The author gratefully acknowledges the technical assistance of the staff of the Cancer Therapeutics and Immunology Department, Southern Research Institute. J. Tubbs assisted with data management, and K. Cornelius prepared the manuscript.

REFERENCES

1. Law LW, Dunn DB, Boyle PJ, Miller JH. Observations on the effect of a folic-acid antagonist on transplantable lymphoid leukemias in mice. *J Natl Cancer Inst* 1949; 10:179–192.
2. Dawe CJ, Potter M. Morphologic and biologic progression of a lymphoid neoplasm of the mouse in vivo and in vitro. *Am J Pathol* 1957; 33:603.
3. Griswold DP Jr, Harrison SD Jr. Tumor models in drug development. *Cancer Metastasis Rev* 1991; 10:255–261.
4. Zubrod CG. Historic milestone in curative chemotherapy. *Semin Oncol* 1979; 6:490–505.
5. Goldin A, Serpick AA, Mantel N. A commentary, experimental screening procedures and clinical predictability value. *Cancer Chemother Rep* 1966; 50:173–218.
6. Carter S. Anticancer drug development progress: A comparison of approaches in the United States, the Soviet Union, Japan, and Western Europe. *Natl Cancer Inst Monogr* 1974; 40:31–42.
7. Goldin A, Venditti JM, Muggia FM, Rozencweig M, DeVita VT. New animal models in cancer chemotherapy. In: Fox BW, ed., *Advances in Medical Oncology, Research and Education*, vol 5. *Basis for Cancer Therapy 1*. New York: Pergamon Press. 1979:113–122.
8. Alley MC, Scudiero DA, Monks A, et al. Feasibility of drug screening with panels of human tumor cell lines using a microculture tetrazolium assay. *Cancer Res* 1988; 48:589–601.
9. Budget cuts to force early end of P388 screening, DTP's Boyd says. *Cancer Lett* 1987; 13:5–7.
10. Skipper HE, Schabel FM Jr, Wilcox WS, Laster WR Jr, Trader MW, Thompson SA. Experimental evaluation of potential anticancer agents. XVII. Effects of therapy on viability and rate of proliferation of leukemic cells in various anatomic sites. *Cancer Chemother Rep* 1965; 47:41–64.
11. Schabel FM Jr, Griswold DP Jr, Laster WR Jr, Corbett TH, Lloyd HH. Quantitative evaluation of anticancer agent activity in experimental animals. *Pharmacol Ther* 1977; 1:411–435.
12. Lloyd HH. Application of tumor models toward the design of treatment schedules for cancer chemotherapy. In: Drewinko B, Humphrey RM, eds., *Growth Kinetics and Biochemical Regulation of Normal and Malignant Cells*. Baltimore: Williams & Wilkins. 1977:455–469.

13. Skipper HE, Schabel FM Jr, Wilcox WS. Experimental evaluation of potential anticancer agents. XXI. Scheduling of arabinosylcytosine to take advantage of its S-phase specificity against leukemia cells. *Cancer Chemother Rep* 1967; 51:125–165.
14. Corbett TH, Valeriote FA, Baker LH. Is the P388 murine tumor no longer adequate as a drug discovery model? *Invest New Drugs* 1987; 5:3–20.
15. Staquet MJ, Byar DP, Green SB, Rozencweig M. Clinical predictivity of transplantable tumor systems in the selection of new drugs for solid tumors: rationale for a three-stage strategy. *Cancer Treat Rep* 1983; 67:753–765.
16. Trader MW, Harrison SD Jr, Laster WR Jr, Griswold DP Jr. Cross-resistance and collateral sensitivity of drug-resistant P388 and L1210 leukemias to flavone acetic acid (FAA, NSC 347512) in vivo (Abstr). *Proc AACR* 1987; 28:312.
17. Wilkoff LJ, Dulmadge EA. Sensitivity of proliferating cultured murine pancreatic tumor cells to selected antitumor agents. *J Natl Cancer Inst* 1986; 77:1163–1169.
18. Schabel FM Jr, Skipper HE, Trader MW, Laster WR Jr, Griswold DP Jr, Corbett TH. Establishment of cross-resistance profiles for new agents. *Cancer Treat Rep* 1983; 67:905–922 (see correction, *Cancer Treat Rep* 1984; 68:453–459).
19. Waud WR, Griswold DP Jr. Therapeutic resistance in leukemia. In: Teicher BA, ed., *Drug Resistance in Oncology*. New York: Marcel Dekker. 1993:227–250.
20. Dykes DJ, Waud WR. Murine L1210 and P388 leukemias. In: Teicher B, ed., *Tumor Models in Cancer Research*. Totowa, NJ: Humana. 2002:23–40.
21. Ho AD, Seither E, Ma DDF, Prentice G. Mitoxantrone-induced toxicity and DNA strand breaks in leukemic cells. *Br J Haematol* 1987; 65:51–55.
22. Nelson EM, Tewey KM, Liu LF. Mechanism of antitumor drug action: poisoning of mammalian DNA topoisomerase II on DNA by 4'-(9-acridinylamino)methanesulfon-*m*-anisidide. *Proc Natl Acad Sci USA* 1984; 81:1361–1365.
23. Rose WC, Huftalen JB, Bradner WT, Schurig JE. In vivo characterization of P388 leukemia resistant to mitomycin C. *In Vivo* 1987; 1:47–52.
24. Eng WK, McCabe FL, Tan KB, et al. Development of a stable camptothecin-resistant subline of P388 leukemia with reduced topoisomerase I content. *Mol Pharmacol* 1990; 38:471–480.

6

In Vivo Methods for Screening and Preclinical Testing

Use of Rodent Solid Tumors for Drug Discovery

Thomas Corbett, PhD, Lisa Polin, PhD, Patricia LoRusso, DO, Fred Valeriote, PhD, Chiab Panchapor, BS, Susan Pugh, BS, Kathryn White, BS, Juiwanna Knight, BA, Lisa Demchik, BS, Julie Jones, BS, Lynne Jones, BS, and Loretta Lisow, BA

CONTENTS

INTRODUCTION
MALIGNANT NEOPLASMS: HOW WIDESPREAD IS THE DISEASE?
HISTORICAL ADVANCES LEADING TO THE DEVELOPMENT OF RODENT
    MODELS
HISTORICALLY USED SOLID TUMOR MODELS
INDICATIONS OF AN IMMUNOGENIC PROBLEM WITH A TUMOR MODEL
NECESSITY FOR A PRESCREEN IN NEW DRUG DISCOVERY
STRATEGIES FOR CONSTRUCTING THE FIRST IN VIVO
    PRIMARY SCREEN FOR NEW DRUG DISCOVERY OF SOLID TUMOR-
    ACTIVE AGENTS
TUMOR MODEL SELECTION FOR IN VIVO PRIMARY SCREENING
PROTOCOL DESIGN CONSIDERATIONS FOR PRIMARY
    SCREENING WITH SOLID TUMORS
MEASURING TUMORS
DISCOVERY GOAL OF PRIMARY SCREENING
WHAT HAPPENS AFTER THE AGENT IS DISCOVERED IN THE PRIMARY
    SCREEN?
FINAL COMMENT

From: *Cancer Drug Discovery and Development:*
Anticancer Drug Development Guide: Preclinical Screening, Clinical Trials, and Approval, 2nd Ed.
Edited by: B. A. Teicher and P. A. Andrews © Humana Press Inc., Totowa, NJ

1. INTRODUCTION

The classic question in the field of drug discovery is: Which tumor model is a satisfactory predictor for cancer in humans? The classic answer is: None of them!

Each independently arising tumor is a separate and unique entity with its own unique histologic appearance, biologic behavior, and drug response characteristics *(1–8)*. This is true even when separate tumors arise in the same birth date batch of inbred mice, in the same organ, induced by the same carcinogen *(1,3–5,9)*. We have often cited the cases of reciprocal drug responses patterns in different colon adenocarcinomas arising in the same birth date batch of inbred mice induced by 1,2-dimethylhydrazine, e.g., Colon-51 is cured by PCNU and is unresponsive to Cytosine Arabinoside; whereas Colon-36 is cured by Cytosine Arabinoside, but unresponsive to PCNU *(1,3,5)*. A similar response reciprocal with DTIC and L-PAM for Colon-06 and Colon-07 has been cited *(1)*. These and other examples dating back over 30 yr *(5,10,11)* have made it clear that drug response characteristics are acquired haphazardly during carcinogenesis and are independent of host factors.

Thus, to expect that one colon tumor of a mouse will perfectly predict for all other colon tumors is unrealistic. Similarly, a clinician seeing an excellent response of one colon cancer patient to 5-FU would not expect all colon cancer patients to have a similar response to 5-FU. Nonetheless, one expects that colon tumors will predict better for other colon tumors than would a leukemia. Clearly the opposite case is well established; leukemias have been markedly more predictive for other leukemias than they have been for various solid tumors *(1)*.

Implied in the above discussion is the fact that none of the drugs thus far discovered are truly "anticancer agents," i.e., active against all malignant tumors *(1)*. Instead, they are antiproliferative agents that have activity against some tumors. These sensitive tumors have acquired a vulnerability that is greater than the vital normal cells of the host (1). These vulnerabilities are usually one or more of the following:

1. Selective uptake of the drug;
2. Selective activation of the drug;
3. Defective catabolism or elimination; or
4. Poor ability to repair the damage, or use an alternate or salvage pathway.

Since none of these biochemical mechanisms of vulnerability are common to all cancer cells, these agents cannot be "cancer-specific." Using supersensitive models (eg., P388 leukemia) with many of these specific vulnerabilities dooms a discovery effort to isolate "more of the same." We like to cite an actual example of the consequence of using a supersensitive tumor strategy (although omitting the name of the company). For several years, Company X supplied 10% or more of the entire P388 screening effort of NCI. Many active agents were found. Analog searches of the inventory at Company X uncovered many more P388 active hits. Analog synthesis efforts at Company X resulted in yet more hits. The leads seemed boundless. Gradually, the leads were subjected to detailed secondary evaluation against solid tumor models and leukemia models that were more challenging. All of the leads eventually vanished. This is not an isolated example, although a few suppliers were more fortunate in eventually obtaining clinically useful agents for their efforts. Two major lessons seem obvious: (1) A supersensitive model will divert and consume resources at an alarming rate. (2) The use of tumor models that have few or none of the vulnerabilities of P388 (and are insensitive to most or all of the currently available agents) may increase the probability of finding agents with activity against a true "cancer target" *(1)*. At the very least, drug-insensitive tumor models will generate novel agents with novel mechanisms and not have the defect of consuming resources with redundant mechanism of action discoveries.

2. MALIGNANT NEOPLASMS: HOW WIDESPREAD IS THE DISEASE?

The experimentalists' definition of a malignant neoplasm is as follows. The neoplasm must be able to carry out both of the following biologic events: (1) The cells must be able to transplant into another animal of the same inbred strain. (2) The cells must grow and kill the new host *(1)*. No normal cell of any adult vertebrate can carry out these functions. Likewise, neoplasms of plants, worms, echinoderms, and other lower life forms cannot carry out these functions. It appears that it is only in the higher life forms that have eyes that malignant neoplasms occur and can be induced by carcinogens. This includes birds, fish, reptiles, amphibians, and mammals *(12)*. The occurrence in arthropods and some mollusks (both of which have different types of eyes than birds, fish, and so forth) is unclear, but likely. Not only is cancer widespread in the animal kingdom, but it is clearly an ancient disease. Evidence of osteogenic sarcomas have been found in bones of dinosaurs that are more than 70 million yr old. Thus, it seems reasonable to assume that many "nonhuman" biological systems could be developed into meaningful models (tools) to study the malignancy processes and perhaps even for drug discovery efforts. Indeed, the simplest systems may be the most enlightening.

3. HISTORICAL ADVANCES LEADING TO THE DEVELOPMENT OF RODENT MODELS

In 1775, Percival Pott called attention to the high incidence of scrotal cancer among chimney sweeps of London, and correctly attributed the cause to continual contact with soot (coal tar) *(13)*. By 1778, workers in some countries (Holland, the first) were required to wear heavy clothing and wash daily. This eventually eliminated the disease. These observations made it clear that coal tar/soot contained a chemical carcinogen.

In 1889–1890, Hanau was the first to transplant spontaneous tumors of the rat with any degree of consistency *(14)*. However, the lack of inbred animals produced erratic results (owing to tumor rejection on the basis of tissue-specific antigens). Nonetheless, the principle of tumor transplantation was established.

Between 1905 and 1915, inbred strains of mice were first developed. An inbred is defined as 20 generations of brother-sister matings with each generation reducing heterozygosity by 19%. Thus, 20 generations of brother-sister matings created a mouse that had > 99% homozygosity. The four most commonly used inbred strains are C3H, C57B1/6, Balb/c, and DBA/2. All of these strains have 150 or more brother-sister matings *(15)*.

In 1915, Yamagawa and Ichikawa reported on the induction of skin tumors with months of applications of coal tar to the ears of rabbits (and later mice) *(16)*. This established that cancer could be induced and that the latency period for induction was long. The effort was then made to discover the active principle of the coal tar.

In 1927, Mayneord discovered that the active principle could be followed by fluorescence and determined that it was a benzanthracene-type structure.

In 1932, the active carcinogen in coal tar (benzo[a]pyrene) was isolated by Cook and coworkers and tested by Kennaway *(17)*. Following this discovery, a wide variety of active synthetic analogs were made. Induction of malignant tumors in many organ systems became routine with these carcinogens. Several tumor models in common use were induced with these carcinogens (e.g., 3-Methylcholantrene was used to induce L1210 [1948], P388 [1956], Pancreatic Ductal Adenocarcinoma 02 and 03 [1979]). Between 1940 and the 1990s, many other carcinogens were identified and used to induce tumors in rodents.

From the 1930s to the 1960s, it slowly became recognized that tumor model systems were most predictive if the tumors arose (or were induced) in inbred mice and were passaged only in the inbred host of origin. In noninbred systems, the immune system would magnify any slight antitumor activity of chemical agents, and in many cases, produce regressions and cures of tumors without therapy (obviously making interpretation of results of testing with potentially useful agents difficult). Today the use of immunogenic systems, such as Sarcoma-180, Walker-256, and Ehrlich Ascites carcinoma, would seem ridiculous. The fact that they were used for so many years was part of the philosophy of using supersensitive models. Among the technical support staff, the old-timers joked about not shutting the doors too hard for fear that it would kill the tumors. However, it should be noted that in a properly controlled trial, nonspecific cytotoxic agents were not active against these immunogenic models (thus, they could be used for primary screening). However, if antitumor activity was found in such a model, the true degree of antitumor activity was almost impossible to determine. This was because of the variable interaction of three different events:

1. The drug acting on the tumor;
2. The immune system acting on the tumor; and
3. The drug acting on the immune system.

Thus, the results obtained from the use of these tumors in secondary drug evaluations were essentially meaningless. The need for compatible tumor-host systems in cancer chemotherapy drug discovery and secondary evaluation has been reviewed *(1,2)*.

The reasons that rodents and rodent tumors became the favored models of cancer researchers are obvious:

1. Ease of handling and housing;
2. Cost; and
3. The induction and transplantation of rodent tumors from many organs systems having been accomplished with consistency.

Transplantable tumors of hamsters, guinea pigs, mice, rabbits, and rats have for many years been supplied by the National Tumor Repository at the NCI Division of Cancer Treatment, Frederick Cancer Research Center in Frederick, MD. However, over the years, the mouse clearly became the favored animal. In drug discovery, cost and the requirement for larger amounts of expensive agents eliminated the larger rodents from most discovery programs by the 1970s (including the NCI program).

4. HISTORICALLY USED SOLID TUMOR MODELS

The number of different rodent tumors that have been used in various discovery efforts is enormous. The following review papers are helpful in documenting various drugs, tumors, and individuals involved, as well as providing specific references (18–25). The following is only a brief summary.

Primary screening efforts began at NCI with Shear in 1934. This laboratory lasted until 1953 (18). Initially, Shear began with mouse Sarcorna-37, looking for necrosis and hemorrhage as an endpoint. The tumor was carried in random bred mice and was therefore immunogenic. In the late 1940s and early 1950s, as many as 100 different tumors from rats, hamsters, and mice were used at various centers, most notable being Memorial Sloan Kettering; University of Columbia; Children's Cancer Research Foundation in Boston; Chester Beatty in England; and University of Tokyo (18). Most were immunogenic systems, since they were derived in or maintained in random bred animals. Some of the more well known were: Yoshida sarcoma of rats, Sarcoma-180 of mice, Walker-256 carcinosarcoma of rats, Ehrlich Ascites carcinoma of mice (all of which were highly immunogenic systems). In 1955, the Cancer Chemotherapy National Service Center (CCNSC) was established. Primary screening in this program was essentially L1210 leukemia prior to 1975 and P388 leukemia after 1975. By 1982, 700,000 materials had been screened (26). Only a few agents entered primary screening with solid tumors in the CCNSC program and only in the first few years. The solid tumors used were mainly Sarcoma-180, Ehrlich Ascites carcinoma, Walker-256, and Carcinoma-755. Of these, only Carcinoma-755 (a metastatic mammary adenocarcinoma, sensitive to purine anti-metabolites) was derived and carried in inbred mice (C57B1/6), and thus was not immunogenic. Several other nonimmunogenic solid tumors were used in the CCNSC program in subsequent years, but always for secondary evaluation and not for primary screening. The most common were: Lewis lung carcinoma (spontaneous [1951], C57BL/6 mouse); B16 Melanoma (spontaneous [1954], C57B1/6 mouse); Colon Carcinoma-26 (nitrosomethyurethane induced [1973], Balb/c mouse); Colon Adeno carcinoma-38 (1,2-dimethylhydrazine induced [1973], C57B1/6 mouse); and CD8F1 spontaneous mammary adenocarcinomas. The CD8F1 tumors were used as first-generation transplants by mixing cells from three or four spontaneous tumors and implanting the cell mixtures. Obviously, the best take-rate, fastest-growing tumor dominated. Cell lines of these CD8F1 mammary tumors were also established and used for secondary evaluation. Various sublines of Lewis lung carcinoma were used and supplied by NCI were highly immunogenic sublines (2). Two agents were sent to the clinic on the basis of curative activity against these immunogenic sub lines, demonstrating the problem of depending on a single tumor model for decision making. The M5076 tumor was also used extensively in the NCI program for secondary evaluation. This was a reticulum cell sarcoma (27). Of interest is the protocol design of many of the NCI drug evaluation assays, commonly known as the ip-tumor, ip-drug "test tube in the mouse" assays. This approach became widely adopted by other investigators. The tumor was prepared as a brei and injected either as a percent-brei (5 or 10% for B16, 1% for Colon-26) or as counted cells. Drug injections started the next day. Obviously, this magnified antitumor activity by 1–3 logs, and also favored agents that crossed physiologic barriers poorly (1). The practice of using ip-implanted tumors and ip-injected drug to eliminate the need for crossing physiologic barriers was part of the supersensitive tumor model strategy *(1)*.

Of the tumor assays routinely used by NCI, only three required the agent to cross physiologic barriers (Colon-38, Lewis Lung, and CD8F1 mammary). The schedules were always fixed, and were often only able to detect schedule independent agents: e.g., 1 × only for CD8F1 or q7d × 2 for Colon-38. The details of the protocols, endpoints used, codes, instructions, and so forth, can be obtained from the Automated Information Section, Drug Evaluation Branch, Drug Research and Development, Division of Cancer Treatment, National Cancer Institute, Building 37, Bethesda, MD 20014.

5. INDICATIONS OF AN IMMUNOGENIC PROBLEM WITH A TUMOR MODEL

Clearly the immunogenic tumors discussed above are only of historic interest. Likewise, many tumors currently being used will phase out of usage as more relevant models become available. NCI has started a program of embryo freezing in an effort to stabilize the genetics of the inbred strains. One of the intentions is to prevent genetic drift that could render many of the existing tumor model systems immunogenic. Obviously, stabilization of the tumor lines by freezing has been standard practice at NCI and elsewhere. Indications of immunogenic behavior of transplantable tumor models used in chemotherapy trials have been published *(2)*. The most obvious clues that signal a problem are:

1. Occurrence of spontaneous tumor regressions in passage or control mice. If the tumor ulcerates, regresses, and regrows, it could be an infection. However, if it ulcerates, regresses to zero, and does not regrow, it is usually an immunogenic problem. If one challenges the animal with 60-mg fragments of the same tumor and they fail to grow, one has essentially absolute proof of an immunogenic system.
2. Cures at more than two dose levels (0.67 decrements) should make one suspect immunologic help in a chemotherapy trial. Cures at four dose levels are essentially impossible without immunologic help with the exception of simple no-takes or staging the tumor very close to the take rate. Rechallenge of the cures with 60-mg fragments will help clarify the situation.
3. If one has a life-span trial and excludes the cures in the %ILS calculation, the %ILS among the survivors should be < 250%. If it is > 250%, one should suspect an immunogenic system.
4. Poor take-rate, no-takes, lack of significant invasion, and metastasis could be a tumor of low malignancy, but could also signal an immunologic problem. In this case, one would need to know the natural history of the tumor.
5. Changes in the drug response profile of a tumor often indicate that an immunogenic system has developed, e.g., excessive responsiveness to an agent that historically was only modestly active *(2)*.
6. Better tumor response for upstaged disease than for early stage disease is a sure indication of an immunogenic system. Historically, a syngeneic tumor model system is more responsive if treatment is started early, soon after implant while the tumor cell burden is small. An immunogenic system is more responsive later, after the immune system has had time to "see" and "process" the antigen (i.e., tissue-specific foreign antigens on the surface of the tumor cells). Thus, an immunogenic system is more responsive if it is allowed to grow for 5–10 d before the start of chemotherapy.

7. Response to Cetus-IL-2 is a quick and relatively inexpensive method of determining an immunologic system (28).

The use of X-ray-killed tumor cells to prime mice twice about 10 d apart and then implanting the live tumor cells in primed and unprimed mice after an additional 10 d is a satisfactory, but more time-consuming and expensive method of detecting an immunologic problem.

The student of history should note that although the noncompatible rodent tumor model systems have been abandoned as senseless and misleading, there is almost universal acceptance of the noncompatible human tumor xenograft systems. Lack of genetic identity between the host (mice) and tumors (human) produces several unusual results and appears to skew the type of antitumor agent discovered. Several of these problems have been recently reviewed *(30)*.

6. NECESSITY FOR A PRESCREEN IN NEW DRUG DISCOVERY

Historically, the first in vivo (whole-animal) test has been referred to as the "primary screen." Any in vitro cellular, or biochemical/molecular target assay is referred to as a "prescreen." Between 1955 and 1985, NCI evaluated over 700,000 materials directly in mice without any prescreen testing. This practice has come to an end. Direct in vivo primary screening (without prescreen information) has essentially been eliminated worldwide over the last 10 yr. The reasons are as follows:

1. Most animal investigation committees have banned primary screening without prescreen information for humane considerations because the discovery rate was excessively low ($< 0.1\%$).
2. Advancements in cellular and biochemical/molecular prescreens have occurred. Cellular prescreens that detect selective cytotoxicity for one tumor type over another, as well as cytotoxicity for tumor cells over normal cell have eliminated 97% or more of the agents evaluated *(29)*. Furthermore, they have improved the discovery frequency to approx 5% for random materials and 25–88% for analogs of previous solid tumor-active agents *(29,30)*.
3. The amount of material needed for a prescreen is usually only a small fraction of the amount required for an in vivo test (in our case 1/80th the amount) *(29)*.

Thus, for expensive agents in limited supply that require resynthesis or natural products that require fractionation and purification, a prescreen can markedly reduce costs and research efforts.

There is scant information on the improvement in the in vivo primary screen discovery rates provided by the various biochemical/molecular target prescreens. In our own case, we found that > 90% of natural products that have been isolated on the basis of certain molecular target prescreens are not even cytotoxic for any of the tumor cells that we use in our cellular assay (indicating that they cannot even cross cell membranes). This is worse than randomly acquired materials. It may be that animal investigation committees will demand cellular prescreen information, unless the hit-rates of biochemical/molecular target screens are better than our limited experience.

7. STRATEGIES FOR CONSTRUCTING THE FIRST IN VIVO PRIMARY SCREEN FOR NEW DRUG DISCOVERY OF SOLID TUMOR-ACTIVE AGENTS

Many ingredients (in addition to the prescreen) are responsible for detecting promising new leads in a primary screen. We will review various aspects of the following two points: (1) tumor model selection and (2) protocol design strategies.

8. TUMOR MODEL SELECTION FOR IN VIVO PRIMARY SCREENING

After an agent passes some prescreen, the first in vivo discovery model (the primary screen) almost totally controls the nature of the agents discovered *(1)*. Further test systems (secondary evaluation) mainly define the strengths and weaknesses of the agents discovered by the primary screen *(1,29)*. Prior to 1985, drug discovery efforts at NCI and elsewhere focused on leukemias as the primary screen *(1)*. The results are now well documented. The agents discovered were markedly more active against leukemias and lymphomas than against solid tumors *(1)*. Furthermore, when a discovery was made, analogs were almost always tested first against these same leukemias, thus selecting agents with more leukemia/lymphoma activity, but not necessarily more useful against any other tumor type. Since 1985, many programs (including the NCI program) have refocused toward solid tumor drug discovery efforts *(1,31)*. This is because leukemias have been unable to detect agents broadly active against common solid tumors and because of the prevalence of solid tumors (>85% of human tumors).

As implied by discussions in the beginning of this chapter, the selection of tumor models is controlled both by the types of agents that one is attempting to find and also by the types of agents that one is attempting to avoid finding (since the latter will needlessly divert and consume resources). We need to emphasize this last point concerning the selection of models to avoid certain types of discoveries with a specific example. For many years, clinicians complained that they were being inundated with alkylating agents from the L1210 and later the P388 leukemia discovery programs. This was clearly true. These tumor models are excessively sensitive to alkylating agents. However, one must be careful not to duplicate the same problem. Switching to one or more poorly chosen solid tumors of rodents or human solid tumors will not necessarily get rid of the problem. For example, the human tumors used by NCI as a group are excessively sensitive to alkylating agents. By far the best agent discovered in the NCI in vivo xenograft panel is Mitomycin-C, an alkylating agent (personal communication of J. Plowman of NCI). Past that, DTIC and BCNU end up near the top of the discovery list. If the aim was to discover alkylating agents, one could go back to screening with L1210 and P388 for a lot less money.

The focus of our particular discovery program is to find new antitumor agents that are broadly active against solid tumors *(1,2,29,30)*. For our search, we began with the following hypothesis: that in order to have broad solid tumor activity (including human solid tumors in humans), it is necessary to have selective cytotoxicity for solid tumor cells at the cellular level, compared to leukemia cells or normal cells. It should be noted that this basic strategy will not miss the elusive, universally active agent should it exist *(1)*, since it includes normal cells in the search. In this prescreen, various solid tumors of mouse and human origin have been used. Selective cytotoxicity for a given solid tumor (seen at the

Table 1a
In Vivo Activity of Standard and Investigational Agents
Against Early Stage Mouse Solid Tumors

In vivo activity	Colon 38	Mam 16/C	Colon 51	Panc 02	Panc 03
Adriamycin	+ +	+ + + +	±	−	+ + +
Taxotere/taxol	+ + + +	+ + + +	+ + +	−	+ + + +
CPT-11	+	+ + +	+	−	+ + + +
VP-16	+ +	+ + +	±	−	+ + + +
VINC	−	+ +	−	−	−
5-FU	+ + +	+ + +	−	−	−
ARA C	+ +	+ +	−	−	−
Cytoxan	±	+ + +	+ +	−	+ +
CisDDPt	±	+	+ +	−	+ +
PZA	+ + + +	+ + + +	+	+ +	+ + + +
CI994	+ +	+ + +	+	+ + + +a	+ + + +
WIN33377	+ + + +	+ + + +	+	+	+ + + +
XK469	+ + + +	+ + + +	+ + +	+ + +	+ + + +
Nanopiposulfan	+	+ + +	+ + + +	±	+ +
DMP840	+	+	±	−	−
Doubling time in days	2.3–3.0	1.0–1.2	2.2–2.9	1.2–1.5	2.3–2.8
Metastatic behavior	Moderate/low	Very high	High	Very high	Moderate
Mouse of origin	C57BL/6	C3H	Balb/C	C57BL/6	C57BL/6

aBased on gross kill of a 37-d schedule, no net kill was obtained.

cellular level) then controls the choice of the in vivo primary screen (in that the same solid tumor is used) (29). The degree of selective cytotoxicity, potency, and number and types of solid tumors in which selective cytotoxicity is obtained in vitro determines the advancement of the agent to mouse testing (29). As may be surmised from the previous discussions, we only use non-immunogenic, drug-insensitive solid tumors (e.g., Pancreatic Ductal Adenocarcinomas-02,03; Colon Adenocarcinoma-38,07,09,26; Mammary Adenocarcinoma-16/C, Mam 16/C/Adr, Mam17, Mam17/Adr; B16 Melanoma [1,29,30]). We also include selected human tumors, e.g., Human Lung H125, Human Colon H116 (neither of which is alkylating agent-sensitive). Examples of some of the in vivo drug response profiles of the mouse solid tumors that we have used (in comparison with L1210 and P388 leukemias) are shown in Table 1. All the tumors can be obtained from the National Tumor Repository at Frederick, MD.

At the present time, our choice of tumors is operational, e.g., in addition to being drug-insensitive and nonimmunogenic, the tumors must have excellent growth in soft agar directly from mice (some need culture adaptation); and must be easy to use in vivo for a primary screen. If selective cytotoxicity at the cellular level is seen against a human tumor, we can almost always find a mouse tumor with the same degree of sensitivity in the culture assay (30). This mouse tumor can then be used for the in vivo primary screen. In this fashion, we can carry out the primary screen for a small fraction of the cost and avoid the pitfalls of new agent screening in xenograft systems (30). As tumors become better characterized in terms of oncogene expression, tumor suppressor gene mutations,

Table 1B
Conversion of Log_{10} Tumor Cell Kill to an Activity Rating

Antitumor activity	Duration of Rx <5 d, log_{10} kill, net	Duration of Rx 5–20 d, log_{10} kill net	gross	Duration of Rx >20d, log_{10} kill net	gross
Highly active					
+ + + +	>2.6	>2.0	>2.8	>0.8	>3.4
+ + +	1.6–2.6	0.8–2.0	2.0–2.8		2.5–3.4
+ +	0.9–1.5		1.3–1.9		1.7–2.4
+	0.5–0.8		0.7–1.2		1.0–1.6
Inactive					
–	<0.5		<0.7		<1.0

An active rating of + + + to + + + + is needed to effect partial (PRs) or complete regressions (CRs) of 100–300 mg size masses of most transplanted solid tumors of mice. Thus, an activity rating of + or + + would not be scored as active by usual clinical criteria.

types of MDR mechanisms, and so forth, the choice of the most appropriate models should become better clarified. At the present time, it seems that any given solid tumor could have defects that will create a drug selection bias. Safeguard strategies include using multiple tumors of different tissues and strains of origin, differing drug response profiles (including MDR tumors and tumors that are among the most drug-insensitive that can be found), requiring selective cellular cytotoxicity for multiple solid tumors in the tissue-culture prescreen, and requiring large degrees of cellular selectivity between the solid tumors and the leukemias or normal cells in the tissue-culture prescreen (29,30). Clearly, using drug-insensitive, nonimmunogenic solid tumor models has decreased redundant discoveries that have plagued previous efforts (30).

9. PROTOCOL DESIGN CONSIDERATIONS FOR PRIMARY SCREENING WITH SOLID TUMORS

9.1. Tumor Stage for Primary Screening Protocols

It has been suggested that since cancer in humans is usually at an advanced stage when first detected and treated, investigators should use advanced-staged tumors for discovery. They argue further that the most clinically useful agents are active against specific advanced-staged tumor models, again suggesting that advanced-staged tumors should be used for primary screening.

Overlooked in these arguments are the practical aspects of laboratory testing. The primary screen is usually carried out with a limited supply of drug that will never be resynthesized unless it is clearly active in the primary screen. Furthermore, the technical support staff doing the screen will never have any advance information regarding toxicity behavior (acute and chronic), optimum doses schedule, optimum formulation, and so forth. Remember, this is the primary screen, not secondary evaluation. If we were to present a limited supply of Taxol, Adriamycin, and VP-16 in a blinded group of drugs and

ask that they be tested against advanced-stage (300–600 mg) Mammary Adenocarci-
noma-16/C (a tumor that is nicely sensitive to each of these agents, even at an advanced
stage), it is unlikely that any investigator in the world would discover any of them. This
is because the optimum dose-schedule and route would need to be injected during the first
2 d of the trial, or it would be too late and the tumors would become too large to respond
(the M16/C Adenocarcinoma has a 1.1-d doubling time). On the other hand, an experienced laboratory staff would easily discover all three if they could start the trial the day
after the tumors were implanted as 30–60 mg size fragments. Two factors need to be
considered: (1) The first discovery screen is never carried out under ideal dose-schedule
conditions with the ideal formulation. (2) In primary screen in vivo, the investigator is
trying to uncover promising leads from which analog search and synthesis efforts will
provide improved agents. Although there are obvious exceptions, the first discovery is
usually not going to be the highly active clinical candidate *(30)*. For example, VP-16 was
approximately the 500th analog examined *(32)*. With solid tumor primary screening,
early stage disease is an ample challenge.

9.2. Tumor Route of Implant for Primary Screening Protocols

Animal investigation committees have been limiting the use of survival assays for
humane considerations. The agent must become a clear clinical candidate to be approved
for survival testing at some institutions. Thus, primary screening protocols that involve
survival endpoints are rapidly vanishing.

There are indications that tumor cells will respond better or worse at various locations
in the body, although $> 1 \log_{10}$ in tumor cell kills are rarely demonstrated. Nonetheless,
the differences have led to orthotopic and various internal site implants being investigated at NCI and elsewhere. An example would be an iv implant with lung colony counts
as an end point. Another example would be a subrenal capsule implant with sacrifice after
treatment and optical measurement of the tumor. Implants have also included tumor cells
sealed in porous plastic tubes. These are removed after treatment, and the cells bioassayed
or counted after staining. The topic is reviewed in Chapter 7 of this book.

The standard site for solid tumors is still the subcutaneous (sc) implant, using either
12-gage trocar implants or counted numbers of cells. The location for the trocar insertion
(swabbed with ethanol) is midway between the axillary and inguinal region along the side
of the mouse. The trocar is slipped approx 3/4 of an inch sc up toward the axilla before
discharging the tumor fragment, and pinching of skin as the trocar is removed. For
primary screening, we follow the British practice of bilateral trocar implants. The two
tumors are added together for each mouse, thus producing a tumor burden per mouse
value for data analysis. The advantage of the British system is reduced mouse-to-mouse
variability and, thus, the ability to reduce the number of animals per group, with five being
sufficient for accurate data analysis of tumor response and evaluation of toxicities. This
presumes that the tumor has an acceptable take-rate and reasonable doubling time. Tumors
that require more than 21 d to reach 1000 mg/mouse tumor burden from trocar fragments
are not acceptable for primary screening because of excessive mouse-to-mouse variability and, thus, a requirement for larger numbers of mice per group. The number of animals
per group has become a major issue with animal investigation committees, to say nothing
of cost and drug supply requirements.

9.3. Schedule of Drug Administration for Primary Screening Protocols

Historically, a wide variety of schedules have been investigated for primary screens, e.g., 1 × only, daily × 4, daily × 9, daily to death, and so forth. For a given tumor and a given protocol design, virtually all primary screening programs use a fixed schedule for all agents being tested. From our perspective, we have always considered this a disaster and responsible for many false negatives (1). Before we can undertake a discussion of a "flexible schedule" approach, the following discussion of schedule and the various schedule categories need to be understood.

We have invariably found that cytotoxic agents fall into one of four different categories (29,33,34).

1. Category 1 (schedule dependent for lethal toxicity): In this category, schedule markedly influences the total dosage that can be administered (33,34). This occurs for most antimetabolites (S-phase-specific, e.g., 6-Thioguanine, Cytosine Arabinoside, and Methotrexate). The total dosage (at the maximum tolerated level) markedly decreases (usually by a factor of 15 or more) as the number of injections increase within a 10-d treatment period (33). The reason for the marked change is well understood. Cytotoxicity (for normal and tumor cells) from these drugs occurs because of inhibition of critical enzymes necessary for DNA synthesis during S phase. In category 1, efficacy (for a sensitive tumor) correlates predominantly with time above a minimum cytotoxic concentration of the drug.

   Interestingly, if the half-life of a schedule-dependent drug is very long, the agent will behave like a schedule-independent agent. An example is the palmatate depot form of Cytosine Arabinoside (Palmo-Ara-C, which has a 27-h half-life). This compound has an LD_{10} of 200 mg/kg regardless of the schedule used.

2. Category 2 (schedule independent for lethal toxicity): This schedule does not appreciably influence the total dosage that can be administered (33,34). Examples include: mitotic inhibitors, DNA binders, alkylating agents, DNA scission agents that produce repairable lesions (VP-16), and some antimetabolites (5-FU). The maximum tolerated total dosage (MTTD) does not change significantly as the number of injections increase in a 10-d time period. In category 2, the antitumor activity for a sensitive tumor correlates with the total dosage (actually the area under the concentration × time curve) that can be administered, and dose splitting does not appreciably change efficacy. As might be expected, drugs in this category are the easiest to discover (especially with a fixed-schedule design used in most primary screening programs).

3. Category 3 (schedule independent with a peak plasma problem): The total dosage at the apparent maximum tolerated level appears to increase as the number of injections increase within the 10-d period (29,34,35). This phenomenon is usually caused by an intolerance to a high plasma level of the drug, and results in immediate postinjection deaths and an erroneous assignment of the MTTD. The schedule producing the immediate deaths is not satisfactory for the evaluation of antitumor activity. In these cases, efficacy and the MTTD can only be determined with a schedule utilizing more frequent injections of lower dosage levels (i.e., individual dosages approx 0.7 × those causing immediate toxicity problems). Frequently, it is necessary to extend the treatment duration (e.g., 3 times/d for 12–15 consecutive days) in order to obtain meaningful toxicity. Category 3 agents are often encountered in new drug discovery programs, but have almost universally been overlooked because of inflexible schedules.

We find that many solid-tumor-selective materials are in this category. Historically, agents in category 3 are rarely evaluated adequately. Very few have reached clinical trials. The problem is mainly a mouse problem. In the human, the drug will produce a much lower peak level at an equivalent area-under-the-plasma-curve. The difference is the 10-fold slower transit time through the liver and kidneys of the human, and the resulting longer half-life. In category 3, the antitumor activity (for a sensitive tumor) correlates with the total dosage (area under the concentration × time curve). There is a subcategory of this type of schedule, which is the toxicity-adapting agents (e.g., Glaucarubinone). In these cases, the mice adapt to the dose-limiting toxicity over a period of several days, and levels can be markedly increased (often greater than sixfold above a dosage that is lethal in unadapted mice).

4. Category 4: The total dose (at the apparent MTTD levels) increases with the dose splitting (opposite category 1), whereas efficacy decreases with dose splitting (unlike categories 2 and 3) *(29)*. As we now understand, this is owing to nonlinear pharmacokinetics and the fact that the agent has peak plasma problems similar to the standard category 3 agent.

Once the laboratory staff understands the various categories and the fact that schedules producing immediate injection deaths cannot be used to assign the MTD value, schedule adjustments and a flexible protocol design are rather easy to carry out. The first step is to determine if the agent produces immediate postinjection deaths in one or two normal mice before the efficacy trial is started *(29)*. If it does, the top dose of the efficacy trial will begin at a level slightly below the level that causes immediate lethality. Furthermore, the agent is injected 2 or 3 times/d, daily until a true dose-limiting toxicity is reached (as judged by weight loss, appearance, or lethality from chronic administration). Thus, a split-dose flexible schedule design will allow the identification of the category 3 agent in a primary screening trial *(29)*. In selected cases, the trial can be repeated with an infusion by a modified Harvard pump or implantable Alzet pumps (if potency, solubility, and drug supply permit).

In general, the laboratory staff needs to understand the intent of the flexible schedule concept, since one has a limited time to administer treatment properly before the tumor becomes too big. This time can be as short as 8 d for a very rapid tumor ($T_d = 1$ d) to 15 d for a slower tumor ($T_d = 2.8$ d). During this time, one is attempting to administer the maximum amount of drug without producing lethality (since in most cases, the antitumor activity is related to the total dose). Host recovery can thus be taken into account. If the weight loss is evident (or appearance and function compromised), injections can be omitted, dosages reduced, and so on. Injections can then be restarted or doses escalated depending on the appearance and weight recovery. Again, the intent is to maximize total dose without killing the animals. Historically, in many animal fixed-schedule screening protocols, the mice were injected if they were breathing (even if they were in the processes of dying). Obviously, this is a waste of valuable drug, to say nothing of humane considerations.

9.4. Dosages in Primary Screening Protocols

As with scheduling, we recommend a flexible protocol design for drug dosages in primary screening. In our case, we use three groups/drug with 50% decrements *(29)*. Again, one needs to understand the intent of the flexible design, i.e., to get the maximum amount of drug into the mice without encountering lethality. Thus, dose escalations and reductions can be carried out anytime depending on weight loss and appearance. The three dose levels are necessary because delayed and cumulative toxicities often cannot be anticipated. In our program, starting dosages are controlled by cytotoxicity obtained in the cellular prescreen, but usually are in the 15–220 mg/kg range for the first day of injection (in the absence of immediate postinjection lethality in the toxicity test) (29).

All clinically useful cytotoxic antitumor agents (with the exception of Hydroxyurea) are active and toxic in mice at < 1100 mg/kg total dose on an optimum schedule (29). Less potent agents (except Hydroxyurea) have universally failed. This is known as the "1100 mg/kg rule," and agents without this degree of potency are not considered of interest. Although we and others do not feel compelled to follow this rule, it is hard to ignore history. Thus, in the primary screen, we attempt to exceed the 1100 mg/kg total dose before giving up on the agent as nontoxic (we usually attempt to reach 2000 mg/kg total if supply permits).

Historically, fixed-dose protocols have been used for primary screening (three to five dose levels). In selected cases, initial toxicity trials were carried out in nontumor mice. If all the animals died in the efficacy trial, it was repeated at lower dosages. If they all lived, it was repeated at higher dose levels or abandoned, depending on the total dose and lack of activity encountered in the first test. An immediate postinjection death was recorded in NCI P388 and L1210 testing as dead the next day. Thus, one cannot tell the drugs that fell into schedule category 3 and were inappropriately evaluated. Obviously, fixed-dose schedule protocols use more mice and consume more drug, in addition to missing category 3 agents. With a flexible-dose schedule, a good evaluation can be carried out with 500 mg of material. Most fixed-dose schedule programs require 2000 mg samples to undertake in vivo testing.

9.5. Drug Route in Primary Screening with Solid Tumors

Historically, all agents that entered primary screening at NCI and elsewhere were injected intraperitoneally (ip) with the agent. This was usually carried out with a 0.5-mL vol/mouse, injected through a 1/4-in. 23-gage needle (to avoid excessive hydraulic forces of small or long needles), with 6-mL plastic syringes. The site was high enough to avoid the bladder, but low enough to avoid the diaphragm, and slightly off midline. This route of delivery is attractive, since it can be accomplished with great fidelity and very quickly (usually 10 mice can be injected in < 30 s). This route was, and still is, used regardless of the route of the tumor, and the nature of the solubility or formulation of the drug.

We are not opposed to the ip route, but do not use it for primary screening ourselves. In most cases, the physical properties of the drug controls the route used in our primary screening trials. If the agent is water-soluble (with pH variation of 4.0–8.5 permitted), the agent is injected intravenously (iv). This simulates the clinical condition, and eliminates the need for the agent to be absorbed and transported into the bloodstream from the ip cavity. Furthermore, humane consideration of injecting a pain-producing agent and tissue-damaging agent is reduced with the iv route (there are no intravascular pain receptors, and rapid dilution, albumin binding, and the nature of the endothelial lining minimize tissue damage). Practiced laboratory staff can carry out 12–18 iv injections in a mouse if the agent is not necrotizing. It is clear that certain agents are difficult to detect if tested only ip against a sc tumor (e.g., Taxol, AMSA, Adriamycin). This is because of poor biodistribution from the ip drug (Taxol or AMSA) or long delayed lethality from wounding (Adriamycin). The iv route obviously requires more technical skill and is more time-consuming (and thus more expensive). In addition, tail vein damage does occur for a portion of the agents, requiring a route change to sc.

In our program, water-insoluble agents are evaluated sc behind the neck; remember the tumor is bilateral along the sides of the animal. If drug supply permits, a water-insoluble agent is also evaluated orally (po) if it is obvious from the structure that the agent is chemically stable to the acid, base, or enzymatic conditions of the gastrointestinal tract. Historically, there was a drug discovery axiom that stated: "If it is not water-soluble, it better be orally active." This is no longer true. Water-insoluble materials can be reduced to nanoparticle size, coated with various surfactant materials, and then injected iv. We have recently published such an example *(30)*. Furthermore, in primary screening, we (and others) are looking for novel new leads with new mechanisms of solid tumor action. Analog search and synthesis can usually deal with the solubility problems. The sc route is not as good as iv for tissue-damaging agents and pain producers. It is, however, far better than ip, since the problem becomes quickly evident and treatments can be discontinued.

The primary screening discovery rate of a water-soluble vs water-insoluble agent is of academic interest. In a review of 1010 solid-tumor-selective agents discovered by our prescreen and tested in mice over a 3-yr period, the following results were obtained: 490 (48.5%) were water-insoluble and could not injected iv. With only a few exceptions, they were tested sc. Of these, 76 (15.5%) were active in mice. Thus, poor water solubility was not a deterrent to discovery either in our prescreen or in our in vivo primary screen. To complete the analysis of the 1010 compounds: 520 (51.5%) were water-soluble and were tested iv with a few exceptions. Of the 520 water-soluble agents tested, 135 (26%) were active in mice. These tabulations include both "random" agents and analogs of previous solid tumor-active hits (natural products and synthetics), which had been selected as solid-tumor-selective by our cellular prescreen. The water-soluble materials were further subdivided: 41 agents required acid to effect solution; of these 15 were in vivo active. Sixty-two required base to effect solution; of these five were in vivo active. The remaining 417 went into solution at pH = 7.0; of these, 115 were in vivo active. The tumors were always sc bilateral implants. Activity was defined as T/C < 42% at a nontoxic dose. Tumor weight (in mg) = $(a \times b^2)/2$, where a and b are the tumor length and width (mm), respectively. Tumor weights are added together for each mouse.

The treatment and control groups are measured when the control group tumors reach approx 700–1200 mg in size (median of group). The median tumor weight of each group is determined (including zeros). The T/C value in percent is an indication of antitumor effectiveness: A T/C ≤ 42% is considered significant antitumor activity by the Division of Cancer Treatment (NCI). A T/C < 10% is an indication of a highly active agent by NCI standards. Other efficacy endpoints are discussed later in this chapter.

9.6. Formulation of New Materials for Primary Screening

It is obviously helpful to have the chemical structure in order to project drug stability in water, acid, base, heat, and so forth, and suggest formulation for the laboratory staff. The laboratory staff can then investigate the solubility with a few crystals on a microscope slide in various solvents, e.g., water, pH 4.0 water, pH 8.0 water, ethanol, propylene glycol, DMSO, as well as in various carriers (agents that have a hydrophylic and a hydrophobic region to hold the drug in solution), e.g., Tween-40 (POE-40), PEG, and Cremophor. In general, DMSO and Cremophor are the most toxic and least desirable. The intention is to effect total solubility, or if solubility cannot be accomplished, a suspension with the smallest crystal size possible. If the agent is not "water-soluble, the following procedures are done in a homogenizer with a Teflon™ pestle: The organic solvent is added first with mixing (making up 3–5% of the total final volume), followed by the carrier with mixing (making up 1–3% of the final volume), followed by the water with mixing. The final preparation is to be injected in a volume of 0.2 mL/mouse (iv, sc, or po).

In certain cases, an agent will be in solution in acid or base, but it is not suitable for iv injection because it will precipitate at physiologic pH and plug the capillaries in the lungs, thus causing a respiratory death. This is easy to check by simply injecting 0.2 mL of the drug preparation into 2 mL of horse serum and looking for precipitation. A 20-g mouse will have approx 2 mL of blood.

9.7. Mouse Weights and Weighing of Mice in Primary Screening Trials

In general, we suggest a slightly higher initial body weight for mice entering into primary screening than NCI, drug supply permitting. Thus, females should be a minimum of 18 g and males a minimum of 19 g. All mice in the trial should be within a 5-g range. Using animals from the oldest stock, 22–26 g average weights are perfectly acceptable. Mice that have been in the laboratory for a longer period of time have adjusted to all the stresses and possible circulating infections.

Mice are group weighed daily during the drug treatment period, including Saturday, Sunday, and holidays, all of which are also drug injection days. These daily weighings are usually the best methods to assess toxicity in a flexible dose-schedule screening trial. Following the last day of drug injection, weighings are continued in each group until full pretreatment body weight is restored (the time to recovery from the weight loss nadir provides an excellent measure of host recovery time) or until it is evident that the agent is clearly inactive.

9.8. Necropsy and Other Toxicity Assessments in Primary Screening Trials

Historically, dead mice were not necropsied even in the leukemia primary screening trials at NCI. In many cases, it was not possible to separate drug deaths from tumor deaths, and impossible to select a true MTD level. Furthermore, it created a lot of unnecessary secondary evaluation testing and favored the selection of agents with long delayed toxicity (1). In our laboratories, we carry out necropsies of all dead mice, assessing spleen size, and appearance of liver, lungs, kidney, GI tract, and so forth. This information is useful for deaths that occur during drug treatments and is critical for identifying slightly delayed drug deaths in the faster-growing solid tumors.

Many other toxicities are encountered in primary screening trials: neurologic (stupor, ataxia, peripheral neuropathy splay-foot-walk, coma, seizures, spasms, tremors, paralysis, unconscious laying on its side, and so forth); respiratory problems; activity level (jumping, running, crouched, no movement, avoidance behavior); grooming or lack thereof, tissue damage, stomatitis; squealing; animals look poorly; and so on. Daily notation on the observation sheets of the trials should include: type of occurrence, severity, and duration (at each dosage level). These notations can save a great deal of time and drug in a secondary evaluation trial if the agent is active. They can also assist in deciding if the agent should be retested, resynthesized, or an analog search be carried out. Notations concerning the drug being well tolerated are also helpful.

9.9. Controls and Parameters of the Primary Screening Trials Using Solid Tumors

The research purist would say that if you need a thousand controls to assure the fidelity of a single group, make sure you have the thousand controls. There are, however, the realities of cost, research time, and unjustified consumption of mice for little or no information. The rationale for shortcutting some of the controls is also the fact that any agent that looks good will be retested in secondary evaluation. Thus, the general strategy in primary screening is to minimize the chance that the agent is truly a promising active and you will miss it (false negatives). The general NCI practice is usually followed in most primary screening trials: The mice are trocared and mixed in a large tub or large cage, and unselectively distributed to the treatment and control groups. Several agents are usually tested in one trial with one no-treatment control. Obviously, it is highly unlikely that all of the agents in the trial will be active. Because of this, it is virtually assured that you will have a negative control built into the trial. These inactive drugs can also double as diluent controls especially at the bottom dose levels. Since there are so many diluent controls in the trial (inactive drugs), the need for large numbers of untreated control mice is unnecessary (since a variance with the diluent controls would be evident). Thus, we use only 5 mice/group in the untreated control, the same as the treatment groups (since all animals are bilaterally implanted with tumor). There is no positive control in the primary screening trials, since the tumors are used so often and are included in secondary evaluation testing also (where there is a positive control). Furthermore, growth/invasion/ metastasis behavior, histology, viral testing, and periodic recovery from frozen storage are done frequently with highly used screening tumors to maintain quality-control standards. All cured mice are rechallenged with the tumor to monitor possible immunologic problems.

10. MEASURING TUMORS

10.1. Endpoints Used to Assess Drug Efficacy in Primary Screening

Historically, in primary screening trials (and even some secondary evaluation trials) with solid tumors, the tumors are measured only once when the controls reach approx 1000 mg; the mice are then sacrificed. Alternately, the mice are all sacrificed when the controls reach approx 1000 mg average; the tumors are removed and weighed. This is known as the "slice-in-time" protocol design with nothing known prior to or after the one time-point. Although cheap, this type of design misses the opportunity to anticipate an active agent. It also misses the opportunity to acquire a great deal more information in the initial screening trial. In our testing, we carry out at least three measurements of all groups. The initial measurement is carried out when the untreated control tumors are approx 150–200 mg in size. At this time, additional treatment decisions can still be made. If treated groups are zeros, one has immediately flagged a potentially active agent. More frequent measurements are then scheduled. This allows the accurate calculation of the exponential doubling time of the tumors. Mice are terminated when each tumor reaches

1200–1500 mg in size. This allows the calculation of the $\log_{10}$ tumor cell kill and allows the accurate determination of the host recovery time (since the weighing of the mice is continued up to the point of full recovery).

Furthermore, any delayed toxicities, if any, become evident since the mice are not prematurely sacrificed.

Thus, in addition to the usual T/C evaluation, the data are available for the calculation of the tumor growth delay and the exponential tumor volume doubling time. This information can then be accurately converted to the log cell kill. These calculations are shown below. Tumor weights are estimated from two-dimensional measurements:

$$\text{Tumor weight (in mg)} = (a \times b2)/2 \tag{1}$$

where a and b are the tumor length and width in (mm), respectively.

10.2. Tumor Growth Delay (T – C Value)

T is the median time (in days) required for the treatment group tumors to reach a predetermined size (e.g., 1000 mg), and C is the median time (in days) for the control group tumors to reach the same size. Tumor-free survivors are excluded from these calculations (cures are tabulated separately). In our judgment, this value is the single most important criterion of antitumor effectiveness, because it allows the quantification of tumor cell kill.

10.3. Calculation of Tumor Cell Kill

For sc growing tumors, the $\log_{10}$ cell kill is calculated from the following formula:

$$\text{The } \log_{10} \text{ cell kill total (gross)} = [\text{T} - \text{C value in days} / (3.32) (T_d)] \tag{2}$$

Where T – C is the tumor growth delay as described before, and T_d is the tumor volume doubling time (in days) estimated from the best-fit straight line from a log-linear growth plot of the control group tumors in exponential growth (100–800 mg range). The conversion of the T – C values to $\log_{10}$ cell kill is possible, because the T_d of tumors regrowing posttreatment (Rx) approximates the T_d values of the tumors in untreated control mice. The calculations for net $\log_{10}$ tumor cell kill are provided by subtraction of the duration of the treatment period from the T – C value and then dividing by 3.32 × T_d (2,29).

11. DISCOVERY GOAL OF PRIMARY SCREENING

At one time, there was a myth in oncology that the first agent discovered in a series was going to be the most active. In actual fact, this is usually not the case. Indeed, in dealing with a large inventory of agents, one should assume that this will not be the case, and should not be the goal of the screening effort. For example, let us propose an inventory of 300,000 agents (a medium-size inventory for a pharmaceutical company), and propose that three novel solid tumor-active clinical candidates exist in that inventory. If we test 5000/yr (slightly below our usual rate), we would encounter a clinical candidate only every 20 yr of testing. However, let us propose that each of the three clinical candidates have 100 analogs each, of which 20 are moderately active (60 additional agents to detect). With totally random selection and testing of the inventory and the same 5000/yr testing rate, we would encounter 1 moderately active/yr. Each hit would lead us to test all the related analogs (which would contain the clinical candidate). Thus, it would take us only

3–4 yr to discover all three clinical candidates from this inventory. Obviously, finding highly active agents leads to analog synthesis programs. In other cases, analog synthesis programs are started around moderately active hits, especially for novel agents with activity against very drug-insensitive solid tumors. Thus, the overall strategy of primary screening is not to uncover the rare clinical winner, but rather to uncover the moderately active agents that will lead to the clinical winner or to a synthesis program that will make a clinical winner.

12. WHAT HAPPENS AFTER THE AGENT IS DISCOVERED IN THE PRIMARY SCREEN?

Historically, this next step is called "development," and varies greatly with the nature of the agent, availability of analogs, drug supply, and criteria established to move the agent toward clinical development. For educational purposes, we often like to start a discussion of secondary evaluation testing with admonitions of "what not to do." In general, a multitude of techniques are available to make marginally active agents look superactive in animal testing. Five simple examples are as follows:

1. Stage the tumor approx three times the take-rate level of the tumor; i.e., each animal will receive three clonogenic cells. All the tumors will grow, but a half a log of tumor cell kill will produce a high percentage of cures (note: half a log kill is considered essentially inactive).
2. Use an immunogenic tumor. Upstage the tumor 5–6 d so that the mouse can process the antigen, and then start treating with the drug. Again, a half a log kill will usually produce cures this time because of immunologic help from the host.
3. Use a superlethal dose. Stage the tumor so that the control tumors will be 800–1000 mg in size a day or two before the mice will die from drug toxicity. Sacrifice all the mice on that day. Do not weigh the mice. Impressive antitumor activity will be seen for marginally active agents. This technique is excellent for agents that have some delayed toxicity.
4. Evaluate an agent against a wide variety of tumors to find the most sensitive. Do all the testing in the highly sensitive tumors; show no other data.
5. Give the drug soon after implantation of the tumor, both given by the same route (e.g., ip). This will magnify the tumor cell kill by 2–4 logs greater than the same design with the drug injected by a route different than the tumor (1).

Likewise, a multitude of techniques are available to make virtually any agent look bad. The following are three examples:

1. Evaluate a variety of tumors. Find three or four tumors that are unresponsive. Use those unresponsive tumors for evaluation; show no other data.
2. Upstage tumors that are sensitive to the drug to the point that a lengthy schedule at the correct total dose will be inactive. The testing looks clean and well run, but the agent will be inactive.
3. Learn the operating characteristics of the agent, schedule category, optimum dose and schedule, and determine the log kill and dose at various dosage levels. Select a tumor with a very rapid doubling time and select the schedule to produce a log kill/dose well below the doubling time replacement of the cells. The total dose will be correct, but it is too little too late for the rapidly growing tumor even if it is highly responsive by the correct dose schedule.

The point of these absurd examples is that the operating conditions of the tumors and the drug needs to be understood in order to obtain a fair and representative evaluation of a new agent. Thus, the following protocol design considerations are suggested:

1. Use nonimmunogenic tumors.
2. Tumors appropriately staged, e.g., more than 3 $\log_{10}$ units above the take-rate for most trials is sufficient; more than 5 logs if a very high cell kill is expected.
3. Tumor and drug are injected by different routes, unless both are iv.
4. Treatment should start day 1 or 2 for rapidly growing tumors (implant day is day 0; T_d for rapid solid tumors = 1.0–1.8 d). At least 60% of the MTD should be injected by day 6. Treatment for slow-growing tumors can start day 3 (T_d = 2.2–2.8 d), and the treatment period can be more prolonged than the fast-growing tumors.
5. A variety of tumors types are selected: fast, slow, range of drug sensitivities, tumors from different tissues of origin and histologic types, tumors derived from different strains of inbred animals, with highly invasive and highly metastatic tumors favored.
6. Determine operating characteristics of the drug: solubility, stability, schedule category, dose/schedule behavior, activity by po, sc, and iv (if soluble). Often the ip route is also evaluated. Dose and schedules are chosen to minimize immediate postinjection toxicities (if any) and maximize the total dosage within the treatment period. Historically, three dose levels of 0.62 or 0.67 decrements are used in secondary evaluation studies.
7. Determine host recovery time, dose-limiting toxicity (acute and chronic), and possible long-delayed toxicity. Long-delayed toxicity evaluations are done in nontumor mice.
8. Include all the necessary controls: proper randomization, and so forth. Historically, if one is unfamiliar with the test model, a positive control, a negative control, a diluent control, and multiple dose levels ranging from toxic to inactive will cover most requirements.
9. Measure all tumors frequently enough to be able to determine the T_d and the tumor growth delay, which can be converted to log cell kill.
10. Confirm results.

We have reviewed these design considerations and others at length (1–7,29,30,33–40). The goal of protocol design for secondary evaluation is simple: to understand the weaknesses and the strengths of each new agent.

As discussed above, only a very small fraction of the initial discoveries progress to clinical trials; in most cases, it is an analog of the initial hit. Thus, it is usual to acquire a limited set of close analogs at the same time that the first hit is entered into evaluations against additional tumors. If more hits are obtained with the analogs, a broader analog search and analog synthesis program is usually started. A rather typical example of an analog search and synthesis program has been published from these laboratories (39,41,42). Eventually, the best analogs progress to detailed secondary evaluation testing. It is usual to include the most active positive control for each tumor model and to have "head-to-head" comparison trials (i.e., same experiment test) of the best analogs. One attempts to identify the active pharmacomorphic pattern in the analog series (minimum active structure, as well as the pattern conferring analogs with the best therapeutic index) (39,41,42). Eventually, using a set of development criteria, one selects the clinical candidate, an immediate backup, and eventually a second- and even third-generation analog to advance to clinical trials. An example of a set of criteria used to advance an agent to clinical development is shown in Table 2. Several examples of secondary evaluation testing using rodent tumors can be examined in the following references (29,34–36,43–45). The heavy emphasis on breadth of activity testing should be noted in these publications.

Table 2
Preclinical Criteria for the Advancement of a Solid Tumor-Active Agent
Toward Clinical Development[a]

Selective cytotoxicity for solid tumors over a leukemia (L1210, P388) or normal cells at the cellular level; a zone differential of > 250 U is required for meaningful selectivity (29); a 250-U zone change (6.5 mm) can, on the average, be produced by a sevenfold change in drug concentration. This requirement is consistent with our hypothesis that broad solid tumor activity in vivo will be attended by solid tumor selectivity at the cellular level.

Activity (defined as < 42% T/C) against one or more human tumors in SCID mice is required; the trials are carried out with bilateral sc tumor implant of 30–60 mg fragments, with the agent injected iv if water-soluble and po if insoluble; we consider the following three tumors most acceptable: Lung H125, Colon 116, and Prostate LNCaP.

At a nontoxic dosage level (LD_{10} or less and <20% body wt loss), the agent should produce greater than a 2-$\log_{10}$ tumor cell kill in two tumor systems from a single course of treatment (10 d or less), with the drug and the tumor administered by a different route, thus requiring the drug to cross multiple physiologic barriers; it must be verified that the responses were obtained in a nonimmunogenic tumor model system (e.g., cured mice reimplanted with 60-mg fragments of the tumor will regrow the tumor with no substantial alteration in the T_d value, or the tumor will not respond to IL-2 treatments); we focus on a set of five tumors for the first evaluations, with two additional MDR tumors given priority also; these are: Colon Adenocarcinoma-38 and 51, Mammary Adenocarcinoma-16/C, Pancreatic Ductal Adenocarcinoma-02 and 03; MDR tumors: Mammary Adenocarcinoma-16/C/Adr (not P-glycoprotein), and Mammary Adenocarcinoma-17/Adr (with P-glycoprotein); a variety of other tumors are also used in special circumstances to evaluate agents against tumors of other tissue types (i.e., undifferentiated Colon-26, B-16 Melanoma, Colon Adenocarcinoma 09). The methods for in vivo evaluation and quantification of tumor cell kill have been previously published (2,29).

In the evaluation of 10 tumor systems (from the list given in the above entry), it is required to have in vivo activity at two nontoxic dosage levels (0.62 decrements) in three tumor models, with the drug administered by a route different than the tumor; activity is defined as T/C values of <42%; the "two-dose-level" requirement is included to exclude agents with exceptionally steep dose-response curves (where only the MTD is active); in clinical trials, an agent is rarely escalated to a dose that is similar to an MTD in a healthy young mouse.

In normal, nontumor mice with MTDs of the agent (i.e., no lethality within 15 d of last treatment), there should be no long delayed lethality (e.g., 30–150 d post last treatment) and a reasonable host recovery time; if the agent has an adequate host recovery time, animals treated with an MTD should regain their pretreatment weights within 12 d of the weight loss nadir and continue to gain both weight and skeletal size thereafter.

It is desirable to have activity against one or more tumors with the MDR phenotype; e.g., activity against Mammary Adenocarcinoma 16/C/Adr and Mammary Adenocarcinoma 17/Adr.

In addition to the criteria discussed above, we consider the following to be important in the development of a new agent.

IV formulation possible: If an agent is water-soluble, it is usually possible for the chemists to design water-soluble analogs; an example of some commonly used groups are:
—NH—$(CH_2)_2$—$N(CH_3)_2$ or   —CH_2—CH_2—CH_2—N—$(CH_3)_2$ or   —CH_2—CH_2—$N(CH_2CH_3)_2$

(continued)

Table 2 (*Continued*)
Preclinical Criteria for the Advancement of a Solid Tumor-Active Agent
Toward Clinical Development[a]

It would be possible to develop a water-insoluble agent for clinical trials if it had oral activity and dependable and consistent absorption. However, if at all possible, it is better to wait for a water-soluble analog because iv delivery reduces the number of physiologic barriers the agent must cross and usually produces a better therapeutic index as a result; in rare cases, water-insoluble agents that are not active orally can be developed to the clinic with the nanoparticle technology developed by Eastman Kodak Nanosystems *(30)*.

Good stability in solution: A half-life of at least 30 min in solution at room temperature is considered necessary for ease of handling and consistent dose delivery; obviously, the greater the stability, the better.

Dosage levels within the limits of the 1100 mg/kg rule *(see text)*.
The agent can be made available in necessary amounts for a reasonable cost: In drug development, these problems have delayed development of some agents for many years (e.g., Taxol), but have rarely terminated development for highly active agents.

Patent protection possible: Companies are usually unwilling to put up developmental costs unless they can obtain patent protection.

[a]Over the last 40 yr, a large number of "antitumor agents" have been advanced to clinical trials and have failed to be useful. Learning from both the clinical successes as well as the failures, we have drafted a set of preclinical criteria that we hope will improve the chances for clinical success. We wish to emphasize that these criteria are only guidelines, and we would in selected cases forego the need for a specific criteria. Obviously, validation of these criteria awaits the testing of sufficient numbers of agents in the clinic.

As stated at the beginning of this chapter, each independently arising tumor (spontaneous or induced) is a separate and unique biologic entity. Thus, the strategy of essentially all investigators in this field is not to depend on any one tumor model. With this in mind, the more tumors that respond, respond at more than one dose level, and respond markedly, the more likely the agent will be clinically useful.

13. FINAL COMMENT

In a review of past practices and models, it is difficult not to make parts of the discussion sound like a condemnation. Such is not the intention, and it is overwhelmingly obvious that the individuals involved were as anxious to find active antitumor agents as current investigators. There is clearly no "absolutely right way to discover antitumor agents," as witnessed by the enormous array of rodent models and protocol designs that have been used in the discovery of agents currently in clinical usage. We simply have our own bias, since we are intimately involved in a discovery program and have had some successes in using these approaches *(30)*. In addition, we are also the benefactors of hindsight, and have seen the problems in dealing with a bewildering array of variable and changeable tumor model systems, as well as a disease entity that is nearly a black box. It is a virtual certainty that the future will reveal that many of our current opinions are highly flawed and that most of the models in use are only partially predictive. We can only marvel at the dedication, perseverance, and hard work that went into the discovery of so many good agents that are responsible for curing some fraction of at least 14 different tumor types in humans.

ACKNOWLEDGMENT

This work was supported by the Barbara Ann Karmanos Cancer Institute and Wayne State University School of Medicine, Detroit, MI.

ADDENDUM

This chapter was published in 1997 (and has been reproduced intact since the general concepts and testing methodology remain unchanged). However, newer agents have been discovered using this methodology. Thus, the following referenced publications are recommended to the reader for an update on the evaluations of these agents (46–56). These newer publications also include additional tumor models that we considered useful secondary evaluation of antitumor agents.

REFERENCES

1. Corbett T, Valeriote F, Baker L. Is the P388 murine tumor no longer adequate as a drug discovery model? *Invest New Drugs* 1987; 5:3–20.
2. Corbett TH, Valeriote FA. Rodent models in experimental chemotherapy, In: Kallman RF, ed. *The Use of Rodent Tumors in Experimental Cancer Therapy: Conclusions and Recommendations*. Pergamon. 1987: 233–247.
3. Corbett TH, Griswold DP Jr, Roberts BJ, Peckham JC, Schabel FM Jr. Evaluation of single agents and combinations of chemotherapeutic agents in mouse colon carcinomas. *Cancer* 1977; 40:2660–2680.
4. Corbett TH, Griswold DP, Roberts BJ, Peckham JC, Schabel FM Jr. Biology and therapeutic response of a mouse mammary adenocarcinoma (16/C) and its potential as a model for surgical adjuvant chemotherapy. *Cancer Treat Rep* 1978; 62:1471–1488.
5. Corbett TH, Roberts BJ, Leopold WR, Peckham JC, Wükoff LJ, Griswold DP Jr, Schabel FM Jr. Induction and chemotherapeutic response of two transplantable ductal adenocarcinomas of the pancreas in C57BL/6 mice. *Cancer Res* 1984; 44:717–726.
6. Corbett TH, Griswold DP Jr, Roberts BJ, Peckham JC, Schabel FM Jr. Tumor induction relationships in development of transplantable cancers of the colon in mice for chemotherapy asays, with a note on carcinogen structure. *Cancer Res* 1975; 35:2434–2439.
7. Corbett TH, Griswold DP Jr, Roberts BJ, Schabel FM Jr. Cytotoxic adjuvant therapy and the experimental model. In: Stoll BA, ed. *New Aspects of Breast Cancer vol. 4. Systemic Therapy in Breast Cancer*. London: William Heinemann Medical Books. 1981:204–243.
8. Pitot HC, Shires TK, Moyer G, Garret CT. Phenotypic variability as a manifestation of translational control. In: Busch H, ed. *The Molecular Biology of Cancer*. London: Academic. 1974: 524–533.
9. Hirshberg E. Patterns of response of animal tumors to anticancer agents: a systematic analysis of the literature in experimental cancer chemotherapy—1945–1958. *Cancer Res* 1963; 23:521–1084.
10. Griswold DG, Laster WR Jr, Snow MY, Schabel FM Jr, Skipper HE. Experimental evaluation of potential anticancer agents. XII. Quantitative drug response of the SA180, CA755, and leukemia L1210 systems to a "standard list" of "active" and "inactive" agents. *Cancer Res* 1963; 23:271–521.
11. Skipper HE, Wilcox WS, Schabel FM Jr, Laster WR Jr, Mattil L. Experimental evaluation of potential anticancer agents. X. A specific test for distinguishing false positives. *Cancer Chemother Rep* 1963; 29:1–62.
12. Heston WE. Genetics: Animal Tumors. In: Becker FF, ed. *Cancer, A Comprehensive Treatise*, vol. 1. New York: Plenum. 1975:33–57.
13. Pott P. Cancer of the scrotum. In: *Chirurgical Observations*. London: Hawkes, Clarke, and Collons. 1775:63–68.
14. Hanau A. Erfolgreiche experimentelle ubertragung von karzinom. *Fortschr Med.* 1889; 9:5–12.

15. Staats J. Standardized nomenclature for inbred strains of mice: eighth listing. *Cancer Res* 1985; 45:945–977.
16. Yamagawa K, Ichikawa K. Experimentelle studie uber die pathogenese der epithelialgeschwulste. *Mitteilungen Med Facultat Kaiserl Univ Tokyo* 1915; 15:295–344.
17. Kennaway E. The identification of a carcinogenic compound in coal-tar. *BMJ* 1975; 2:749–752.
18. Zubrod CG. Historic milestones in curative chemotherapy. *Semin Oncol* 1979; 6:490–505.
19. Goldin A, Schepartz SA, Venditti JM, DeVita VT. Historical development and current strategy of the National Cancer Institute drug development program, Chapter V. *Methods in Cancer Res* 1979; 16:165–245.
20. Schabel FM Jr. Laboratory methods for the detection and development of clinically useful anticancer drugs. In: Burchenal JH, Oettgen HF, eds. *Cancer: Achievements, Challenges, and Prospects for the 1980's*, vol. 2. New York: Grüne & Stratton. 1981: pp. 9–26.
21. Venditti JM. The National Cancer Institute antitumor drug discovery program, current and future perspectives: a commentary. *Cancer Treat Rep* 1983; 67:767–772.
22. Venditti JM, Wesley RA, Plowman J. Current NCI preclinical antitumor screening in vivo: results of tumor panel screening, 1976-1982, and future directions. In: Garattini S, Coldin A, Hawking F, eds. *Advances in Pharmacology and Chemotherapy*, vol. 20. Orlando, FL: Academic. 1984:1–20.
23. Zee-Cheng RKY, Cheng CC. Screening and evaluation of anticancer agents. *Methods Findings Exp Clin Pharmacol* 1988; 10:67–101.
24. Boyd MR. Status of the NCI preclinical antitumor drug discovery screen. *Principles Prac Oncol* 1989; 3:1–12.
25. Boyd MR. The future of new drug development. In: Neiderhuber JE, ed. *Current Therapy in Oncology*. Philadelphia: B.C. Decker. 1993: 11–22.
26. Frei E HI. The national cancer chemotherapy program. *Science* 1982; 217:600–606.
27. Han IR, Talmadge JE, Fidler IJ. Metastatic behavior of a murine reticulum cell sarcoma exhibiting organ-specific growth. *Cancer Res* 1981; 41:1281–1287.
28. LoRusso PM, Polín L, Aukerman SL, Redman BG, Valdivieso M, Biernat L, Corbett TH. Antitumor efficacy of Interleukin-2 alone and in combination with Adriamycin and Dacarbazine in murine solid tumor systems. *Cancer Res* 1990; 50:5876–5882.
29. Corbett TH, Valeriote FA, Polin L, et al. Discovery of solid tumor active agents using a soft agar colony formation disk-diffusion assay. In: Valeriote, FA Corbett TH, Baker LH, eds. *Cytotoxic Anticancer Drugs: Models and Concepts/ok, Drug Discovery and Development*. Boston/Dordrecht, London: Kluwer Academic Publishers. 1992: 33–87.
30. Corbett TH, Valeriote F, LoRusso P, Polin L, et al. Tumor models and the discovery and secondary evaluation of solid tumor active agents. *Int J Pharmacognosy* 1995; 33(suppl.):102–122.
31. Grindey GB. Current status of cancer drug development: failure or limited success? *Cancer Cells* 1990; 2:163–171.
32. Stahelin H, von Wartburg A. The chemical and biological route for Podophyllotoxin Glucoside to Etoposide: Ninth Cain Memorial Award Lecture. *Cancer Res* 1991; 51:5–15.
33. Corbett TH, Leopold WR, Dykes DJ, Roberts BJ, Griswold DP Jr, Schabel FM Jr. Toxicity and anticancer activity of a new triazine antifolate (NSC-127755). *Cancer Res* 1982; 42:1707–1715.
34. Corbett TH, Bissery M-C, LoRusso P-M, Polin L. 5-Fluorouracil containing combinations in murine tumor systems. *Invest New Drugs* 1989; 7:37–49.
35. LoRusso PM, Wozniak AJ, Polin L, Capps D, Leopold WR, Werbel LM, Biernat L, Dan ME, Corbett TH. Antitumor efficacy of PD115934 (NSC 366140) against solid tumors of mice. *Cancer Res* 1990; 50:4900–4905.
36. Corbett TH, Roberts BJ, Trader MW, Laster WR Jr, Griswold DP Jr, Schabel FM Jr. Response of transplantable tumors of mice to anthracenedione derivatives alone and in combination with clinically useful agents. *Cancer Treat Rep* 1982; 66:1187–1200.
37. Schabel FM Jr, Skipper HE, Trader MW, Laster WR Jr, Griswold DP Jr, Corbett TH. Establishment of cross-resistance profiles for new agents. *Cancer Treat Rep* 1983; 67:905–922.
38. Schabel FM Jr, Griswold DP Jr, Corbett TH, Laster WR Jr, Mayo JC, Lloyd HH. Testing therapeutic hypotheses in mice and man. Observations on the therapeutic activity against advanced solid tumors of mice treated with anticancer drugs that have demonstrated or potential clinical utility for treatment of advanced solid tumors of man. In: Busch H, DeVita V Jr, eds. *Cancer Drug Development. PartB. Methods in Cancer Research*, vol. 17. New York: Academic. 1979:3–51.

39. Corbett T, Lowichik N, Pugh S, et al. Antitumor activity of N-[[l-[[2-(diethylamino)ethyl] amino]-9-oxo-9H-Thioxanthen-4-yl]methyl]methanesulfonamide (WIN33377) and analogs. *Exp Opin Invest Drugs* 1994; 3:1281–1292.

40. Corbett TH, Roberts BJ, Lawson AJ, Leopold WR III. Curative chemotherapy of advanced and disseminated solid tumors of mice. In: Jacobs JR, Al-Sarraf M, Crissman J, Valeriote F, eds. *Scientific and Clinical Perspectives in Head and Neck Cancer Management: Strategies for Cure.* New York: Elsevier Scientific Publishing. 1987:175–192.

41. Wentland MP, Perni RB, Powles RG, Hlavac AG, Mattes KC, Corbett TH, Coughlin SA, Rake JB. Anti-solid tumor efficacy and preparation of N-[[l-[[2-(Diethylamino)ethyl]amino] -9-Oxo-9H-Thioxanthen-4-Yl]methyl]methanesulfonamide (Win 33377) and related derivatives. *Bioorganic Med Chem Lett* 1994; 4(4):609–614.

42. Horwitz JP, Massova I, Wiese TE, Besler BH, Corbett TH. Comparative molecular field analysis of the tumor activity of 9H-Thioxanthen-9-one derivatives against pancreatic ductal carcinoma 03. *J Med Chem* 1994; 37:781–786.

43. LoRusso PM, Polín L, Biernat LA, Valeriote FA, Corbett TH. Activity of detallilptinium (NSC 311152) against solid tumors of mice. *Invest New Drugs* 1990; 8:253–261.

44. Bissery M-C, Gurnard D, Gueritte-Voegelein F, Lavelle F. Experimental antitumor activity of taxotere (RP 56976, NSC-628503), a Taxol analog. *Cancer Res* 1991; 51:4845–4852.

45. Annual Progress Report to Division of Cancer Treatment, National Cancer Institute on Primary Screening and Development and Application of Secondary Evaluation Procedures for Study of New Materials with Potential Anticancer Activity. Section 21. Evaluation of Single Agents and Combinations of Chemotherapeutic Agents in Mouse Colon Carcinomas. Southern Research Institute, Contract NO1-CM-43756, March 15, 1982.

46. Corbett TH, Valeriote FA, Demchik L, et al. Preclinical anticancer activity of cryptophycin-8. *J Exp Ther Oncol* 1996; 1:95–108.

47 Polin L, Valeriote F, White K, et al. Treatment of human prostate tumors PC-3 and TSU-PR1 with standard and investigational agents in SCID mice. *Invest New Drugs* 1997; 15:99–108.

48. Corbett TH, Valeriote FA, Demchik L, et al. Discovery of cryptophycin-1 and BCN-183577: Examples of strategies and problems in the detection of antitumor activity in mice. *Invest New Drugs* 1997; 15:207–218.

49. Corbett TH, LoRusso P, Demchik L, et al. Preclinical antitumor efficacy of analogs of XK-469:Sodium-(2-{4-[(7-chloro-2-quinoxalinyl)oxy]phenoxy}propionate. *Invest New Drugs* 1998; 16:129–139.

50. Corbett TH, Panchapor C, Polin L, et al. Preclinical efficacy of thioxanthone SR-271425 against transplanted solid tumors of mouse and human origin. *Invest New Drugs* 1999; 17:17–27.

51. Corbett TH, Polin L, Roberts BJ, et al. Transplantable syngeneic rodent tumors: solid tumors of mice. In: Teicher B, ed. Tumor Models in Cancer Research. Totowa, NJ: Humana Press Inc. 2001:41–71.

52. Hazeldine ST, Polin L, Kushner J, et al. Design, synthesis and biological evaluation of some analogues of the antitumor agent 2-{4-[(7-chloro-2 quinoxalinyl)oxy]phenoxy}propionic acid (XK469). *J Med Chem* 2001; 44:1758–1776.

53. Polin L, White K, Kushner J, et al. Preclinical efficacy evaluations of XK-469: Dose schedule, route and cross-resistance behavior in tumor bearing mice. *Invest New Drugs* 2002; 20:13–22.

54. Hazeldine ST, Polin L, Kushner J, et al. II. Synthesis and biological evaluation of some bioisosteres and congeners of the antitumor agent, 2-{4-[(7-chloro-2 quinoxalinyl)oxy]phenoxy}propionic acid (XK469). *J Med Chem* 2002; 45:3130–3137.

55. Corbett TH, White K, Polin L, et al. Discovery and preclinical antitumor efficacy evaluations of LY32262 and LY33169. *Invest New Drugs* 2003; 21:33–45.

56. Liang J, Moore RE, Moher E, et al. Cryptophycin-309 and other cryptophycin analogs: Preclinical efficacy studies with mouse and human tumors. *Invest New Drugs* 2003; accepted.

7

Human Tumor Xenograft Models in NCI Drug Development

Michael C. Alley, PhD,

Melinda G. Hollingshead, DVM, PhD,

Donald J. Dykes, BS, and William R. Waud, PhD

CONTENTS

INTRODUCTION
HISTORICAL DEVELOPMENT OF NCI SCREENS
HUMAN TUMOR XENOGRAFT MODELS IN CURRENT USE
STRATEGY FOR INITIAL COMPOUND EVALUATION IN VIVO
STRATEGY AND EXAMPLES OF DETAILED DRUG EVALUATION
ALTERNATIVE MODELS: NEW APPROACHES TO IN VIVO DRUG TESTING
CONCLUSIONS

1. INTRODUCTION

The methods used by the National Cancer Institute (NCI) for in vivo preclinical development of anticancer drugs were described in detail in the first edition of this book (1). In addition, a series of review articles have charted the evolution of the overall NCI drug discovery process, which began in 1955 (2–12). Although the methodologies associated with xenograft model testing have remained fundamentally the same, during the past 10 yr a series of improvements to preclinical drug testing to expedite in vivo drug development have been made that now precede the employment of xenograft models in the in vivo drug development process. These specialized assays are described in Chapter 8. For the sake of completeness, the present chapter provides (1) a brief history of the in vivo screens used by the NCI, (2) a description of the human tumor xenograft systems that are employed in preclinical drug development, and (3) a discussion of how these xenograft models are employed for both initial efficacy testing as well as detailed drug evaluations.

From: *Cancer Drug Discovery and Development:*
Anticancer Drug Development Guide: Preclinical Screening, Clinical Trials, and Approval, 2nd Ed.
Edited by: B. A. Teicher and P. A. Andrews © Humana Press Inc., Totowa, NJ

2. HISTORICAL DEVELOPMENT OF NCI SCREENS

Analyses of various screening methods available prior to 1955 indicated that (1) nontumor systems were incapable of replacing tumor systems as screens and (2) no single tumor system was capable of detecting all active antitumor compounds *(13)*. Since that time, the preclinical discovery and development process of potentially useful anticancer agents by the NCI has utilized a variety of animal and human tumor models, not only for initial screening but also for subsequent studies designed to optimize antitumor activity of a lead compound or class of compounds. Although the various preclinical data review steps and criteria have remained essentially the same throughout the years, the modes and rationale of in vivo testing employed by the NCI have evolved significantly.

2.1. Murine Tumor Screens, 1955–1975

In 1955, the NCI initiated a large-scale in vivo anticancer drug screening program utilizing three murine tumor models: sarcoma 180, L1210 leukemia, and carcinoma 755. By 1960, in vivo drug screening was performed in L1210 and in two additional rodent models selected from a battery of 21 possible models. In 1965, screening was limited to the use of two rodent systems, L1210 and Walker 256 carcinosarcoma. In 1968, synthetic agents were screened in L1210 alone, whereas natural product testing was conducted in both L1210 and P388 leukemias. A special testing step was added to the screen in 1972 to evaluate active compounds against B16 melanoma and Lewis lung carcinoma. It is noteworthy that this first 20 yr of in vivo screening relied heavily on testing conducted in the L1210 model.

2.2 Prescreen and Tumor Panel, 1976–1986

In late 1975, the NCI initiated a new approach that involved prescreening of compounds in the ip-implanted murine P388 leukemia model, followed by evaluation of selected compounds in a panel of transplantable tumors *(14)*. The tumors in the panel were chosen as representative of the major histologic types of cancer in the United States and, for the first time in NCI history, included human solid tumors. The latter was made possible through the development of immunodeficient athymic (nu/nu) mice and transplantable human tumor xenografts in the early 1970s *(15,16)*. Beginning in 1976, the tumor panel consisted of paired murine and human tumors of breast (CD8F$_1$ and MX-1), colon (colon 38 and CX-1 [the same as HT29]), and lung (Lewis and LX-1), together with the B16 melanoma and L1210 leukemia used in previous screens.

Most of the early NCI testing conducted with the human tumors used small fragments growing under the renal capsule of athymic mice. This subrenal capsule (src) technique and assay were developed by Bogden and associates *(17)*. Although it is labor-intensive, the src assay provided a rapid means of evaluating new agents against human tumor xenografts at a time when the testing of large numbers of compounds against sc xenografts seemed untenable. As experience was gained with the husbandry of athymic mice, longer duration sc assays became manageable.

A detailed evaluation of the sensitivities of individual tumor systems employed from 1976 to 1982 revealed a wide range in sensitivity profiles as well as "yield" of active compounds *(14)*. The data clearly indicated that rodent models may not be capable of detecting all compounds with potential activity against human malignancies and also indicated that the best strategy for testing is to employ a combination of tumor systems to minimize the loss of potentially useful compounds. These findings prompted the NCI in 1982 to develop a strategy for testing compounds that involved a sequential process of "progressive selection": the NCI continued to use the P388 leukemia as a prescreen, but subsequent evaluation of selected agents was conducted in a modified tumor panel composed of "high-yield" models from the original panel (i.e., src-implanted MX-1 mammary carcinoma and ip-implanted B16 melanoma and L1210 leukemia) and a new model, the ip-implanted M5076 sarcoma. Thereafter, evaluation of selected compounds would be compound-oriented and would use protocols and models, selected on the basis of prior testing results and known properties of each compound, that would present the compound with increased biological and pharmacological challenge.

Alternate approaches to in vivo drug evaluation have been prompted by investigations on the metastatic heterogeneity of tumor cell populations. During the 1980s, several investigators associated with the NCI conducted studies to assess the metastatic potential of selected murine and human tumor cell lines (B16, A-375, and LOX-IMVI melanomas and PC-3 prostate adenocarcinoma) and their suitability for experimental drug evaluation *(18–21)*. A series of investigations by Fidler and associates *(22,23)* has demonstrated that metastasis is not random, but selective, and that metastasis consists of a progression of sequential steps the pattern of which is dependent on the injection site. Such findings support the establishment of in vivo models by implantation of tumor material into host tissues that are anatomically correct, e.g., colon tumors are implanted into the colon, giving "seed" and "soil" compatibility. Such "orthotopic" models have been developed and utilized to study lung cancer *(24)*, breast cancer *(25)*, and prostate cancer *(26)*. Routine application of these models is often limited by the greater costs, both in time and resources, that are required. Thus, the NCI does not routinely employ them in the initial steps of in vivo drug evaluations. However, these models are employed for subsequent, more detailed evaluations of compounds that exhibit activity in preliminary assays. One notable feature of the orthotopic models, is their superiority in some efficacy trials when the pharmacodynamic behavior of a compound suggests poor distribution to the subcutaneous tissues. Metastases and orthotopic models are discussed in greater detail in Chapters 8 and 9.

2.3. Human Tumor Colony Formation Assay, 1981–1985

Based on initial reports by Salmon and colleagues *(27,28)*, various clinical investigators working with fresh human tumor samples from patients and/or with early-passage human tumor xenograft materials utilized various culture techniques to identify chemotherapeutic agents active against human malignancies *(29,30)*. The NCI sponsored a pilot drug screening project using a human tumor colony-forming assay (HTCFA) at multiple clinical cancer centers. Although it was possible to identify unique antitumor drug "leads" using such a technique, the HTCFA could be employed only for a limited number of tumor types and was not suitable for large-scale drug screening *(31)*.

2.4. Human Tumor Cell Line Screen, 1985–present

In 1985, the NCI initiated a new project to assess the feasibility of employing human tumor cell lines for large-scale drug screening *(12; see also* Chapter 24 of this monograph). Cell lines derived from seven cancer types (brain, colon, leukemia, lung, melanoma, ovarian, and renal) were acquired from a wide range of sources, cryopreserved, and subjected to a battery of in vitro and in vivo characterizations, including testing in drug sensitivity assays. The approach was deemed suitable for large-scale drug screening in 1990 *(1)*. With the implementation of a 60-member cell line in vitro screen, in vivo testing procedures were substantially altered, as discussed below.

3. HUMAN TUMOR XENOGRAFT MODELS IN CURRENT USE

The new in vitro human tumor cell line screen shifted the NCI screening strategy from a compound-oriented to a disease-oriented process of drug discovery *(12)*. Compounds of interest, identified by the screen (e.g., those demonstrating disease-specific differential cytotoxicity), were considered *leads*, requiring further preclinical evaluation to determine their therapeutic potential. As part of this follow-up testing, the antitumor efficacy of the compounds was to be evaluated in in vivo tumor models derived from the in vitro tumor lines used in the screen. Although only a subset of cell lines, selected on the basis of in vitro sensitivity, would be used for each agent, it was anticipated that a selected compound might require any of the 60 cell lines as a xenograft model. To accomplish such an objective, a concerted developmental effort was required to establish a battery of human tumor xenograft models. As discussed in the next section and elsewhere *(32)*, tumorigenicity was established for most of the tumor lines utilized in the in vitro screen that became fully operational in April 1990 *(1)*. Then, in 1993, the composition of the cell line screen was modified: cell lines with variable growth characteristics, and those providing redundant information, were replaced by groups of prostate and breast tumor lines. As a consequence, additional xenograft development was initiated for prostate and breast cancers.

3.1. Development of Human Tumor Xenografts

Efforts focused on the establishment of sc xenografts from human tumor cell culture lines obtained from the NCI tumor repository at Frederick, MD. The approach is outlined in Fig. 1. The cryopreserved cell lines were thawed, cultured in RPMI-1640 medium supplemented with 10% heat-inactivated fetal bovine serum (HyClone), and expanded until the population was sufficient to harvest $\geq 10^8$ cells. Cells were harvested and then implanted sc into the axillary region of ten athymic NCr nu/nu mice (1.0×10^7 cells/0.5 mL/ mouse) obtained from the NCI animal program, Frederick, MD. Mice were housed in sterile, polycarbonate, filter-capped Microisolator™ cages (Lab. Products), maintained in a barrier facility on 12-h light/dark cycles, and provided with sterilized food and water *ad libitum*. The implanted animals were observed twice weekly for tumor appearance. Growth of the solid tumors was monitored using *in situ* caliper measurements to determine tumor mass. Weights (in mg) were calculated from measurements (in mm) of two perpendicular dimensions (length and width) using the formula for a prolate ellipsoid and assuming a specific gravity of 1.0 g/cm^3 *(33)*. Fragments of these tumors were subjected to histological, cytochemical, and ultrastructural examination to monitor the characteristics of the in vivo material and to compare them with those of the in vitro lines and, where possible, with those reported for initial patient tumors *(34)*. Both in vitro and in vivo tumor materials exhibited characteristics consistent with tissue type and tumor of origin. However, not unexpectedly, differences in the degree of differentiation were noted between some of the cultured cell lines and corresponding xenograft materials.

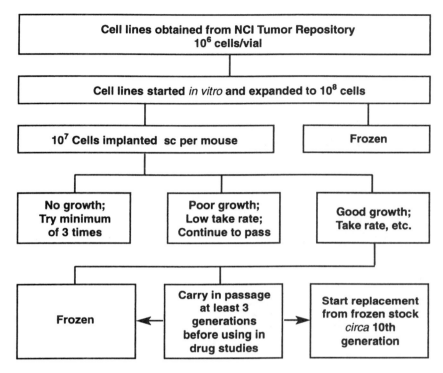

Fig. 1. Schematic of the development of in vivo models for drug evaluation.

The initial solid tumors established in mice were maintained by serial passage of 30–40-mg tumor fragments implanted sc near the axilla. There was an apparent cell population selection occurring in some of the tumors as they adapted to growth in animals during early in vivo passage, with growth rates increasing appreciably in sequential passages *(32)*. Thus, xenografts were not utilized for drug evaluation until the volume-doubling time stabilized, usually around the fourth or fifth passage. The doubling time of xenografts derived from tumor cell lines constituting both the initial (1990) and the modified (1993) human tumor cell line screens, plus three additional breast tumors, is presented in Table 1. Also provided in the table is information on the take rate of the tumors and the experience of the NCI in the use of the tumors as early-stage sc models. The doubling times were determined from vehicle-treated control mice used in drug evaluation experiments (only data for passage numbers 4–20 have been included). For each experiment, the doubling time is the median of the time interval for individual tumors to increase in size from 200 to 400 mg (usually a period of exponential growth). Both ranges and mean values are provided to demonstrate the inherent variability of growth for some of the xenograft materials even after a period of stabilization. Mean doubling times range from <2 d for five tumors (SF-295 glioblastoma, MOLT 4 leukemia, DMS 273 small-cell lung tumor, LOX-IMVI, and SK-MEL-28 melanomas) to >10 d for the MALME-3M and M19-MEL melanomas.

Difficulty was experienced in establishing and/or using some of the sc models. For example, even though HOP-62 nonsmall-cell lung tumors exhibited good growth rates, poor take rates of 70, 50, 64, and 30% attained in the second through fifth passages,

Table 1
Growth Characteristics of sc-Implanted Human Tumor Xenografts

Tumor origin	Line	In vitro panel status		Mean volume doubling time (range) in days[a]	Take rate[b]	Opinion for use as early-stage sc model
		1990	2002			
Colon	SW-620	Yes	Yes	2.4 (1.7–3.9)	Good	Good
	KM12	Yes	Yes	2.4 (1.9–3.3)	Good	Good
	HCT-116	Yes	Yes	2.6 (1.8–3.4)	Good	Good
	HCT-15	Yes	Yes	3.4 (1.8–5.0)	Good	Good
	HCC-2998	Yes	Yes	3.5 (2.4–7.7)	Good	Acceptable
	DLD-1	Yes	No	3.8 (3.1–5.5)	Good	Acceptable
	KM20L2	Yes	No	3.9 (2.5–5.4)	Good	Acceptable
	COLO 205	Yes	Yes	4.3 (2.4–8.9)	Good	Acceptable
	HT29	Yes	Yes	5.1 (2.4–7.6)	Good	Acceptable
CNS	SF-295	Yes	Yes	1.4 (1.0–2.0)	Good	Good
	SNB-75	Yes	Yes	3.1 (2.0–4.6)	Good	Good
	U251	Yes	Yes	4.3 (2.4–8.9)	Good	Good
	XF 498	Yes	No	4.4 (2.6–8.3)	60–70%	Not acceptable
	SNB-19	Yes	Yes	6.9 (3.1–4.4)	60–70%	Not acceptable
	SF-539	Yes	Yes	8.4 (one only)	70%	Not acceptable
	SF-268	Yes	Yes	NA	Minimal growth	NA
	SNB-78	Yes	No	NA	No growth	NA
Leukemia	MOLT-4	Yes	Yes	1.2 (2.0–5.6)	80–100%	Acceptable
	HL-60(TB)[c]	Yes	Yes	3.3 (2.1–4.9, ip)	85–100% (ip)	Good (ip)
	CCRF-CEM	Yes	Yes	4.6 (4.3–4.6)	60–80%	Acceptable
	SR	Yes	Yes	5.1 (one only)	80%	Not acceptable
	RPMI-8226	Yes	Yes	NA	Minimal growth	NA
	K-562	Yes	Yes	NA	Minimal growth	NA

Lung, nonsmall cell	NCI-H460	Yes	Yes	2.1 (1.3–3.0)	Good	Good
	NCI-H522	Yes	Yes	2.3 (1.0–3.4)	Good	Good
	HOP-62	Yes	Yes	3.6 (3.3–3.8)	30–65%	Not acceptable
	NCI-H23	Yes	Yes	3.7 (2.0–6.4)	Good	Good
	NCI-H322M	Yes	Yes	4.0 (2.7–5.9)	Good	Acceptable
	EKVX	Yes	Yes	5.5 (3.5–7.9)	Good	Acceptable
	HOP-92	Yes	Yes	6.0 (5.1–8.4)	Good	Acceptable
	A549/ATCC	Yes	Yes	8.4 (5.8–10.9)	70–80%	Not acceptable
	HOP-18	Yes	No	NA	Minimal growth	NA
	NCI-H266	Yes	Yes	NA	Minimal growth	NA
Lung, small cell	DMS273	Yes	No	1.7 (1.6–2.1)	Good	Good
	DMS114	Yes	No	4.8 (2.8–7.5)	75–90%	Acceptable
Mammary	ZR-75-1	No	No	1.8 (1.5–1.9)	Good	Good
	MX-1	No	No	2.7 (2.2–3.0)	Good	Good
	UISO-BCA-1	No	No	4.1 (2.8–4.8)	Good	Acceptable
	MDA-MB-231/ATCC	No	Yes	4.4 (2.7–7.7)	Good	Acceptable
	MCF-7^d	No	Yes	4.5 (2.2–8.0)	Good	Acceptable
	MCF-7/ADR-RES	No	Yes	6.1 (4.2–7.9)	Good	Acceptable
	MDA-MB-435^e	No	Yes	6.6 (2.8–13.6)	Good	Acceptable
	MDA-N	Yes	No	7.9 (4.5–10.2)	Good	Acceptable
	HS578T	No	Yes	NA	Minimal growth	NA
	BT-549	No	Yes	NA	No growth	NA
	T-47D	No	Yes	NA	No growth	NA
Melanoma	LOX-IMVI	Yes	Yes	1.5 (1.1–2.1)	Good	Good
	SK-MEL-28	Yes	Yes	1.9 (1.1–2.5)	Good	Good
	UACC-62	Yes	Yes	2.8 (1.8–4.2)	70–80%	Not acceptable
	UACC-257	Yes	Yes	5.4 (3.8–7.7)	Good	Acceptable
	SK-MEL-2	Yes	Yes	5.7 (4.8–6.6)	80–90%	Not acceptable
	M14	Yes	Yes	6.7 (2.8–12.7)	Good	Acceptable
	SK-MEL-5	Yes	Yes	7.3 (5.1–8.2)	Good	Acceptable
	MALME-3M	Yes	Yes	11.2 (7.1–16.9)	80–90%	Not acceptable
	M19-MEL	Yes	No	12.3 (8.7–16.8)	60–90%	Not acceptable

(Continued)

131

Table 1

Growth Characteristics of sc-Implanted Human Tumor Xenografts

Tumor origin	Line	In vitro panel status 1990	In vitro panel status 2002	Mean volume doubling time (range) in days[a]	Take rate[b]	Opinion for use as early-stage sc model
Ovarian	OVCAR-5	Yes	Yes	3.3 (2.2–4.3)	Good	Good
	SK-OV-3	Yes	Yes	3.4 (2.6–4.9)	Good	Good
	OVCAR-3[f]	Yes	Yes	5.5 (5.0–5.9)	Good	Acceptable
	OVCAR-4	Yes	Yes	6.2 (one only)	70–100%	Acceptable
	IGROV1	Yes	Yes	6.4 (5.3–8.6)	Good	Acceptable
	OVCAR-8	Yes	Yes	12.2 (11.2–13.0)	70%	Not acceptable
Prostate	PC-3	No	Yes	2.4 (1.5–3.9)	Good	Good
	DU-145	No	Yes	4.4 (2.0–7.9)	Good	Acceptable
Renal	CAKI-1	Yes	Yes	2.1 (1.3–2.5)	Good	Good
	RXF 631	Yes	No	3.3 (1.5–6.8)	Good	Acceptable
	A498	Yes	Yes	3.4 (2.2–4.3)	Good	Acceptable
	RXF 393	Yes	Yes	3.4 (2.3–5.7)	Good	Good
	SN12C	Yes	Yes	5.6 (3.2–11.4)	Good	Acceptable
	786-0	Yes	Yes	6.7 (one only)	80%	Not acceptable
	ACHN	Yes	Yes	NA	Minimal growth	NA
	UO-31	Yes	Yes	NA	Minimal growth	NA
	TK-10	Yes	Yes	NA	No growth	NA

ABBREVIATIONS: CNS, central nervous system; NA, not applicable.

[a]Time for tumors to increase in size from 200 to 400 mg. Data are compiled from experiments using passage numbers 4–20. Tumors are listed in order of increasing mean doubling time per histologic type.

[b]Good: reproducible take rate of ≥90%.

[c]Based on ip implant of 1.0×10^7 cells.

[d]MCF7 growth in athymic NCr nu/nu mice requires 17β-estradiol supplementation.

[e]NCI 60-cell line panel revealed that the pattern of gene expression for this cell line more closely resembles that of melanoma cell lines than that of other breast tumor cell lines (65,66).

[f]Limited sc data obtained from implant of 0.5 mL 25% brei derived from ip-passaged tumor: poor growth is attained with serial passage of fragments from sc tumors.

respectively, precluded their use for experimental drug testing. Although serial passage of OVCAR-3 ovarian tumors from sc-implanted fragments was difficult, tumors grew more readily from sc implants of brei derived from ip-passaged material. Growth characteristics of sc-implanted RXF 393 renal tumors are perhaps more suited for evaluation of a survival endpoint than for measurements of tumor size. Although demonstrating good initial growth, the RXF 393 tumors cause death in mice with low tumor burden, probably owing to paraneoplastic mechanisms. Other cell lines failed to become functional in vivo tumors, including two central nervous system (CNS), two nonsmall-cell lung, three breast and three renal tumor lines, and two leukemias, although minimal in vivo growth was observed with 9 of these 12 cultured lines (Table 1). With more extensive studies, it might be possible to attain improved tumor take rates and growth by implanting tumors in severe combined immunodeficient (SCID) mice (scid/scid) (35). As discussed below, tumor take rates for some human lymphoma lines were markedly superior in SCID mice compared with athymic (nu/nu) (36) or triple-deficient BNX (bg/nu/xid) mice (37).

Establishment of breast tumor xenografts in vivo raised issues concerning hormonal requirements for growth of these tumors. For example, the importance of hormones in the growth of MCF7 breast carcinoma cells as solid tumors in athymic mice has been described (38). Our experience with this tumor has also shown the importance of 17β-estradiol supplementation for the growth of the sc-implanted MCF7. Growth of the remaining breast tumor xenografts can be achieved independently of estradiol supplements, although some lines may perform better in the presence of estradiol supplementation since the in vitro cell lines have been characterized as estrogen receptor (ER)+ (39).

The in vivo growth characteristics of the xenografts determine their suitability for use in the evaluation of test agent antitumor activity, particularly when the xenografts are utilized as early-stage sc models. For the purposes of the current discussion, the latter model is defined as one in which tumors are staged to 63–200 mg prior to the initiation of treatment. Our experience with the suitability of the xenografts as early-stage models is listed in Table 1. Growth characteristics considered in rating tumors include take rate, time to reach 200 mg, doubling time, and susceptibility to spontaneous regression. As can be noted, the faster growing tumors tend to receive the higher ratings.

Since non-Hodgkin's lymphoma is one of the two principal malignancies occurring in the growing population of HIV-infected persons (40), the Developmental Therapeutics Program (DTP) also established a group of human lymphoma xenografts for evaluating potential chemotherapeutic agents (41). This includes an Epstein-Barr virus (EBV)-positive, HIV-negative Burkitt's lymphoma derived from an AIDS patient (AS283) (42); an EBV-negative pediatric Burkitt's lymphoma (KD488) (43–46); and a diffuse, small noncleaved B-cell lymphoma (RL) (47). These lines grow sc with take rates in excess of 90% in SCID mice, whereas much lower take rates occur in athymic or triple-deficient BNX mice. Our finding of greater take rates for the human leukemias/lymphomas in SCID mice compared with athymic mice is consistent with the known capacity of SCID mice to support xenografts of normal human hematopoietic cells (48).

3.2. Advanced-Stage sc Xenograft Models

Advanced-stage sc-implanted tumor xenograft models were established originally for use in evaluating the antitumor activity of test agents so that clinically relevant parameters of activity could be determined, i.e., partial and complete regressions, and durations of remission *(49–51)*. Tumor growth is monitored, and test agent treatment is initiated when tumors reach a weight range of 100–400 mg (staging day, median weights approx 200 mg), although, depending on the xenograft, tumors may be staged at larger sizes. Tumor size and body weights are obtained approx two times per week and entered into the DTP's VAX alpha 10,000 computer. Through software programs developed by staff of the Information Technology Branch of the DTP, in particular by David Segal and Penny Svetlik, data are stored, various parameters of effect are calculated, and data are presented in both graphic and tabular formats. Parameters of toxicity and antitumor activity are defined as follows.

1. *Parameters of toxicity.* Both drug-related deaths (DRDs) and maximum percent relative mean net body weight losses are determined. A treated animal death is presumed to be treatment-related if the animal dies within 15 d of the last treatment and either its tumor weight is less than the lethal burden in the control mice, or its net body weight loss at death is 20% greater than the mean net weight change of the controls at death or sacrifice. Other experimental observations may result in a death being designated a DRD by the investigator. To determine weight changes, the mean net body weight of each group of mice on each observation day is compared with their mean net body weight on the staging day. Any weight change that occurs is calculated as a percent of the staging day weight. These calculations are also performed for the control mice since tumor growth of some xenografts has an adverse effect on the weight of the mice.

2. *Optimal % T/C.* Changes in tumor weight (delta weights) for each treated (T) and control (C) group are calculated for each day tumors are measured by subtracting the median tumor weight on the day of first treatment (staging day) from the median tumor weight on the specified observation day. These values are used to calculate a percent T/C as follows:

$$\% \text{ T/C} = (\text{delta T/delta C}) \times 100 \qquad \text{where delta T} > 0, \text{ or}$$

$$= (\text{delta T/}T_I) \times 100 \qquad \text{where delta T} < 0$$

and T_I is the median tumor weight at the start of treatment. The optimum (minimum) value obtained after the end of the first course of treatment is used to quantitate antitumor activity.

3. *Tumor growth delay.* This is expressed as a percentage by which the treated group weight is delayed in attaining a specified number of doublings (from its staging day weight) compared with controls using the formula

$$[(\text{T} - \text{C})/\text{C}] \times 100$$

where T and C are the median times in days for treated and control groups, respectively, to attain the specified size (excluding tumor-free mice and DRDs). The growth delay is expressed as a percentage of control to account for the growth rate of the tumor since a growth delay based on T – C alone varies in significance with differences in tumor growth rates.

4. *Net log cell kill.* An estimate of the number of $\log_{10}$ units of cells killed at the end of treatment is calculated as

$$\frac{[(\text{T} - \text{C}) - \text{duration of treatment})] \times 0.301}{\text{median doubling time}}$$

where the doubling time is the time required for tumors to increase in size from 200 to 400 mg, 0.301 is the $\log_{10}$ of 2, and T and C are the median times in days for treated and control tumors to achieve the specified number of doublings. If the duration of treatment is 0, then it can be seen from the formulae for net log cell kill and percent growth delay that log cell kill is proportional to percent growth delay. A log cell kill of 0 indicates that the cell population at the end of treatment is the same as it was at the start of treatment. A log cell kill of +6 indicates a 99.9999% reduction in the cell population.

5. *Tumor regression.* The importance of tumor regression in animal models as an endpoint of clinical relevance has been propounded by several investigators *(49–51)*. Regressions are defined as partial if the tumor weight decreases to 50% or less of the tumor weight at the start of treatment without dropping below 63 mg (5×5-mm tumor). Both complete regressions (CRs) and tumor-free survivors are defined by instances in which the tumor burden falls below measurable limits (< 63 mg) during the experimental period. The two parameters differ by the observation of either tumor regrowth (CR) or no regrowth (tumor-free) prior to the final observation day. Although one can measure smaller tumors, the accuracy of measuring an sc tumor smaller than 4×4 or 5×5 mm (32 and 63 mg, respectively) is questionable. Also, once a relatively large tumor has regressed to 63 mg, the composition of the remaining mass may be only fibrous material/scar tissue. Measurement of tumor regrowth following cessation of treatment provides a more reliable indication of whether or not tumor cells survived treatment.

Most xenografts that grow sc are amenable to use as an advanced-stage model, although for some tumors the duration of the study may be limited by tumor necrosis. As mentioned previously, this model enables the investigator to measure clinically relevant parameters of antitumor activity, and provides a wealth of data on the effects of the test agent on tumor growth. Also, by staging day, the investigator knows that angiogenesis has occurred in the area of the tumor, and staging enables no-takes to be eliminated from the experiment. However, the model can be costly in terms of time and mice. For the more slowly growing tumors, the passage time required before sufficient mice can be implanted with tumors may be at least 3–4 wk, and an additional 2–3 wk may be required before the tumors can be staged. To stage tumors, more mice than needed for actual drug testing must be implanted, often 50%, and sometimes 100%, more.

3.3. Early-Treatment and Early-Stage sc Xenograft Models

Early-treatment and early-stage sc models are similar to the advanced-stage model, but, because treatment is initiated earlier in the development of the tumor, the models are not suitable for tumors that have less than a 90% take rate or have a greater than 10% spontaneous regression rate. We define the early-treatment model as one in which treatment is initiated before tumors are measurable, i.e., <63 mg, and the early-stage model as one in which treatment is initiated when tumor size ranges from 63 to 200 mg. The 63-mg size is used as an indication that the original implant of approx 30 mg has demonstrated some growth. Parameters of toxicity are the same as those for the advanced-stage model; parameters of antitumor activity are similar. Percent T/C values are calculated directly from the median tumor weights on each observation day instead of as changes (delta) in tumor weights, and growth delays are based on the time in days after implant for the tumors to reach a specified size, e.g., 500 or 1000 mg.

Tumor-free mice are recorded but may be designated no-takes or spontaneous regressions if the vehicle-treated control group contains more than 10% mice with similar growth characteristics. A no-take is a tumor that fails to become established and grow progressively. A spontaneous regression (graft failure) is a tumor that, after a period of growth, decreases to 50% or less of its maximum size. Tumor regressions are not normally recorded as they are not always a good indicator of antineoplastic effects in the early-stage model. For those experiments in which treatment is initiated when tumors are 100 mg or less, only a minimal reduction in tumor size may bring the tumor below the measurable limit; for some small tumors early in their growth, reductions in tumor size may reflect erratic growth rather than a true reflection of a cell killing effect. Advantages of the early-treatment model are the lower challenge level that a nonoptimized experimental agent has to impact for activity to be observed and the ability to use all implanted mice. The latter is the reason a good tumor take rate is required, and in practice the tumors most suitable for this model tend to be the faster growing ones.

3.4. Challenge Survival Models

Although they are not utilized to a significant degree in the current NCI program, a few studies are conducted that depend on determining the effect of human tumor growth on the life span of the host. Three tumors have been used as ip-implanted models: the HL-60 (TB) promyelocytic leukemia, the LOX-IMVI melanoma, and the OVCAR-3 ovarian carcinoma. Other challenge survival models include SF-295 and U251 glioblastomas implanted intracerebrally and various tumor cell lines administered intravenously. All mice dying, or sacrificed because of a moribund state or extensive ascites, prior to the final observation day are used to calculate median days of death for treated (T) and control (C) groups. These values are used to calculate a percent increase in life span (ILS) as follows:

$$\% \text{ ILS} = [(T - C)/C] \times 100.$$

Wherever possible, titration groups are included to establish a tumor doubling time for use in $\log_{10}$ cell kill calculations. Laboratory personnel may designate a death (or sacrifice) as drug-related based on visual observations and/or the results of necropsy. Otherwise, treated animal deaths are designated as treatment-related if the day of death precedes the mean day of death of the controls minus 2 standard deviations, or if the animal dies without evidence of tumor within 15 d of the last treatment.

3.5. Response of Xenograft Models to Standard Agents

The drug sensitivity profiles for the advanced-stage sc xenograft models in our program have been established using 12 clinical antitumor drugs (Tables 2 and 2A). Each of these agents, obtained from the Drug Synthesis and Chemistry Branch, DTP, was evaluated following ip administration at multiple dose levels. The activity ratings are based on the optimal effects attained with the maximally tolerated dose ($<LD_{20}$) of each drug for the treatment schedule shown. The latter were selected on the basis of the doubling time of a given tumor, with longer intervals between treatments for more slowly growing tumors. Apparent inconsistencies between the doubling times shown in Table 1 and selected schedules in Tables 2 and 2A are owing to increased tumor growth rates for some tumors in the later studies depicted in Table 1. In later chemotherapeutic trials with breast tumors, paclitaxel was included in the clinical drugs evaluated, and drug characteristics were considered to some extent in the selection of treatment regimens (Table 3).

Table 2
Response of Staged sc-Implanted Human Tumor Xenografts to 12 Clinical Anticancer Drugs[a,b]

Tumor	Ip treatment schedule	Alkylating Agents						DNA binders			Antimetabolites		Mitotic inhibitor
		L-PAM	CYT	DTIC	BCNU	MMC	DDPt	Act D	ADR	BLEO	MTX	5-FU	VBL
Colon													
SW-620	q7dx3	1	0	4	3	4	1	0	0	1	0	0	0
KM12	q4dx3	NA	NA	0	1	NA	0	0	NA	1	0	0	0
HCT-116	q4dx3	NA	0	0	0	1	0	1	0	1	0	0	0
HCT-15	q7dx3	1	0	0	0	1	0	1	0	0	0	0	0
HCC-2998	q4dx3	0	0	0	0	4	0	0	0	1	0	0	0
KM20L2	q4dx3	0	1	0	0	1	1	0	0	0	0	1	0
COLO 320DM	q4dx3	0	0	3	0	0	NA	0	0	0	0	1	1
COLO 205	q4dx3	1	0	0	0	3	1	1	0	0	0	1	1
HT29	q4dx3	0	0	0	0	2	2	0	0	1	0	0	0
CNS													
SF-295	q4dx3	0	1	0	1	0	1	0	0	0	0	0	4
U251	q4dx3	0	2	4	4	3	3	1	0	0	0	0	1
XF 498	q7dx3	0	0	4	3	1	1	0	1	0	0	0	0
SNB-19	q4dx3	1	2	3	NA	3	NA	0	NA	NA	0	0	1
Lung, nonsmall cell													
NCI-H460	q4dx3	0	0	NA	NA	4	0	0	0	1	0	0	0
NCI-H522	q4dx3	1	0	0	NA	≥2	1	NA	1	NA	NA	0	NA
HOP-62	q4dx3	2	NA	NA	NA	1	1	0	1	1	0	0	1
NCI-H23	q4dx3	3	1	0	0	4	4	1	1	1	1	1	0
NCI-H322M	q7dx3	0	0	0	0	4	1	0	0	0	0	1	0
EKVX	q4dx3	1	1	1	0	1	0	0	0	1	0	0	1
HOP-92	q4dx3	1	0	4	2	0	1	0	1	0	0	0	1
Lung, small cell													
DMS 273	qdx4	1	1	0	0	1	0	1	0	1	1	1	2
DMS 114	q4dx3	0	1	0	1	1	0	0	0	0	0	0	1
NCI-H69	q4dx3	4	1	3	4	2	0	0	0	0	0	1	0

(Continued)

Table 2 (*Continued*)

Response of Staged sc-Implanted Human Tumor Xenografts to 12 Clinical Anticancer Drugs[a,b]

Tumor	Ip treatment schedule	Alkylating Agents						DNA binders			Antimetabolites		Mitotic inhibitor
		L-PAM	CYT	DTIC	BCNU	MMC	DDPt	Act D	ADR	BLEO	MTX	5-FU	VBL
Melanoma													
LOX-IMVI	qdx5	1	2	2	2	2	1	0	1	0	1	0	2
SK-MEL-28	q4dx3	0	1	0	0	1	0	0	0	0	0	0	0
UACC-62	q7dx3	0	0	1	1	1	1	1	1	1	0	0	1
SK-MEL-31	q4dx3	0	0	0	NA	1	1	1	0	NA	0	0	NA
UACC-257	q7dx3	0	0	4	1	2	1	1	1	0	0	1	0
SK-MEL-2	q7dx3	1	0	0	0	1	1	1	0	1	0	1	2
M14	q4dx3	0	0	0	0	0	0	0	1	1	0	1	0
MALME-3M	q4dx3	1	0	4	1	1	1	1	0	1	0	0	0
Ovarian													
SK-OV-3	q7dx3	0	0	0	0	1	0	0	0	1	0	0	0
IGROV1	q4dx3	1	0	0	0	1	1	1	0	1	1	1	0
OVCAR-5	q7dx3	0	0	2	0	2	2	0	2	1	0	0	2
OVCAR-8	q7dx3	0	0	0	0	1	1	0	1	0	0	0	0
Prostate													
PC-3	qdx4	1	0	1	0	0	0	0	0	1	1	0	0
DU-145	q4dx3	0	1	0	NA	NA	1	0	NA	NA	1	0	0
Renal													
CAKI-1	q7dx3	1	1	0	0	1	1	1	1	0	0	1	0
SN12K1	q7dx3	0	0	0	0	4	0	0	0	0	0	0	1
A498	q7dx3	0	0	1	1	1	1	0	1	1	0	0	0
RXF 393	q4dx3	1	1	1	1	2	1	0	1	1	0	0	1
SN112C	q7dx3	0	0	0	1	0	0	0	0	1	0	0	0
786-0	q7dx3	0	NA	NA	NA	1	1	0	NA	NA	0	NA	NA

[a]Standard agents are melphalan (L-PAM), cytoxan (CYT), dacarbazine (DTIC), 1,3-bis (2-chloroethyl)-1-nitrosourea (BCNU), mitomycin C (MMC), cisplatin (DDPt), actinomycin D (act D), doxorubicin (ADR), bleomycin (BLEO), methotrexate (MTX), 5-fluorouracil (5-FU), and vinblastine (VBL). NA, not applicable.

[b]Activity rating based on optimal % delta T/delta C attained after treatment had ended:

0 = inactive, % T/C > 40

1 = tumor inhibition, % T/C range 1 to 40

2 = tumor stasis, % T/C range 0 to −49

3 = tumor regression, % T/C range −50 to −100

4 = % T/C range −50 to −100 and >30% tumor-free mice at experiment end.

Table 2A
Response of Early-Stage sc-Implanted Human Leukemia and Lymphoma Xenografts to 12 Clinical Anticancer Drugs[a,b]

Tumor	Alkylating agents						DNA binders			Antimetabolites		Mitotic inhibitor
	L-PAM	CYT	DTIC	BCNU	MMC	DDPt	Act D	ADR	BLEO	MTX	5FU	VBL
Leukemia and lymphoma												
MOLT-4 adv-st	4	1	0	0	1	1	0	1	1	1	0	0
MOLT-4 early-st	4	1	0	0	NA	1	0	0	1	1	0	0
CCRF-CEM	4	1	0	1	NA	1	0	NA	0	1	1	1
RPMI-8226[c]	1	1	1	0	NA	1	1	1	1	1	1	1
SR	4	4	4	4	NA	1	4	1	1	NA	0	4
K-562	1	0	1	0	NA	0,1	0	0	1	NA	NA	0
AS-283	4	4	1	0	NA	1	0	0	0	4	0	1
PA-682	1	0	4	1	NA	1	1	NA	1	4	0	1
SU-DHL-6	1	1	4	0	NA	0	0	1	1	0	0	0
SU-DHL-7	4	4	4	4	NA	0	0	0	0	1	0	1

[a]See footnotes to Table 2 for description of agents and activity ratings.
[b]Treatment regimens were ip qd×5 for MTX and 5FU, ip q4d×3 for L-PAM, CYT, DTIC, BCNU, MMC, DDPt, Act D, BLEO and VBL, iv q4d×3 for ADR.
[c]Myeloma

139

Table 3
Response of Advanced-Stage sc-Implanted Breast Tumor Xenografts to 13 Clinical Anticancer Drugs[a,b]

Tumor	Alkylating agents						DNA binders			Antimetabolites		Mitotic inhibitors	
	L-PAM	CYT	DTIC	BCNU	MMC	DDPt	Act D	ADR	BLEO	MTX	5-FU	VBL	PAC
ZR-75-1	1	1	4	1	1	1	1	3	1	0	0	1	1 (ES[c])
MX-1	4	4	0	1	4	4	0	2	1	1	0	0	4
UISO-BCA-1	0	0	1	0	NA	0	0	0	0	NA	0	0	3
MCF7	1	0	1	1	1	0	0	0	1	0	0 (ES)	0	0
MDA-MB-435[d]	1	0	4	3	NA	0	0 (ES)	0	1	0 (ES)	0	1	4

[a]Clinical drugs include those listed in Table 2. In addition, paclitaxel (PAC) was tested with an iv qd×5 treatment regimen.
[b]For definitions and explanation of activity ratings, *see* footnotes to Table 2.
[c]ES refers to use of early-stage model for the testing of this agent.
[d]Recent experimental evidence for melanoma characteristics of this model: *see* Table 1 footnote.

With the caveat that no attempts were made to optimize drug administration in each model, it can be seen that at least minimal antitumor effects (% T/C ≤ 40) were produced in each tumor model by at least 2, and as many as 10, clinical drugs (Table 4). The number of responses appeared to be independent of doubling time and histological type with a range in the number of responses observed for tumors in each subpanel. When the responses are considered in terms of the more clinically relevant endpoints of partial or complete tumor regression, it can be seen that the tumor models were quite refractory to standard drug therapy, with 30 of 48 (62.5%) not responding to any of the drugs tested (Table 4). As tested, the clinical drugs producing the highest response rates (number of tumors responding [% T/C ≤ –50%]/total tumors evaluated) were DTIC (11/44) and mitomycin C (9/45; Tables 2 and 3). Paclitaxel was not evaluated in most tumors, but it demonstrated excellent activity in four of five breast tumor models (Table 3).

4. STRATEGY FOR INITIAL COMPOUND EVALUATION IN VIVO

The in vitro primary screen provides the basis for selection of the most appropriate lines to use for the initial follow-up in vivo testing, with each compound tested against xenografts derived from cell lines demonstrating the greatest sensitivity to the agent in vitro. Our early strategy for in vivo testing emphasized the treatment of animals bearing advanced-stage tumors. Further studies resulted in a change of approach such that early evaluations are often conducted in early-stage tumors with follow-up testing conducted in the more rigorous advanced-stage tumors.

The strategy for in vivo testing has undergone some modifications over the last several years based on several changes in the NCI approaches to cancer drug discovery and development within the DTP and Cancer Therapy Evaluation Program (CTEP), as recently described (52). The DTP and CTEP now facilitate the anticancer drug discovery and development process through the Rapid Access to Intervention Development (RAID) and Rapid Access to NCI Development (RAND) initiatives as well as compound entry to phase I and phase II clinical trials via a Drug Development Group (DDG) review process (as further described at http://dtp.nci.nih.gov). In most cases, dose range finding studies in non-tumor-bearing mice are conducted for new compounds identified by the in vitro screen or received through other input mechanisms (e.g., RAID, RAND, DDG). Unless information is available to guide dose selection, single mice are treated with single ip bolus doses of 400, 200, and 100 mg/kg and observed for 14 d. Sequential three-dose studies are conducted as necessary, until a nonlethal dose range is established. The highest dose not producing mortality or a >20 % body weight loss is defined as the maximum tolerated dose (MTD). The MTD is used to select dose levels for the initial animal efficacy studies.

For compounds with no prior in vivo efficacy data, the first assay conducted is the hollow fiber assay. This assay allows preliminary assessment of a compound's in vivo efficacy potential without excessive expenditures of resources. Alternatively, for compounds presented to the program with pre-existing evidence of in vivo activity, or with defined mechanisms of action, the first in vivo efficacy trials may involve classical syngeneic or xenogeneic tumor studies. Compounds selected for efficacy studies through the Biological Evaluation Committee (BEC) or DDG process are generally evaluated in one or more early-stage xenograft models using standard protocols. Generally, the compounds are administered ip, often as suspensions, on schedules based, with some excep-

Table 4
Response of Staged sc Human Tumor Xenografts to Clinical Anticancer Drugs

Panel	Tumor	No. of drugs active[a]	
		Minimal activity[b]	Tumor regression[c]
Colon	SW-620	6	3
	KM12	2/8	0/8
	HCT-116	3/11	0/11
	HCT-15	3	0
	HCC-2998	2	1
	KM20L2	4	0
	COLO 320DM	2/11	0/11
	COLO 205	6	1
	HT29	3	0
CNS	SF-295	4	1
	U251	7	4
	XF 498	5	2
	SNB-19	5/8	2/8
Lung, Nonsmall cell	NCI-H460	2/9	1/9
	NCI-H522	4/7	0/7
	HOP-62	5/9	0/9
	NCI-H23	9	3
	NCI-H322M	3	1
	EKVX	6	0
	HOP-92	6	1
Lung, small cell	DMS 273	8	0
	DMS 114	4	0
	NCI-H69	6	3
Mammary	ZR-75-1	10	2
	MX-1	9	5
	UISO-BCA-1	2/11	1/11
	MCF7	5	0
	MDA-MB-435	6/10	3/10
Melanoma	LOX-IMVI	9	0
	SK-MEL-28	2	0
	UACC-62	8	0
	SK-MEL-31	3/9	0/9
	UACC-257	7	0
	SK-MEL-2	7	0
	M14	3	0
	MALME-3M	7	1

(*continued*)

tions, on the mass doubling time of the tumor. For doubling times of 2.5 d or less, the schedule is daily for five treatments (qdx5); tumors with doubling times of greater than 2.5 d are treated every fourth day for three treatments (q4dx3). For most tumors, the interval between individual treatments approximates the doubling time of the tumors, and the treatment period allows a 0.5–1.0 $\log_{10}$ unit of control tumor growth. For tumors staged

Table 4 (*Continued*)
Response of Staged sc Human Tumor Xenografts to Clinical Anticancer Drugs

| Panel | Tumor | No. of drugs active[a] | |
		Minimal activity[b]	Tumor regression[c]
Ovarian	SK-OV-3	2	0
	IGROV1	7	0
	OVCAR-8	3	0
Prostate	PC-3	4	0
	DU-145	3/6	0/6
Renal	CAKI-1	7	0
	SN12K1	2	0
	A498	6	0
	RXF 393	9	0
	SN12C	2	0
	786-0	2/5	0/5

[a]Except where noted, the number of clinical drugs evaluated was 12 for the tumors listed in Table 2 and 13 for the breast tumors listed in Table 3.
[b]% T/C ≤ 40, ratings 1–4 in Tables 2 and 3.
[c]% T/C ≤ –50, ratings 3 and 4 in Tables 2 and 3.

at 100 to 200 mg, the tumor sizes of the controls at the end of treatment range from 500 to 2,000 mg, which allows sufficient time after treatment to evaluate the effects of the test agent before it becomes necessary to sacrifice mice because of tumor size.

5. STRATEGY AND EXAMPLES OF DETAILED DRUG EVALUATION

Once a compound has been identified that demonstrates some in vivo efficacy in initial evaluations, more detailed studies can be designed and conducted in human tumor xenograft models to explore the compound's therapeutic potential further. By varying the concentration and exposure time of the tumor cells (in vitro time-course assays; *see* Chapter 8) and the host to the drug (in vivo range finding test in non-tumor-bearing mice), it is possible to devise and recommend treatment strategies designed to optimize antitumor activity.

As many of the initial in vivo studies deliver suspensions of the compound into the peritoneal cavity, it is unlikely that the sc tumors receive optimal concentrations of, and exposure to, test agents. The early preclinical antitumor evaluation of paclitaxel illustrates this problem. In NCI studies, prior to its clinical evaluation, paclitaxel had demonstrated its best effects against ip-implanted tumors, and no activity was observed in sc models following ip administration as a suspension *(53,54)*. Later investigations demonstrated that sc-implanted MX-1 mammary carcinoma xenografts were highly responsive to treatment with iv solutions of paclitaxel *(55)*, although they had failed to respond to treatment with ip suspensions *(54)*. As illustrated in Table 5, iv solutions of paclitaxel administered on either a daily or intermittent schedule produced complete tumor regressions in most treated mice. Some of these mice remained tumor-free for 24–28 d after the last treatment, and tumor growth delays in the remaining mice were excellent. In contrast, only modest

Table 5
Effect of Route of Administration on the Activity
of Paclitaxel Against Staged sc-Implanted MX-1 Mammary Carcinoma Xenografts

Route schedule	Opt. Dose $(mg/kg/d)^a$	Complete regressions /total	Tumor-free on d 40	Minimum % T/C^b (d)	Growth delay $[\% (T - C)/C]^c$	Net log cell kill
iv, d8–12	22.5	1/9	8	−100 (15)	449	2.9
ip, d8–12	15.0	2/9	1	28 (19)	29	−0.2
iv, d8,12,16	22.5	6/9	2	−100 (15)	357	2.1
ip, d8,12,16	30	0/9	0	20 (22)	70	−0.3

^{a}Paclitaxel was administered as a solution in 12.5% ethanol/12.5% cremophor/75% normal saline at multiple dose levels. Data from doses ($\leq LD_{10}$) producing the optimal effects are shown.
^{b}See Subheading 3.2. for an explanation of the parameters of antitumor effects. Number in parentheses indicates the observation day on which data were entered.
^{c}Based on an endpoint of two doublings, C = 7–1 d. Tumor-free mice and mice dying of apparent drug-related effects were excluded from the calculations.

antitumor effects were observed following the ip administration of paclitaxel solutions. Pharmacokinetic data obtained in mice indicated only 10% bioavailability of paclitaxel from ip administration (56).

To interpret better the results of detailed efficacy studies on new compounds, it is important to employ the drug sensitivity profile of individual tumor xenograft systems to clinical anticancer drugs as benchmarks. It is also important to relate the effective dose to the MTD in a given tumor model to ascertain that the agent exhibits a therapeutic index. An example of such a detailed drug study can be found in the recent preclinical drug development of 2-chloroethyl-3-sarcosinamide-1-nitrosourea (SarCNU, NSC 364432).

Initial testing by the NCI demonstrated activity against P388 leukemia and also striking activity against three early-stage sc-implanted human brain tumor xenograft models, SNB-75, SF-295, and U-251, using both ip and iv routes of administration (57). Although a related compound, BCNU, was also highly effective against SNB-75 and U-251 tumor systems, BCNU was minimally active against the SF-295 tumor system. Under optimal experimental conditions, six of six SNB-75, six of six U-251, and four of six SF-295-bearing animals were tumor-free following ip SarCNU administration. In subsequent detailed drug studies, BCNU at 0.67 × MTD displayed moderate growth-inhibitory activity (T/C of 15%), whereas SarCNU at 0.67 × MTD showed exceptional growth-inhibitory activity (T/C of −100%). Treatment with BCNU produced neither partial or complete remissions nor tumor-free animals, as shown in Fig. 2A; the drug produced a tumor growth delay of approx 200% over that of the control group. In contrast, SarCNU produced three tumor-free animals and four tumor regressions and a tumor growth delay of approx 560%. At lower dosages of SarCNU in which tumor-free status was not achieved, partial and complete tumor regressions were observed.

Further detailed drug testing showed that oral SarCNU treatment leads to the greatest efficacy and least toxicity of all routes tested. For example, as shown in Fig. 2B, 100% tumor-free status against SF-295 was achieved by SarCNU dosages that are half to two-thirds of the MTD. By contrast, BCNU at best produced a tumor growth delay of approx 266% at a dosage approximating the LD_{25}; no tumor-free animals or tumor regressions were seen with BCNU treatment. In contrast, SarCNU produced eight of eight tumor-free animals at a dose approx 0.8 × the MTD and five tumor regressions at a dose 0.52 × MTD.

An additional study was performed to define more precisely the effective dose range of oral SarCNU. This study revealed one partial tumor regression at 0.45 × MTD, six tumor-free animals at 0.6 × MTD, and eight of eight tumor-free animals at 0.8 × MTD. This study also showed that the protective effect of SarCNU against tumor growth was maintained for up to 5 wk following cessation of treatment. It is highly noteworthy that SF-295 is a very unresponsive tumor model, i.e., it exhibits minimal growth inhibition (and no tumor-free responses) to only 2 of 12 clinical agents and a limited number of experimental agents. In fact, SarCNU is the only agent tested by the NCI to date that is capable of inducing a high incidence of complete tumor regressions and/or tumor-free status in this model.

It is noteworthy that SarCNU also produced a moderate to good antitumor effect in non-CNS tumor systems as well, e.g., A498 renal cell carcinoma and SW-620 colon adenocarcinoma. The results shown in Fig. 2C are typical of the antitumor activity in non-CNS tumor models. At comparable dosages (0.8 × MTD), BCNU treatment conferred 2/10 complete regressions with an average growth delay of 192%. By contrast, SarCNU produced 10/10 complete regressions, with an average growth delay of 426%. These and other in vivo results demonstrate that (1) SarCNU is highly active yet exhibits selectivity among a variety of human solid tumors and that (2) SarCNU is consistently more effective than BCNU.

In addition to comparisons of the relative efficacy of SarCNU and BCNU, both agents were compared with respect to their therapeutic indices (58). SarCNU exhibits optimal efficacy and the least toxicity on a q4d×3 schedule in mice. Oral SarCNU is clearly more efficacious than oral BCNU and this is accompanied by a more favorable TI (>3.95 vs 1.33), where the TI is defined as the highest dose producing less than 20% body weight loss. Although SarCNU is highly active by several routes of administration in seven human xenograft models, oral therapy confers the best activity and least toxicity (TI_{po} = 3.95 vs TI_{iv} = 2.22). The TI value for SarCNU given po is a low estimate because at the dose defined as the MTD, only an 8% body weight loss is observed, and at the next highest dose level, the body weight loss is only 15%. The TI with oral administration is clearly superior to that with iv administration, suggesting that the oral route is the most optimal route of administration.

6. ALTERNATIVE MODELS: NEW APPROACHES TO IN VIVO DRUG TESTING

As mentioned earlier, the DTP has adopted a variety of alternative models for assessing specific tumor sensitivities. A useful model for assessing the antitumor activity of compounds for treating breast tumors is the orthotopic mammary fat pad (MFP) tumor implant model. For this, the tumor cells are injected directly into the MFP, most commonly the number 4 MFP, which is readily accessed by a small surgical incision. This model is associated with spontaneous tumor metastases similar to the natural history of breast cancer in humans. Tumor growth can be monitored as for sc-implanted tumors;

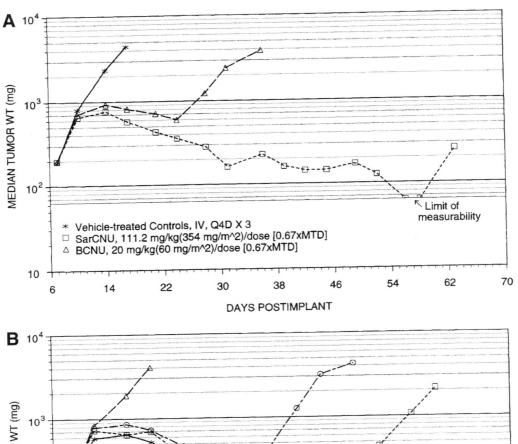

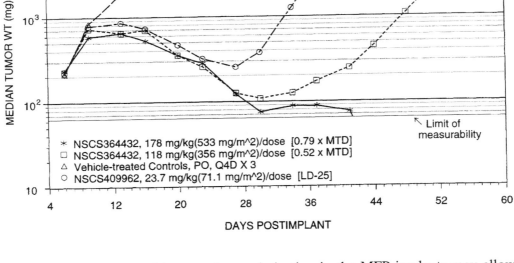

however, the presence of improved vascularization in the MFP implants may allow activity to be detected in this model that would not be observed in the sc model.

Another model that allows assessment of the impact of the blood-brain barrier on treating CNS tumors is the orthotopic implantation of CNS tumor lines directly into the brain via a needlestick placed through the sutures of the skull. Assessing the antitumor effect in this model is dependent on observing a prolongation in the life span of the treated mice compared with the controls.

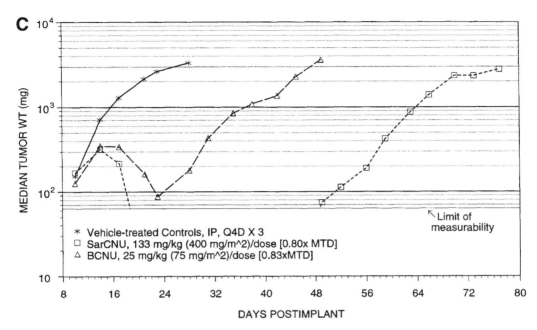

Fig. 2. Responses of advanced-stage human tumor xenografts to 2-chloroethyl-3-sarcosinamide-1-nitrosourea (SarCNU, NSC 364432) and 1,3-*bis*-chloro(2-chloroethyl)-1-nitrosourea (BCNU, NSC 409962). All SarCNU solutions were prepared fresh in 0.01 *M* sodium acetate/saline (pH 5), and all BCNU solutions were prepared fresh in 2% EtOH/saline; each was administered to mice within 30 min of preparation. There were 20 mice in each vehicle control group and 10 mice in each treated group in each of three efficacy experiments. (**A**) Mice bearing SF-295 glioblastoma xenografts received intermittent iv bolus treatments (q4d × 3) of SarCNU at 33.0, 49.5, 74.2, 111, and 167 mg/kg/dose or BCNU at 8.90, 13.4, 20.0, and 30.0 mg/kg/dose. (**B**) Mice bearing SF-295 glioblastoma xenografts received intermittent oral bolus treatments (q4d×3) of SarCNU at 118.5, 178, 267, and 400 mg/kg/dose or BCNU at 23.7, 35,5, 53.3, and 80 mg/kg/dose. (**C**) Mice bearing SW-620 colon carcinoma xenografts received intermittent iv bolus treatments (q4d×3) of SarCNU at 39.6, 59.4, 89.0, 133.4, and 200 mg/kg/dose or BCNU at 7.41, 11.11, 16.67, and 25.0 mg/kg/dose.

The impact of treatment on tumors growing in the liver can be assessed by injecting tumor cells into the spleen and allowing the tumor cells to distribute to the liver. Tumors established in this manner cause a measurable increase in the weight of the liver approx 30–40 d post injection and provide adequate sample volumes for good immuno-histochemical or molecular biology analyses. This model allows a compound to be tested for efficacy against liver tumors, both primary and secondary, which may have significance in many cases because of the greater vascularity of the liver compared with the sc site.

An orthotopic model that has proved useful in assessing agents targeted at renal cancer is direct injection of tumor cells into the caudal pole of the kidney. Appropriate tumor cell lines will establish viable tumors and produce significant increases in kidney weight in the tumor-bearing kidney compared with the non-tumor-bearing kidney. This can be further analyzed by immunohistochemistry and molecular techniques.

For assessing purported antiangiogenic agents, the DTP has used syngeneic models, primarily mouse B16F10 melanoma and Lewis lung carcinoma. The choice of syngeneic

Table 6

Alternative Models for Assessing the Efficacy of Purported Antitumor Agents[a]

Models	Endpoints	Suitable cell lines	Histology	Applications
Intravenous	Morbidity/mortality Histology Tumor metastastis counts	LOX IMVi HL-60 (TB) AS-283 B16	Human amelanotic melanoma Human promyelocytic leukemia Human lymphoma Murine melanoma	Disseminated disease; different tumor lines localize to lungs, brain, liver
Intracranial	Morbidity/mortality Histology	U-251 SF-295 U-87MG	Human glioblastoma Human glioblastoma Human glioblastoma	Impact of the blood-brain barrier on drug distribution
Intrarenal	Kidney weight Histology	RXF 393 CaKi-1 SN12K1	Human hypernephroma Human renal clear cell carcinoma Human renal cell carcinoma	Evaluate impact of pharmacokinetics on drug activity
Mammary fat pad	Tumor volume	MDA-MB-231 MCF-7 ZR-75-1 MX-1	Human breast adenocarcinoma Human breast adenocarcinoma Human breast ductal carcinoma Human breast carcinoma	Some tumors metastasize; tumor may be more vascular than a subcutaneous tumor
Intrahepatic	Liver weight Histology	AsPC-1 KM12 MHC 1544 M5076 B16	Human pancreatic adenocarcinoma Human colon carcinoma Human colon carcinoma Murine sarcoma Murine melanoma	Evaluate impact of pharmacokinetics on drug activity
Angiogenesis	Tumor volume Metastatic lesions Vascular density	B16F10 Lewis Lung MHEC5-T	Murine melanoma Murine lung carcinoma Murine hemangioendothelioma	Evaluate impact of treatment on tumor microenvironment including vascularity

[a]All tumor cell lines evaluated to date are verified to meet basic quality assurance criteria and to show suitable growth characteristics under in vitro/in vivo maintenance and assay conditions; they are prepared for histological and cytochemical evaluations using standardized procedures (34).

models for these studies was based on the probability that mouse endothelium would probably respond to mouse tumor signaling more easily than to human tumor signaling. This decision is supported by the finding of other researchers that syngeneic tumors appear to respond differently than do xenogeneic tumors *(14,33,59–64)*. Table 6 provides a list of these implant sites with tumor lines known to work in these models. Although these models depend on classical diagnostic techniques including mass and histologic evaluations, it is worth noting that the introduction of new technologies (including high-performance CCD camera systems in conjunction with green fluorescent protein or luciferase-transfected cell lines) is opening the frontiers for novel models with exceptional potential in the foreseeable future.

7. CONCLUSIONS

The discovery and development of potential anticancer drugs by the NCI is based on a series of sequential screening and detailed testing steps to identify new, efficacious lead compounds and to eliminate nonactive and/or highly toxic materials from further consideration. Past experience in large-scale screening with a wide variety of animal and human tumor systems and the management of disease-free athymic mouse facilities has proved to be highly valuable for the recent characterization, calibration, and utilization of newly acquired human tumor xenograft models. Furthermore, the DTP's experience with computer programming has enabled the development and implementation of specialized analytical software that permits acquisition, storage, and presentation of data in readily accessible tabular and graphic formats. Many of the human tumor xenografts have been employed to test a variety of distinct chemical compound classes over the past 5 yr. Thus, the in vivo drug sensitivity profiles of these human tumor xenografts are well suited to serve as benchmarks for the testing of newly synthesized agents as well as agents isolated from natural product sources currently under investigation.

In addition to standard models of in vivo testing, the NCI has implemented a hollow fiber-based assay to allow rapid assessment of a compound's potential for in vivo activity. This has reduced the time and costs required to develop early in vivo evidence of efficacy. Additionally, the DTP has used human and rodent tumor cell lines to develop and implement alternate assay systems, e.g., metastatic, orthotopic, and angiogenesis-related models.

REFERENCES

1. Grever MR, Schepartz SA, Chabner BA. The National Cancer Institute: cancer drug discovery and development program. *Semin Oncol* 1992; 19:622–638.
2. Zubrod CG, Schepartz S, Leiter J, Endicott KM, Carrese LM, Baker CG. The chemotherapy program of the National Cancer Institute: history, analysis and plans. *Cancer Chemother Rep* 1966; 50:349–540.
3. Goldin A, Schepartz SA, Venditti JM, DeVita VT Jr. Historical development and current strategy of the National Cancer Institute Drug Development Program. In: DeVita VT Jr, Busch H, eds. *Methods in Cancer Research*, vol XVI. New York: Academic, 1979:165–245.
4. DeVita VT Jr, Goldin A, Oliverio VT, et al. The drug development and clinical trials programs of the Division of Cancer Treatment, National Cancer Institute. *Cancer Clin Trials* 1979; 2:195–216.
5. Goldin A, Venditti JM. The new NCI screen and its implications for clinical evaluation. In: Carter SK, Sakurai Y, eds. *Recent Results in Cancer Research*, vol 70. Berlin: Springer-Verlag. 1980:5–20.
6. Venditti JM. Preclinical drug development: rationale and methods. *Semin Oncol* 1981; 8:349–361.
7. Frei E. The national chemotherapy program. *Science (Wash DC)* 1982; 217:600–606.

8. Venditti JM. The National Cancer Institute antitumor drug discovery program, current and future perspectives: a commentary. *Cancer Treat Rep* 1983; 67:767-772.

9. Driscoll J. The preclinical new drug research program of the National Cancer Institute. *Cancer Treat Rep* 1984; 68:63–76.

10. Goldin A. Screening at the National Cancer Institute: basic concepts. In: Hellman K, Carter SK, eds. *Fundamentals of Cancer Chemotherapy*. New York: McGraw-Hill. 1987:141–149.

11. Suffness M, Newman DJ, Snader K. Discovery and development of antineoplastic agents from natural sources. In: Scheuer P, ed. *Bioorganic Marine Chemistry*, vol 3 Berlin: Springer-Verlag. 1989:131–168.

12. Boyd MR. Status of the NCI preclinical antitumor drug discovery screen. In: DeVita VT Jr, Hellman S, Rosenberg SA, eds. *Cancer: Principles and Practice of Oncology, Updates*, vol 3. Philadelphia: Lippincott. 1989:1–12.

13. Gellhorn A, Hirschberg E. Investigation of diverse systems for cancer chemotherapy screening. *Cancer Res* 1955; 15 (suppl 3):1–125.

14. Venditti JM, Wesley RA, Plowman J. Current NCI preclinical antitumor screening in vivo: results of tumor panel screening, 1976–1982, and future directions. In: Garrattini S, Goldin A, Hawking F, eds. *Advances in Pharmacology and Chemotherapy*, vol 20. Orlando, FL: Academic. 1984:1–20.

15. Rygaard J, Povlsen CO. Heterotransplantation of a human malignant tumor to "nude" mice. *Acta Pathol Microbiol Scand* 1969; 77:758–760.

16. Giovanella BC, Stehlin JS. Heterotransplantation of human malignant tumors in "nude" thymusless mice. I. Breeding and maintenance of "nude" mice. *J Natl Cancer Inst* 1973; 51:615–619.

17. Bogden A, Kelton D, Cobb W, Esber H. A rapid screening method for testing chemotherapeutic agents against human tumor xenografts. In: Houchens D, Ovejera A, eds. *Proceedings of the Symposium on the Use of Athymic (nude) Mice in Cancer Research*. New York: Gustav Fischer, 1978:231–250.

18. Fidler IJ, Kripke ML. Metastasis results from preexisting variant cells within a malignant tumor. *Science* 1977; 197:893–895.

19. Kozlowski JM, Fidler IJ, Campbell D, Xu Z, Kaighn ME, Hart IR. Metastatic behavior of human tumor cell lines grown in the nude mouse. *Cancer Res* 1984; 44:3522–3529.

20. Dykes DJ, Shoemaker RH, Harrison SD, et al. Development and therapeutic response of a spontaneous metastasis model of a human melanoma (LOX) in athymic mice. *Proc Am Assoc Cancer Res* 1987; 28:431.

21. Shoemaker RH, Dykes DJ, Plowman J, et al. Practical spontaneous metastasis model for in vivo therapeutic studies using a human melanoma. *Cancer Res* 1991; 51:2837–2841.

22. Fidler IJ. Rationale and methods for the use of nude mice to study the biology and therapy of human cancer metastasis. *Cancer Metastasis Rev* 1986; 5:29–49.

23. Fidler IJ, Wilmanns C, Staroselsky A, Radinsky R, Dong Z, Fan D. Modulation of tumor cell response to chemotherapy by the organ environment. *Cancer Metastasis Rev* 1994; 13:209–222.

24. McLemore TL, Liu MC, Blacker PC, et al. A novel intrapulmonary model for the orthotopic propagation of human lung cancers in athymic nude mice. *Cancer Res* 1987; 47:5132–5140.

25. Leone A, Flatow U, VanHoutte K, Steeg PS. Transfection of human nm23-H1 into the human MDA-MB-435 breast carcinoma cell line: effects on tumor metastatic potential, colonization and enzymatic activity. *Oncogene* 1993; 8:2325–2333.

26. Carter CA, Dykes, DJ. Characterization of tumor growth and drug sensitivity for human prostate tumors implanted orthotopically. *Proc Am Assoc Cancer Res* 1994; 35:280.

27. Hamburger AW, Salmon SE. Primary bioassay of human tumor stem cells. *Science (Wash DC)* 1977; 197:461–463.

28. Salmon SE, Hamburger AW, Soehnlen B, Durie BGM, Alberts DS, Moon TE. Quantitation of differential sensitivity of human tumor stem cells to anticancer drugs. *N Engl J Med* 1978; 298:1321–1327.

29. Taetle R, Koessler AK, Howell SB. In vitro growth and drug sensitivity of tumor colony-forming units from human tumor xenografts. *Cancer Res* 1981; 41:1856–1860.

30. Salmon SE, Trent J, eds. *Human Tumor Cloning*. New York: Grune & Stratton, 1984.

31. Shoemaker RH, Wolpert-DeFilippes MK, Kern DH, et al. Application of a human tumor colony forming assay to new drug screening. *Cancer Res* 1985; 45:2145–2153.

32. Dykes DJ, Abbott BJ, Mayo JG, et al. Development of human tumor xenograft models for in vivo evaluation of new antitumor drugs. In: Huber H, Queißer W, eds. *Contributions to Oncology*, vol 42. Basel: Karger. 1992:1–12.

33. Geran RI, Greenberg NH, MacDonald MM, Schumacher AM, Abbott BJ. Protocols for screening chemical agents and natural products against animal tumors and other biological systems. Cancer Chemother Rep 1972; 3:51.

34. Stinson SF, Alley MC, Koop WC, et al. Morphological and immunocytochemical characteristics of human tumor cell lines for use in a disease-oriented anticancer drug screen. *Anticancer Res* 1992; 12:1035–1054.

35. Boxma GC, Custer RP, Bosma MJ. A severe combined immunodeficiency mutation in the mouse. *Nature* 1983; 301:527–530.

36. Fogh J, Fogh JM, Orfeo, T. One hundred and twenty-seven cultured human tumor cell lines producing tumors in nude mice. *J Natl Cancer Inst* 1977; 59:221–225.

37. Andriole GL, Mule JJ, Hansen DT, Linehan WM, Rosenberg SA. Evidence that lymphokine-activated killer cells and natural killer cells are distinct based on an analysis of congenitally immunodeficient mice. *J Immunol* 1985; 135:2911–2913.

38. Shafle SM, Grantham FH. Role of hormones in the growth and regression of human breast cancer cells (MCF-7) transplanted into athymic nude mice. *J Natl Cancer Inst* 1981; 67:51–56.

39. Engel LW, Young NA, Tralka TS, Lippman ME, O'Brien SJ, Joyce MJ. Establishment and characterization of three new continuous cell lines derived from human breast carcinomas. *Cancer Res* 1978; 38:3352–3364.

40. Boyle MJ, Sewell WA, Milliken ST, Cooper DA, Penny R. HIV and malignancy. *J Acquir Immune Defic Syndr* 1993; suppl 1:S5–9.

41. Grever MR, Giavazzi R, Anver M, Hollingshead MG, Mayo JG, Malspeis L. An in vivo AIDS-related lymphoma model for assessing chemotherapeutic agents. *Proc Am Assoc Cancer Res* 1994; 35:369.

42. Personal communication: Dr. Ian Magrath, Pediatrics Branch, Division of Cancer Treatment, NCI.

43. Magrath IT, Pizzo RA, Whang-Peng J, et al. Characterization of lymphoma-derived cell lines: Comparison of cell lines positive and negative for Epstein-Barr virus nuclear antigen. I. Physical cytogenetic, and growth characteristics. *J Natl Cancer Inst* 1980; 64:465–476.

44. Magrath IT, Freeman CB, Pizzo P, et al. Characterization of lymphoma-derived cell lines: Comparison of cell lines positive and negative for Epstein-Barr virus nuclear antigen. II. Surface markers. *J. Natl Cancer Inst* 1980; 64:477–483.

45. Magrath I, Freeman C, Santaella M, et al.Induction of complement receptor expression in cell lines derived from human undifferentiated lymphomas. II. Characterization of the induced complement receptors and demonstration of the simultaneous induction EBV receptor. *J Immunol* 1981; 127:1039–1043.

46. Benjamin D, Magrath IT, Maguire R, Janus C, Todd HD, Parson RG. Immunoglobulin secretion by cell lines derived from African and American undifferentiated lymphomas of Burkitt's and non-Burkitt's type. *J Immunol* 1982; 129:1336–1342.

47. Beckwith M, Urba WJ, Ferris DK, et al. Anti-IgM-mediated growth inhibition of a human B lymphoma cell line is independent of phosphatidylinositol turnover and protein kinase C activation and involves tyrosine phosphorylation. *J Immunol* 1991; 147:2411–2418.

48. Mosier DE, Gulizia RJ, Baird SM, Wilson DB. Transfer of a functional human immune system to mice with severe combined immunodeficiency. *Nature* 1988; 335:256–259.

49. Martin DS, Stolfi RL, Sawyer RC. Commentary on "clinical predictivity of transplantable tumor systems in the selection of new drugs for solid tumors: rationale for a three-stage strategy." *Cancer Treat Rep* 1984; 68:1317–1318.

50. Martin DS, Balis ME, Fisher B, et al. Role of murine tumor models in cancer treatment research. *Cancer Res* 1986; 46:2189–2192.

51. Stolfi RL, Stolfi LM, Sawyer RC, Martin DS. Chemotherapeutic evaluation using clinical criteria in spontaneous, autochthonous murine breast tumors. *J Natl Cancer Inst* 1988; 80:52–55.

52. Sausville EA, Feigal E. Evolving approaches to cancer drug discovery and development at the National Cancer Institute, USA. *Ann Oncol* 1999; 10:1287–1291.

53. Suffness M, Cordell G. Antitumor alkaloids. In: Brossi A, ed. *The Alkaloids*, vol XXV. New York: Academic. 1985:1–355.

54. Rose WC. Taxol: a review of its preclinical in vivo antitumor activity. *Anticancer Drugs* 1992; 3:311–321.

55. Plowman J, Dykes DJ, Waud WR, Harrison SD Jr, Griswold DP Jr. Response of murine tumors and human tumor xenografts to Taxol (NSC 125973) in mice. *Proc Am Assoc Cancer Res* 1992; 33:514.

56. Eiseman JL, Eddington N, Leslie J, et al. Pharmacokinetics and development of a physiologic model of taxol in CD2F1 mice. *Proc Am Assoc Cancer Res* 1993; 34:396.
57. Marcantonio, D, Panasci, LC, Hollingshead, MG, et al. 2-Chloroethyl-3-sarcosinamide-l-nitrosourea, a novel chloroethylnitrosourea analogue with enhanced antitumor activity against human glioma xenografts. *Cancer Res* 1997; 57:3895–3898.
58. Tomaszewski JE, Donohue SJ, Brown AP, et al. Preclinical efficacy and toxicity of (2-chloroethyl)-3-sarcosinamide-l-nitrosourea (SarCNU, NSC 364432). *Ann Oncol* 1998; 9(suppl. 2):202.
59. Mayo JG, Laster WR Jr, Andrews CM, Schabel FM Jr. Success and failure in the treatment of solid tumors. III. "Cure" of metastatic Lewis lung carcinoma with methyl-CCNU (NSC-95441) and surgery-chemotherapy. *Cancer Chemother Rep* 1972; 56:183–95.
60. Bertalanffy FD, Gibson MH. The in vivo effects of arabinosylcytosine on the cell proliferation of murine B16 melanoma and Ehrlich ascites tumor. *Cancer Res* 1971; 31:66–71.
61. Fidler IJ. Biological behavior of malignant melanoma cells correlated to their survival in vivo. *Cancer Res* 1975; 35:218–224.
62. Houchens DP, Ovejera AA, Sheridan MA, Johnson RK, Bogden AE, Neil GL. Therapy for mouse tumors and human tumor xenografts with the antitumor antibiotic AT-125. *Cancer Treat Rep* 1979; 63: 473–476.
63. Bouis D, Hospers GA, Meijer C, Dam W, Peek R, Mulder NH. Effects of the CDT6/ANGX gene on tumour growth in immune competent mice. *In Vivo* 2003; 17:157–161
64. Raso E, Paku S, Kopper L, Timar J. Trace elements improve survival of DTIC-treated mice with overt liver metastases of Lewis lung carcinoma. *Pathol Oncol Res* 2003; 9:96–99.
65. Ross DT, Scherf U, Eisen MB, et al. Systematic variation in gene expression patterns in human cancer cell lines. *Nat Genet* 2000; 24:227–235.
66. Ellison G, Klinowska T, Westwood RF, Docter E, French T, Fox JC. Further evidence to support the melanocytic origin of MDA-MB-435. *Mol Pathol* 2002; 55:294–299.

8

NCI Specialized Procedures in Preclinical Drug Evaluations

Melinda G. Hollingshead, DVM, PhD,
Michael C. Alley, PhD, Gurmeet Kaur, MS,
Christine M. Pacula-Cox, MS,
and Sherman F. Stinson, PhD

CONTENTS

INTRODUCTION
HOLLOW FIBER ASSAYS: FIRST-STAGE IN VIVO EFFICACY TESTING
  AND SPECIALIZED TESTING
IN VITRO/IN VIVO ANGIOGENESIS ASSAY
IN VITRO PHARMACOLOGIC CHARACTERIZATION
  OF EXPERIMENTAL AGENTS
CONCLUSIONS

INTRODUCTION

Agents now come to the U.S. National Cancer Institute (NCI) from many sources for preclinical evaluation and/or potential development *(1)*. In most cases, experimental agents have limited antiproliferative data against a broad spectrum of human cancers, and these agents usually are then tested in the NCI's in vitro anticancer drug screen. Data from the screen permits the identification of agents that exhibit differential activity among multiple tumor cell line panels and/or that exhibit patterns of in vitro anticancer drug activity that may correspond to novel molecular targets *(2)*. Agents that exhibit differential or novel patterns of in vitro activity are subsequently tested in vivo using the hollow fiber assay to assess their potential for in vivo activity in minimum challenge models. Some agents that cause differentiation, inhibit angiogenesis, and/or work in combination with other experimental or known anticancer agents are also submitted to NCI for preclinical evaluation. Such agents often require alternative and/or specialized in vitro or in vivo evaluation procedures to confirm initial experimental findings and to further support the rationale for development of potential new drug therapies.

From: *Cancer Drug Discovery and Development:*
Anticancer Drug Development Guide: Preclinical Screening, Clinical Trials, and Approval, 2nd Ed.
Edited by: B. A. Teicher and P. A. Andrews © Humana Press Inc., Totowa, NJ

2. HOLLOW FIBER ASSAYS: FIRST-STAGE IN VIVO EFFICACY TESTING AND SPECIALIZED TESTING

2.1. Methodology

The hollow fiber assay was the result of an effort to develop a method for prioritizing compounds for testing in the xenograft models and to improve the probability of rapidly identifying those compounds with the greatest potential for in vivo efficacy *(3)*. The criteria used during assay development were as follows: (1) a minimal challenge, (2) high volume capacity, (3) short assay time, (4) conservative compound consumption, and (5) low false-negative rate.

In brief, tumor cells are inoculated into polyvinylidene fluoride (PVDF) hollow fibers (1-mm internal diameter), and the fibers are heat-sealed and cut at 2-cm intervals. These samples are cultivated for 24–48 h in vitro and then implanted into athymic (nu/nu) mice. At the time of implantation, a representative set of fibers is assayed for viable cell mass by 3-(4,5-dimethylthiazol-2-yl)-2,5-diphenyl tetrazolium bromide (MTT) dye conversion to determine the time 0 cell mass for each cell line. The mice are treated with experimental therapeutic agents once daily for 4 d (qd×4), and the fibers are collected 6–8 d post implantation. At collection, the quantity of viable cells contained in the fibers is measured by the stable endpoint MTT dye conversion assay. The cytostatic and/or cytocidal antitumor effects of the test agent are determined from the changes in viable cell mass in the fibers collected from compound-treated and diluent-treated mice as well as the time 0 viable cell mass afforded by the "stable endpoint" feature of the MTT assay *(4)*. Using this technique, three different tumor cell lines can be grown concurrently in two physiologic sites, intraperitoneally (ip) and subcutaneously (sc) within each experimental mouse. This allows a test agent to be administered ip (or by other routes) for simultaneous evaluation against tumor cells growing in both sites. With the simultaneous assessment of multiple tumor cell lines grown in two physiologic compartments, it is possible to rapidly identify lead compounds with the greatest promise of in vivo activity, as summarized previously *(3,5,6)*.

2.2. Routine Screening

A selection of standard hollow fiber screening panels was established to accommodate testing agents with different expected activities. The standard assay uses 12 tumor cell lines selected because they are among the most sensitive in the in vitro 60-cell line screen. This screen consists of the following tumor cell lines: MDA-MB-231 human breast tumor, MDA-MB-435 human breast tumor (melanoma-like; *see* refs. *7* and *8*), U251 human glioma, SF-295 human glioma, OVCAR-3 human ovarian tumor, OVCAR-5 human ovarian tumor, COLO-205 human colon tumor, SW-620 human colon tumor, LOX-IMVI human melanoma, UACC-62 human melanoma, NCI-H23 human lung tumor, and NCI-H522 human lung tumor. A panel of six human leukemia/lymphoma tumor lines is applied to compounds that have a greater selectivity against the leukemia panel of the NCI in vitro screen. The tumor lines used are HL-60, MOLT-4, AS-283, KD488, SR, and RPMI-8226. For melanoma-directed agents, a panel of six melanomas, in addition to the two melanomas in the standard panel, is evaluated. The melanoma lines tested include MALME-3M, M14, SK-MEL-2, SK-MEL-5, SK-MEL-28, and UACC-257. There are also prostate and renal panels, each composed of three cell lines. The prostate lines are JCA-1, DU-145, and PC-3. The renal lines are RXF-393, A498, and CaKi-1.

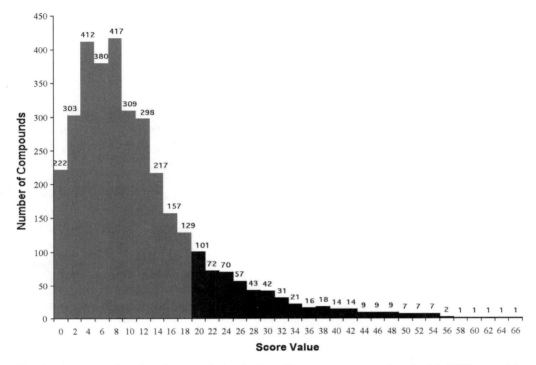

Fig. 1. Histogram showing the cumulative hollow fiber scores accumulated with 3398 tests. The scores are the total obtained by summing the sc and the ip score from a single compound test. Of the tested compounds, 16.3% (554) had a total score of 20 or greater. Paclitaxel, the positive control compound, routinely scores 34 in the standard hollow fiber assay following ip administration. The compounds scoring 60 and 64 are NSC 327993 (verrucarin A derivative) and NSC 123976 (neriifolin), respectively. The compounds scoring 58, 62, and 66 are discreet.

To simplify evaluation of the hollow fiber assay, a scoring system was developed in which a compound is given 2 points each time there is a 50% or greater reduction in net cell growth in the treated samples compared with the controls. The scores obtained with the ip and sc fibers are recorded individually and then summed to obtain the total score. In addition, the capacity of the compound to produce cell kill, defined as a lower viable cell mass at the end of the incubation compared with time 0, is also recorded. In this scoring system the maximum total score a compound can achieve in the standard hollow fiber assay is 96 (48 test combinations × 2 points/positive), and the maximum single-site score is half of that, or 48 (24 test combinations × 2 points/positive). The 48 test combinations result from having 12 cell lines grown in two sites, and these are tested against two compound dose levels (12 × 2 × 2 = 48). For the other panels, the total possible score is reduced since there are fewer cell lines and thus fewer combinations for each test agent (e.g., 6 cell lines × 2 sites × 2 doses = 24).

There have been 3398 tests conducted with the hollow fiber assay. The number of occurrences of each possible score is shown graphically in Fig. 1. The minimum score used as a selection cutoff can be manipulated to increase or decrease the number of referrals obtained. Our program determined that a minimum total score of 20 would be the selection criteria for the standard hollow fiber assay. To date, 16.3% (554) of the tests completed have a score of 20 or greater. Obviously, shifting the stringency of the selection criteria readily modulates the number of referrals.

2.3. Molecular Target Screening

Additional applications for the hollow fiber approach have been developed. Since the tumor cells are trapped within a readily retrieved implantable device, it is possible to collect tumor cells after exposure to physiologically achievable drug concentrations. Although this can be achieved using classical tumor xenograft material, the presence of host stroma within the xenograft cannot be readily avoided. This is not an issue with the hollow fiber approach since the fibers contain only the tumor cell lines inoculated into them. Hall and coworkers (9), using cells collected from hollow fibers, demonstrated the impact of treatment with cisplatin on proliferating cell nuclear antigen and retinoblastoma protein expression by Western blot analyses on the post-treatment fiber contents. Similar work is being pursued against additional targets. The tumor cells within the fiber can be collected for use in assays such as Western blotting, and the entire fiber with its cellular content can be fixed, sectioned, and subjected to immunohistochemical stains to determine the level of target expression in the treated cells.

2.4. Luciferin-Based Technologies

The introduction of high-sensitivity charge-coupled device (CCD) camera systems capable of detecting light emission from luciferase-transfected cell lines is further expanding the application of hollow fiber-based assays. First, it is possible to monitor the viable cell mass in the fibers without need for removal from the host. Figure 2 shows the photon emission from luciferase-transfected U251 human glioma cells (10) contained within hollow fibers implanted in an athymic mouse. If cell lines with responsive elements are used, then it is possible to determine whether compounds have targeted the responsive element by simply imaging the mice after fiber implantation and drug treatment. Our program is actively pursuing this technology. One result of using the luciferase detection system is the demonstration that hollow fibers, whether implanted ip or sc, are oxygenated and receive rapid exposure to luciferin following ip injections. The luciferase enzyme, using Mg^{2+} as a cofactor, catalyzes the reaction:

$$luciferin + O_2 + ATP \rightarrow oxyluciferin + AMP + CO_2 + light\ emission$$

Since the reaction is dependent on the presence of all reactants, we can conclude that light emission from cells entrapped in hollow fibers demonstrates the presence of these reactants at the hollow fiber implant site. Figure 3 shows the light emission curve for a set of hollow fibers that were implanted sc in mice. These mice received a single ip injection of luciferin at 150 mg/kg and were imaged every 2 min for 1/2 h. As seen, light emission is detectable within 6 min following luciferin administration and plateaus at approx 1 h post administration. Phillips et al. (11) suggested that the sc implanted hollow fibers used by the NCI screening program are not valid because they are not vascularized. The light emission occurring from luciferase-transfected cell lines implanted sc demonstrates that vascularization is not critical to the hollow fiber assay since chemicals (e.g., luciferin) injected ip obviously reached these fibers within 6 min post injection. Furthermore, the presence of light emission also demonstrates that cells within the sc hollow fibers have sufficient O_2 and ATP present to be metabolically active and are thus susceptible to antitumor agents.

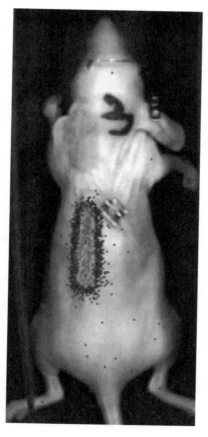

Fig. 2. A single hollow fiber containing U251-pGL3, the human glioma U251 stably transfected with a constitutive luciferase gene, was implanted into this mouse. Three hours post implantation the mouse received 150 mg/kg luciferin (Xenogen) intraperitoneally. The mouse was anesthetized and imaged for 30 s in a Xenogen IVIS® system 20 min post luciferin administration. The light emission detected from the hollow fiber-entrapped cells is readily seen on the dorsum of the mouse just lateral to the spinal column.

3. IN VITRO/IN VIVO ANGIOGENESIS ASSAYS

3.1. In Vitro Assays

Vascularization in the vicinity of transplanted tumors was described by Goldman as early as 1907 *(12)*, with further characterization in the mid-20th century by Ide, Green, Coman, Sheldon, Merwin, Algire, Goodall, and their coworkers *(13–17)*. In 1966, Folkman et al. *(18)* proposed that tumors are dependent on capillary formation and are limited to a size of 1–2 mm in the absence of vascularization. This led to the concept of inhibiting blood vessel development as a therapeutic modality for cancer. Since then, many approaches to cancer therapy based on antiangiogenic concepts have been actively pursued. Broadly, target categories have included agents that inhibit angiogenic growth factors including basic fibroblast growth factor (bFGF) and vascular endothelial growth factor (VEGF); matrix metalloproteinase inhibitors (MMPIs); agents that target receptors (e.g., integrins); and others with poorly defined mechanisms *(19)*.

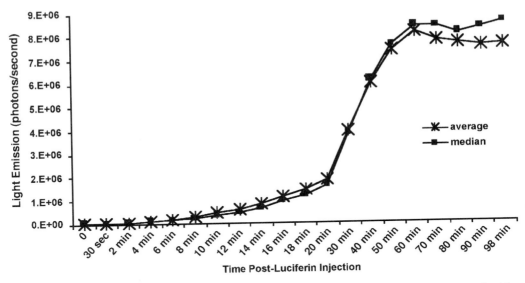

Fig. 3. Hollow fibers containing U251-pGL3, the human glioma U251 stably transfected with a constitutive luciferase gene, were implanted into 5 athymic mice. Three hours post implantation the mice received a single ip dose of 150 mg/kg luciferin. The mice were anesthetized with isoflurane and sequentially imaged in a Xenogen IVIS system over the course of 98 min. Each image was the result of a 30-s exposure; $n = 5$ mice, each containing one hollow fiber.

The interest in developing antiangiogenic therapies suggested a need for our program to provide support for these efforts. As part of this goal, a repository to provide human umbilical vein endothelial cells (HUVECs) to qualified researchers, as well as a series of assays intended to identify and aid in the development of new therapies, was implemented (*see* Angiogenesis Resource Center at http://dtp.nci.nih.gov). For in vitro studies, these include a panel of standard assays: growth inhibition, cord formation, chemotaxis (motility), and the aortic ring assay. A brief description of these assays is given here.

3.1.1. GROWTH INHIBITION ASSAY

Growth inhibition assays are designed to measure the capacity of a test agent to reduce the proliferation capacity of endothelial cells. These assays are conducted in a 96-well plate format using HUVECs as the target. The routine protocol for this assay uses growth medium containing a full complement of growth factors including bFGF, VEGF, insulin-like growth factor (IGF), and epithelial growth factor (EGF). This can be modified to use only a single growth factor (e.g., bFGF or VEGF) if the test compound is expected to target one pathway specifically. The routine assay uses HUVECs, but it is possible to study other endothelial cells (e.g., microvascular, bovine aortic endothelial cells) as appropriate for the test agent. HUVECs are plated in 96-well plates at a density of 2500 cells/well in a volume of 100 µL of EBM-2 medium (Clonetics). Twenty-four hours after plating, 100 µL of medium containing a 2× concentration of the test agent are added per well. Initial testing is routinely conducted using serial 10-fold dilutions of the agent, with each concentration assessed in triplicate. At the time compounds are added to the test plates, a time 0 plate is stained using 0.5% crystal violet. The remaining, compound-treated, plates are incubated at 37°C for 24, 48, or 72 h as desired. After incubation the

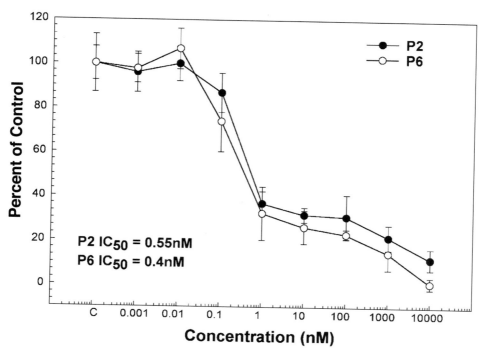

Fig. 4. Growth inhibition assay. HUVECs (2.5×10^3) were plated in a 96-well plate in 100 μL of EGM-2 medium. After 24 h, TNP-470 was added to each well at 2× the final concentration along with proper vehicle controls. Cells were incubated for 72 h, and growth was determined using the crystal violet assay. This graph is representative of the growth curve of HUVEC from several experiments.

plates are stained with 0.5% crystal violet, rinsed, and allowed to air dry. The stain is eluted from the test and time 0 plates with an ethanol/citrate solution, and the absorbance is measured at 540 nm in a 96-well plate reader (Dynex MRX® Microplate Reader). The growth inhibition is calculated from the absorbance measurements using the averages of the replicate time 0 (T_z), growth control (T_C), and test wells (T_i) in the formula $[(T_i-T_z)/(T_c-T_z)] \times 100$. The 50% inhibitory concentration (IC_{50}) is calculated. The fumagillin analog TNP-470 (AGM-1470; NSC 642492; *see* ref. *30*) is the positive control for this assay. TNP-470 inhibits endothelial cell proliferation and migration through a mechanism that is mediated, at least in part, by covalent binding to a metalloproteinase, methionine aminopeptidase 2 *(20)*. The effects of a 48-h exposure to TNP-470 on HUVEC growth at passage 2 (P2) and at passage 6 (P6) are shown in Fig. 4. The IC_{50} is 0.55 n*M* and 0.4 n*M* at P2 and P6, respectively.

3.1.2. Cord Formation Assay

The cord formation assay assesses the impact of a test agent on the natural capacity of endothelial cells to line up and form organized tubular structures when plated on a matrix. The surface of 96-well plates is coated with Matrigel®, a basement membrane complex derived from Engelbreth-Swarm-Holm (EHS) sarcoma. Following gelling of the matrix, a suspension of HUVECs in medium containing the full complement of growth factors (e.g., BFGF, VEGF, IGF, EGF) is mixed with the test agent and added to each well (2 ×

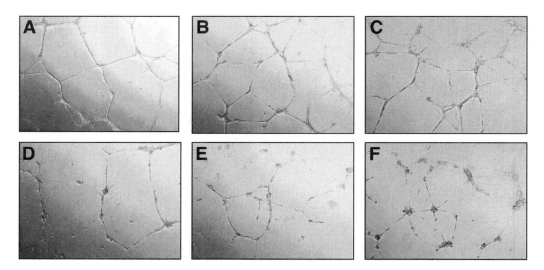

Fig. 5. Effect of a drug treatment on cord formation. Untreated control (200 μL of 1 × 10⁵) (**A**) or drug-treated HUVECs (**B–F**) were plated on Matrigel in a 96-well plate. After 18 h the cells were visualized under a microscope, and three pictures were taken from each well. Cord lengths and numbers of junctions were disrupted in a concentration-dependent manner. (**A**) Vehicle control. NSC 712305 at (**B**) 5 ng/mL, (**C**) 10 ng/mL, (**D**) 25 ng/mL, (**E**) 50 ng/mL and (**F**) 100 ng/mL.

10^4 cells/well). The plates are incubated for 18–24 h at 37°C in a humidified CO_2 incubator. The cords are observed under magnification, and photographic images are collected for analysis. Figure 5 shows the cords produced in control and NSC 713205-treated HUVECs. The control sample (Fig. 5A) demonstrates the normal cord formation seen with HUVECS. The graded doses of NSC 713205 (Fig. 5B–F) show a significant impact on cord formation without even necessitating comparison of the actual junction numbers or length between junctions.

The number of junctions and the tube length (in mm) between junctions is determined using an image analysis system. Figure 6A and B demonstrates how the cord lengths and junctions are measured, respectively. The impact of treatment is then determined by comparing the counts from treated samples with those from vehicle control samples. Figure 6C shows the results of treatment on the cord length as well as the number of junctions for the compound shown in Fig. 5. There is complete loss of cord formation at 30 nM. It is important when assessing cord formation to verify that the effect is not a result of simple cytotoxicity by conducting appropriate growth inhibition assays.

3.1.3. CHEMOTAXIS ASSAY

Chemotaxis (motility) assays measure the response of HUVECs to chemoattractants (e.g., VEGF, BFGF), in that HUVECs migrate toward the concentration gradient created by these agents. These assays are performed in a 96-well migration plate (Neuro Probe) that allows cells on one side of a permeable membrane to be exposed to the chemoattractant on the other side of the membrane. In response to this gradient, the HUVECs migrate through pores (8 μm) in the membrane and are found on the chemoattractant side of the membrane following a suitable incubation. The membrane is coated with collagen

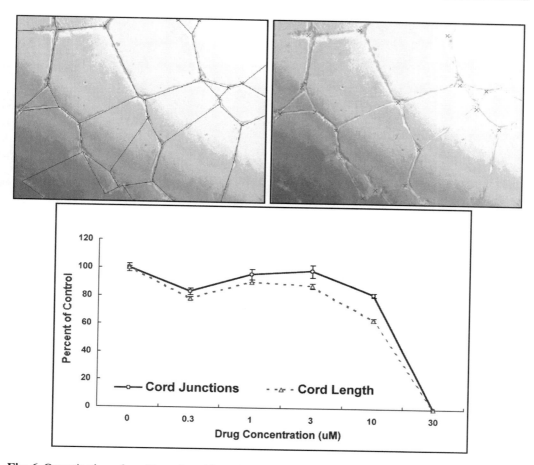

Fig. 6. Quantitation of cord length and junctions. Cord lengths and junctions were measured using a Bioquant Image Analysis system. Cord length was overlaid (**A**), total length was measured in millimeters, and cord junctions were counted (**B**) for each picture. Data were plotted (six replicates at each point), and the IC_{50} was calculated.

to provide a suitable attachment and migration surface for the cells. The membrane separates a lower chamber containing the chemoattractant or control solution and an upper surface bearing the HUVECs in suspension with the test agent. A 4–6 h incubation at 37°C in a humidified 5% CO_2 incubator allows migration of the HUVECs. Following incubation, the membrane is removed, fixed, and stained with a differential stain (e.g., Diff Quik®). The membrane is rinsed and the cells are wiped off the side of the membrane against which they were originally placed. The opposite side is quantitated for the number of cells/microscope field. The number of cells migrating in the compound treated well is compared with the control wells containing no compound treatment. Figure 7 graphically presents the results obtained with TNP-470 and Taxol® in the motility assay. The higher dose of each compound (1 μM) inhibits the number of cells migrating through the membrane by approx 50%.

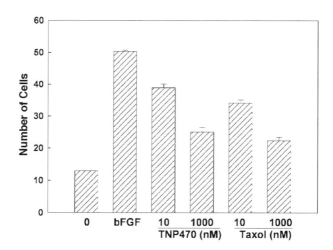

Fig. 7. Chemotaxis/motility/cell migration. The effects of TNP-470 and Taxol were assessed on migration of HUVECS using basic fibroblast growth factor (bFGF; 5 ng/mL) as a chemoattractant in 96-well ChemoTex® disposable plates (Neuro Probe). The data represent three fields (400× magnification) counted for each replicate with four replicates per dose.

3.1.4. Aortic Ring Assays

Another assay that assesses endothelial cell growth and migration under more physiologic conditions is the rat or embryonic chicken aortic ring assay. For this, aortas are retrieved from young rats or 12- to 14-d-old chicken embryos, and the aortas are sterilely stripped of extraneous connective tissue using a dissecting microscope as necessary. The aorta is cut into thin rings that are placed onto a layer of polymerized Matrigel, and then the ring is sealed in place with an overlay of Matrigel. In both instances the Matrigel is growth factor-depleted to avoid confounding the results. Once the Matrigel has polymerized, the sample is overlaid with medium containing the desired growth factors, e.g., VEGF, bFGF, endothelial cell growth supplement (ECGS; Collaborative Research) and the test compound. At the end of the incubation period (8–10 d for rat; 24–48 h for chick), the aortic rings are imaged. The effect is measured by determining the length of vessels (rat) and area of sprouting (chick) around the ring (Fig. 8G). A representative sample of chick embryo aortic rings treated with TNP-470 (NSC 642492) or Taxol (paclitaxel; NSC 125973) is given in Fig. 8. The negative control (Fig. 8A) shows a lack of sprouting that occurs if no growth factors are included in the medium. The 50 μg/mL ECGS image (Fig. 8B) demonstrates the sprouting that occurs in the presence of growth factors. The 1.0 μM NSC 642492 (Fig. 8D) shows a good effect on sprouting; however, the 25 nM concentration of Taxol (Fig. 8F) is significantly more active in that it shows essentially complete inhibition of sprouting.

3.1.5. Conclusions

To date, 176 compounds have been evaluated in these assays. Table 1 presents a summary of the results obtained for these compounds with respect to how many compounds were positive in each combination of possible outcomes (e.g., positive and negative in the assays). The compounds are considered active with an IC$_{50}$ of <25 μM or <50 μg/mL in growth inhibition, cord formation, or migration assay. No correlation has

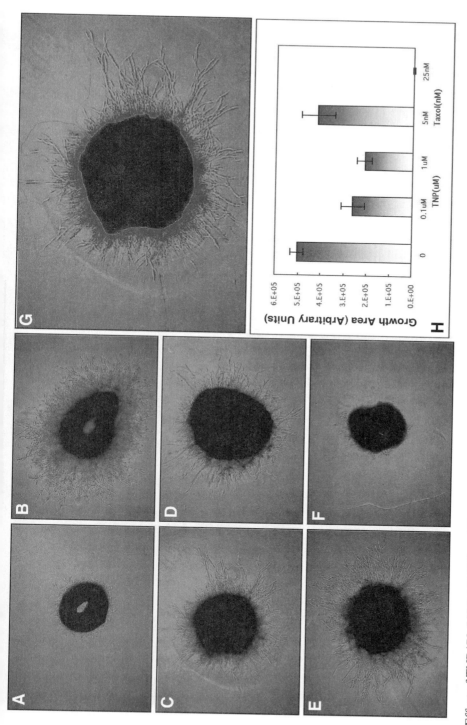

Fig. 8. Effect of TNP470 (NSC 642492) and Taxol (NSC 125973) on chick aortic ring assay. Aortic arches were isolated from 12-d old embryonated eggs, and the aortic rings were placed in Matrigel in a 48-well plate. Rings were treated for 48 h with medium without growth factors (**A**, negative control), with 50 µg/mL of ECGS (**B**, untreated control), 0.1 µM TNP-470 in 50 µg/mL of ECGS (**C**), 1 µM TNP-470 in 50 µg/mL ECGS (**D**), 5 nM Taxol in 50 µg/mL ECGS (**E**), and 25 nM Taxol in 50 µg/mL ECGS (**F**). The growth area for each ring is quantitated by calculating the sprouts around each aortic ring (**G**, dark gray) with the area of the ring (black area) excluded. The data are plotted for the net growth by subtracting the negative control from each value for the untreated control and the drug-treated rings (**H**).

Table 1
Compound Activity in the Standard Anti-Angiogenesis Screens

Growth inhibition	Tube formation	Migration	No. of compounds
+	+	+	38
+	+	−	14
+	−	+	14
+	−	−	67
−	−	−	26
−	+	+	4
−	−	+	10
−	+	−	3

been found between the structural character of the compounds and their activity or lack of activity in each of the assays evaluated. The largest single category for the various combinations of outcomes was compounds that only had growth-inhibitory activity. These represented a total of 38% of the compounds screened. The lowest percentage, 1.7%, occurred in compounds that only inhibited tube formation.

The assays described here evaluate the impact of compound on HUVECs; however, it is important to determine whether this effect is specific to HUVECs or is more broadly representative of mammalian cells in general. Compounds assessed in these assays are also assessed for activity against the NCI 60-cell line in vitro tumor panel. If the compound is more active against the HUVECs than the tumor cells, then some specificity is suggested. More specialized assays applicable to specific compounds and/or mechanisms of action, e.g., integin expression, impact of growth factors (VEGF, BFGF) on compound activity, and time-dose exposure requirements further aid in determining the specificity of activity on HUVECs compared with other cell types.

3.2. In Vivo Assays

3.2.1. MATRIGEL® PLUG ASSAY

Compounds with results suggesting antiangiogenic activity are evaluated in animal models designed to assess the activity. A common model for this purpose is the Matrigel plug assay. For this, Matrigel is mixed with growth factors (VEGF or bFGF) and injected sc into mice. Following a 7-d incubation, the Matrigel plugs are collected from the mice, homogenized, and analyzed for the presence of hemoglobin as an indicator of the presence of new blood vessel growth. This can be confirmed histologically by staining sections of the plug for endothelial cell markers. A section through a Matrigel plug following trichrome staining to reveal the full character of the sample is given in Fig. 9. The overlying skin at the top of the image and the underlying muscle at the bottom produce a sandwich in which the Matrigel (marked by the arrow) is trapped between the skin and the muscle. Vessels and cells can be seen penetrating the Matrigel matrix. Special stains for endothelial cell markers are required to discern which penetrating cells are endothelial in origin.

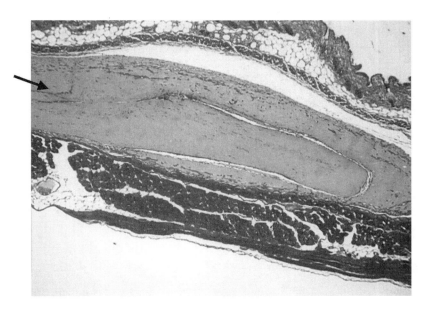

Fig. 9. Trichrome stain of Matrigel plug. This is a 50× magnification of a Matrigel plug fixed en bloc with the surrounding tissues. The Matrigel was injected subcutaneously on the ventral abdominal surface just caudal to the xyphoid process. Ten days post injection, the Matrigel plug and surrounding tissues were excised, fixed in 10% buffered formalin, processed, and stained by the trichrome technique. The epidermis and loose connective tissue can be seen at the top of the image, and the deeper muscular layer can be seen at the lower side of the image. The Matrigel plug stains a uniform pale blue with many penetrations by ingrowing cells. The arrow indicates the Matrigel plug portion of the image.

3.2.2. Syngeneic Tumor Models

For evaluations in a more physiologic environment, the compounds are tested in mouse tumor models. The most commonly used models are syngeneic, as this provides a physiologically more relevant microenvironment. Two commonly used models for this are B16F10 murine melanoma B16F10 *(21)* and murine Lewis lung carcinoma models. The B16F10 tumor is syngeneic in C57Bl/6 mice and grows rapidly following inoculation by the sc route. The tumor has been well characterized, so a large body of data is available with regard to its drug sensitivity and its physiologic characteristics and behavior. Routine assays of antiangiogenic compounds are conducted using sc B16F10 tumors. Generally, 5×10^4 tumor cells are inoculated in the axillary region, and treatment is begun 1–3 d post injection. Routinely, treatments are continued for about 10 d, with tumor length and width measurements collected every 2–3 d until they reach 20 mm in diameter. The positive control compound, TNP-470 (NSC 642492), is included for comparison in all assays. The routine dose, route, and schedule for this compound is a 30 mg/kg/ dose given every 48 h for a minimum of six doses by the sc route. The median tumor weights for each group are determined and used to calculate the percent test/control (% T/C) at each time point. Historically, a % T/C of 40% or less was suggestive of activity

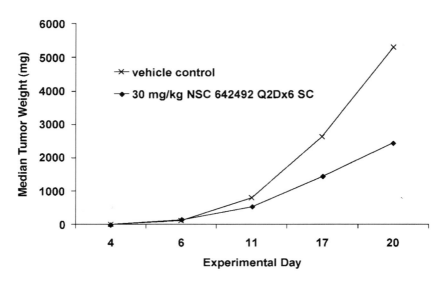

Fig. 10. TNP-470 vs. B16F10 murine melanoma. B16F10 murine melanoma cells (5×10^4) were injected subcutaneously in C57Bl/6 mice, and treatment was initiated on d 4 post tumor injection. TNP-470 was administered once every other day for a total of six doses. The administration route was sc. The optimal % T/C for the TNP-470 treatment was 46.5%.

with cytotoxic agents. Antiangiogenic compounds may not produce a % T/C in this range, so caution must be exercised when selecting compounds for further development. Generally, a reproducible % T/C in the 60% range may indicate that further evaluations are in order, particularly if dose, route, and schedule issues have not been resolved. The results of evaluating TNP-470 in a subcutaneously implanted B16F10 tumor are shown in Fig. 10. In this instance the optimal % T/C is 47%.

Subcutaneously implanted Lewis lung carcinoma *(22)*, which is also syngeneic in the C57Bl/6 mouse, can be evaluated in the same manner. The advantage with this model is that spontaneous metastases to the lung occur following sc implantation. Metastasis occurs early in the tumor growth so the impact of treatment on primary as well as meta-static tumor growth can be readily assessed. The assays are conducted similarly to the B16F10 assay. The median tumor weights obtained following treatment with TNP-470 are shown in Fig. 11. The optimal % T/C in this model was 20% when the TNP-470 was administered sc every 2 d for 7 doses (q2d×7).

3.2.3. TNP-470 (NSC 642492) Activity in Xenograft Models

In addition to syngeneic tumors, TNP-470 has been evaluated in a large number of xenograft models with evidence of differential sensitivity. Whether this sensitivity is directly correlated with vascular density remains to be determined. Table 2 presents the optimal % T/C obtained with a 30 mg/kg/injection dose of TNP-470 given sc on a repeating every other day (q2d) schedule. The median tumor weight at the beginning of therapy was not identical for each tumor; however, it is reasonable to conclude that the mouse tumors may be slightly more sensitive than the human tumors as a rule. Several possibilities exist to explain the difference in sensitivity among the tumors. Obviously, there are some differences among the tumors because of the weight the tumor had achieved

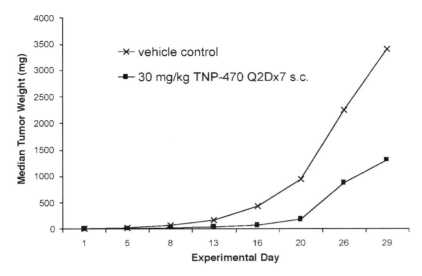

Fig. 11. TNP-470 vs. Lewis lung carcinoma. Lewis lung carcinoma tumor fragments in the fifth in vivo passage were inoculated sc into C57Bl/6 mice, and 24 h later the mice began receiving treatment with TNP-470 on an every second day schedule for a total of seven doses. The route was sc. The optimal % T/C for the TNP-470 treatment was 20%.

at the start of treatment as well as the number of doses administered in each tumor model. Less obvious, but more provocative, is the possibility that differences in vascular density exist among the various tumors. In our experience mouse tumors are generally more vascularized than human tumor xenografts. The vascular densities of the tumors presented in Table 2 have not been fully characterized, so the impact of vascularity on the differences in xenograft sensitivity cannot be defined.

4. IN VITRO PHARMACOLOGIC CHARACTERIZATION OF EXPERIMENTAL AGENTS

From in vitro screening results and initial in vivo hollow fiber assay testing, it is usually possible to identify a number of tumor cell lines that are sensitive to a given experimental agent. However, from such initial in vitro and in vivo screening data, one cannot ascertain the minimum exposure required for a given agent to achieve in vivo activity, nor can one gauge what treatment regimens would confer antitumor efficacy in a group of in vivo xenograft models. In addition, one cannot identify optimal treatment regimens for subsequent in vivo efficacy testing in xenograft models without preliminary pharmacologic information.

For these reasons, hollow fiber assay-active agents are tested in specialized in vitro pharmacology assays to identify the most sensitive group of tumor cell line targets, and to identify the minimum *concentration × time* exposures required to achieve anticancer effect(s), and to characterize the in vitro *concentration × time* exposures required to achieve some degree of activity not only in the most sensitive tumor cell lines, but also in alternate, lesser responsive models that may nevertheless serve as in vivo sensitive targets. In addition, other specialized in vitro pharmacology assays can be performed to

Table 2
Optimal %T/C for TNP-470 Tested Against Various Tumor Models

Tumor	Species of origin	Tumor type	Implant site	Median tumor weight (mg)	Treatment schedule	% T/C
B16F10	Mouse	Melanoma	sc	<63	q2d×6	29
Lewis lung	Mouse	Lung	sc	<63	q2d×9	31
UACC-62	Human	Melanoma	sc	94	q2d×9	33
E-END-1	Mouse	Endothelioma	sc	<63	q2d×6	35
MDA-MB-435	Human	Breast	MFP	<63	q2d×22	35
M5076	Mouse	Sarcoma	sc	<63	q2d×10	39
CCRF-CEM	Human	Leukemia	sc	<63	q2d×10	42
MX-1	Human	Breast	sc	126	q2d×10	48
JURKAT	Human	Leukemia	sc	63	q2d×12	52
10.5	Human	Pancreas	sc	126	q2d×6	54
KS Y-1	Human	Kaposi's sarcoma	sc	<63	q2DX6	55
SW-620	Human	Colon	sc	146	q2d×5	56
U251	Human	CNS	sc	106	q2d×10	56
RPMI-8226	Human	Myeloma	sc	83	q2d×6	57
SF-295	Human	CNS	sc	159	q2d×6	57
MDA-MB-361	Human	Breast	MFP	<63	q2d×10	58
HCT-116	Human	Colon	sc	111	q2d×6	60
ASPC-1	Human	Pancreas	sc	184	q2d×21	61
COLO 205	Human	Colon	sc	78	q2d×6	62
H5V	Mouse	Endothelioma	sc	<63	q2d×6	67
HT-29	Human	Colon	sc	196	q2d×6	72
A498	Human	Renal	sc	<63	q2d×8	75
Caki-1	Human	Renal	sc	148	q2d×6	78
ECV-304	Mouse	Endothelioma	sc	146	q2d×6	80
HL-60	Human	Leukemia	sc	129	q2d×6	80
6.03	Human	Pancreas	sc	144	q2d×6	85
SR	Human	Leukemia	sc	91	q2d×6	91
MCF7	Human	Breast	sc	126	q2d×6	99
H209	Human	Small-cell lung	sc	148	q2d×6	100
H510A	Human	Small-cell lung	sc	117	q2d×6	100

ABBREVIATIONS: CNS, central nervous system; MFP, mammary fat pad; % T/C, % test/control.

measure stability of an experimental agent and to determine whether a compound's effective *concentration × time* can be achieved in vivo in non-tumor-bearing mice administered maximum tolerated dosages. With in vitro pharmacology bioassays, one can (1) identify pharmacologic characteristics of a given agent or series of experimental agents quickly and with a minimum amount of material as well as (2) choose which agents and models are most likely to be suitable for preclinical development without incurring the time and expense of large-scale comparative in vivo efficacy testing of all candidate agents.

4.1. Methodologies

The various specialized assays described below utilize similar steps methodologies. These assays share the same steps of (1) cell culture inoculation, (2) analysis of "stable endpoint" MTT formazan colorimetry, and (3) computerized calculations, data uploading, and storage. The assays differ in terms of the methods of experimental agent preparation and application, in the modes of specialized computer calculations, tabulation, and graphical representations of concentration-effect relationships, as well as in how results are interpreted with respect to other biologic and pharmacologic information.

4.1.1. In Vitro Time Course Assays

Methods for cell culture, drug preparations, and conventional in vitro drug sensitivity testing have been described previously *(23)*. The concentration ranges of experimental agents to be evaluated in the more specialized *concentration × time* assays are chosen on the basis of 60-cell line screening data and/or from testing in an abbreviated set of 48/72- and 144/168-h assays in selected cell lines.

As described elsewhere *(24)*, the concurrent testing of an experimental agent or group of agents in replicate culture plates permits quantitation of drug activity conferred by each of several exposure durations ranging from ≤ 1 h to 144 h. In addition, use of "proliferation control" plates stained at the time of drug addition (drug addition T_0) permits the determination of multiple pharmacologic indices (50% growth inhibition [GI_{50}], total growth inhibition [TGI], and 50% lethal concentration [LC_{50}]) for each duration of drug exposure.

From the plotting of composite *concentration × time* data, one can readily determine the minimum exposure conditions (both concentration and time) required to achieve cytostatic and/or cytocidal activity in a given cell line for each compound or group of compounds. Such in vitro data are plotted as *concentration × time* bar graphs from which one can readily determine the minimal exposure conditions required for a given agent to achieve cytostatic and/or cytocidal activity. This data format of composite *concentration × time* data presentation permits (1) a comparison of the effects of multiple agents in a given cancer cell line or (2) a comparison of the activities of a given agent in multiple cell lines under conditions of specific, controlled in vitro exposure.

4.1.1.1. In Vitro *Concentration × Time* Drug Exposure Assay. For the in vitro *concentration × time* drug exposure assay, cells cultivated in standard culture medium (RPMI-1640 supplemented with 20% defined fetal bovine serum [Hyclone] and 2 m*M* L-glutamine without antibiotics) are inoculated into replicate 96-well PVDF membrane plates (Millipore MAHVS45; one plate for each duration of drug treatment to be tested) in 100-µL volumes using multichannel electronic pipets (programmable Impact and

Impact 2). Following overnight incubation (37°C, 5% CO_2, 100% humidity) 100 µL of culture medium, culture medium containing drug, or culture medium containing drug vehicle are dispensed within appropriate wells (vehicle control group, $n = 6$; each drug treatment group, $n = 3$). Following each duration of drug treatment (i.e., usually 0.75, 1.5, 3, 6, 12, 24, 48, and 144 h—unless shorter or longer exposures are required), the culture medium containing drug is removed from the plate wells by vacuum using the Millipore multiscreen filtration system (cat. no. MAVM0960R) and replaced with 200 µL of fresh culture medium.

Following drug treatments and rinses, the whole set of plates is then incubated for the remainder of the 7-d culture duration and then stained with MTT. Fifty microliters of MTT working solution is added to each culture well (resulting in 100 µg MTT/250 µL total medium volume), and cultures are incubated at 37°C for 4 h. At the end of the MTT incubation, all culture supernatant is removed by vacuum, and wells are rinsed twice with 300 µL 2.5% protamine sulfate (Sigma P4380) buffer following overnight incubations at 4°C in the dark. Use of protamine sulfate rinses provides a "stable MTT formazan" endpoint and very low media background levels (3,4). Finally, plates are vacuum-aspirated and dried. MTT formazan is solubilized with dimethyl sulfoxide (DMSO) (200 µL/well); 150 µL amounts are transferred to fresh plates, and absorbances are measured at 540 nm using a plate colorimeter (MRX Dynex Technologies). Subsequently, data are uploaded to a VAX alpha 10,000 computer for processing and storage. Through software programs developed in collaboration with staff of the DTP Information Technology Branch (in particular, David Segal and Marie Hose), experimental information and comparative data are then further processed using Microsoft Excel® programs to retrieve, assemble, tabulate, scale, and plot datasets.

4.1.1.2. In Vitro *Concentration* × *Time* Drug Stability Assay. Cells are inoculated in replicate 96-well PVDF membrane plates, and drug is diluted into culture medium in the same manner as for the in vitro *concentration* × *time* drug exposure assay. However, to assess the stability of drug in culture medium, solutions are preincubated at 37°C over a range of durations prior to their addition to cell culture plates (i.e., usually preincubations are performed over the course of 0, 0.75, 1.5, 3, 6, 12, 24, and 48 h). The whole set of plates is then incubated until the end of the assay (7-d total culture duration) and then stained with MTT, rinsed, dried, extracted, and analyzed in the same manner as for other in vitro assays. In addition to evaluating stability of the experimental agent in culture medium, one can also assay the stability of drug stocks following preparation and storage in selected solvents or vehicles at room temperature, 4°C, and –70°C over the course of days, weeks, or months. Such procedures are useful when one needs a biological index of the stability of new experimental agents. One can employ the same method to test the biological stability and/or activity of experimental agents incubated in fresh plasma derived from laboratory animals.

4.1.2. Ex Vivo Pharmacology Bioassay

4.1.2.1. Testing Strategy. Identify sensitive tumor cell line target(s) based on the in vitro time-course assays. Determine effective dose range and maximum tolerated dose from hollow fiber assay and/or initial testing in xenograft models. Perform initial ex vivo pharmacology bioassay following single drug injection at the maximum tolerated dose MTD as previously described (25). Compare drug activity in mouse plasma following in vivo treatments with that of the drug activity in pooled mouse plasma to which the same compound stock was added ex vivo. Perform subsequent ex vivo pharmacology bioassay on mice or rats receiving drug by alternate dose, route, and/or schedule. Determine which treatment regimens yield the most favorable drug disposition.

4.1.2.2. Operational Steps. Formulate compound for both in vitro time-course assay and ex vivo pharmacology bioassay. Administer compound to replicate mice or rats and collect heparinized whole blood on ice at relevant intervals: (iv route at 3.25, 7.5, 15, 30, and 60 min; ip and sc routes at 15, 30, 60, 120, and 240 min). Isolate and dilute plasma samples in culture medium containing 20% pooled mouse serum and sterile-filter samples. Apply diluted samples to PVDF filter plates containing cells inoculated in culture medium containing 20% defined FBS, incubate for 6 d, and then analyze viable cell mass using the same procedures as for the in vitro time-course assay. Calculate the in vivo plasma concentrations of the test agent based on measuring the plasma content required to produce GI_{50} activity equivalent to the activity measured in replicate cultures exposed to mouse serum supplemented in vitro with known concentrations of test agent.

4.2. Prototypic Examples of Experimental Agents Evaluated in Specialized In Vitro Pharmacology Assays

4.2.1. Assessment of In Vitro and In Vivo Pharmacology of a Tricyclic Thiophene

Results of testing a substituted thiophene structure (NSC 652287) in the in vitro anticancer drug screen (48-h drug exposure, 72-h culture duration) are depicted in Fig. 12. The averaged mean graph of 60-cell line drug sensitivities exhibits a multilog differential pattern of activity. This pattern is highly unusual compared with standard anticancer agents. The agent was highly active in hollow fiber assays (16 ip + 12 sc = 28 total score with two cell lines killed) and was prioritized for in vivo efficacy evaluation in multiple human tumor xenograft models.

In vivo efficacy evaluations of this agent administered ip were performed in mice bearing early-staged tumors of HCC-2998, UACC-62, UACC-257, OVCAR-3, OVCAR-5, A-498, and CaKi-1. Intraperitoneal treatment demonstrated efficacy against OVCAR-3 and UACC-257 and prominent regressions in the A-498 model; however, no antitumor activity was observed against HCC-2998, UACC-62, and CaKi-1 models, with equivocal antitumor activity against the OVCAR-5 model using the same ip treatment protocol. Intravenous administration of this agent exhibited even greater activity in the A-498 model and good, but not curative, activity against CaKi-1 xenografts.

A lack of activity of this agent in the majority of xenograft models of "sensitive cancer" cell lines prompted our program to compare in vitro *concentration × time* assay endpoints with the measurement of in vivo plasma pharmacokinetic profiles of this agent in mice. Results of testing this experimental agent in *in vitro concentration × time* drug exposure assays of 10 sensitive tumor cell lines are shown in Fig. 13. Of the cell lines tested, A-498 was the most sensitive in terms of both concentration and time responsiveness: LC_{50} levels of activity were achieved readily with less than a *3 h × 100 n*M exposure. OVCAR-3, OVCAR-5, and NCI-H226 were also moderately sensitive, with LC_{50} activity achieved with less than a *3 h × 300 n*M exposure. CaKi-1, LXFL-529, and UACC-257 required significantly higher drug concentrations and/or longer exposures, with TGI activity requiring on the order of *3 h × 400–600 n*M exposures. By contrast, HCC-2998, UACC-

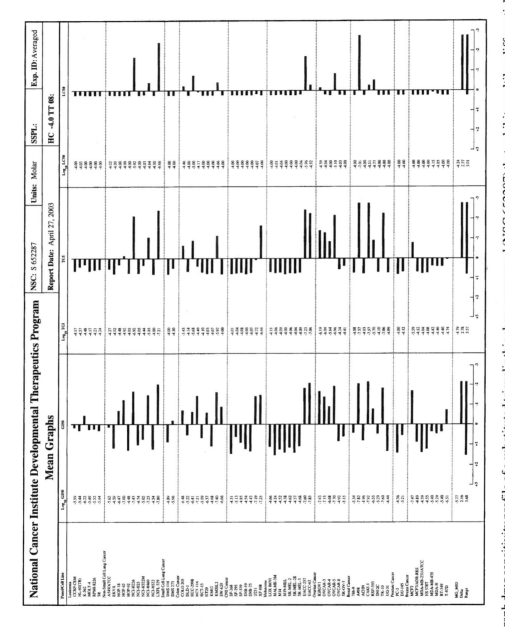

Fig. 12. Mean graph drug sensitivity profile of a substituted tricyclic thiophene compound (NSC 652287) that exhibits multilog differential effect among cell lines and a "unique" pattern of activity (COMPARE negative to standard agents) in the NCI in vitro cancer screen. Depicted in the figure are mean log GI$_{50}$, TGI, and LC$_{50}$ indices derived from eight separate assays.

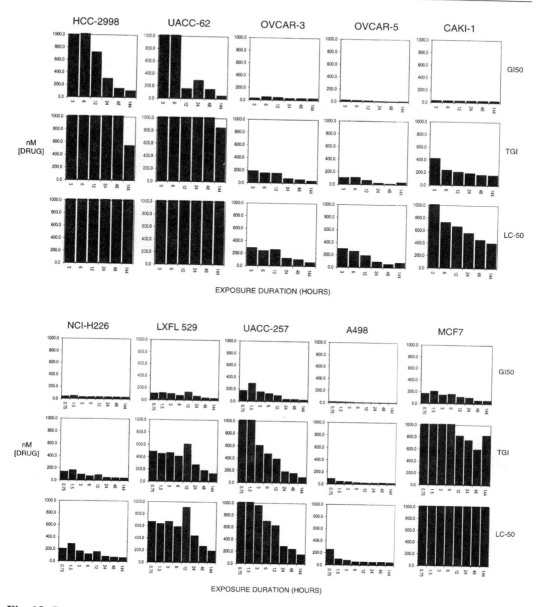

Fig. 13. Comparative in vitro *concentration × time* profiles of NSC 652287 in selected "sensitive" human tumor cell lines.

62, and MCF-7, although among the sensitive series of cell lines in the cancer screen, nevertheless exhibited far less sensitivity to this agent with *> 6 h × >1000 n*M required to achieve GI_{50} or TGI activity in the in vitro *concentration × time* assay.

The pharmacokinetics of NSC 652287 were examined following administration employing doses and routes similar to those used during in vivo efficacy studies. Plasma samples were collected at scheduled intervals of 8 (iv) or 24 (ip and po) h, and concentrations were analyzed by high-performance liquid chromatography (HPLC) *(26)*. Plasma

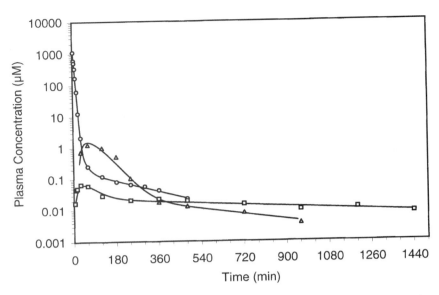

Fig. 14. Plasma concentrations and line of best fit obtained following iv administration of 100 mg/kg NSC 652287 to CD2F1 mice as a short (1-min) infusion (circles), or 200 mg/kg by ip injection (triangles) or po dosing (squares). Each point represents the geometric mean of samples collected from a minimum of three mice. The line of best fit was determined by nonlinear regression analysis.

concentration vs time profiles were constructed and the pharmacokinetics evaluated as previously described *(27)*. Plasma levels of NSC 652287 declined in a triexponential manner after iv injection of 100 mg/kg (Fig. 14). Concentrations initially (2 min) exceeded 1000 μM, but fell rapidly ($t_{1/2}$ = 3 min) to 250 nM by 1 h, and then decreased at a slower rate ($t_{1/2}$ = 2.6 h) through 8 h to 23 nM. Following ip injection at a dose of 200 mg/kg, plasma concentrations of NSC 652287 were between 500 and 1300 nM from 30 min through 3 h, decreased to 18 nM at 6 h, and further fell to 4 nM by 16 h. The same dose given orally (intragastric intubation) produced plasma levels of NSC 652287 between 20 and 70 nM from 5 min until 8 h, which gradually declined to 8 nM by 24 h. The bioavailability of NSC 652287 was very low (<5%) when administered by either the ip or oral routes. This is probably owing to rapid hepatic metabolism from direct absorption into the hepatic portal circulation. In support of this, plasma levels of a metabolite (identified as the carboxylic acid derivative *[28]*) greatly exceeded those of the parent in samples from these studies.

It is clear that effective concentrations (as indicated by the LC_{50} or TGI levels from in vitro *concentration × time* assays) are achieved for A498 by all three routes of administration. Levels required for activity against OVCAR-3 and OVCAR-5 are achieved by the iv or ip routes. The in vivo responsiveness of the CaKi-1 model is marginal; effective plasma concentrations appear to be achieved for a TGI level of activity with ip administration; however, results obtained for the iv route are less clear. Levels required for TGI of UACC-257 are approached by ip administration. In summary, most of the in vitro and in vivo pharmacologic findings are consistent with the results of in vivo efficacy testing performed in mice.

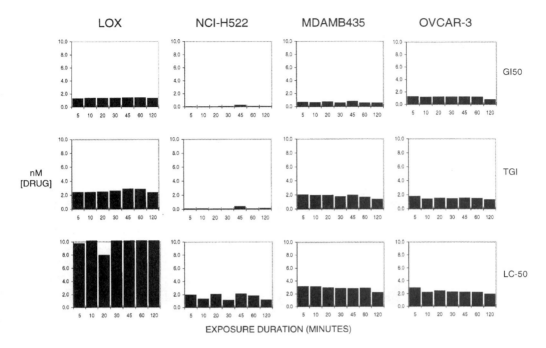

Fig. 15. Comparative in vitro *concentration × time* profiles for very brief exposures of (NSC 609395) in selected human tumor cell lines.

This particular thiophene analog was pursued vigorously as a preclinical drug development candidate until it became clear that effective *concentration × time* levels could not be achieved in nonrodent species without substantial toxicity. Results of in vitro *concentration × time* testing and pharmacokinetic analyses on this particular agent prompted our program to consider alternate thiophene analogs that may possess more favorable pharmacologic profiles than NSC 652287 in mice and nonrodent species. To date we have not encountered a more efficacious and/or less toxic thiophene structure.

4.2.2. In Vitro Stability Time-Course Assays of Halichondrin B

Natural products that are highly potent in vitro, available in very limited supply, and exhibit in vivo antitumor efficacy at or near the maximum tolerated dosages present major challenges to preclinical drug development. This was especially true in the case of Halichondrin B (NSC 609395), which also defied the development of analytical methods of analysis in biological specimens. In vitro pharmacology bioassays proved to be important demonstrations of activity during the early preclinical development of this agent because they demonstrated that this particular agent possessed a number of unusual but useful therapeutic attributes. Namely, as shown in Fig. 15, the agent was highly active in multiple cell lines at low nanomolar concentrations and near-maximum and irreversible activity could be achieved with as little as 5-min exposures to this agent. This profile is very unusual, since most anticancer drugs usually require ≥6 h to achieve near-maximum activities against human solid tumor cell lines. Furthermore, although halichondrin B is inactivated in the presence of fresh mouse serum, as shown in Fig. 16 (approx 25%

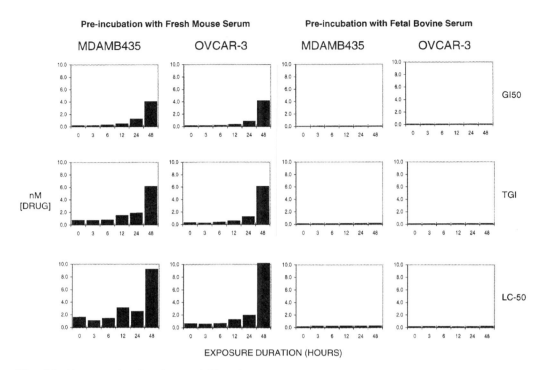

Fig. 16. Comparative in vitro stability time-course assays of Halichondrin B (NSC 609395) preincubated in fresh mouse serum and in fetal bovine serum.

in 6 h, 44% in 12 h, and 86% in 24 h), the agent is more active on a molar basis in both fetal bovine serum and human serum (Fig. 17). Loss of activity occurs far more slowly in fetal bovine serum (2.64% in 12 h and 11.5% in 24 h) and inappreciably in serum samples from healthy volunteers. Even though no drug activity could be detected in ex vivo pharmacology bioassays sampled at 3.25 or 7.5 min post iv injection or at 15 or 30 min post ip injection, the agent was active in each of five treatment regimens: qd×5 ip and iv, q4d×3 ip and iv, and qd×9 ip, with the intermittent iv regimen resulting in the highest frequency of complete regressions (8/10), as described previously (29).

4.2.3. Ex Vivo Pharmacology Bioassay and Analytical Characterizations of Phenylurea Thiocarbamate

Phenylurea thiocarbamate (PTC, NSC 161128) was originally selected as a candidate for preclinical development based on the activity shown in the NCI-sponsored in vitro prostate cancer screen at Stanford University. Subsequently, PTC was found to exhibit differential activity and antileukemia activity in the NCI in vitro 60-cell line cancer screen and to have in vivo efficacy in the DU-145 prostate cancer xenograft model. On the basis of these experimental findings, its unique chemical structure, and its potentially novel mechanism of action, PTC was approved by NCI for stage IIa preclinical development.

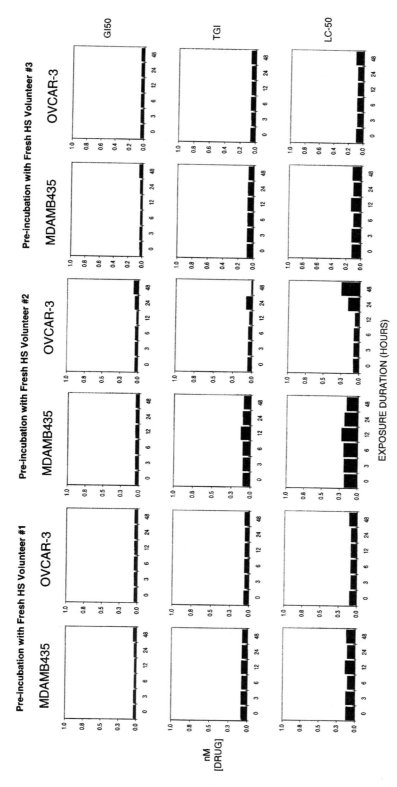

Fig. 17. Comparative in vitro stability time-course assays of NSC 609395 preincubated in fresh human serum samples collected from three healthy human volunteers.

177

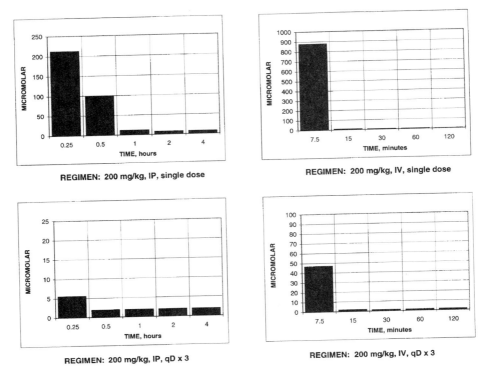

Fig. 18. Ex vivo pharmacology bioassay of non-tumor-bearing mice treated with phenylurea thiocarbamate (PTC; NSC 161128) ip or iv at 200 mg/kg/dose. Plasma samples from groups of mice ($n = 6$) were collected at each of five time intervals post treatment, processed, and applied to OVCAR-3 cell cultures as described in the methods section. In vivo plasma drug concentrations were calculated from the GI_{50} equivalence of responses in the ex vivo treated and in vitro treated cultures.

In vivo studies showed that a dose of 200 mg/kg/dose, qd×5, resulted in minimal-to-moderate anticancer activity (optimal T/C values of 25, 28, 36, and 57%) in the DU-145 xenograft model. However, equivocal results or no activity were observed in LNCaP and PC-3 prostate xenograft models, and no activity was observed in CCRF-CEM, HL-60 TB, K-562, and AS-283 xenografts. Analytical studies demonstrated a correlation between antineoplastic activity and metabolism of PTC. These studies also showed marked variability in the metabolic profile of PTC within a given laboratory animal species. PTC was observed to be sparingly soluble in conventional vehicles and initially was thought to be metabolized only to inactive metabolites.

Subsequent testing of PTC in in vitro *concentration × time* assays and ex vivo pharmacology bioassays demonstrated that single-dose ip treatment produced plasma PTC levels that readily exceeded the minimum effective *concentration × time* level for several tumor cell lines. Subsequent bioassays and analytical measurements of PTC and a principle metabolite revealed unexpected findings for single vs repeated ip and iv administrations of PTC. Although repeated daily ip PTC dosage was presumed to produce a drug depot and sustained blood levels in vivo, subsequent ex vivo bioassays revealed *reduced* plasma levels and a more rapid decrease in residual drug activity following three daily injections compared with that of single injections. Moreover, companion ex vivo bioas-

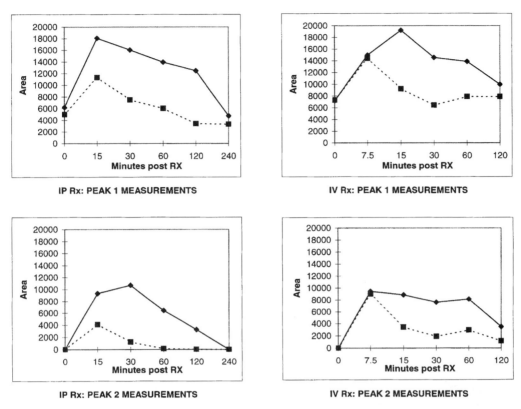

Fig. 19. Analytical measurements of ex vivo plasma samples derived from non-tumor-bearing mice treated with phenylurea thiocarbamate (PTC; NSC 161128) ip or iv at 200 mg/kg/dose. Aliquots of the same plasma samples collected and analyzed in the ex vivo pharmacology bioassay depicted in Fig. 18 were analyzed for chromatographic peak areas associated with PTC parent structure (peak 1) and also the principle metabolite (peak 2). Profiles measured following single dose treatments (diamonds) are compared with profiles measured following repeated treatments (squares).

says following iv drug injections likewise demonstrated that a single injection was accompanied by effective drug activity for 60 min, whereas multiple injections led to ineffective activity within 15 min following injection as shown in Fig. 18.

Analytical measurements of the parent compound (peak 1) and the principle metabolite (peak 2) in replicate serum samples collected for ip and iv ex vivo bioassays further confirmed the occurrence of altered drug disposition in mice receiving single vs multiple injections for both ip and iv routes of administration (Fig. 19). Although analytical measurements indicate that the parent compound and principle metabolite persist in plasma longer following iv treatment than following ip treatment, it is noteworthy that antitumor activity observed in the ex vivo bioassay suggests that a single ip treatment resulted in a more sustained level of activity than single or multiple iv treatments. These results suggested that the disposition and metabolism of PTC may be very complicated and that multiple reactive species in low concentration may be formed but escape analytical detection. Nevertheless, based on the limited and nonreproducible in vivo activity and the unfavorable pharmacokinetic behavior of the parent compound, including extensive metabolism and variable metabolic profiles among animal species, PTC (NSC 161128) was dropped from active preclinical development.

5. CONCLUSIONS

The various specialized in vitro/in vivo testing procedures described in this chapter provide means to evaluate the biological and pharmacologic properties of potentially new anticancer therapies. The procedures, coupled with a few prototypic examples of their use, have been provided in an effort to demonstrate how such testing can facilitate a preclinical drug development process. Although there are, no doubt, other procedures that are useful, we have simply summarized the procedures that we have developed and found helpful to better characterize anticancer drug activity with calibrated and objective endpoints. Hopefully these procedures will serve as useful indicators of in vitro and in vivo drug activity.

Preliminary screening in *hollow fiber assays* allows rapid selection of lead compounds in a short time frame. The space required to house animals for these studies is less demanding than that required for housing subcutaneous tumor implant models and thus puts less demand on resources. The assay will not identify every potentially valuable compound, but it does improve the probability of finding good leads when one is screening batteries of compounds or comparing the products of lead optimization studies, e.g., analog or prodrug programs.

Screening of compounds through *angiogenesis assays* does not provide the level of throughput possible with classical tumor cell screens. The HUVECs are more fastidious than most tumor cell lines, and they are a limited resource because of the need for a continuing supply. However, they are excellent tools to address the activity of lead compounds that are expected to impact vascularization processes. Follow-up evaluations in the rodent models give further insight into the potential value of the lead compounds.

The in vitro *concentration × time drug exposure assay* readily enables the concurrent evaluation of a multiplicity of tumor cell lines each exposed to a range of treatment regimens for a given compound. Results permit (1) determinations of effective concentration range and minimum exposure times required to achieve cytostatic and/or cytocidal effects for each cell line and (2) the ranking of cell line sensitivities on the basis of time-relevant drug exposure conditions.

In a similar fashion, the in vitro *drug stability assay* provides useful indices regarding storage and biological stability of new experimental agents. One can employ the same method to test the activity of experimental agents incubated in fresh plasma derived from laboratory animals and humans.

Ex vivo pharmacology bioassays provide important information regarding which of several potential treatment regimens yield the most favorable drug disposition for subsequent, more detailed, in vivo efficacy studies. In combination with initial in vivo hollow fiber assays, in vitro time-course assays, and/or analytical drug measurements, the ex vivo pharmacology bioassay is anticipated to facilitate the interpretation of in vivo drug efficacy arising from multiple active drug species as well as to help decipher and improve marginal in vivo drug activities.

Together, the specialized in vitro/in vivo procedures provide objective experimental endpoints that help to guide the preclinical anticancer drug development process. It is important to ask the right questions regarding the activity and status of a given candidate compound in pre-clinical development, to employ technically sound methodologies to answer those questions, and then to be careful and decisive regarding how to proceed at each step of preclinical drug development.

REFERENCES

1. Sausville EA, Feigal E. Evolving approaches to cancer drug discovery and development at the National Cancer Institute, USA. *Ann Oncol* 1999; 10:1287–1291.
2. Sausville EA, Johnson JI. Molecules for the millennium: how will they look? New drug discovery year 2000. *Br J Cancer* 2000; 83:1401–1404.
3. Hollingshead MG, Alley MC, Camalier RF, et al. *In vivo* cultivation of tumor cells in hollow fibers. *Life Sci* 1995; 57: 131–141.
4. Alley MC, Pacula-Cox CM, Hursey ML, Rubinstein LR, Boyd MR. Morphometric and colorimetric analyses of human tumor cell line growth and drug sensitivity in soft agar culture. *Cancer Res* 1991; 51:1247–1256.
5. Hollingshead MG, Grever MR, Alley MC, et al. *In vivo* evaluations of compounds with in vitro activity against breast cancer. *Proc Amer Assoc Cancer Res* 1994; 35:428.
6. Plowman J, Dykes DJ, Hollingshead MG, Simpson-Herren L, Alley MC. Human tumor xenograft models in NCI drug development. In Teicher BA, ed., *Anticancer Drug Development Guide: Preclinical Screening, Clinical Trials, and Approval*. Totowa, NJ: Humana. 1997:101–125.
7. Ross DT, Scherf U, Eisen MB, et al. Systematic variation in gene expression patterns in human cancer cell lines. *Nat Genet* 2000; 24:208–209.
8. Ellison G, Klinowska T, Westwood RF, Docter E, French T, Fox JC. Further evidence to support the melanocytic origin of MDA-MB-435. *Mol Pathol* 2002; 55:294–299
9. Hall L-AM, Krauthauser CM, Wexler RS, Hollingshead MG, Slee AM, Kerr JS. The hollow fiber assay: continued characterization with novel approaches. *Anticancer Res* 2000; 20:903–912.
10. Rapisarda A, Uranchimeg B, Scudiero DA, et al. Identification of small molecule inhibitors of hypoxia-inducible factor 1 transcriptional activation pathway. *Cancer Res* 2002; 62:4316–4324.
11. Phillips RM, Pearce J, Loadman PM, et al. Angiogenesis in the hollow fiber tumor model influences drug delivery to tumor cells: implications for anticancer drug screening programs. *Cancer Res* 1998; 58:5263–5266.
12. Goldman E. The growth of malignant disease in man and the lower animals with special reference to the vascular system. *Lancet* 1907; 2:1234–1240.
13. Ide AG, Baker NH, Warren SL. Vascularization of the Brown-Pearce rabbit epithelioma transplant as seen in the transparent ear chamber. *AJR* 1939; 42:891–899.
14. Greene HS. Heterologous transplantation of mammalian tumors. I. The transfer of rabbit tumors to alien species. *J Exp Med* 1941; 73:461–473.
15. Coman DR, Sheldon WF. The significance of hyperemia around tumor implants. *Am J Pathol* 1946; 33:821–831.
16. Merwin RM, Algire GH. The role of graft and host vessels in the vascularization of grafts of normal and neoplastic tissue. *J Natl Cancer Inst* 1956; 17:23–33.
17. Goodall CM, Sanders AG, Shubik P. Studies of vascular patterns in living tumors with a transparent chamber inserted in hamster cheek pouch. *J Natl Cancer Inst* 1965; 35:497–521.
18. Folkman J, Cole P, Zimmerman S. Tumor behavior in isolated perfused organs: in vitro growth and metastases of biopsy material in rabbit thyroid and canine intestinal segment. *Ann Surg* 1966; 164: 491–502.
19. McKenna S, Eatock M. The medical management of pancreatic cancer: a review. *Oncologist* 2003; 8:149–160.
20. Sin N, Meng L, Wang MQW, Wen JJ, Bornmann WG, Crews CM. The anti-angiogenic agent fumagillin covalently binds and inhibits the methionine aminopeptidase, MetAP-2. *Proc Natl Acad Sci USA* 1997; 94:6099–6103.
21. Fidler IJ, Nicolson GL. Organ selectivity for implantation survival and growth of B16 melanoma variant tumor lines. *J Natl Cancer Inst* 1976; 57:1199–1202.
22. Mayo JG, Laster WR Jr, Andrews CM, Schabel FM Jr. Success and failure in the treatment of solid tumors. 3. Cure of metastatic Lewis lung carcinoma with methyl-CCNU (NSC-95442) and surgery-chemotherapy. *Cancer Chemother Rep* 1972; 56: 183–195.

23. Alley MC, Scudiero DA, Monks A, et al. Feasibility of drug screening with panels of human tumor lines using a microculture tetrazolium assay. *Cancer Res* 1988; 48:589–601.

24. Alley MC, Pacula-Cox CM, Hollingshead MG, et al. Utility of a PVDF filter plate assay to facilitate selection of tumor cell lines for *in vivo* drug testing. *Proc Am Assoc Cancer Res* 1995; 36:305.

25. Alley MC, Pacula-Cox CM, Stinson SF, et al. Applications of an *ex vivo* pharmacology bioassay to measure activity of experimental anticancer compounds in the plasma of athymic mice. *Proc Amer Assoc Cancer Res* 1997; 38:605.

26. Rivera MI, Stinson SF, Vistica DT, Jorden JL, Kenney S, Sausville EA. Selective toxicity of the tricyclic thiophene NSC 652287 in renal carcinoma cell lines. *Biochem Pharmacol* 1999; 57:1283–1295.

27. Stinson SF, House T, Bramhall C, Saavedra JE, Keefer LK, Nims RW. Plasma pharmacokinetics of a liver-selective nitric oxide-donating diazeniumdiolate in the male C57BL/6 mouse. *Xenobiotica* 2002; 32:339–347.

28. Philips LR, Jorden JL, Rivera MI, Upadhyay K, Wolfe TL, Stinson SF. Identification of the major metabolite of 2, 5-bis(5-hydroxymethyl-2-thienyl)furan, an antitumor agent, in the S9 subcellular fraction of dog liver cells. *J Chromatogr B* 2002; 767:27–33.

29. Alley MC, Dykes DJ, Waud WR, et al. Efficacy evaluations of halichondrin B in selected xenograft systems. *Proc Amer Assoc Cancer Res* 1998; 39:226.

30. Abe J, Zhou W, Takuwa N, et al. A fumagillin derivative angiogenesis inhibitor, AGM-1470, inhibits activation of cyclin-dependent kinases and phosphorylation of retinoblastoma gene product but not protein tyrosyl phosphorylation or protooncogene expression in vascular endothelial cells. *Cancer Res* 1994; 54:3407–3412.

9

Patient-Like Orthotopic Metastatic Models of Human Cancer

Robert M. Hoffman, PhD

Contents

INTRODUCTION
EARLY STUDIES OF TUMOR TRANSPLANTATION
USE OF IMMUNODEFICIENT RODENTS FOR TUMOR TRANSPLANTATION
USE OF ATHYMIC NUDE MICE FOR TUMOR HETEROTRANSPLANTATION
ORTHOTOPIC TRANSPLANT MODELS UTILIZING HUMAN TUMOR TISSUE
    IN NUDE MICE: ENHANCED METASTATIC POTENTIAL
POSSIBLE MECHANISMS OF ENHANCED METASTASIS
    OF HETEROTRANSPLANTED TUMORS AT THE ORTHOTOPIC SITE
EXPERIMENTAL PROOF OF PAGET'S SEED AND SOIL HYPOTHESIS
    WITH METAMOUSE MODELS
DRUG DISCOVERY WITH PATIENT-LIKE MOUSE MODELS OF CANCER
NEW DIRECTIONS

1. INTRODUCTION

In 1889, Paget formulated the seed and soil hypothesis of cancer metastasis. Since that time there have ben major efforts to develop animal models of cancer to test and investigate the hypothesis of Paget as well as for treatment and drug discovery. Thus, there has been a critical need in cancer treatment and research for rodent models that are clinically relevant. Ideal models would allow the transplantation of the majority of human tumors such that the tumor would behave in the rodent in a similar manner as it did in the patient. Such models would be useful for individual patient treatment design and for evaluation of new antineoplastic agents and procedures. This review traces the development of rodent animal models from the first transplantation experiments over 100 yr ago to the present era. The present era is one of great promise, with the use of immunodeficient rodents, which accept foreign tissues for human tumor transplantation. The modern era is characterized by new orthotopic transplant methodologies that allow human tumors to express their metastatic potential, especially the models developed in our laboratory that

From: *Cancer Drug Discovery and Development:*
Anticancer Drug Development Guide: Preclinical Screening, Clinical Trials, and Approval, 2nd Ed.
Edited by: B. A. Teicher and P. A. Andrews © Humana Press Inc., Totowa, NJ

are constructed by surgical orthotopic implantation with intact tumor tissue. The use of tumors expressing green fluorescent protein and other fluorescent proteins for external whole-body imaging has enabled imaging of tumor growth and metastasis even on internal organs. The SOI models have allowed experimental confirmation of Paget's seed and soil hypothesis of 1889. The use of SOI models for discovery of antimetastatic and antiangiogenesis agents is discussed. The exciting possibility of the use of the SOI models for discovery of antitumor and antimetastatic genes is also discussed.

2. EARLY STUDIES OF TUMOR TRANSPLANTATION

Early studies of transplantation of human tumors to animals ended in failure, including attempts to transplant human tumors to higher primates (1). Ewing (1) has described the following historical developments: For example, Sticker tried to transplant a dog lymphosarcoma to foxes in 1904 (2). Experiments such as these had limited success. Transplantation of sarcoma was attempted between dogs by Novinsky in 1876, who had only two successes in 42 attempts (3). Hanau in 1889 had greater success in transplanting a vulva epidermoid carcinoma from a rat to other rats (4). The first systematic study of transplanted tumors was that of Morau in 1894, who transplanted a cylindrical-cell carcinoma of a mouse for a number of generations (5). Loeb in 1901 and 1902 in the United States passaged a cystic sarcoma of the thyroid between rats for 40 generations with maintenance of structure, but no metastases were observed (6,7). Jensen in 1902 and 1903 passaged a mouse sarcoma through 19 generations of mice, again without noting metastases (8,9). Ewing noted that with regard to therapeutics, transplantable tumors "opened up many new trails which unfortunately have led mostly astray" (1).

With regard to metastases, Bashford et al. (10) noted local infiltration and metastases in the Jensen tumor, and Apolant (11) showed that infiltrative and metastatic growth most frequently occurred when the tumor invaded dense resisting tissues. Many other tumor types have been described in rodents that have long been extensively transplanted. Rous described three chicken sarcomas that were transplantable and showed that cell-free extracts of the spindle cell sarcoma could serve as the agent to induce further tumors in other animals (12).

It was shown that in animals inoculated with the cell-free "juice," as Ewing described it (1), tumors developed at the point of inoculation but always more slowly than when animals were inoculated with tumor cells themselves. Filtrates from Rous' spindle-cell tumor and condroma gave rise to similar tumors from the tumor in which the filtrates were obtained. We now know that the filtrate contained the Rous sarcoma virus, which is one of the most characterized of all tumor viruses.

Ewing noted that nearly all experiments found difficulty in getting the original tumor to engraft in another animal, but subsequent passages usually occurred at higher rates and some tumors such as the buffalo rat sarcoma have eventually been able to be passed at a 100% take rate (1). Ehrlich proposed that tumors, after passage, became increasingly virulent (13). As Ewing noted, among the passaged tumors, the subcutaneous tissue was the site ordinarily used for transplantation. However, internal organs, especially the spleen, have been used for implantation but have proved, according to Ewing, less susceptible (1).

In the early transplantation experiments, it was found that not only was the same species of animal required in transplantation of tumor from one animal to another, but the results were more successful between animals of exactly the same color and antecedent as Ewing described *(1)*. This is owing, of course, to what we now know to be the rejection of transplants from nongenetically identical animals. Ewing noted that Beebe and Van Alstyne *(14)* observed that a carbohydrate-free diet made buffalo rats highly refractory to the buffalo sarcoma and that even the progression of this tumor was retarded by carbohydrate-free diets but was accelerated by butyrates.

Ewing *(1)* stated that many tumors maintained a uniform histology through many generations but that some carcinomas changed greatly through passaging. He also noted that the most striking change induced by the passageable tumors was the induction of malignant sarcoma properties in the normal host stroma. This was first observed by Ehrlich *(13)* and Apoland *(11)* in the 10th generation of passage of a mouse adenocarcinoma. Both the passaged tumor and a now-malignant stroma could persist together or as separate strains of sarcoma and carcinoma. The rate of growth of mixed tumors appears to be enhanced. It was concluded that the sarcoma was caused by a neoplastic transformation of the stroma of the host induced by the stimulation of the stromal cells by the malignant epithelium *(11,13)*. Ewing *(1)* noted another possibility, that the spindle-like cells of the stroma might be in reality altered epithelium; it had been shown repeatedly that animals resisting engraftment of passaged tumors may often develop spontaneous tumors (and vice versa), so Ewing concluded that the problem of continued growth of an engrafted tumor is quite different from "spontaneous" tumor development.

As mentioned above, with regard to heterotransplantation in the early days, it was difficult to find tumors that could be consistently transplanted between different strains of even the same species. The Ehrlich tumor in mice, however, was found to be readily transplantable. The Ehrlich tumor was originally a mammary tumor that transformed into the ascites form and could be transplanted into outbred Swiss mice by even a few cells *(15)*. Researchers then tried to advance heterotransplantation by finding what we now consider potentially immunologically privileged sites in the animal such as the anterior chamber of the eye, the cheek pouch, and the brain, all of which had many limitations *(15)*. Greene *(16)*, for example, used the eye of rabbits and guinea pigs to grow human tumors. as mentioned above,

3. USE OF IMMUNODEFICIENT RODENTS FOR TUMOR TRANSPLANTATION

Another approach to tumor heterotransplantation has been the use of immunoincompetent animals. For example, tumors have been successfully grown in newborn mice and fetuses, which are naturally immunoincompetent *(17,18)*. The fetuses and the newborns, however, become immunocompetent and eventually can reject the transplanted tumor.

Attempts were then made to immunosuppress adult animals such as with whole body radiation and steroids *(19,20)*. This treatment, however, is very damaging to the animal. As Giovanella and Fogh *(15)* point out, the observations that the thymus is critical in rejection allowed heterotransplantation studies to proceed at a faster rate using, for example, thymectomy or antilymphocyte (ALS) or antithymocyte serum (ATS) *(21–26)*. Giovanella and Fogh *(15)* noted that the most effective combination treatment for immunosuppression of animals to be used as hosts for tumor passaging is thymectomy at birth with total body radiation and later a reconstitution with syngeneic bone marrow *(25,27,28)*. All these procedures are difficult, however, and involve serious side effects.

4. USE OF ATHYMIC NUDE MICE
FOR TUMOR HETEROTRANSPLANTATION

4.1. Subcutaneous Implant Tumor Models

A new era was opened with the isolation and identification of genetically immunosuppressed animals. In particular, in 1966 Flannigan *(29)* identified the nude mouse mutant. In 1968, Pantelouris *(30)* showed that this animal was athymic and lacked T cells and therefore could not reject foreign tissue. If the nude mice are kept in a germ-free environment, the life span can be increased to almost the normal length, thereby making them useful experimental animals. The first reported xenograft in nude mice was a subcutaneously implanted human colon adenocarcinoma *(31)*. In 1972, Giovanella et al. *(32)* inoculated a cell line of a human melanoma in nude mice and obtained an invasive tumor. The most frequently occurring tumors have been successfully xenografted subcutaneously in nude mice *(33)*. Fogh et al. *(34)* successfully subcutaneously xenografted 381 tumors in 6–8-wk-old nude mice from 14 categories of cancer. With regard to take rate they found that the melanomas and colon tumors had the highest take ratio, with breast and lymphoreticular tumors having the lowest. The percentage of takes for the total series was 28%. The take rate was 50% for recurrent tumors, 38% for metastases, and 21% for primary site tumors, *(34)*. One-third of the transplants could be established as lines. If the xenografts could be carried beyond passage three, they had a 90% probability of becoming established as lines. Fogh et al. *(34)* noted that there was a variability in the growth rate of the transplanted tumors in nude mice. Gynecological tumors and colon tumors grew rapidly, and germ cell and bone tumors grew slowly. Metastases and recurrent tumors were found to grow faster than tumors from primary sites, and the less differentiated tumors were more easily established as lines and grew faster *(15)*. Giovanella et al. *(32)* used cultured cells for the first time to initiate tumors in nude mice. This approach was used to assay the tumorigenicity of the cell lines *(35)*. However, it became apparent that some highly malignant-appearing cultured lines formed tumors at a low rate after transplantation into nude mice *(15)*.

Sharkey et al. *(36)* reported that about one-third of the tumors studied in their series increased their differentiation status after growing as xenografts in nude mice. It was also shown that in some human malignant glial tumors implanted in the brains of nude mice, new histological patterns occurred *(37)*. A similar observation was made in a study of 12 human melanomas grown in nude mice *(38)*. Pancreatic adenocarcinomas in nude mice produced many of the pancreatic-specific enzymes, but digestive enzymes were not being produced *(39)*.

In a large series of subcutaneous implantation of surgical specimens Shimosato et al. *(40)* obtained 58 tumor takes out of 243 attempts. Most difficult to implant successfully were breast carcinomas. Rae-Venter and Reid *(41)* have shown that subcutaneous growth of a number of human breast tumors was enhanced by implantation of estrogen. Shafie and Grantham *(42)* have demonstrated with the MCF-7 human breast carcinoma cell line a lack of growth in animals without functional ovaries and a pancreas, the results of which could be reversed by estrogen and insulin.

A number of models for prostate cancer have been developed including the Dunning R-3327 hormonally dependent rat prostatic adenocarcinoma *(43)*. A number of cell lines from human prostatic carcinoma that grow in athymic nude mice, including the LNCaP line, which is androgen-dependent *(44)*, and the androgen-independent cell lines Du145 *(45)* and PC-3 *(46,47)*, have also been isolated. The usual mode of in vivo growth of the human prostate carcinoma lines has been after subcutaneous transplantation. The use of extracellular matrix proteins such as Matrigel seems to enhance the take rate of subcutaneously implanted tumors *(48)*. However, intrasplenic injection *(49)* has also been used, which may result in more metastatic activity. The PC-3 line has been injected into the tail vein of nude mice while the inferior vena cava was occluded, which allowed tumor growth in the lumbar vertebrae, pelvis, and femur *(50)*. When PC-3 cells were injected into the peritoneal cavity, intra-abdominal growth resulted *(51)*. When they were injected into the spleen, liver metastases resulted, and when they were injected into the seminal vesicles, large tumors developed there *(51)*. However, none of these models is representative of the clinical course of growth of prostate carcinoma and are not of use for predicting the clinical course or response to treatment of individual patients. Shroeder *(52)* implanted flat pieces of prostate tumor directly into exposed subcutaneous muscle where the muscular fascia was scraped away. The PCA-2 human prostrate carcinoma has been serially transplanted in male nude mice but would not grow tumors in female nude mice and regressed after castration or estrogen treatment of the male, thereby demonstrating its hormone dependency *(53)*.

Bullard and Bigger *(54)* and Shapiro et al. *(55)* were successful in growing craniopharyngiomas, glioblastomas, and astrocytomas directly in the brain or in subcutaneous tissue. Schackert et al. *(56)* found that carcinomas of the colon, breast, kidney, and lung, when injected into the cerebrum carotid arteries, produced brain tumors.

A number of investigators have been quite successful in growing bladder carcinoma subcutaneously in nude mice. Sufrin et al. *(57)* succeeded in growing 8 of 20 human transitional cell carcinomas, and Naito et al. *(58)* successfully implanted 8 of 31 human urinary cancers. All these studies were done at the subcutaneous site in the nude mice. Mattern et al. *(59)* were able to implant and passage 22 human lung tumors. Many other human tumor types have now been grown subcutaneously in nude mice including a wide range of sarcomas, lymphomas, leukemias, testicular carcinomas, mesotheliomas, hepatomas, pancreatic carcinomas, and squamous cell carcinomas of the head and neck *(15)*.

Giovanella et al. *(60)* have found that malignancies of many cell types may be expressed only in nude mice that have been further immunosuppressed, for example by ALS or X-ray irradiation. This has been shown for human bladder carcinomas and a human osteosarcoma, which in control nude mice did not form tumors but grew after subcutaneous implantation in X-ray-treated mice. Two-week-old mice have also been proved to be better than 6- to 8-wk-old mice, since the younger mice are more immunoincompetent. The young mice have allowed certain tumors to grow that could not grow in older animals, such as tumors of the bladder and thyroid and glioblastomas.

With regard to enhancement of tumor growth in nude mice, it has recently been shown that Matrigel significantly accelerated small-cell lung carcinoma cell line growth after the cells and Matrigel were coinjected subcutaneously in nude mice (61). Other human and murine tumor types were found to have their growth stimulated by coinjection of the cells with Matrigel (62).

Sharkey and Fogh (63) have shown that it is necessary to demonstrate that the tumors growing in nude mice are of human origin. It has been demonstrated by Giovanella and Fogh (15) that the nude mouse stromal elements can be converted by xenografted carcinomas to malignant sarcoma-producing nude mouse tumors, as mentioned above in early studies described by Ewing (1).

A number of more recent studies have shown that the implantation of tumors but not tumor cell lines from humans induced a transformation of murine stromal cells. For example, the transformed stromal cells, after short-term culture in vitro, could produce sarcomas in other nude mice (64,65).

Studies have been done with human premalignant tissue, but such tissue has been difficult to xenograft successfully (15). However, Bhargava and Lipkin (66) were able to demonstrate that benign polyps of the colon could survive for up to 28 d implanted in kidney capsules in nude mice. Normal tissue from fetuses can be implanted in nude mice (67), and human adult tissue can be quite normal after implantation in nude mice (68,69).

Metastases have not been observed in most tumor transplantation experiments in nude mice using the subcutaneous site. However, with regard to melanomas, when the primary tumor was surgically resected, the animals could live longer and could subsequently develop distant metastases, sometimes 7–12 mo after the tumor inoculations (70). Three amelanotic human melanomas cell lines, when injected intradermally, produced metastases in the regional lymph nodes and in one case lymphatics in the lungs (71). Recent studies with another amelanotic melanoma cell line termed LOX (72,73), as well as pigmented melanoma cell lines, have also demonstrated growth and metastasis after subcutaneous or subdermal implantation. Recently, Van Muijen et al. (74) showed that by first passaging a human melanoma three times in nude mice and then establishing a cell line, subcutaneous implantation of the cell line caused 90% of the nude mice to demonstrate lung metastases. In the series of Sharkey and Fogh (75), 106 malignant human tumor cell lines were xenografted to 1045 nude mice. Metastases were observed in only 14 animals, involving 11 different tumor lines. Breast tumor cell lines metastasized at the highest frequency, but none of the sarcoma lines metastasized, which was quite different from the human patient situation. These investigators found that deep penetration of the body wall during tumor growth correlated with the occurrence of metastases.

The human tumor lines in the study of Sharkey and Fogh (75) included carcinomas in the breast, lung, and gastrointestinal and urogenital tracts, as well as tumors of unknown primary sites. Metastatic sites included local lymph nodes in two cases, distant lymph nodes in two cases, and a spleen and mediastinum in one case each. Metastatic and non-metastatic tumors from the patient population metastasized equally poorly in the nude mice in this series (15). A renal cell adenocarcinoma in some instances metastasized to axillary and inguinal lymph nodes after subcutaneous inoculation (76). The SW480 cultured colon carcinoma was seen to metastasize to the regional lymph nodes after subcutaneous implantation, and when the tumor was implanted intraperitoneally, metastasis to the lymph nodes and lungs was seen (77).

Shimosato et al. *(40)* found that after subcutaneous inoculation, an acute lymphocytic leukemia as well as a number of breast cancers metastasized to regional lymph nodes. Kyriazis et al. *(77)* have shown that in addition to the cultured colon carcinoma, transitional cell carcinomas of the bladder and adenocarcinoma of the pancreas could invade and even metastasize to the lymph nodes of the lung after subcutaneous implantation. Neulat-Duga et al. *(78)* found metastasis in 30% of 63 human tumors implanted subcutaneously.

Therefore, although metastases can occur from subcutaneously growing tumors in nude mice in a number of different tumor types and studies, this is rather rare. Giovanella and Fogh *(15)* emphasize that if the animals bearing the subcutaneously growing tumors can be kept alive for long periods, such as by resecting the primary tumors described above, the probability of metastasis can be raised. Provoked local recurrences at the site of a subcutaneous growth such as reimplantation of tumor fragments or fragments left in the animal following reduction of a tumor load can induce massive lung metastases from xenografted cell lines derived from mammary tumors, colon carcinomas, melanomas, and prostate tumors *(15)*.

4.2. Effect of Implant Site on Tumor Growth

Early studies showed that the site of implantation could influence the growth rate, invasiveness, and metastatic behavior of the resulting tumors. For example, Hajdu et al. *(87)* found that subcutaneously growing tumors were better differentiated than the same tumors growing intraperitoneally in nude mice. Kyriazis and Kyriazis *(79)* noted that tumor growth in the anterior lateral thoracic wall was faster than in the posterior aspect of the trunk. With regard to human small-cell carcinoma, intracranial injection was found to be superior to the subcutaneous or subdermal site. At the intracranial site, takes of 100% with small-cell carcinomas were observed by Chambers et al. *(80)*, with one-tenth of those cells required to produce subdermal tumors. The latent time for tumor growth was shorter in the intercranial site than in the subdermal site. Importantly, the tumors grew in the meninges and subsequently invaded and destroyed the brain, in contrast to the subcutaneously growing tumors, which were not invasive. In addition, the MCF-7 cell line grew well in the mammary fat pad, indicating the importance of the orthotopic site *(81,82)* *(see* Subheading 5.). The mammary fat pad was also shown to be a preferential site for growth and metastasis for estrogen receptor-negative human breast cancer cell lines *(83)*. As mentioned above, the mammary fat pad was shown to be a superior implantation site for tumor growth and metastasis for hormone-independent human breast cancer cells *(42,83)*. As with the small-cell carcinoma, the MCF-7 carcinoma was highly invasive after intracranial inoculation *(84)*. When transplanted into the intracranial region, lymphoma and leukemia cells and cell lines derived even from normal donors produced tumors *(60,85)*. The subrenal capsule site developed by Bogden et al. *(86)* as a means of implanting tumors in nude mice has allowed the growth of many different types of tumors; some of them were shown to be invasive even if they were not implanted at the subcutaneous site. Kyriazis and Kyriazis *(79)* showed that when some tumors were implanted intraperitoneally, the neoplastic growth in the peritoneal cavity was malignant, including the ability to invade various organs by lymphatic and hematogenous routes.

5. ORTHOTOPIC TRANSPLANT MODELS UTILIZING HUMAN TUMOR TISSUE IN NUDE MICE: *ENHANCED METASTATIC POTENTIAL*

In the last 20 years it has thus become clear that orthotopic sites of implantation are critical to the metastatic capability of the transplanted tumors in nude mice *(88)*. With regard to colon carcinoma, when the cecum and spleen were used as sites of implantation of colon tumor cell lines or disaggregated tumor tissue, metastasis occurred including that to liver as opposed to the subcutaneous site, which allowed primary growth to occur but not metastasis *(89–95)*. Inoculation of tumor cell lines into the descending portion of the large bowel allowed micro- and macroinvasive behavior of the cells via infiltration of the various layers of the mouse colonic wall, in particular the muscularis propria *(89–94)*. This behavior was contrasted to melanoma cell lines implanted into the colon, which exhibited limited invasiveness compared with the colon carcinomas *(94)*.

5.1. Colon Tumor Models

In our laboratories, histologically intact human colon tumor fragments directly derived surgically from patients were transplanted by surgical orthotopic implantation (SOI) to either the colon or the cecum of nude mice. SOI for colon tumor involves suturing the tumor tissue on the serosa of these organs. We have achieved extensive orthotopic growth in more than 50 cases of patient colon tumors with subsequent regional, lymph node, and liver metastasis, depending on the case. Similar results were found with SOI of intact tissue from a human colon cancer xenograft line, including liver metastasis. Thus, a patient-like model for human colon cancer has been developed that can be used for research into the biology of colon cancer metastases, for the potential prediction of clinical course, for drug response testing of the disease in individual patients, and for the discovery of new therapeutics *(96)*. In a comparison between SOI of intact colon tumor tissue and orthotopic injection of cell suspensions derived from the colon tumor tissue, Furukawa et al. *(97)* observed that SOI performed in intact tissue resulted in high metastatic rates, and the cell suspension injections resulted in no metastases.

Partial hepatectomy has been widely employed in clinical practice as the therapy of choice for primary and metastatic liver tumors. However, the recurrence rate after the treatment remains high, probably because of the growth of residual microscopic lesions. We have observed the effect of partial hepatectomy on the growth of two human colon cancers (Co-3 and AC3603) implanted in the liver of nude mice using SOI. Our results showed a dramatic acceleration of tumor growth following 30% partial hepatectomy, which resembles clinical procedures. Tumor volumes were assessed with calipers on d 15 by abdominal palpation and on d 30 at autopsy by direct measurement. For both Co-3 and AC3603, tumor volumes in the hepatectomized animals were significantly larger than the control at the above two time points ($p < 0.001$). The results demonstrate the stimulating effect of partial hepatectomy directly on the tumor growth in the liver. Furthermore, since conservative partial hepatectomy (30%) is normally used in clinical practice for surgical treatment of liver metastasis, this animal model should be useful for the clinical investigation of the high recurrence rate of liver metastasis following partial hepatectomy *(98)*.

5.2. Bladder Tumor Models

With regard to bladder carcinomas, Ahlering et al. *(99)* found that two human bladder transitional cell carcinoma lines, when injected transurethrally into the urinary bladders of athymic nude mice, invaded the mouse bladder and metastasized to the lung. Subcutaneous inoculation of these cell lines allowed tumor growth but very little local invasion and no metastases. Theodorescu et al. *(100)* confirmed the results of Ahlering et al. with respect to the RT-4 human bladder carcinoma cell line. Theodorescu et al. found, however, that when a mutated *H-ras* oncogene was transfected into RT-4 such that overexpression of this gene occurred in the selected cell line RT-4-mr-10, the cell line became more invasive after transurethral inoculation. Areas of invasion of transitional cell carcinoma deep into the muscularis propria of the bladder occurred that in some instances extended into the surrounding adipose tissue and vascular spaces. However, no continuous or metastatic spread of RT-4-mr-10 occurred. These findings are in contrast to the effects of subcutaneous injection of these cell lines, which showed no evidence of tissue invasion *(100)*.

In our laboratories, the ras-transfected human bladder RT-4 carcinoma tissue cell line RT-4-mr-10 just described was transplanted by SOI as histologically intact tissue to the nude mouse bladder. Extensive invasive orthotopic growth and local invasion occurred as well as multiorgan metastases in the liver, pancreas, spleen, lung, ovary, kidney, ureter, and lymph nodes. The results for the implanted RT-4-mr-10 cells are in striking contrast to the experiments described above in which RT-4-mr-10 injected transurethrally as disaggregated cells exhibited only local invasion and no distant metastasis. These results further indicate the potential of the intact tissue SOI model to allow full expression of the metastatic capacity of human cancer in the nude mouse *(101,102)*. We have recently demonstrated that the RT-4 parental bladder tumor line is highly metastatic when implanted orthotopically as histologically intact tissue, thereby showing that the *ras* gene had no effect *(103)*.

5.3. Pancreatic Tumor Models

Vezeridis et al. *(104)* reported that the fast-growing variant of the human pancreatic carcinoma COLO 357, when injected as disaggregated cells into the spleen of the nude mice, resulted in metastases to the liver and lungs of the animal. The authors stated, however, that this study bypasses invasion and generates seeding and colonization rather than metastases. A subsequent study was carried out *(105)* using the COLO 357 and L3.3 human pancreatic tumors to compare orthotopic transplantation with subcutaneous inoculation. These authors took tumors that were subcutaneously grown and harvested and sectioned them into 2 × 2 pieces. Xenografts were first attached to the exteriorized pancreas. The pancreas was then wrapped around the xenograft to cover it completely. The edges of the fatty tissue surrounding the pancreas were sutured such that the xenograft would remain covered upon the return of the pancreas to the peritoneal cavity. It was found that most of the animals produced tumors at the orthotopic site of transplantation. Metastasis occurred in the liver, lung, regional lymph nodes, and distant lymph nodes. The authors felt that by using tumor pieces as xenografts rather than injecting tumor cells into the pancreas, the probability of injecting tumor cells into the circulation with subsequent seeding and colonization was eliminated. They emphasized that their model was similar to the human situation of pancreatic cancer: the retroperitoneal nodes, liver, and lungs become involved.

Marincola et al. *(106)* also orthotopically implanted human pancreatic cancer cell lines, in their case in the doudenal lobe of the pancreas for comparison with heterotopic implantation at the hepatic and subcutaneous sites. Intrapancreatic tumor growth was occasionally associated with liver metastases in the animals that were killed after 28 d, 17.8% in young animals and 22.2% in adult animals. However, after more than 45 d of tumor growth, the incidence of hepatic metastases increased to 57.1%. Direct extension of the tumor into surrounding tissues was frequently observed, with involvement of the duodenum of 84% in growing tumors, the kidneys in 31%, and other intra-abdominal organs in 44%. Subcutaneously growing tumors did not give rise to detectable metastases.

In our laboratories, we have implanted histologically intact human pancreatic tumor tissue in the pancreas of the nude mouse and have achieved tumor growth in six of six patient cases *(107)*. Extensive local growth occurred in all cases, with regional extension and frequent metastases to Iymph nodes and visceral organs *(107)*.

We evaluated the efficacy of mitomycin C (MMC) and 5-fluorouracil (5-FU) against the human pancreatic adenocarcinoma cell line PAN-12-JCK in an SOI human metastatic pancreatic cancer nude mice model. Implantation was in the tail portion of the pancreas near the spleen. The PAN-12-JCK cells grew very aggressively in the control group of nude mice, with extensive local invasion and distant metastases to various organs; a propensity for metastasis to the lung was seen, but other organs were involved as well, including the liver, kidney, and regional and distant lymph nodes. Remarkably, none of the mice in the MMC-treated group developed tumors. Although mice in the 5-FU-treated group survived statistically significantly longer than those in the untreated control, the overall incidence of metastasis in these mice was equivalent to those in the control group. However, no liver or kidney metastases were found in the 5-FU-treated animals, perhaps accounting in part for their longer survival. This clinical nude mouse model of highly metastatic pancreatic cancer can now be used to discover new effective agents for this disease *(108)*.

After SOI of the human tumor xenograft PAN-12-JCK into the tail of the nude mouse pancreas, MMC and cisplatin (DDP) were administered intraperitoneally at doses of 4 and 6 mg/kg, respectively, on d 7. The mice were observed for 95 d. There was a statistically significant increase in disease-free and overall survival rates in the MMC and MMC + DDP-treated groups. Local tumor growth was eliminated only in the group treated with MMC + DDP. Hepatic metastasis and peritoneal disseminations were completely inhibited by MMC but not DDP. This study demonstrated the usefulness of the SOI model of pancreatic cancer for studying the differential efficacy of agents affecting primary tumor growth metastasis and survival *(109)*.

Two human pancreatic cancer cell lines expressing green fluorescent protein (GFP), MIA-PaCa2 and BxPC-3, were studied in SOI models. BxPC-3-GFP tumors developed rapidly in the pancreas and spread regionally to the spleen and retroperitoneum as early as 6 wk. Distant metastases in BxPC-3-GFP lines were rare. In contrast, MIA-PaCa-2-GFP lines grew more slowly in the pancreas but rapidly metastasized to distant sites including liver and portal lymph nodes. Regional metastases in MIA-PaCa-2-GFP lines were rare. These studies demonstrate that pancreatic cancers have highly specific and individual "seed-soil" interactions governing the chronology and sites of metastatic targeting (110).

Two GFP-expressing pancreatic tumor cell lines, BXPC-3 and MiaPaCa-2, were implanted by SOI as tissue fragments in the body of the pancreas of nude mice. Whole-body optical images visualized real-time primary tumor growth and formation of metastatic lesions that developed in the spleen, bowel, portal lymph nodes, omentum, and liver. Intravital images in the opened animal confirmed the identity of whole-body images. The whole-body images were used for real time quantitative measurement of tumor growth in each of these organs. Intravital imaging was used for quantification of growth of micrometastasis on the liver and stomach. Whole-body imaging was carried out with either a transilluminated epifluorescence microscope or a fluorescence light box, both with a thermoelectrically cooled color CCD camera. The simple, noninvasive, and highly selective imaging made possible by the strong GFP fluorescence allowed detailed simultaneous quantitative imaging of tumor growth and multiple metastasis formation of pancreatic cancer. The GFP imaging affords unprecedented continuous visual monitoring of malignant growth and spread within intact animals without the need for anesthesia, substrate injection, contrast agents, or restraint of animals required by other imaging methods. The GFP imaging technology will facilitate studies of modulators of pancreatic cancer growth including inhibition by potential chemotherapeutic agents (111).

Parathyroid hormone-related protein (PTHrP) is an oncoprotein that regulates the growth and proliferation of many common malignancies including pancreatic cancer. Previous studies have shown that PTHrP is produced by human pancreatic cancer cell lines, can be seen in the cytoplasm and nucleus of paraffin-embedded pancreatic adenocarcinoma tumor specimens, and is secreted into the media of cultured pancreatic adenocarcinoma cells. We hypothesized that PTHrP could serve as a tumor marker for the growth of pancreatic cancer in vivo. To test this hypothesis, we used the SOI model of the human pancreatic cancer line BxPC-3. This tumor was stably transduced with GFP to facilitate visualization of tumor growth and metastases. At early (5 wk) and late (13 wk) time points after SOI, serum PTHrP was measured, and primary and metastatic tumor burden was determined for each mouse by GFP expression. By 5 wk after SOI (early group), the mean serum PTHrP level was 32.7 pg/mL. In contrast, at 13 wk post SOI (late group), the mean serum PTHrP level increased to 155.8 pg/mL. These differences were highly significant ($p < 0.001$, Student's t-test). Numerous metastatic lesions were readily visualized by GFP in the late group. Serum PTHrP levels measured by immunoassay correlated with primary pancreatic tumor weights ($p < 0.01$). PTHrP levels were not detectable (<21 pg/mL) in any of the 10 control mice with no tumor. Western blotting of BxPC-3-GFP tumor lysates confirmed the presence of PTHrP. BxPC-3-GFP tumor tissue stained with antibody to PTHrP. These results indicate that PTHrP has a high potential as a useful tumor marker for clinical pancreatic adenocarcinoma in the future (112).

5.4. Head and Neck Tumor Models

With regard to head and neck tumors, Dinesman et al. (113) implanted 42 nude mice with laryngeal squamous cell carcinoma cell lines on the floor of the mouth. Pulmonary metastases were noted in 44%, bone invasion in 80%, angioinvasion in 76%, and soft tissue invasion in 96% of the animals, thereby mimicking the clinical state. In the head and neck study, lymph node metastasis was seen in only 2 of the 42 animals. In comparison, the subcutaneous model of transplantation for head and neck tumors has not resulted in metastases of tumors that did eventually take, which was at a low rate. For example, Brackhuis et al. *(114)* implanted 130 head and neck carcinomas in subcutaneous tissues of nude mice with a 26% take rate and no observed metastases.

Our laboratory has utilized tumor material directly from surgery from human head and neck cancer patients, including metastatic tongue and laryngeal tumors, and implanted them as histologically intact tissue into the muscles of the floor of the mouth including the mylohyoid muscle as further examples of the SOI technique. We have observed subsequent invasions into the structures of the head (X. Fu and R.M. Hoffman, unpublished observations). When the same tumor tissue was implanted subcutaneously, even in the neck area, extensive tumor growth occurred without subsequent invasion.

5.5. Stomach Tumor Models

The human gastric cancer cell line G/F was implanted either subcutaneously or into the stomach wall of nude mice *(115)*. The G/F tumor implanted in the stomach wall showed a slower growth rate than when the tumor was implanted subcutaneously. Importantly, the tumor implanted in the stomach wall grew and invaded the surrounding tissues and metastasized to the regional lymph nodes and distant organs such as the lung and liver in 27 of 43 mice. In contrast, the tumors growing subcutaneously were highly encapsulated, and metastasis to other organs was not observed. Thus the stomach wall provided a superior microenvironment for the G/F gastric cancer to express its metastatic properties.

SOI of human stomach cancer tissue fragments derived from cell lines resulted in the formation of metastases in 100% of the mice, with extensive primary growth to the regional lymph nodes, liver, and lung. In contrast, when cell suspensions were used to inject stomach cancer cells at the same site, metastases occurred in only 6.7% of the mice with local tumor formation, emphasizing the importance of using intact tissue to allow full expression of metastatic potential. Injuring the serosa, as occurs in intact tissue transplantation, did not increase the metastatic rate after orthotopic injection of cell suspensions of stomach tumor cells. This intact tissue orthotopic implantation model should allow development of new treatment modalities and further study of the biology of human stomach cancer *(116)*.

Fresh surgical specimens derived from 36 patients with advanced stomach cancer were transplanted in nude mice using SOI. Twenty of 36 patient tumors gave rise to locally growing tumors in the mice. All 20 patients whose stomach tumors resulted in local growth in the nude mice had clinical lymph node involvement, whereas 8 of the other 16 patients whose tumors were rejected had lymph node involvement. There was a statistical correlation ($p < 0.01$) between local tumor growth in nude mice and clinical lymph node involvement. Of the 20 cases resulting in local growth in the nude mice, 5 had clinical liver metastases and all 5 cases resulted in liver metastases in the nude mice. Of the 20 cases, 6 had clinical peritoneal involvement of their tumor; of these, 5 resulted in peritoneal metastasis in the nude mice. Of the 15 patients without liver metastases whose primary tumor grew locally in the mice, only one case gave rise to a liver metastasis in a mouse. There were statistical correlations ($p < 0.01$) for both liver metastases and peritoneal involvement between patients and mice. These results indicate that, after orthotopic transplantation of histologically intact stomach cancers from patients to nude mice, the subsequent metastatic behavior of the tumors in the mice closely correlated with the course of the tumors in the patients *(117)*.

GFP gene was administered to intraperitoneally growing human stomach cancers in nude mice to visualize future regional and distant metastases. GFP retroviral supernatants were injected ip from d 4 to d 10 following ip implantation of the cancer cells. Tumor and metastasis fluorescence was visualized every other week with the use of fluorescence optics via a laparotomy on the tumor-bearing animals. Two weeks after retroviral GFP delivery, GFP-expressing tumor cells were observed in gonadal fat, greater omentum, and intestine, indicating that these primary intraperitoneally growing tumors were efficiently transduced by the GFP gene and could be visualized by its expression. At the second and third laparotomies, GFP-expressing tumor cells were found to have spread to lymph nodes in the mesentery. At the fourth laparotomy, widespread tumor growth was observed. No normal tissues were found to be transduced by the GFP retrovirus. Thus, reporter gene transduction of the primary tumor allowed detection of its subsequent metastasis. This gene therapy model could be applied to primary tumors before resection or other treatment for a fluorescence early detection system for metastasis and recurrence *(118)*.

5.6. Lung Tumor Models

Recent studies have demonstrated that inoculation of human lung tumor cell lines intrathoracically or intrabronchially into nude mice *(120,121)* results in orthotopic growth.

SOI was used for lung tumor implantation in the left lung in nude and SCID mice by a thoracotomy procedure we have developed. Results thus far *(122)* indicate that this method not only allows extensive local growth in nude and SCID mice but also allows development of regional and distant metastases as described above.

When a poorly differentiated large cell squamous cell patient tumor was transplanted orthotopically to the left lung as histologically intact tissue directly from surgery, five of five mice produced locally grown tumors. Opposite lung metastases occurred, as well as lymph node metastases. When grown subcutaneously, this tumor grew locally, but no metastases were found *(122)*.

When the human small-cell lung carcinoma cell line Lu-24 was transplanted histologically intact into the left lung of nude mice via thoracotomy after harvesting of subcutaneously growing tissue from nude mice, five of five mice produced locally growing tumors averaging 10 mm in diameter within 24 d. All five mice produced regional metastases including tumor invasion of the mediastinum, the chest wall, and the pericardium and distant metastases including the right lung, esophagus, diaphragm, parietal pleura, and lymph nodes. These five mice were implanted with only one 1.5-mm³ piece of tissue. Three SCID mice were also implanted orthotopically with histologically intact Lu-24 tissue via thoracotomy. All three animals produced locally growing tumors averaging 7.5 mm in diameter within 17 d. All three SCID mice also developed regional metastases including the mediastinum, left chest wall, and pericardium and distant metastases including the opposite lung, lymph nodes, parietal pleura, and diaphragm. The time when symptoms could be observed in the nude mice after transplantation of Lu-24 via thoracotomy was 24 d, as mentioned above; in the SCID mice, it was only 17 d, with the tumor seemingly growing and metastasizing more rapidly in the SCID mice *(122)*.

Similar results were found after orthotopically transplanting histologically intact tissue of human small-cell lung carcinomas Lu-130 and H-69; very large local growth and metastases to the opposite lung and distant lymph nodes were seen. These results contrast with the orthotopic injection of a suspension of small-cell carcinoma cells in nude rats, resulting in poor local growth and no metastases (123,124).

By implantation of histologically intact human tumor tissue in the parietal or visceral pleura of nude mice, we were able to construct models of early and advanced pleural cancer, respectively. Symptoms and survival of pleural-implanted mice closely resemble the clinical situation, showing a statistically significant difference in survival between parietal- and visceral-pleural implanted mice, the latter representing an advanced stage cancer. Thus such models, reflecting clinical features, should be of great value in the development of new drugs and treatment strategies (125).

Human malignant pleural mesothelioma is an aggressive cancer with no effective treatment. A relevant animal model is needed for studying the biology and for discovery of effective treatment. To meet this need, we have developed an orthotopic transplant model of human malignant pleura mesothelioma in nude mice that closely mimics the pattern found in the mesothelioma patient. Fresh specimens derived from four patients with malignant mesothelioma were implanted on the parietal pleural of nude mice. All patient tumors gave rise to locally growing tumors in the mice. The transplanted mice presented with symptoms of malignancy such as decrease in physical activity and signs of tumor-related respiratory distress. These animals were shown to have extensive tumor spread in the ipsilateral as well as contralateral pleural cavity and mediastinal lymph nodes. When the lesions were still confined to the ipsilateral parietal pleura, the implanted animals were asymptomatic. The macroscopic features usually found in the patients were also found in the implanted animals such as nodules and masses as well as pleural thickness owing to tumor spread. Histological examination revealed malignant mesothelioma similar to that from which the original tumor specimen was derived. Orthotopic parietal-pleura implantation of fresh histological human malignant mesothelioma thus allows mesothelioma growth in an animal model that very closely mimics the clinical pattern of the human disease. This model provides for the first time a useful human model for biological studies of this disease and for developing effective treatment (126–129).

To understand the skeletal metastatic pattern of nonsmall-cell lung cancer, we developed a stable high-expression GFP transductant of the human lung cancer cell line H460 (H460-GFP). The GFP-expressing lung cancer was visualized to metastasize widely throughout the skeleton when implanted orthotopically in nude mice. H460 was tranduced with the pLEIN retroviral expression vector containing the GFP gene and the neomycin (G418) resistance gene. A stable high GFP-expressing clone was selected in vitro using 800 µg/mL G418. Stable high-level expression of GFP was maintained in subcutaneously growing tumors formed after injecting H460-GFP cells in nude mice. To utilize H460-GFP for visualization of metastasis, fragments of subcutaneously growing H460-GFP tumors were implanted by SOI in the left lung of nude mice. Subsequent micrometastases were visualized by GFP fluorescence in the contralateral lung, and plural membrane and widely throughout the skeletal system including the skull, vertebra, femur, tibia, pelvis, and bone marrow of the femur and tibia. The use of GFP-expressing H460 cells transplanted by SOI revealed the extensive metastatic potential of lung cancer in particular to widely disseminated sites throughout the skeleton. This new metastatic model can play a critical role in the study of the mechanism of skeletal and other metastases in lung cancer and in screening of therapeutics that prevent or reverse this process *(130)*.

The Lewis lung carcinoma has been widely used for many important studies. However, the subcutaneous transplant or orthotopic cell suspension injection models have not allowed expression of it's full metastatic potential. A powerful new highly metastatic model of the widely used Lewis lung carcinoma was developed using SOI tumor fragments and enhanced GFP transduction of the tumor cells. To achieve this goal, we first developed in vitro a stable high-expression GFP transductant of the Lewis lung carcinoma with the pLEIN retroviral expression vector containing the GFP gene. Stable high-level expression of GFP was maintained in vivo in subcutaneously growing Lewis lung tumors. The in vivo GFP-expressing tumors were harvested and implanted as tissue fragments by SOI in the right lung of additional nude mice. This model resulted in rapid orthotopic growth and extensive metastasis visualized by GFP expression. In all, 100% of the animals had metastases on the ipsilateral diaphragmatic surface, contralateral diaphragmatic surface, contralateral lung parenchema, and mediastinal lymph nodes. Heart metastases were visualized in 40%, and brain metastases were visualized in 30% of the SOI animals. Mice developed signs of respiratory distress between 10 and 15 d post tumor implantation and were sacrificed. The use of GFP-transduced Lewis lung carcinoma transplanted by SOI reveals for the first time the high malignancy of this tumor and provides an important useful model for metastasis, angiogenesis, and therapeutic studies *(131)*.

5.7. Prostate Tumor Models

The human hormone-independent prostate cancer lines Du145 and PC-3 were transplanted into nude mice using SOI. The tumor grew locally and became invasive and metastatic. The tumor invaded the lamina propria of the mouse urinary bladder. The local large tumor growth on the prostate of the mice caused urinary obstruction and hydronephrosis, and local and distal lymph node and lung metastases were observed *(132,133)*.

Intact tissue of the androgen-dependent human prostate cancer cell line LNCaP was implanted on the ventral lateral lobes of the prostate gland by SOI in a series of 20 nude mice. Mice were autopsied, and histopathological examination of primary tumors and relevant organs was performed to identify and quantitate micrometastasis. Eighteen of 20 animals transplanted with LNCaP by SOI had tumor growth. Mean primary tumor weight in the prostate was 9.24 g at time of necropsy. Sixty-one percent of the transplanted animals had lymph node metastasis. Forty-four percent had lung metastasis. Mean survival time was 72 d, indicating a high degree of malignancy of the tumor. The extensive and widespread lung metastasis as well as lymph node metastasis following orthotopic implantation of LNCaP in nude mice and the short survival time provide a high-malignancy nude model of the LNCaP human prostate tumor *(134)*.

A fluorescent spontaneous bone metastatic model of human prostate cancer was developed by SOI of GFP-expressing prostate cancer tissue. A high-GFP-expression PC-3 human prostate cancer clone was injected subcutaneously in nude mice, and stable high-level expression of GFP was maintained in the growing tumors. To utilize GFP expression for metastasis studies, fragments of the fluorescent subcutaneously growing tumor were implanted by SOI in the prostate of nude mice. Subsequent micrometastases and metastases were visualized by GFP fluorescence throughout the skeleton including the skull, rib, pelvis, femur, and tibia. The central nervous system was also involved with tumor, including the brain and spinal cord as visualized by GFP fluorescence. Systemic organs including the lung, plural membrane, liver, kidney, and adrenal gland also had fluorescent metastases *(135)*.

5.8. Ovarian Tumor Models

Three examples of human ovarian cancer were transplanted by SOI into the ovarian capsule into nude mice in our laboratory *(136)*. In three cases, we observed three completely different patterns of tumor growth. In the first case, a highly encapsulated tumor developed measuring 33 × 23 mm with watery fluid. No rupture or intraperitoneal seeding was observed. This tumor grew with a cystadenocarcinoma growth pattern. During autopsy, a very small metastatic nodule on the lung of the mouse was observed. In the second case, extensive primary tumor growth was observed. Extensive seeding on the colon and parietal peritoneum of the nude mouse was also found.

The nude mouse models of human ovarian carcinoma described above therefore have the following characteristics:

1. They can be constructed directly from patient tumor specimens.
2. The tumors grow locally in the ovary.
3. The tumors can metastasize to the lung, can seed and grow in the peritoneal wall, and can involve critical organs such as the colon, all of which reflects the clinical situation.

An ovarian tumor line (RMG-1: human clear cell carcinoma of the ovary) previously grown subcutaneously was implanted orthotopically as intact tissue into the ovarian capsule of 22 nude mice. The tumors showed progressive growth at the orthotopic site in all animals. The tumor marker tumor-associated serum galactosyltransferase (GAT) tended to be positive in all nude mice. The tumors invaded or metastasized to the contralateral ovary (1/22), retroperitoneum (6/22), mesentery (2/22) and peritoneum (1/22), and omentum (6/22) and metastasized to the subcutaneous tissue (1/22), lymph nodes (9/22), and distant organs including the liver, kidney, pancreas, and diaphragm. In striking contrast, subcutaneous transplantation of this tumor resulted in growth in only two of five animals, with local lymph node and kidney involvement but no retroperitoneal or peritoneal involvement. These findings suggest that orthotopic implantation provides a suitable microenvironment in which ovarian cancer can express its intrinsic clinically relevant properties. This approach is relevant to the clinical features of ovarian cancer and is thought to be a useful model for studies of therapy for this cancer *(137)*.

5.9. Breast Tumor Models

Histologically intact patient breast tumor tissue was transplanted as intact tissue to the mammary fat pad of nude mice where the tumor tissue grew extensively and metastasized to the lung *(138)*.

We developed an optically imageable orthotopic metastatic nude mouse model of the human breast cancer line MDA-MB-435 expressing GFP. We have demonstrated fluorescent imaging of primary and metastatic growth in live tissue and in intact animals. Fragments of tumor tissue expressing GFP were sutured into the pocket in the right second mammary gland using SOI. Tumor tissue was strongly fluorescent, allowing whole-body imaging of tumor growth by wk 5. Neovascularization of the primary tumor was also visualized by whole-body imaging by contrast of the vessels to the fluorescent tumor. At autopsy, MDA-MB-435-GFP cells were found to have metastasized to various organs, including the lung in 15%, the lymph nodes in 55% (including axillary nodes), and the liver in 10% of the animals. These metastases could be visualized in fresh tissue by fluorescence imaging. Detailed fluorescence analysis visualized extensive metastasis in the thoracic cavity and the lymphatic system. Large metastatic nodules in the lung involved most of the pulmonary parenchyma in all lobes. Lymph node metastasis was found mainly in the axillary area. In the liver, fluorescent macroscopic metastatic nodules were found under the capsule. The metastatic pattern in the model thus reflected clinical metastatic breast cancer and provides a powerful model for drug discovery for this disease *(139)*.

5.10. GFP Models

Mouse models of metastatic cancer with genetically fluorescent tumor cells that can be imaged in fresh tissue, *in situ* as well as externally, have been developed. These models have opened many new possibilities including real-time tumor progression and metastasis studies on internal organs and real-time drug response evaluations. The GFP gene, cloned from bioluminescent organisms, has now been introduced into a series of human and rodent cancer cell lines in vitro to express GFP stably in vivo after transplantation to metastatic rodent models. Techniques were also developed for transduction of tumors by GFP in vivo. With this fluorescent tool, tumors and metastasis in host organs can be imaged down to the single cell level. GFP tumors on the colon, prostate, breast, brain, liver, lymph nodes, lung, pancreas, bone, and other organs have also been visualized externally (transcutaneously by quantitative whole-body fluorescence imaging). Real-time angiogenesis has also been imaged and quantified using GFP technology. The GFP technology allows a fundamental advance in the visualization of tumor growth and metastasis in real time in vivo *(140–179)*.

6. POSSIBLE MECHANISMS OF ENHANCED METASTASIS OF HETEROTRANSPLANTED TUMORS AT THE ORTHOTOPIC SITE

As to why orthotopically growing tumors metastasize to a much greater extent than ectopically growing tumors, Reid and Zvibel *(180)* indicated that investigators have identified a number of parameters: (1) anatomy, which determines the local microenvironment including the location of an available capillary bed; (2) formation of tumor emboli; (3) molecules that specify attachment of tumor cells to particular cells or to extracellular matrix molecules that are tissue-specific; (4) local growth factors; and (5) local matrix chemistries.

Colon tumor cells implanted intracecally grew and produced metastases and also produced higher levels of heparinase and 92- and 64-kDa species of type IV collagenase than the same tumors planted subcutaneously, which did not metastasize *(181)*. Nakajima et al. *(181)* speculate that these enzymes are critical for the enhanced metastatic capability of the orthotopically implanted tumor.

Leighton *(182)* postulated that fibroblasts can orient and mediate the directionality of cell spread in metastases. Thus, the stromal elements at the orthotopic site such as fibroblasts might be more interactive with the organ-specific tumor epithelium, with regard to directing cellular invasion, than at ectopic sites.

We have demonstrated that hormone-refractory PC-3 human prostate carcinomas growing orthotopically produce viable circulating metastasis cells. Using a dual-color tumor model in vivo, we showed that viable circulating human prostate carcinoma cells have increased metastatic propensity and, therefore, can be defined as a precursor of metastatic lesions. This study shows the critical role played by the orthotopic microenvironment in enabling the primary tumor to produce viable circulating metastatic cells. These findings explain why orthotopic tumors producing viable circulating carcinoma cells frequently metastasize and small-cell tumors very infrequently metastasize *(183)*.

7. EXPERIMENTAL PROOF OF PAGET'S SEED AND SOIL HYPOTHESIS WITH METAMOUSE MODELS

Tumors that metastasize do so to preferred target organs. More than 100 yr ago, Paget formulated his seed and soil hypothesis to explain this apparent specificity, i.e., the cells from a given tumor would "seed" only favorable "soil" offered by certain groups. The hypothesis implies that cancer cells must find a suitable "soil" in a target organ, i.e., one that supports colonization, for metastasis to occur. The ability of human colon cancer cells to colonize liver tissue governs whether a particular colon cancer is metastatic. In the model used in this study, human colon tumors are transplanted into the nude mouse colon as intact tissue fragments by SOI. These implanted tumors closely simulate the metastatic behavior of the original human patient tumor and are clearly metastatic or nonmetastatic to the liver. Both classes of tumors are equally invasive locally into tissues and blood vessels. However, the cells from each class of tumor behave very differently when directly injected into nude mouse livers. Only cells from metastasizing tumors are competent to colonize after direct intrahepatic injection. Also, tissue fragments from metastatic tumors affixed directly to the liver resulted in colonization, whereas no colonization resulted from nonmetastatic tumor tissue fragments even though some growth occurred within the tissue fragments themselves. Thus, local invasion (injection) and even adhesion to the metastatic target organ (fragments) are not sufficient for metastasis. The results suggest that the ability to colonize the liver is the governing step in the metastasis of human colon cancer *(184)*.

To understand further the role of the host organ in tumor progression, we have transplanted into nude mice histologically intact human colon cancer tissue on the serosal layers of the stomach (heterotopic site) and the serosal layers of the colon (orthotopic site). The xenograft lines Co-3, which is well differentiated, and COL-3-JCK, which is poorly differentiated, were used for transplantation. After orthotopic transplantation of the human colon tumors on the nude mouse colon, the growing colon tumor resulted in macroscopically extensive invasive local growth in 4 of 10 mice, serosal spreading in 9 of 10 mice, muscularis propria invasion in 1 of 10 mice, submucosal invasion in 3 of 10 mice, mucosal invasion in 3 of 10 mice, lymphatic duct invasion in 4 of 10 mice, regional lymph node metastasis in 4 of 10 mice, and liver metastasis in 1 of 10 mice. In striking contrast, after heterotopic transplantation of the human colon tumor on the nude mouse stomach, a large growing tumor resulted but with only limited invasive growth and without serosal spreading, lymphatic duct invasion, or regional lymph node metastasis. It has become clear from these studies that the orthotopic site, in particular the serosal and subserosal transplant surface, is critical to the growth, spread, and invasive and metastatic capability of the implanted colon tumor in nude mice. These studies suggest that the original host organ plays the same critical role in tumor progression *(185)*.

We have found an exquisite specificity of metastasis in that a metastatic human colon tumor transplanted to the liver of nude mice specifically "reverse metastasized" to the colon of the mouse. The results demonstrate the selective affinity of cancer to the matched soils of the primary and metastatic organs *(186)*.

8. DRUG DISCOVERY WITH PATIENT-LIKE MOUSE MODELS OF CANCER

Matrix metalloproteinases (MMPs) have been implicated in the growth and spread of metastatic tumors. This role was investigated in an orthotopic transplant model of human colon cancer in nude mice using the MMP inhibitor BB-94 (batimastat). Fragments of human colon carcinoma (1–1.5 mm) were surgically implanted orthotopically on the colon in 40 athymic nu/nu mice. Administration of BB-94 or vehicle (phosphate-buffered saline, pH 7.4, containing 0.01% Tween 80) commenced 7 d after tumor implantation (20 animals/group). Animals received 30 mg/kg BB-94 ip once daily for the first 60 d and then three times weekly. Treatment with BB-94 caused a reduction in the median weight of the primary tumor from 293 mg in the control group to 144 mg in the BB-94-treated group ($p < 0.001$). BB-94 treatment also reduced the incidence of local and regional invasion, from 12 of 18 mice in the control group (67%) to 7 of 20 mice in the treated group (35%). Six mice in the control group were also found to have metastases in the liver, lung, peritoneum, abdominal wall, or local lymph nodes. Only two mice in the BB-94 group had evidence of metastatic disease, in both cases confined to the abdominal wall. The reduction in tumor progression observed in the BB-94-treated group translated into an improvement in the survival of this group, from a median survival time of 110 d in the control group to a median survival time of 140 d in the treated group ($p < 0.01$). Treatment with BB-94 was not associated with any obvious toxic effect, and these results suggest that such agents may be effective as adjunctive cancer therapies *(187)*.

CT1746, an orally active synthetic MMP inhibitor, has a greater specificity for gelatinase A, gelatinase B, and stromelysin than for interstitial collagenase and matrilysin. CT1746 was evaluated in a nude mouse model that better mimics the clinical development of human colon cancer. The model is constructed by SOI of the metastatic human colon tumor cell line Co-3. Animals were gavaged with CT1746 twice a day at 100 mg/kg for 5 d after the SOI of Co-3 for 43 d. In this model, CT1746 significantly prolonged the median survival time of the tumor-bearing animals from 51 to 78 d. Significant efficacy of CT1746 was observed on primary tumor growth (32% reduction in mean tumor area at d 36), total spread, and metastasis (6/20 treated animals had no detectable spread and metastasis at autopsy compared with 100% incidence of metastasis in control groups). CT1746 was also efficacious in reducing tumor spread and metastasis to individual organ sites such as the abdominal wall, cecum, and lymph nodes compared with vehicle and untreated controls. We conclude that chronic administration of a peptidomimetic MMP inhibitor via the oral route is feasible and results in inhibition of solid tumor growth, spread, and metastasis with increase in survival in this model of human cancer, thus converting aggressive cancer to a more controlled indolent disease *(188)*.

The effects of a new selective MMP inhibitor, MMI-166, were evaluated on tumor growth, angiogenesis, and metastasis in an SOI liver metastatic model of human colon cancer (TK-4) *(193,194)*. Also investigated were the synergistic effects of MMI-166 and a conventional cytotoxic agent, MMC, in this model. Mice transplanted orthotopically with TK-4 were divided into four groups: a control group treated with vehicle solution, an MMI-166 group in which MMI-166 was administered orally at a dose of 200 mg/kg, 6 d/wk for 5 wk, an MMC group in which MMC was administered intraperitoneally at a dose of 2 mg/kg/wk for 5 wk, and a combination group treated with MMI-166 and MMC. MMI-166 did not inhibit transplanted tumor growth but significantly inhibited liver metastasis compared with the control group and the MMC group ($p < 0.01$). Significant antitumor and antimetastatic effects of the combination therapy were demonstrated. These results suggest that MMI-166 has potential antimetastatic ability and a synergistic effect with MMC *(193,194)*.

An SOI model of the human colon cancer cell line Co-3 in nude mice was treated with two doses of the new platinum analogs (Pt[cis-dach][DPPE] · 2NO$_3$) and (Pt[trans-dach][DPPE] · 2NO$_3$). The analogs were evaluated for antimetastatic efficacy in comparison with two doses of cisplatinum. Unlike the untreated control group, there were no mesenteric lymph node metastases in the groups treated with the high or low doses of both forms of new DPPE platinum analogs as well as the cisplatinum-treated group. However, much more body weight loss occurred in the cisplatinum-treated group than the DPPE-treated groups. The results obtained with the SOI animal model of colon cancer demonstrated that both *cis*- and *trans*-forms of DPPE had as strong an inhibitory effect on metastasis as that of cisplatinum, but with much less toxicity. Thus, the new platinum analogs appears to have promising clinical potential *(189)*.

An SOI model of the human RT-4 bladder tumor in nude mice resulted in local growth, invasion, regional extension, and metastases as well as distant metastases to other organ sites and lymph nodes, thus mimicking the bladder cancer patient. This metastatic bladder tumor animal model was treated with two doses of the new platinum analog (Pt[cis-dach][DPPE] · 2NO$_3$) for the evaluation of antimetastatic efficacy compared with two doses of cisplatinum. Unlike the untreated control group or the group treated with the low dose of cisplatinum, there were no metastases in either the high- or low-dose platinum analog-treated groups and the high-dose cisplatinum-treated group. The results obtained with this patient-like nude-mouse model of bladder cancer indicate that the new platinum analog appears to be a valuable lead compound with antimetastatic efficacy and clinical potential *(190)*.

Gemcitabine is a promising new agent that has recently been studied for palliation of advanced (stage IV) unresectable pancreatic cancer. We hypothesized that adjuvant gemcitabine would reduce recurrence and metastases following surgical resection of pancreatic cancer. To test this hypothesis, we evaluated gemcitabine on a GFP transductant of the human pancreatic cancer cell line BxPC-3 (BxPC-3-GFP) using SOI in mice. GFP allowed high-resolution fluorescence visualization of primary and metastatic growth. Five weeks after SOI, the mice were randomized into three groups. Group I received exploratory laparotomy only. Group II underwent surgical resection of the pancreatic tumor without further treatment. Group III underwent tumor resection followed by adjuvant treatment with gemcitabine, 100 mg/kg every 3 d for four doses, starting 2 d after resection. The mice were sacrificed at 13 wk following implantation, and the presence and location of recurrent tumor were recorded. Gemcitabine reduced the recurrence rate to 28.6% compared with 70.6% with resection only ($p = 0.02$) and reduced metastatic events 58% in the adjuvant group compared with resection only. This study, demonstrating that gemcitabine is effective as adjuvant chemotherapy post pancreatectomy, suggests a new indication of the drug clinically (150).

MIA-PaCa-2 was engineered to express stably high levels of the *Discosoma species* coral red fluorescent protein (RFP). Orthotopic implantation of highly red fluorescent human pancreatic tumor fragments onto the pancreas spontaneously yielded extensive, locoregional, primary tumor growth and the development of distant metastases. The primary and metastatic tumors were visualized, tracked, and imaged in real time by noninvasive whole-body imaging using selective tumor RFP fluorescence. Treatment with two well-described therapeutic agents, gemcitabine and CPT-11, demonstrated that gemcitabine highly improved survival (72 days, $p = 0.004$) by inducing transient tumor regression over the first 3 wk. However, at this time, growth and dissemination occurred despite continued treatment, suggesting the development of tumor resistance (205).

We have examined the ability of orally administered cytosine analogue CS-682 to both inhibit metastasis and prolong survival in an aggressive, orthotopic model of human MIA-PaCa-2 pancreatic cancer that selectively expresses high level of *Driscosoma sp.* RFP. Tumor RFP fluorescence facilitated real-time, sequential imaging and quantification of primary and metastatic growth and dissemination in vivo. Mice were treated with varying oral doses of CS-682 on a five times per week schedule until death. At a dose of 40 mg/kg, CS-682 prolonged survival compared to untreated animals (median survival 35 d vs. 17 d, $p = 0.0008$). At nontoxic doses, CS-682 effectively suppressed the rate of primary tumor growth. CS-682 also decreased the development of malignant ascites and the formation of metastases, which were significantly reduced in number in the diaphragm, lymph nodes, liver and kidney (206).

We determined the antitumor and antimetastatic efficacy of the camptothecin analog DX-8951f in an SOI metastatic mouse model of pancreatic cancer. DX-8951f showed efficacy against two human pancreatic tumor cell lines in this model. These cell lines were transduced with GFP, allowing high-resolution visualization of tumor and metastatic growth in vivo. The DX-8951f studies included both an early and advanced cancer model. In the early model, utilizing the human pancreatic cancer lines MIA-PaCa-2 and BxPC-3, treatment began when the orthotopic primary tumor was approx 7 mm in diameter. DX-8951f was significantly effective against both MIA-PaCa-2 and BxPC-3 cells. In contrast, gemcitabine, the standard treatment for pancreatic cancer, did not have significant efficacy against MIA-PaCa-2 cells. Although gemcitabine showed significant activity against BxPC-3 primary tumor growth, it was not effective in metastasis. In the model of advanced disease, utilizing BxPC-3, treatment started when the orthotopic primary tumor was 13 mm in diameter. DX-8951f was significantly effective in a dose-response manner on the BxPC-3 primary tumor. DX-8951f also demonstrated antimetastatic activity in the late-stage model, significantly reducing the incidence of lymph node metastasis while eliminating lung metastasis. In contrast, gemcitabine was only moderately effective against the primary tumor and ineffective against metastasis at both sites in the late-stage model. Therefore, DX-8951f was highly effective against primary and metastatic growth in this very difficult-to-treat disease and showed significantly higher efficacy than gemcitabine, the standard treatment for pancreatic cancer. DX-8951f, therefore, has important clinical promise and has more positive features than the currently used camptothecin analog CPT-11, which requires metabolic activation and is toxic (187).

We have examined the ability of orally administered cytosine analogue CS-682 to both inhibit metastasis and prolong survival in an aggressive, orthotopic model of human MIA-PaCa-2 pancreatic cancer that selectively expresses a high level of *Driscosoma sp.* RFP. Tumor RFP fluorescence facilitated real-time, sequential imaging and quantification of primary and metastatic growth and dissemination in vivo. Mice were treated with varying oral doses of CS-682 on a five times per week schedule until death. At a dose of 40 mg/kg, CS-682 prolonged survival compared to untreated animals (median survival 35 d vs. 17 d, $p = 0.0008$). At nontoxic doses, CS-682 effectively suppressed the rate of primary tumor growth. CS-682 also decreased the development of malignant ascites and the formation of metastases, which were significantly reduced in number in the diaphragm, lymph nodes, liver and kidney (206).

The efficacy of recombinant human interferon-γ (rh IFN-γ) was evaluated for the treatment of human pleural adenocarcinoma in an SOI model of the human nonsmall-cell lung cancer cell line H-460. IFN-γ was tested in three different dosages (25,000, 50,000, and 100,000 U) vs an untreated control through ip injection twice a day for 5 d, which was started 48 h after SOI. The results showed that IFN-γ can prolong the survival time of the tumor-bearing animals. The symptoms and signs of hypoxia, such as restricted physical activity and cyanosis owing to primary tumor growth in the thoracic cavity, as well as cachexia, developed much earlier in the control than in the IFN-γ-treated mice. The mice in the control group had succumbed by d 23 after tumor implantation. However, at that time 67% of the mice in the 100,000 U-treated group, 15% of the mice in the 50,000 U-treated group, and 16% of the mice in the 25,000 U-treated group were still alive. The orthotopically transplanted tumor grew rapidly and metastasized to the lung and liver in the untreated control. In the IFN-γ-treated groups, both primary tumor growth and metastasis were reduced, probably accounting for the increased survival rate. The results demonstrated dose-dependent efficacy of IFN-γ in suppressing symptomology, primary tumor growth, invasiveness, and metastasis of the human lung cancer cell line H 460, as well as increased survival of the tumor-bearing animals. These results suggest that clinical trials of IFN-γ should begin for treatment of pleural adenocarcinoma, for which there is no current effective therapy (191).

We examined the importance of interleukin-8 receptor B (IL-8RB) mRNA expression in the growth of non small-cell lung cancer. Using the antisense oligonucleotide ICN 197, we were able to inhibit IL-8RB mRNA expression in vitro. The sequence-specific effect of antisense oligonucleotide and downregulation of IL-8RB mRNA was shown by reverse transcription-polymerase chain reaction (RT-PCR) and Southern blot analysis. The proliferation of treated cells was measured by ^{3}H-thymidine incorporation. We found that treatment of these cells caused reversible growth inhibition and reversible downregulation of IL-8RB mRNA. Furthermore, we observed that treatment of nude mice with oligonucleotide ICN 197 inhibited the growth of tumors developed from nonsmall-cell lung cancer cells injected subcutaneously. Our in vitro data suggest that IL-8RB mRNA expression is required to maintain the proliferative rate of these cells. Based on the data in vivo, oligonucleotide ICN 197 may be considered for the development of novel therapeutic treatment for lung cancer (192).

The efficacy of a (phosphorothioate) antisense oligonucleotide for KDR/Flk-1 (KDR/Flk-1-ASO), an endothelial cell-specific vascular endothelial growth factor (VEGF) receptor, was investigated on the metastasis dissemination and angiogenesis of a human gastric cancer cell line in nude mice. GFP-transduced NUGC-4 (NUGC-4-GFP) human gastric cancer cells were implanted into the peritoneal cavity of nude mice. KDR/Flk-1-ASO, -SO, or PBS were administered from d 7 to d 14, 200 µg/mouse, once a day. The mice were sacrificed on d 28. Disseminated peritoneal tumor nodules expressing GFP were visualized by fluorescence microscopy. KDR/Flk-1-ASO significantly decreased the extent of peritoneal dissemination of the tumors. The number of cells undergoing apoptosis was significantly increased in the KDR/Flk-1-ASO-treated tumors. Microvessel density (MVD) was significantly reduced in the KDR/Flk-1-ASO-treated tumor nodules. The KDR/Flk-1 antisense strategy, therefore, decreases tumor dissemination apparently by inhibiting angiogenesis *(119)*.

Doxorubicin (DOX) was encapsulated in a galactose-conjugated hepatotropic liposome (hLip-DOX), and its ability to enhance the antitumor effect while reducing toxicity was compared with that of free DOX and a control Lip-DOX (cLip-DOX). An SOI model of human colon cancer xenograft TK-4 was used to induce liver metastases in mice. Liver metastasis occurred in 0/11 rats given hLip-DOX, whereas liver metastases developed in 10 of 12 mice in the control group and in 5 of 12 mice given cLip-DOX. Liposomal DOX did not have a significant inhibitory effect on transplanted tumor growth assessed 6 wk after transplantation. These findings indicate that hLip-DOX may be an effective strategy for inhibiting liver metastases from human colon cancer *(195)*.

Tanaka et al. *(196)* established a mouse primary tumor resection model in which a transplanted tumor was resected after an SOI of colorectal cancer tissue to estimate the therapeutic effect of an angiogenesis inhibitor on metastasis. The angiogenesis inhibitor FR-118487 is a member of the fumagillin family. One mg/kg/d of FR-118487 was subcutaneously administered to nude mice for 1, 2, or 4 wk through an osmotic pump. Liver metastasis developed in seven of nine control mice, two of six mice that underwent the tumor resection 2 wk after transplantation (early resection), and in all seven of the mice that underwent the tumor resection 4 wk after transplantation (late resection). FR-118487 administration immediately after early resection completely inhibited both hepatic and peritoneal metastases, whereas its administration after late resection had no effect on liver metastasis. In the prolonged treatment trial, inhibitory effects of prolonged treatment with FR-118487 on both hepatic and peritoneal metastases after late resection were clearly demonstrated. The mice in the resection-alone group all died within 106 d after tumor inoculation, owing to metastases. In contrast, half of the mice that underwent resection and then received antiangiogenic therapy were alive (160 days after transplantation) *(196)*.

S-1 (1 M tegafur [FT]/0.4 M 5-chloro-2,4-dihydroxypyridine [CDHP]/1 M potassium oxonate [Oxo]) is an oral agent that modulates 5-FU by CDHP and Oxo. The therapeutic effect of S-1 on human colon cancer xenografts (TK-13) with high metastatic potential to the liver was evaluated. Fragments of TK-13 were sutured into the cecal wall of 52 nude mice using SOI. The animals were randomly divided into three groups (control [$n = 17$], UFT [combination of 1 M FT and 4 M uracil] [$n = 18$], and S-1 [$n = 17$]). S-1 or UFT was administered orally at an equitoxic dose (S-1, 7.5 mg/kg; UFT, 17.5 mg/kg as FT) for 37 consecutive days beginning 10 d after the transplantation. S-1 showed higher tumor growth inhibition than UFT ($p < 0.05$) and also showed a significant liver antimetastatic efficacy, whereas UFT did not. Liver metastasis developed in only 2 of the 17 mice (12%) in the S-1 group, whereas it developed in 9 of the 17 (53%) and 7 of the 18 (39%) in the control and UFT groups, respectively *(197)*.

The efficacy of the combination of vascular endothelial growth factor neutralizing antibody (VEGFAb) and MMC was demonstrated on MT-2, a human gastric cancer xenograft. Fragments of MT-2 were transplanted by SOI into 62 nude mice where liver metastasis developed 6 wk after transplantation. The VEGFAb (100 µg/mouse) was administered ip in the VEGFAb group ($n = 14$) and the combination group ($n = 16$) twice a week starting after transplantation. MMC (2 mg/kg) was administered in the MMC group ($n = 16$) and the combination group ($n = 16$) on d 10, 17, and 24 after transplantation. Compared with the control group, in which saline solution was administered ip, all three treatments inhibited tumor growth significantly. Liver metastases were also significantly inhibited by the administration of VEGFAb alone, MMC alone, or combination therapy. Liver metastasis developed in nine mice of the control group, three of the VEGFAb group, and four of the MMC group, but no mice had liver metastasis in the combination therapy group. However, a significant body weight loss and a decrease in spleen weight were observed in the MMC and combination groups, with no significant difference between the two groups *(198)*.

The therapeutic effect of VEGFAb on liver metastasis of an endocrine neoplasm was demonstrated. Cecal transplantation into nude mice of small pieces of EN-1, a xenotransplanted human intestinal endocrine neoplasm, resulted in liver metastasis. A treated group ($n = 19$) received 100 µg/mouse of VEGFAb intraperitoneally on alternate days from d 10 after tumor transplantation, and the control group ($n = 19$) received saline. Five of the 19 control mice died of tumor progression. The cecal tumor weighed 6316 ± 2333 mg ($n = 17$) in the control group and 1209 ± 837 mg ($n = 19$) in the treated group ($p < 0.01$) 6 wk after transplantation. Liver metastasis developed in 16 of 17 control mice and in 2 of 19 treated mice ($p < 0.01$). The VEGF level of the whole cecal tumor in the control group was significantly higher than that in the treated group (305.1 ± 174.1 vs 54.7 ± 41.2 mg; $p < 0.001$). VEGFAb did not cause any body weight loss (28.52 ± 1.63 in the control vs 28.44 ± 1.71 g in the treated group). These results indicate that VEGFAb may be a novel therapeutic agent for endocrine neoplasm with distant metastasis *(199)*.

To evaluate VEGFAb further, four human carcinoma xenografts, two human colon carcinomas (TK4 and TK 13), and two gastric carcinomas (MT2 and MT5) were transplanted by SOI into nude mice. The anti-VEGF antibody (VEGFAb, 100 µg/mouse) or the same volume of saline was administered ip on alternative days starting from d 10 after transplantation. With each of the four xenografts, administration of VEGFAb significantly inhibited not only primary tumor growth but also macroscopic liver metastasis, although the growth rate varied. The inhibitory effect of VEGFAb on primary tumor growth appeared to have no correlation with the level of VEGF in the tumor. Body weight gain in each treated group was comparable to that in the control group. No toxicity of the antibody was observed. These results suggest that an anti-VEGF antibody can be effective against a wide variety of cancers and that VEGF may be a possible target for cancer therapy *(200)*. A similar VEGFAb, called Avastin, has shown significant clinical efficacy in colon cancer *(207)* demonstrating the predictivity of the SOI model.

The effect of an angiogenesis inhibitor, TNP-470, on primary tumor growth, liver metastasis, and peritoneal dissemination of gastric cancer was investigated using the SOI model of two human gastric cancers, MT-2 and MT-5. TNP-470 showed a significant inhibitory effect on the growth of primary tumors after orthotopic transplantation of both xenografts when given at a dose of 30 mg/kg on alternate days from d 7 after transplantation. However, growth of the MT-2 primary tumor was not inhibited by administration from d 14 after transplantation. Liver metastasis was significantly prevented by the early treatment of TNP-470. In particular, early treatment of MT-2 completely inhibited the development of macroscopic foci in the liver and was significantly more effective than late treatment. Peritoneal dissemination was also inhibited *(201)*.

The colon tumor xenograft TK-4 was transplanted by SOI and treated with TNP-470. Treatment was with 30 mg/kg of TNP-470 on alternate days starting from after d 10 transplantation. The rate of hepatic metastases from orthotopically transplanted tumors of five strains was 38–79%. TK-4 has *K-ras* and *p53* mutations, and overexpression of p53 induced hepatic metastases from both orthotopic (79%) and subcutaneous tumors (44%). Although TNP-470 only significantly inhibited subcutaneous tumor growth, its antimetastatic effect was significantly demonstrated on the hepatic metastases *(202)*.

The antimetastatic effect of TNP-470 was investigated further in nude mice in SOI models with human colon cancer. Tumors from three established human colon cancer cell lines (TK-3, TK-4, and TK-9), which were maintained in nude mice, were implanted into the cecal wall of nude mice via a small incision in the serosa. TNP-470 (20 or 30 mg/kg) was given sc every other day starting from after d 10 implantation, and the mice were sacrificed after 6 wk. There was no difference in the weight of the implanted tumors (control group: 0.45 ± 0.29 g vs treated group: 0.49 ± 0.27 g). An antimetastatic effect of TNP-470 was clearly demonstrated in a dose-dependent manner. In the mice given 20 mg/kg TNP-470, liver metastasis developed in 3 of 10 cases. In the 30-mg/kg group, metastasis developed in only 1 of 17 mice, whereas it developed in 22 of 32 mice of the control group. The number of metastatic foci was significantly less in the treated groups. TNP-470 prevented liver metastasis, but had no effect on the growth of the primary tumor *(203)*.

The antitumor and antimetastatic efficacy of TNP-470 and MMC were investigated in the SOI model of human colon cancer, TK-4. Mice were randomly divided into three groups; a control group given saline solution, a group receiving TNP-470 and a group receiving MMC. TNP-470 was given subcutaneously on alternate days for 5 wk starting from d 10 after cecal transplantation, and MMC was administered intraperitoneally once a week from d 10 after cecal transplantation. MMC significantly inhibited cecal tumor growth. In the control group, liver metastases developed in 9 of 10 mice, including 3 with more than 20 metastatic foci. Liver metastasis also developed in 8 of 10 mice receiving MMC, 2 of which had many metastases. In contrast, liver metastasis developed in only two of eight mice in the TNP-470 group, and neither of these animals had numerous metastases *(204)*.

9. NEW DIRECTIONS

9.1. Dual-Color Imaging of Tumor-Host Interaction

We have established a dual-color fluorescence imaging model of tumor-host interaction based on a red fluorescent protein (RFP)-expressing tumor growing in GFP transgenic mice. This model allowed visualization of the tumor-stroma interaction including tumor angiogenesis and infiltration of lymphocytes in the tumor. Transgenic mice, expressing the GFP under the control of a chicken β-actin promoter and cytomegalovirus enhancer, were used as the host. All the tissues from this transgenic line, with the exception of erythrocytes and hair, fluoresce green under blue excitation light. B16F0 mouse melanoma cells were transduced with pLNCX2-DsRed-2-RFP plasmid. The B16F0-RFP tumor and GFP-expressing stroma could be clearly imaged simultaneously in excised tissue. Dual-color imaging allowed resolution of the tumor cells and the host tissues down to the single cell level. Tumor stroma included fibroblast cells, tumor-infiltrating lymphocytes, blood vessels, and capillaries, all expressing GFP. GFP stromal cells were readily distinguished from the RFP-expressing tumor cells. This dual-color fluorescence imaging system should facilitate studies for understanding tumor-host interaction during tumor growth and tumor angiogenesis. The dual-color system also provides a powerful tool to analyze and isolate tumor-infiltrating lymphocytes and other host stromal cells interacting with the tumor for therapeutic and diagnostic/analytic purposes *(208)*.

REFERENCES

1. Ewing J, ed. *Neoplastic Diseases. A Treatise on Tumors*, 3rd ed. Philadelphia: WB Saunders. 1928.
2. Sticker A. In: Ewing J, ed. *Neoplastic Diseases. A Treatise on Tumors*, 3rd ed. Philadelphia: WB Saunders. 1928:1049–1051.
3. Novinsky M. *Cent Med Wissenschr* 1876; 14:790.
4. Hanau A. In: Ewing J, ed. *Neoplastic Diseases. A Treatise on Tumors*, 3rd ed. Philadelphia: WB Saunders. 1928:1049–1051.
5. Morau. *Arch Med Exper* 1984; 6:677.
6. Loeb J. *J Med Res* 1901; 6:28.
7. Loeb J. In: Ewing J, ed. *Neoplastic Diseases. A Treatise on Tumors*, 3rd ed. Philadelphia: WB Saunders. 1928:1049–1051.
8. Jensen C. In: Ewing J, ed. *Neoplastic Diseases. A Treatise on Tumors*, 3rd ed. Philadelphia: WB Saunders. 1928:1049–1051.
9. Jensen C. In: Ewing J, ed. *Neoplastic Diseases. A Treatise on Tumors*, 3rd ed. Philadelphia: WB Saunders. 1928:1049–1051.
10. Bashford EE, Murray LA, Cramer W. *Imp Cancer Res Fund* 1905; 2.
11. Apoland MW. *Arb Konigl Inst Exper Ther* 1906; I; 1907; 60.2:1720; 1908; 3:61.
12. Rous J. *Exp Med* 1911; 13:248, 239. *Soc Exp Biol* 1910; 12:696; Ibid., 1911; 8:603. JAMA 1910; 55:342, 1805; Ibid., 1911; 56:198, 714; Ibid., 1912; 58.
13. Ehrlich ZK. *Arb Konigl Inst Exper Ther* 1906; I:65,79; 1907; 5:70.
14. Beebe SP, Van Alstyne EVN. *J Med Res* 1914; 29:217.
15. Giovanella BC, Fogh J. *Adv Cancer Res* 1985; 44:69–120.
16. Greene HS. *Science* 1938; 88:357–358.
17. Gallagher EW, Korson R. *Proc Soc Exp Biol Med* 1959; 100:805–807.
18. Levin AG, Friberg S Jr, Klein E. *Nature* 1969; 222:997–998.
19. Toolan HW. *Proc Soc Exp Biol Med* 1951; 77:572–578.
20. Toolan HW. *Cancer Res* 1957; 17:418–420.
21. Osoba D, Auersperg NJ. *Nad Cancer Inst* 1966; 36:523–527.
22. Phillips B, Gazet JC. *Nature* 1967; 215:548–549.
23. Davis RC, Lewis JL. *Surg Forum* 1967; 18:229–231.
24. Cobb LM. *Br J Cancer* 1972; 26:183–189.
25. Castro JE. *Nature New Biol* 1972; 239:83–84.
26. Arnstein P, Taylor DO, Nelson-Rees WA, Huebner RJ, Lennette EH. *J Natl Cancer Inst* 1974; 52:71–84.
27. Cobb LM. *Br J Cancer* 1973; 28:400–411.
28. Pickard RG, Cobb LM, Steel GG. *Br J Cancer* 1975; 31:36–45.
29. Flanagan SP. *Genet Res* 1966; 8:295–309.
30. Pantelouris EM. *Nature* 1968; 217:370–371.
31. Rygaard J, Povlsen C. *Acta Pathol Microbiol Scand* 1969; 77:758–760.
32. Giovanella BC, Yim SO, Stehlin JS, Williams LJ. *J Natl Cancer Inst* 1972; 48:1531–1533.
33. Povlsen C, Rygaard J, Fogh J. In: Fogh J, Giovanella BC, eds., *The Nude Mouse in Experimental and Clinical Research*. New York: Academic. 1982:79–93.
34. Fogh J, Dracopoli N, Loveless JD, Fogh H. *Prog Clin Biol Res* 1982; 89:191–223.
35. Fogh J, Fogh JM, Orfeo T. *J Natl Cancer Inst* 1977; 59:221–226.
36. Sharkey FE, Fogh JM, Hajdu SI, Fitzgerald PJ, Fogh J. In: Fogh J, Ciovanella BC, eds., *The Nude Mouse in Experimental and Clinical Research*. New York: Academic. 1978:187.
37. Horten BC, Basler GA, Shapiro WR. *J Neuropathol Exp Neurol* 1981; 40:493–511.
38. Rofstad EK, Fodstad O, Lindmo T. *Cell Tissue Kinet* 1982; 15:545–554.

39. Grant AG, Duke D, Hermon-Taylor J. *Br J Cancer* 1979; 39:143–151.
40. Shimosato Y, Kameya T, Hrrohashi S. *Pathol Annu* 1979; 14:251–257.
41. Rae-Venter B, Reid LM. *Cancer Res* 1980; 40:95–100.
42. Shafie SM, Grantham FH. *J Natl Cancer Inst* 1981; 67:51–56.
43. Dunning WE. *Natl Cancer Inst Monogr* 1963; 12:351–369.
44. Horoszewicz J, Leong S, Kawinski E, et al. *Cancer Res* 1983; 43:1809–1818.
45. Stone KR, Mickey D, Wunderli H, Mickey G, Paulson D. *Int J Cancer* 1978; 21:274, 281.
46. Kaighn M, Narayan K, Ohnuki Y, Lechner J, Jones LW. *Invest Urol* 1975; 17:16, 23.
47. Kozlowsh J, McEvan L, Keer H, et al. In: Fidler IJ, Nicholson G, eds., *Tumor Progression and Metastasis*. New York: Alan R. Liss. 1988:189–231.
48. Pretlow T, Delmoro C, Dilley G, Spadafora C, Pretlow T. *Cancer Res* 1991; 51:3814–3817.
49. Sherwood E, Pitt Ford J, Lee L, Kozlowski J. *Biol Res Med* 1990; 9:44–52.
50. Shevrin D, Kukreja S, Ghosh L, Lad T. *Clin Exp Metastasis* 1988; 6:401–409.
51. Shevrin D, Gorny K, Kukreja S. *Prostate* 1989; 15:187–194.
52. Schroeder FH. *Natl Cancer Inst Monogr* 1978; 49:71.
53. Hoehn W, Schroeder EH, Riemann JE, Joebsis AC, Hermanek P. *Prostate* 1980; 1:95–104.
54. Bullard DE, Bigner DD. *Neurosurgery* 1979; 4:308–314.
55. Shapiro WR, Basler GA, Chernik NL, Posner JB. *J Natl Cancer Inst* 1979; 62:447–453.
56. Schackert G, Price JE, Bucana CD, Fidler IJ. *Int J Cancer* 1989; 44:892–897
57. Sufrin G, McGarry MP, Sandberg AA, Murphy GR. *J Urol* 1979; 121:159–161.
58. Naito S, Iwakawa A, Tanaka K, et al. *Invest Urol* 1980; 18:285–288.
59. Mattem J, Wayss K, Haag D, Toomes H, Volm M. *Eur J Cancer* 1980;16.
60. Giovanella BC, Stehlm JS, Shepard RC, Williams LJ. *Cancer Res* 39 (1979) 2236–2241.
61. Fridman R, Giaccone G, Kanemoto T, Martin G, Gazdar A, Mulshine J. *Proc Natl Acad Sci USA* 1990; 87:6698–6702.
62. Fridman R, Kibbey M, Royce L, et al. *J Natl Cancer Inst* 1991; 83:769–774.
63. Sharkey FE, Fogh J. *Fed Proc* 1979; 38:921.
64. Goldenberg DM, Pavia RA. *Science* 1981; 212:65–67.
65. Bowen JM, Cailleau R, Giovanella BC, Pathak S, Siciliano MJ. *In Vitro* 1983; 19:635–641.
66. Bhargava DK, Lipkin M. *Digestion* 1981; 21:225–231.
67. Bastert G, Schmidt-Matthiesen H, Althoff P, Usadel KH, Fortmeyer HP. *Naturwissenschaften* 1976; 63:438–439.
68. Reed ND, Manning DD. *Proc Soc Exp Biol Med* 1973; 143:350–353.
69. Rygaard J. *Acta Pathol Microbiol Scand A* 1974; 82:105–112.
70. Wilson LE, Garther Campbell JAH. Dowdle EB. *Proceedings of the 4th International Workshop on Immune Deficient Animals* 1984:357–361.
71. Giovanella BC, Yim SO, Morgan AC, Stehlin JS, Williams LJ Jr. *J Natl Cancer Inst* 1973; 50: 1051–1053.
72. Shoemaker R, Dykes D, Plowman J, et al. *Cancer Res* 1991; 51:2837–2841.
73. Kerbel R, Man M, Dexter D. *J Natl Cancer Inst* 1984; 72:93–108.
74. Van Muijen G, Jansen K, Cornelissen I, Smeets D, Beck J, Ruiter D. *Int J Cancer* 1991; 48:85–91.
75. Sharkey FE, Fogh J. *Int J Cancer* 1979; 24:733–738.
76. Hoehn W, Schroeder FH. *Invest Urol* 1978; 16:106–112.
77. Kyriazis AP, DiPersio L, Michael GJ, Pesce AJ, Stinnett JD. *Cancer Res* 1978; 38:3186–3190.
78. Neulat-Duga I, Sheppel A, Marty C, et al. *Invasion Metastasis* 1984; 4:209–224.
79. Kyriazis AA, Kyriazis AP. *Cancer Res* 1980; 40:4509–4511.
80. Chambers WF, Pettengill OS, Sorenson GD. *Exp Cell Biol* 1981; 49:90–97.
81. Miller FR, Medina D, Heppner GH. *Cancer Res* 1981; 41:3863–3867.
82. Miller FR. *Invasion Metastasis* 1981; 1:220–226.
83. Price J, Polyzos A, Zhang RD, Daniels LM. *Cancer Res* 1990; 50:717–721.
84. Levy JA, White AC, McGrath CM. *Br J Cancer* 1982; 45:375–383.
85. Schaadt M, Kirchner H, Fonatsch C, Diehl V. *Int J Cancer* 1979; 23:751–761.
86. Bogden AE, Houchens DP, Ovejera AA, Cobb WR. In: Fogh J, Giovanella BC, eds. *The Nude Mouse in Experimental and Clinical Research*. NewYork: Academic. 1982:367–400.
87. Hajdu SI, Lemos LB, Kozakewich H, Helson L, Beattie EJ Jr. *Cancer* 1981; 47:90–98.
88. Fidler IJ. *Cancer Res* 1990; 50:6130–6138.

89. Giavazzi R, Campbell D, Jessup J, et al. *Cancer Res* 1986; 46:1928–1933.
90. Morikawa K, Walker SM, Jessup JM, Fidler IJ. *Cancer Res* 1988; 48:1943–1948.
91. Morikawa K, Walker SM, Nakajima M, et al. *Cancer Res* 1988; 48:6863–6871.
92. Schackert HK, Fidler IJ. *Int J Cancer* 1989; 44:177–181.
93. Sordat B, Ueyama Y, Fogh J. In: Fogh J, Giovanella BC, eds. *The Nude Mouse in Experimental and Clinical Research*. New York: Academic. 1982:95–147.
94. Sordat B, Wang WR. *Behring Inst Mitt* 74 (1984) 291–300.
95. Bresalier RS, Raper SE, Hujanen ES, Kim YS. *Int J Cancer* 1987; 39:625–630.
96. Fu XY, Bestemman JM, Monosov A, Hoffman RM. *Proc Natl Acad Sci USA* 1991; 88:9345–9349.
97. Furukawa T, Kubota T, Watanabe M, et al. *Surg Today* 1993; 23:420–423.
98. Rashidi B, An Z, Sun F-X, et al. *Clin Exp Metastasis* 1999; 17:497–500.
99. Ahlering T, Dubeau L, Jones PA. *Cancer Res* 1987; 47:6660–6665.
100. Theodorescu D, Cornil L, Fernandez B, Kerbel R. *Proc Natl Acad Sci USA* 1990; 87:9047–9051.
101. Fu X, Theodorescu D, Kerbel R, Hoffman RM. *Proc Am Assoc Cancer Res* 1991; 32:71.
102. Fu X, Theodorescu D, Kerbel RS, Hoffman RM. *Int J Cancer* 1991; 49:938–939.
103. Fu X, Hoffman RM. *Int J Cancer* 1992; 51:989–991.
104. Vezeridis MR, Tumer MR, Kajiji S, Yankee R, Meitner R. *Proc Am Assoc Cancer Res* 1985; 26:53.
105. Vezeridis M, Doremus C, Tibbetts L, Tzanakakis G, Jackson B. *J Surg Oncol* 1989; 40:261–265.
106. Marincola F, Drucker BJ, Siao D, Hough K, Holder WD Jr. *J Surg Res* 1989; 47:520–529.
107. Fu X, Guadagni E, Hoffman RM. *Proc Natl Acad Sci USA* 1992; 89:5645–5649.
108. An Z, Wang X, Kubota T, Moossa AR, Hoffman RM. *Anticancer Res* 1996; 16:627–631.
109. Tomikawa M, Kubota T, Matsuzaki SW, et al. *Anticancer Res* 1997; 17:3623–3625.
110. Bouvet M, Yang M, Nardin S, et al. *Clin Exp Metastasis* 2000; 18:213–218.
111. Bouvet M, Wang J, Nardin SR, et al. *Cancer Res* 2002; 62:1534–1540.
112. Bouvet M, Nardin SR, Burton DW, et al. *Pancreas* 2002; 24:284–290.
113. Dinesman A, Haughey B, Gates G, Aufdemorte T, Von Hoff D. *Otolaryongol Head Neck Surg* 1990; 103:766–774.
114. Braakhuis B, Sneeuwloper G, Snow GB. *Arch Otorhinolaryngol* 1984; 239:69–79.
115. Yamashita T. *Jpn J Cancer Res* 1988; 79:945–951.
116. Furukawa T, Fu X, Kubota T, et al. *Cancer Res* 1993; 53:1204–1208.
117. Furukawa T, Kubota T, Watanabe M, Kitajima M, Hoffman RM. *Int J Cancer* 1993; 53:608–612.
118. Hasegawa S, Yang M, Chishima T, Shimada H, Moossa AR, Hoffman RM. *Cancer Gene Ther* 2000; 7:1336–1340.
119. Kamiyama M, Ichikawa Y, Ishikawa T, et al. *Cancer Gene Ther* 2002; 9:197–201.
120. McLemore T, Liu M, Blacker P, et al. *Cancer Res* 1987; 47:5132–5140.
121. McLemore T, Eggleston J, Shoemaker R, et al. *Cancer Res* 1988; 48:2880–2886.
122. Wang X, Fu X, Hoffman RM. *Int J Cancer* 1992; 51:992–995.
123. Howard R, Chu H, Zeligman B, et al. *Cancer Res* 1991; 51:3274–3280.
124. Mulvin D, Howard R, Mitchell D, et al. *J Natl Cancer Inst* 1992; 84:31–37.
125. Astoul P, Wang X, Kubota T, Hoffman RM. (Review) *Int J Oncology* 1993; 3:713–718.
126. Colt HG, Astoul P, Wang X, Yi ES, Boutin C, Hoffman RM. *Anticancer Res* 1996; 16:633–639.
127. Astoul P, Wang X, Colt HG, Boutin C, Hoffman RM. *Oncol Rep* 1996; 3:483–487.
128. Hoffman RM. Clinically accurate orthotopic mouse models of cancer. In: Brooks S, Schumacher U, eds. *Metastasis Research Protocols*. Vol. 2. *Cell Behavior* In Vitro *and* In Vivo. *Methods in Molecular Medicine*, vol. 58, Totowa, NJ: Humana. 2001:251–275.
129. Hoffman RM. Metastatic mouse models of lung cancer. In: Driscoll B, ed. *Methods in Molecular Medicine*, Vol. 74: *Lung Cancer*, Vol. 1: *Molecular Pathology Methods and Reviews*. Totowa, NJ: Humana. 2002:457–464.
130. Yang M, Hasegawa S, Jiang P, et al. *Cancer Res* 1998; 58:4217–4221.
131. Rashidi B, Yang M, Jiang P, et al. *Clin Exp Metastasis* 2000; 18:57–60.
132. Fu X, Herrera H, Hoffman RM. *Int J Cancer* 1992; 52:987–990.
133. An Z, Wang X, Geller J, Moossa AR, Hoffman RM. *Prostate* 1998; 34:169–174.
134. Wang X, An Z, Geller J, Hoffman RM. *Prostate* 1999; 39:182–186.
135. Yang M, Jiang P, Sun FX, et al. *Cancer Res* 1999; 59:781–786.
136. Fu X, Hoffman RM. *Anticancer Res* 1993; 13:283–286.
137. Kiguchi, K., Kubota, T., Aoki, D., et al. *Clin Exp Metastasis* 1998; 16:751–756.
138. Fu X, Le P, Hoffman RM. *Anticancer Res* 1993; 13:901–904.

139. Li X-M, Wang J, An Z, et al. *Clin Exp Metastasis* 2002; 19:347–350.
140. Chishima T, Miyagi Y, Wang X, et al. *Cancer Res* 1997; 57:2042–2047.
141. Chishima T, Miyagi Y, Wang X, et al. *Clin Exp Metastasis* 1997; 15:547–552.
142. Chishima T, Miyagi Y, Wang X, Tan Y, Shimada H, Moossa AR, Hoffman RM. *Anticancer Res* 1997; 17:2377–2384.
143. Chishima T, Yang M, Miyagi Y, et al. *Proc Natl Acad Sci USA* 1997; 94:11,573–11,576.
144. Chishima T, Miyagi Y, Li L, et al. *In Vitro Cell Dev Biol Anim* 1997; 33:745–747.
145. Hoffman RM. *Cancer Metastasis Rev* 1998–99; 17:271–277.
146. Hoffman RM. Green fluorescent protein to visualize cancer progression and metastasis. In: Conn PM, ed. *Methods in Enzymology, Green Fluorescent Protein*, vol. 302. San Diego: Academic. 1999:20–31.
147. Naumov GN, Wilson SM, MacDonald IC, et al. *J Cell Sci* 1999; 112:1835–1842.
148. Yang M, Chishima T, Baranov E, Shimada H, Moossa AR, Hoffman RM. In: *Proceedings of the SPIE Conference on Molecular Imaging: Reporters, Dyes, Markers, and Instrumentation.* 1999; 3500: 117–124.
149. Yang M, Jiang P, An Z, et al. *Clin Cancer Res* 1999; 5:3549–3559.
150. Yang M, Chishima T, Wang X, et al. *Clin Exp Metastasis* 1999; 17:417–422.
151. Hoffman RM. Visualization of metastasis in orthotopic mouse models with green fluorescent protein. In: Fiebig HH, Burger AM, eds. *Relevance of Tumor Models in Anticancer Drugs Development*, vol. 54. Dordrecht, The Netherlands: Kluwver Academic Publishers. 1999:81–87.
152. Yang M, Baranov E, Jiang P, et al. *Proc Natl Acad Sci USA* 2000; 97:1206–1211.
153. Dove A. *Nature Biotechnol* 2000; 18:261.
154. Hoffman RM. *J Natl Cancer Inst* 2000; 92:1445–1446.
155. Yang M, Baranov E, Shimada H, Moossa AR, Hoffman RM. In: *Proceedings of the SPIE Conference.* 2000:256–259.
156. Corrigendum BioFeedback. *BioTechniques* 2000; 29:544.
157. Yang M, Baranov E, Moossa AR, et al. *Proc Natl Acad Sci USA* 2000; 97:12,278–12,282.
158. Yang M, Baranov E, Li X-M, et al. *Proc Natl Acad Sci USA* 2001; 98:2616–2621.
159. Robinson K. Imaging system captures whole-body GFP images. *Biophotonics Int* 2001; April:54–55.
160. Pfeifer A, Kessler T, Yang M, et al. *Mol Ther* 2001; 3:319–322.
161. Hoffman RM. *BioTechniques* 2001; 30:1016–1026.
162. Hutchinson E. *Lancet Oncol* 2001; 2:254.
163. McCann J. *J Natl Cancer Inst* 2001; 93:976–977.
164. Lee NC, Bouvet M, Nardin S, et al. *Clin Exp Metastasis* 2001; 18:379–384.
165. Zhao M, Yang M, Baranov E, et al. *Proc Natl Acad Sci USA* 2001; 98:9814–9818.
166. Hoffman RM. Green fluorescent protein for metastasis research. In: Brooks SA, Schumacher U, eds. *Methods in Molecular Medicine*, vol. 58: *Metastasis Research Protocols*, vol. 2: *Cell Behavior* In Vitro and In Vivo. Totowa, NJ: Humana. 2001:285–298.
167. Hoffman RM. GFP-expressing metastatic-cancer mouse models. In: Teicher B, ed. *Tumor Models in Cancer Research*. Totowa, NJ: Humana. 2002:99–112.
168. Yang M, Baranov E, Wang J-W, et al. *Proc Natl Acad Sci USA* 2002; 99:3824–3829.
169. Hoffman RM. *Lab Animal* 2002; 31:34–41.
170. Schmitt CA, Fridman JS, Yang M, et al. *Cancer Cell* 2002; 1:289–298.
171. Schmitt CA, Fridman JS, Yang M, et al. *Cell* 2002; 109:335–346.
172. Hoffman RM. *Trends Mol Med* 2002; 8/7:354–355.
173. Hoffman RM. Whole-body fluorescence imaging with Green Fluorescence Protein. In: Hicks BW, ed. *Methods in Molecular Biology*, vol. 183: *Green Fluorescent Protein: Applications and Protocols.* Totowa, NJ: Humana. 2002; 135–148.
174. Hoffman RM. *Cell Death Differ* 2002; 9:786–789.
175. Zhou J-H, Rosser CJ, Tanaka M, et al. *Cancer Gene Therapy* 2002; 9:681–686.
176. Hoffman RM. *Lancet Oncol* 2002; 3:546–556.
177. Saito N, Zhao M, Li L, et al. *Proc Natl Acad Sci USA* 2002; 99:13,120–13,124.
178. Sun F-X, Tohgo A, Bouvet M, et al. *Cancer Res* 2003; 63:80–85.
179. Wang J-W, Yang M, Wang X, et al. *Anticancer Res* 2003; 23:1–6.
180. Reid LM, Zvibel I. *J Natl Cancer Inst* 1990; 82:1866.
181. Nakajima M, Morikawa K, Fabra A, Bucana C, Fidler J. *J Natl Cancer Inst* 1990; 82:1890–1898.
182. Leighton, J. *Spread of Human Cancer.* New York: Academic. 1967.
183. Glimskii VB, Smith BA, Jiang P, et al. *Cancer Res* 2003; 63:4239–4243.

184. Kuo T-H, Kubota T, Watanabe M, et al. *Proc Natl Acad Sci USA* 1995; 92:12,085–12,089.
185. Togo S, Shimada H, Kubota T, et al. *Cancer Res* 1995; 55:681–684.
186. Togo S, Wang X, Shimada H, et al. *Anticancer Res* 1995; 15:795–798.
187. Wang X, Fu X, Brown PD, et al. *Cancer Res* 1994; 54:4726–4728.
188. An Z, Wang X, Willmott N, et al. *Clin Exp Metastasis* 1997; 15:184–195.
189. Rho Y-S, Lee K-T, Jung J-C, et al. *Anticancer Res* 1999; 19:157–162.
190. Chang S-G, Kim JI, Jung J-C, et al. *Anticancer Res* 1997; 17:3239–3242.
191. An Z, Wang X, Astoul P, Danays T, Moossa AR, Hoffman RM. *Anticancer Res* 1996; 16:2545–2551.
192. Olbina G, Cieslak D, Ruzdijic S, et al. *Anticancer Res* 1996; 16:3525–3530.
193. Ohta M, Konno H, Tanaka T, et al. *Jpn J Cancer Res* 2001; 92:688–695.
194. Oba K, Konno H, Tanaka T, et al. Prevention of liver metastasis of human colon cancer by selective matrix metalloproteinase inhibitor MMI-166. *Cancer Lett* 2002; 10:45–51.
195. Matsuda I, Konno H, Tanaka T, Nakamura S. *Surg Today* 2001; 31:414–420.
196. Tanaka T, Konno H, Baba S, et al. *Jpn J Cancer Res* 2001; 92:88–94.
197. Konno H, Tanaka T, Baba M, et al. *Jpn J Cancer Res* 1999; 90:448–453.
198. Matsumoto K, Konno H, Tanaka T, et al. *Jpn J Cancer Res* 2000; 91:748–752.
199. Konno H, Arai T, Tanaka T, et al. *Jpn J Cancer Res* 1998; 89:933–939.
200. Kanai T, Konno H, Tanaka T, et al. *Int J Cancer* 1998; 77:933–936.
201. Kanai T, Konno H, Tanaka T, et al. *Int J Cancer* 1997; 71:838–841.
202. Konno H, Tanaka T, Kanai T, et al. *Cancer* 1996; 77:1736–1740.
203. Tanaka T, Konno H, Matsuda I, et al. *Cancer Res* 1995; 55:836–839.
204. Konno H, Tanaka T, Matsuda I, et al. *Int J Cancer* 1995; 61:268–271.
205. Katz M, Takimoto S, Spivac D, et al. *J. Surg Res* 2003; 113:151–160.
206. Katz M, Bouvet M, Takimoto, et al. *Cancer Res* 2003; 63:5521–5525.
207. Yang JC, Haworth L, Sherry RM, et al. *N Engl J Med* 2003; 349;427–434.
208. Yang M, Li L, Jiang P, et al. *Proc Natl Acad Sci USA*, in press, 2003.

10 Preclinical Models for Combination Therapy

Beverly A. Teicher, PhD

CONTENTS

INTRODUCTION
ENDPOINTS
TUMOR EXCISION ASSAY
COMBINATION METHODS
THE STEM-CELL SUPPORT MODEL
SCHEDULING AND SEQUENCING OF HIGH-DOSE THERAPIES
CONCLUSIONS

1. INTRODUCTION

The scientific study of cancer therapy relevant to the high-dose setting has required the development of preclinical models that go beyond the conventional dose endpoints of increase in life span and tumor growth delay. High-dose therapy can be modeled using the tumor cell survival assay, which allows tumor-bearing animals to be treated with "supralethal" doses of anticancer treatments with a quantitative measure of tumor cell killing. Furthermore, a stem-cell support regimen in mice has recently been developed in a murine system allowing observation of regression and regrowth of tumors after high-dose therapy. The ability to determine whether combination therapies, especially chemotherapy combinations, retain increasing efficacy in the high-dose setting is critical to the development of new treatment regimens and is an issue best addressed in the laboratory.

2. ENDPOINTS

The earliest in vivo preclinical tumor models were leukemias grown as ascites tumors. The endpoint of experiments with these tumors was most often increase in life span. As solid tumor models were developed, the appropriate endpoints devised were tumor growth delay or tumor control of a primary implanted tumor. These assays require that drugs be administered at doses producing tolerable normal tissue toxicity, so that response of the tumor to the treatment can be observed for a relatively long period. These endpoints

From: *Cancer Drug Discovery and Development:*
Anticancer Drug Development Guide: Preclinical Screening, Clinical Trials, and Approval, 2nd Ed.
Edited by: B. A. Teicher and P. A. Andrews © Humana Press Inc., Totowa, NJ

cannot be applied to the high-dose setting in which normally lethal doses of anticancer therapies can be administered with normal tissue support, such as bone marrow transplantation. Response to high-dose therapies can be assessed by use of excision assays (1–3).

One important difference between excision assays and the *in situ* assays of increase in life span, tumor growth delay, or local tumor control is that excision assays require removal of the tumor from the environment in which it was treated. This difference and the nature of the assay procedure lead to a number of advantages and disadvantages in using excision assays rather than *in situ* assays. The ability to measure cell survival directly is important, because it provides basic information about what is perhaps the ultimate definitive cellular effect. Tumor excision assays also allow greater accuracy and finer resolution between various therapeutic regimens than do the *in situ* assays. Supralethal treatments can be tested. Perhaps the greatest disadvantage of excision assays is that extended treatment regimens cannot be used owing to tumor cell loss and tumor cell proliferation over the treatment time. Thus, an excision assay provides a static picture of tumor response at a short time after treatment (2).

The survival of tumor cells from tumors treated in vivo and then excised is often determined by in vitro colony formation. This requires use of tumor models that grow well in vivo and also have a high plating efficiency in vitro (ideally on the order of 20%). However, in vivo colony formation, such as spleen colony formation for leukemias, is also often used as an excision assay endpoint. The use of excision assays to determine survival of tumor cells after treatment in vivo with a range of drug or agent doses can provide insights concerning both treatment efficacy and tumor biology (2,3).

3. TUMOR EXCISION ASSAY

Historically, clonogenicity, that is, the ability of single cells to proliferate to form a colony of at least 50 cells, has been used to determine the effectiveness of different types of antitumor therapies since the seminal publication of the method by Hewitt and Wilson (4). As the focus of preclinical research evolved from the leukemias and lymphomas to solid tumors, several tumor systems were developed that grew well in vivo and had plating efficiencies (10–20%) from in vivo implants into cell culture suitable for colony-forming assays (3–13). The tumor excision/colony-forming assay has been a highly effective tool for understanding dose response of chemotherapeutic agents as well as radiation therapy, hyperthermia, and so forth in vivo. Until now, the tumor cell survival assay has been applied almost exclusively to the response of the primary tumor to therapy. Recently, however, tumor cell survival assay has been applied to the detection of metastatic disease as well as to the therapeutic response of tumor in several organs.

These studies were performed in the EMT-6/Parent murine mammary carcinoma tumor line that was originally developed as an in vivo/in vitro line by Rockwell et al. (2) and the EMT-6 in vivo alkylating agent-resistant sublines of the original tumor developed by Teicher et al. (13). The in vivo alkylating agent-resistant EMT-6 murine mammary tumors were made resistant to cis-diamminedichloroplatinum (II) (cisplatin; CDDP), carboplatin, cyclophosphamide, or thiotepa in vivo treatment of tumor-bearing animals with the drug during a 6-mo period (13). In spite of high levels of in vivo resistance, no significant resistance was observed when the cells from these tumors were exposed to the drugs in vitro in monolayer culture. The pharmacokinetics of cisplatin and cyclophosphamide were altered in animals bearing the respective resistant tumors. The resistance of all tumor lines, except for the EMT-6/thiotepa, decreased during 3–6 mo of in vivo passage in the absence of drug treatment. These studies indicated that very high levels of resistance to anticancer drugs can develop through mechanisms that are expressed in vivo, but not in monolayer culture *(13–15)*.

The survival of bone marrow granulocyte-macrophage colony-forming units (GM-CFU), an alkylating agent-sensitive normal tissue, was assessed in mice bearing the EMT-6/Parent tumor or the in vivo resistant EMT-6/CDDP, EMT-6/CTX, EMT-6/Thio, and EMT-6/carboplatin tumors *(14)*. The survival pattern of the bone marrow GM-CFU recapitulated the survival of the tumor cells, mimicking the development of resistance and reversion to sensitivity on removal of the selection pressure for each of the four alkylating agents. When the EMT-6/Parent tumor was implanted in the opposite hindlimb of animals bearing the EMT-6/CDDP or EMT-6/CTX tumor, the survival of the parental tumor cells after treatment of the animals with the appropriate antitumor alkylating agent was enhanced. The EMT-6/CDDP tumor was crossresistant to cyclophosphamide and high-dose melphalan, whereas the EMT-6/CTX tumor was somewhat resistant to CDDP and markedly sensitive to etoposide (VP-16). In each case, the survival pattern of the bone marrow GM-CFU reflected the survival of the tumor cells. These results indicated that the presence of an alkylating agent-resistant tumor in a host can affect drug response of tissues distal to that tumor *(14)*.

The expression of several early response genes and genes associated with malignant disease was assessed in the EMT-6/Parent tumor and the EMT-6/CTX and EMT-6/CDDP in vivo resistant tumor lines growing as tumors or as monolayers in culture *(15)*. In the absence of treatment, mRNA levels for the genes *c-jun*, *c-fos*, *c-myc*, *Ha-ras*, and *p53* were increased in the EMT-6/CTX and EMT-6/CDDP tumors compared with the EMT-6/Parent tumor, whereas expression of erb-2 was similar in all three tumors. Although the cells from each of the three tumors showed increased expression of early response genes after exposure to cisplatin (100 μM, 2 h) or 4-hydroperoxycyclophosphamide (100 μM, 2 h) in culture, in mRNA extracted from tumor tissue, these changes were absent or very small. *c-jun* and *erb-2* were detectable in liver. There was increased expression of both of these genes in the livers of tumor-bearing animals compared with non-tumor-bearing animals. The highest expression of both *c-jun* and *erb-2* occurred in the livers of animals bearing the EMT-6/CDDP tumor.

Treatment of the animals with cisplatin or cyclophosphamide in general resulted in increased expression of both genes 6 h post treatment. The increased expression of these genes may impart metabolic changes in the tumors and/or hosts that contribute to the resistance of these tumors to specific antitumor alkylating agents *(15)*. Although the EMT-6/Parent tumor is estrogen receptor-positive, the EMT-6/CTX and EMT-6/CDDP tumors are estrogen receptor-negative. The resistant tumor lines are also much more aggressively metastatic than the EMT-6/Parent tumor line.

The initial study of the response of metastatic tumor to high-dose alkylating agent therapy was carried out in animals bearing the EMT-6/Parent tumor implanted subcutaneously in the hind leg of mice using cyclophosphamide as the treatment agent. The tumor-bearing animals were treated with cyclophosphamide (300 or 500 mg/kg) by intraperitoneal injection on d 8 post tumor cell implantation when the primary tumors were about 200 mm^3 in volume. On d 9, the animals were sacrificed, and tumor, liver, lungs, blood, bone marrow, brain, and spleen were removed from the animals. The tissues were minced with crossed scalpels and then treated with DNase and collagenase to

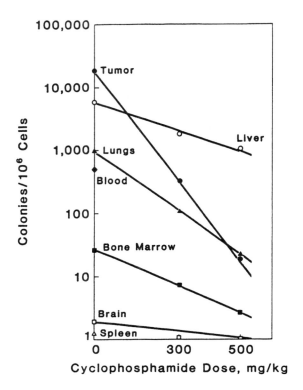

Fig. 1. Colonies/10^6 cells from tissues of animals bearing EMT-6/Parent tumors either without treatment or after cyclophosphamide (300 or 500 mg/kg). The animals were treated on d 7 post tumor implant, and tissues were excised on d 8.

disaggregate the tissues into single cells. The enzyme exposure time was varied depending on the tissue to optimize cell yield from each tissue. Known numbers of nucleated cells from each tissue were plated in monolayer culture under conditions suitable for tumor cell proliferation. After 10 d, colonies were stained and counted.

In Fig. 1, the resulting data are expressed as colonies per 10^6 cells plated from each tissue. In the absence of treatment, the primary tumor produced 2×10^4 colonies per 10^6 cells, whereas about 6000, 1000, and 500 tumor cell colonies grew from liver, lungs, and blood per 10^6 cells, respectively. Many fewer colonies—about 25, 2, and 1.5—grew from the bone marrow, brain, and spleen per 10^6 cells, respectively. These data, then, indicate the relative abundance of viable malignant cells in the respective normal tissues of the host.

Next, the response to therapy of tumor depending on the organ in which the tumor was located was determined. Figure 2 presents these data traditionally as surviving fraction vs dose of cyclophosphamide. The blood and spleen are shown on the lower axis, because no colonies grew from these tissues at either dose of cyclophosphamide. On the other hand, although the number of tumor cells in the brain was relatively few, most of them survived treatment of the host with cyclophosphamide. Tumor metastatic to the liver, bone marrow, and lungs was also less responsive to treatment with cyclophosphamide than the primary tumor.

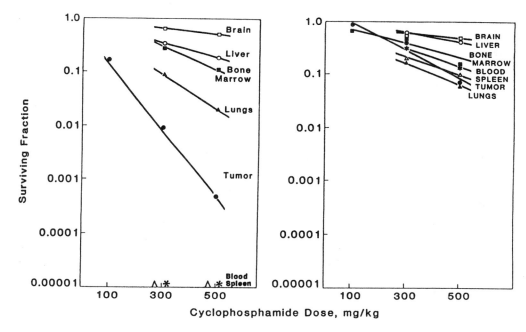

Fig. 2. Survival of EMT-6/Parent or EMT-6/CTX cells from various tissues of animals treated with various doses of cyclophosphamide.

The reasons for the differential responsiveness of the EMT-6/Parent tumor depending on location of the tumor in the host are manifold. The first is the great heterogeneity of drug distribution throughout the host. The second may be the capacity of the surrounding normal tissue to detoxify the drug. The third may be differences in the expression of genes involved in drug detoxification in the tumor cells depending on the molecular environment (organ or tissue) in which they are located. Figure 2 also shows the response of the primary tumor and metastatic disease in animals bearing the EMT-6/CTX tumor after treatment with cyclophosphamide. As was seen with animals bearing the EMT-6/Parent tumor, tumor cells in the blood and spleens were eradicated by the drug treatment. Response of tumor in the other organ sites followed a pattern similar to that of the EMT-6/ Parent tumor; however, relative treatment resistance was clear in both primary and metastatic disease (16,17).

Understanding the mechanisms involved in the sensitivity/resistance of tumors to chemotherapy, coupled with the development of a clinically relevant means of ensuring tumor sensitivity to treatment, is an important continuing endeavor. To explore the mechanisms of drug resistance, transcriptional profiling was performed on Affymetrix 6500 and 19K Murine GeneChip arrays using RNA from EMT-6/CDDP, EMT-6/CTX and parental EMT-6 tumors (18). RNA was extracted from three independent tumors for each line, and these samples were each hybridized to microarrays independently. Assuming the global mean hybridization intensity from chip to chip was the same, hybridization intensities were normalized to permit direct comparisons between samples. One and two percent of the genes in the EMT-6/CDDP and EMT-6/CTX tumors, respectively, showed at least twofold changes in mean hybridization intensities in comparison with parental tumor samples ($p < 0.05$). Although cyclophosphamide and cisplatin have different mechanisms of action, a small subset of genes had significant expression changes in both resistant tumor lines *(18)*. Independently, Brandes et al. *(19)* performed expression analysis of stress-treated EMT-6 cells using the Affymetrix GeneChip. The data showed that hypoxia resulted in enhanced expression of transforming growth factor-β (TGF-β) and decreased expression of the platelet-derived growth factor receptor PDGFRα and the mitogen-activated protein kinase (MAPK) MEK1.

Western blot analysis confirmed that TGF-β protein levels were enhanced and PDGFRα levels were diminished by hypoxic stress. Total MEK1 protein levels did not change with hypoxic stress; however, Western blot analysis with an antibody selective for phosphorylated MEK showed that hypoxia resulted in reduced levels of phosphorylated MEK protein. In vitro studies showed that treatment with TGF-β or the MEK inhibitor U0126 was sufficient to cause resistance to etoposide in both EMT-6 and MDA-MB231 cells *(19)*. These results provided evidence for TGF-β upregulation and PDGFRα/MAPK signaling pathway downregulation in the development of stress-induced tumor drug resistance *(19)*.

4. COMBINATION METHODS

In the study of multimodality therapy or combined chemotherapy, it is of interest to determine whether the combined effects of two agents are additive or whether their combination is substantially different than the sum of their parts *(20,21)*. Although controversy and discussion continue and new methodologies are being developed, two methods for the determination of synergy/additivity have emerged over the past 10 yr as the main functional systems for the experimentalist and investigator in cancer. These are the median effect/combination index method and the isobologram method *(22,33)*. This chapter discusses these methods and provide examples but does not delve into the mathematical derivations associated with each. Both methods have been widely applied. One or the other method may be more applicable to the drug interaction being studied; often this can not be determined until after the experiment is done. Unfortunately, the method for determination of synergy/additivity must be selected before the experiment is performed since each method requires attention to experimental design. Some investigators have applied both the median effect/combination index and the isobologram analyses to their work.

The median-effect and combination index method for the determination of additivity/synergy in experiments involving two-agent combinations in cancer research has been popularized by the work of Chou and Talalay *(22–26)*, who not only described this approach to the assessment of additivity to the cancer research community but also provided a user-friendly computer program for analyzing data by this method *(27–31)*. The median-effect principle was obtained from the derivation of enzyme reaction rate equations and concentration or dose-effect relationship equations. The median-effect equation can be used to describe many biological systems such as Michaelis-Menton and Hill enzyme kinetic relationships, the Langmuir physical adsorption isotherm, the Henderson-Hasselbach pH ionization relationship, the Scatchard equilibrium binding equation, and the many compound-receptor interactions *(22)*.

Chou and Talalay *(23,25)* derived equations to describe two compound situations. For two compounds having similar modes of action in which the effects of both compounds are mutually exclusive (i.e., parallel median effect plots for parent compounds and their mixtures) and for two compounds in which the effects are mutually nonexclusive (i.e., two compounds having different modes of action or acting independently). From this analysis the combination index (CI) for quantifying synergism (greater-than-additive), summation (additive) and antagonism (less-than-additive) effects can be derived for mutually exclusive compounds and for mutually nonexclusive compounds *(24,25)*. CI values that are smaller than 1 indicate synergism (greater-than-additive) effect of the two agents, a combination index equal to 1 indicates summation (additivity) of the two agents, and a combination index value greater than 1 indicates antagonism (less-than-additive) effect of the two agents.

Although the median effect analysis has been the subject of some controversy, as have other methods for assessment of additivity/synergy such as the isobologram method, it has gained widespread use since it can be readily applied to many laboratory systems. Application of the median effect/combination index method requires that the two agents being tested be combined in a constant ratio of doses or concentrations *(30)*. The level of synergy/antagonism at various concentration or dose ratios for the two agents can be determined from the CI calculation. The same can be done for different effect levels.

Gemcitabine (LY18801; 2',2'-difluorodeoxycytidine) is an analog of the natural pyrimidine *(34–36)*. In cell culture, gemcitabine causes accumulation of cells in the S phase of the cell cycle *(34,37,38)*. Gemcitabine is active against a number of solid tumor cells in vitro and has demonstrated activity against many solid tumor models including the CX-1 human colon cancer xenograft and the LX-1 human lung carcinoma xenograft in nude mice *(36–39)*. In phase II human trials, gemcitabine demonstrated activity against small cell lung, nonsmall-cell lung, breast, ovarian, pancreatic, myeloma, prostatic, renal, and bladder cancer *(40,41)*. Mitomycin C is the prototype bioreductive alkylating agent *(42–48)*. Combinations of gemcitabine and mitomycin C in various concentration ratios representing various levels of cytotoxicity were analyzed using a standard clonogenic assay according to the median effect method *(25)*. The interaction of the two chemotherapeutic agents was quantified assuming a mutually nonexclusive interaction in calculating the CI. Aung et al. *(49)* found that a marked synergism (CI = 0.5–0.7) was produced by concurrent exposure to gemcitabine and mitomycin C. In contrast, sequential exposure led to additivity.

Gemcitabine and cisplatin have different and potentially complementary mechanisms of action and thus are attractive candidates for drug combinations. Cisplatin is among the most widely used anticancer drugs, with a broad spectrum of activity *(50–53)*. Studies have shown a schedule-dependent interaction between gemcitabine and cisplatin ranging from antagonism to synergy *(54–58)*. In anaplastic thyroid carcinoma cell lines, Voigt et al. *(59)* found that the combination of gemcitabine and cisplatin produced additive cytotoxicity when gemcitabine exposure preceded cisplatin exposure (CI = 1.0) and antagonism when cisplatin exposure preceded gemcitabine exposure (CI > 1.0). Van Moorsel et al. *(60)* examined interactions between gemcitabine and cisplatin in human ovarian and nonsmall-cell lung cancer cell lines exposed to the combination for 4, 24, and 72 h, and synergy/additivity was assessed using median-effect analysis and calculating a CI. With cisplatin at an inhibitory concentration of 25% (IC_{25}) the average CIs calculated for the combination at IC_{50}, IC_{75}, IC_{90}, and IC_{95} after 4, 24, and 72 h of exposure were < 1.0, indicating synergism. With gemcitabine at IC_{25}, the CIs for the combinations with cisplatin after 24 h were < 1.0 in each cell line, except for the H322 nonsmall-cell lung cancer cell line, which showed an additive effect. At 72 h of exposure, all the CIs were < 1.0.

Irinotecan (7-ethyl-10-[4-{1-piperidino}-1-piperidino]carbonyloxycamptothecin; CPT-11) is a water-soluble camptothecin analog with a broad spectrum of antitumor activity including activity against multidrug-resistant tumors (61–65). Bahadori et al. (66) applied both isobologram analysis and median effect analysis to growth-inhibitory combinations of gemcitabine and irinotecan in human MCF-7 breast carcinoma cells and human SCOG small-cell lung carcinoma cells. By isobologram analysis, the growth inhibition of the combination of gemcitabine and irinotecan exhibited synergy over a wide concentration range (gemcitabine: 0.1–3.0 μM; irinotecan: 5–60 μM). By median effect/combination index analysis (concentration ratio 1:1), the growth inhibition produced by gemcitabine and irinotecan was synergistic at lower concentrations (<0.1 μM) of the compounds in MCF-7 cells but in SCOG cells synergy was achieved at concentrations greater than 1 μM (1–10 μM).

Etoposide (VP-16), a widely used anticancer drug, inhibits the nuclear enzyme topoisomerase II, forming a cleavage complex with the protein and DNA and resulting in double-strand breaks in the DNA (67–69). The interaction between gemcitabine and etoposide was examined by van Moorsel et al. (70) using median effect analysis with either a fixed molar ratio of the compounds or with a variable compound ratio. In the Lewis lung murine carcinoma cell line, the combination of gemcitabine and etoposide at a constant molar ratio (gemcitabine/etoposide = 1:4 or 1:0.125 after 4 or 24 h of exposure, respectively) was synergistic (CI calculated at 50% cell growth inhibition = 0.7 and 0.8, respectively). When cells were exposed to a combination of gemcitabine and etoposide for 24 or 72 h, with etoposide at its IC_{25} and gemcitabine over a concentration range, additivity was found in both the Lewis lung cells and the H322 cells; synergism was observed in the A2780 cells and the ADDP cells. Schedule dependency was found in the Lewis lung cancer cells such that when cells were exposed to gemcitabine 4 h prior to etoposide (constant molar ratio, total exposure time 24 h) synergism was found (CI = 0.5); however, additivity was seen when cells were exposed to etoposide prior to gemcitabine (CI = 1.6).

Paclitaxel, one of the most widely used anticancer agents, is an antimicrotubule agent (71–76). Working in the human T24 bladder cancer cell line, Cos et al. (77) found that for the drug combination of paclitaxel and methotrexate, if cells were exposed to paclitaxel for 24 h and then to methotrexate for 24 h or if cells were exposed to methotrexate for 24 h and then to paclitaxel for 24 h, the cytotoxicity was found to be synergistic by the CI method. A study from McDaid and Johnston (78) explored the interaction between 8-Cl-cAMP (8-chloro-adenosine 3',5'-monophosphate), a cAMP analog, and paclitaxel. The 8-Cl-cAMP/paclitaxel fixed molar ratios were 6.25:1 for A2780 cells and 3448:1 for OAW42 cells. Simultaneous exposure of either cell line to 8-Cl-cAMP and paclitaxel resulted in a high level of synergism, with CIs between 0.18 and 0.62 for A2780 cells and between 0.001 and 0.18 for OAW42 cells.

The combination of paclitaxel and etoposide was examined in three human tumor cell lines, A549 nonsmall-cell lung carcinoma, and MDA-231 and MCF-7 breast carcinoma (79). The single-agent IC_{50} values for each compound in each cell line were used to design the ratios for the combination treatment regimens. The data were analyzed using the median-effect/CI method. The simultaneous exposure results were less-than-additive cytotoxicity in two of the three cell lines. The sequential regimens and the sequential regimen with the intervening 24-h period resulted in synergistic cytotoxicity when either paclitaxel or etoposide exposure occurred first.

Vinblastine, an anticancer vinca alkaloid compound, like paclitaxel, is described as an antitubulin agent but, unlike paclitaxel, vinblastine inhibits tubulin polymerization *(80,81)*. Giannakakou et al. *(82)* maintained a constant concentration ratio of 1:1 for a study of the combination of paclitaxel and vinblastine in human KB epidermoid carcinoma cells and human MCF-7 breast carcinoma cells. Cytotoxicity studies carried out using the median effect method and the CI analysis showed synergism when vinblastine and paclitaxel exposure occurred sequentially and antagonism for simultaneous exposure.

The isobologram method is a generally valid procedure for analyzing interactions between agents irrespective of their mechanisms of action or the nature of their mechanisms of action or the nature of their concentration- or dose-response relations *(32)*. As with the median-effect method, three possible conclusions can be drawn from the isobologram analyses, they are that the agents have zero interaction (additivity), that the agents exhibit synergy (greater-than-additivity), or that the agents exhibit antagonism (less-than-additivity). The isobologram method requires that if a combination is represented by a point and if the axes on the graph represent the two agents in the combination, then the point lies on a straight line connecting the points where each of the two agents is present in zero concentration if the agents are non-interactive *(32)*. In many situations in cancer research, either the response to an agent or its logarithm is linear with the logarithm of the concentration or dose of the agent *(83–90)*.

Several attempts have been made to simplify or modify the isobologram approach to provide for efficient experimental designs and observation over a wide range of effects. Tallarida et al. *(91)* presented a method employing a design in which the dose- or concentration-effect relation for each agent was used to generate theoretical composite additive total dose combinations in fixed agent proportions. This composite additive dose-effect relation is then compared with the data from the actual agent combination in the same proportion. Another simplified conceptual foundation for this form of analysis was developed and popularized by Steel and Peckman *(92)*, based on the construction of an envelope of additivity in an isoeffect plot (isobologram). This approach provides a rigorous basis for defining regions of additivity, supra-additivity, and subadditivity and protection. This method of analysis is based on a clear conceptual formulation of the way that drugs or agents can be expected to show additivity. The first form of additivity is more conceptually simple and is defined as Mode 1 by Steel and Peckham *(92)*. For a selected level of effect (survival in this case) on a log scale, the dose of Agent A to produce this effect for the survival curve is determined. A lower dose of Agent A is then selected, the difference in effect from the isoeffect level is determined, and the dose of Agent B needed to make up this difference is derived from the survival curve for Agent B. For example, 3 mg of Agent A may be needed to produce 0.1% survival (3 logs of kill), the selected isoeffect. A dose of 2.5 mg of Agent A produces 1.0% survival (2 logs of kill). The Mode I isoeffect point for Agent B would thus be the level of Agent B needed to produce 1 log of kill, to result in the same overall effect of 3 logs of kill. In this instance, we might find that 4 mg of Agent B are needed to produce 1 log of kill.

Mode II additivity is conceptually more complex but corresponds to the notions of additivity and synergy discussed in detail by Berenbaum *(32,33)*. For any given level of effect, the dose or concentration of Agent A needed to produce this effect is determined from the survival relationship. The isoeffect dose or concentration of Agent B is calculated as the amount of Agent B needed to produce this effect, determined from the survival relationship. The isoeffect dose or concentration of Agent B is calculated as the amount of Agent B needed to produce the given effect starting at the level of effect produced by Agent A. For example, 3 mg of Agent A may be needed to produced 0.1% survival (3 logs of kill). A dose of 2.5 mg of Agent A produces 1.0% (2 logs of kill). A dose of 6 mg of Agent B is needed to produce 3 logs of kill, and 2 logs of kill are obtained with Agent B at 5 mg. Thus, the Mode II isoeffect point with Agent A at 2.5 mg is equal to the amount of Agent B needed to take Agent B from 2 logs of kill to 3 logs of kill (6 mg – 5 mg = 1 mg). This can be conceptualized by noting that Agent A should produce 2 logs of kill and is, in this case, equal to 5 mg of Agent B. If Agent A + Agent B are identical in their mode of action, then 1 mg more of Agent B should then be equivalent in effect to 6 mg of Agent B. Graphically, on a linear dose scale, Mode II additivity is defined as the straight line connecting the effective dose or concentration of Agent A alone and the effective dose or concentration of Agent B alone. Overall, combinations that produce the desired effect that are within the boundaries of Mode I and Mode II are considered additive. Those displaced to the left are greater-than-additive and those displaced to the right are less-than-additive. Combinations that produce effect outside the rectangle defined by the intersections of A_e and B_e are protective.

This type of classical isobologram methodology is cumbersome to use experimentally as each combination must be carefully titrated to produce a constant level of effect. Dewey et al. *(93)* described an analogous form of analysis for the special case in which the dose of one agent was held constant. Using full survival curves of each agent alone, this method produces envelopes of additive effect for different levels of the variable agent. It is conceptually identical to generating a series of isoeffect curves and then plotting the survivals from a series of these at constant dose of Agent A on a log effect by dose of Agent B coordinate system *(94)*. This approach can often be applied to the experimental situation in a more direct and efficient manner, and isobolograms can be derived describing the expected effect (Mode I and Mode II) for any level of the variable agent and constant agent combinations.

It has been recognized that the schedule and sequence of drugs in combination can affect therapeutic outcome. Over the last 15 yr the definition of additivity and therapeutic synergism has evolved with increasing stringency. In the work by Schabel et al. *(95–100)*, Corbett et al. *(101,102)*, and Griswold et al. *(103,104)*, therapeutic synergism between two drugs was defined to mean that "the effect of the two drugs in combination was significantly greater than that which could be obtained when either drug was used alone under identical conditions of treatment." Using this definition, the combination of cyclophosphamide and melphalan administered simultaneously by intraperitoneal injection every 2 wk was reported to be therapeutically synergistic in the Ridgeway osteosarcoma growth delay assay *(95–99)*. Similarly, the combination of cyclophosphamide and melphalan has been reported to be therapeutically synergistic in L1210 and P388 leukemias *(100)*. Cyclophosphamide plus a nitrosourea (BCNU, CCNU, or MeCCNU) have also been reported to be therapeutically synergistic in increase-in-life span and growth-delay assays using this definition *(100)*.

In the EMT-6 murine mammary carcinoma in vivo, the maximum tolerated combination therapy of thiotepa (5 mg/kg × 6) and cyclophosphamide (100 mg/kg × 3) produced

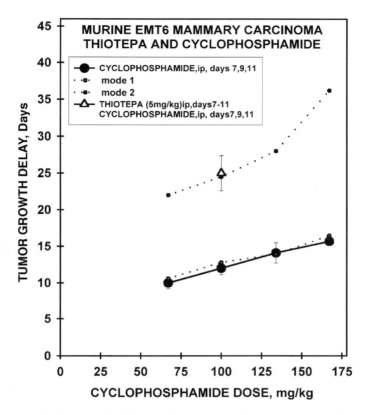

Fig. 3. Isobologram for the growth delay of the EMT6 murine mammary carcinoma treated with combinations of thiotepa and cyclophosphamide. Tumor treatments with cyclophosphamide alone. The dotted area represents the envelope of additivity for treatments with thiotepa and cyclophosphamide. Combination treatment of 5 mg/kg thiotepa x 6 plus 100 mg/kg cyclophosphamide x 3. Points represent three independent experiments (7 animals/group; 21 animals/point); bars represent the SEM. (Adapted from ref. *105.*)

about 25 d of tumor growth delay, which was not significantly different than expected for additivity of the individual drugs (Fig. 3) *(105–109)*. The survival of EMT-6 tumor cells after treatment of the animals with various single doses of thiotepa and cyclophosphamide was assayed. Tumor cell killing by thiotepa produced a very steep linear survival curve through 5 logs. The tumor cell survival curve for cyclophosphamide out to 500 mg/kg gave linear tumor cell kill through almost 4 logs. In all cases, the combination-treatment tumor cell survivals fell well within the envelope of additivity (Fig. 4). Both of these drugs are somewhat less toxic toward bone marrow cells by the GM-CFU in vitro assay method than to tumor cells. The combination treatments were subadditive or additive in bone marrow GM-CFU killing. When bone marrow is the dose-limiting tissue, there is a therapeutic advantage to the use of this drug combination *(105–109)*.

The Lewis lung carcinoma was among the earliest transplantable tumors used to identify new anticancer agents *(110–116)*. This syngeneic tumor system mimics the human disease in that from the primary tumor it metastasizes to lungs, bone, and liver. It is nonimmunogenic and is grown in a host with a fully functional immune system. The rate of tumor growth is relatively rapid, with a tumor volume doubling time of 2.5 d and

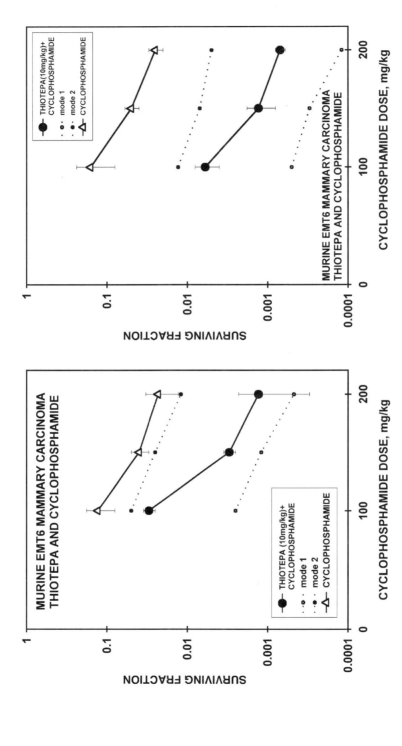

Fig. 4. Isobolograms for the combination treatment of the EMT6 tumor in vivo with 10 or 15 mg/kg thiotepa and various doses of cyclophosphamide. Survival curve for EMT6 tumors exposed to cyclophosphamide only. The dotted area represents the envelope of additivity for the combination treatment. Tumor cell survivals for the combination treatments. (Adapted from ref. *105*.)

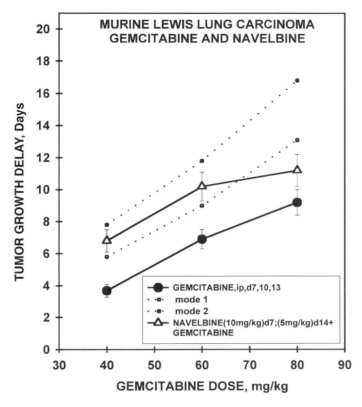

Fig. 5. Growth delay of the Lewis lung carcinoma produced by a range of doses of gemcitabine alone or along with navelbine (15 mg/kg total dose). The dotted area is the envelope of additivity determined by isobologram analysis. The bars are SEM.

it is lethal in 21–25 d. Although this growth rate is rapid, it is in line with the life span of the host, which is about 2 yr.

Vinorelbine (navelbine) is a new, semisynthetic vinca alkaloid whose antitumor activity is related to its ability to depolymerize microtubules that dissolve the mitotic spindles *(117–122)*. Phase II human trials employing weekly schedules of vinorelbine have demonstrated activity against small-cell lung cancer, nonsmall-cell lung cancer, and ovarian and breast cancer *(121–125)*. Gemcitabine was an active anticancer agent in animals bearing the Lewis lung carcinoma and was well tolerated by the animals over the dosage range from 40 mg/kg × 3 to 80 mg/kg × 3 (Fig. 5). Navelbine was administered in three different well-tolerated regimens with total doses of 10, 15, and 22.5 mg/kg. Both gemcitabine and navelbine produced increasing tumor growth delay with increasing dose of the drug. To assess the efficacy of the drug combination, the intermediate dosage regimen of navelbine was combined with each dosage level of gemcitabine. These combination regimens were tolerated, and the tumor growth delay increased with increasing dose of gemcitabine. Isobologram methodology *(20,21,32,33)* was used to determine whether the combinations of gemcitabine and navelbine achieved additive antitumor activity (Fig. 5). At gemcitabine doses of 40 and 60 mg/kg, the combination regimens achieved additivity, with the experimental tumor growth delay falling within the calculated envelope of additivity. At the highest dose of gemcitabine, the combination regimen produced less-than-additive tumor growth delay *(21)*.

The untreated control animals in this study had a mean number of 35 lung metastases on d 20. Gemcitabine was highly effective against disease metastatic to the lungs such that the mean number of lung metastases on d 20 was decreased to 1.0 to 1.5 or 3 to 4% of the number found in the untreated controls. Each of the navelbine regimens decreased the number of lung metastases on d 20 to 10 or 11 or to about 30% of the number found in the untreated control animals. The combination regimens were highly effective against Lewis lung carcinoma metastatic to the lungs, with a mean number of <1–0 metastases found on d 20. These results support the notion that gemcitabine and navelbine may be an effective anticancer drug combination against nonsmall-cell lung cancer *(21)*.

The human HCT116 colon carcinoma was selected for the initial study of ALIMTA in combination treatment because the HCT116 tumor is responsive to ALIMTA and because antitumor activity of ALIMTA has been observed in patients with colon cancer *(126–130)*. Treatment of nude mice bearing subcutaneously implanted HCT116 colon tumors with ALIMTA (100 mg/kg) twice daily for 5 d produced a tumor growth delay of 2.7 ± 0.3 d. Irinotecan administered daily for 5 d produced increasing tumor growth delay with increasing dose of the drug (Fig. 6) *(131)*. Treatment of HCT116 tumor-bearing animals with ALIMTA and irinotecan resulted in greater-than-additive tumor growth for the two drugs, reaching 27 d when the irinotecan dose was 30 mg/kg. No toxicity was observed when a full standard dose of ALIMTA was administered with a full standard dose of irinotecan.

Irinotecan (CPT-11) is a synthetic analog of the plant alkaloid camptothecin that exerts its antitumor activity through inhibition on the DNA unwinding enzyme topoisomerase I, resulting in a strand break in the DNA *(132,133)*. Cell culture studies have shown that combinations of raltitrexed and SN-38, the active metabolite of irinotecan, resulted in tumor cell killing *(134)*. The combination of ALIMTA and irinotecan, can result in synergistic antitumor effect against the human HCT116 colon carcinoma across all the doses of irinotecan examined. In general terms, this may reflect the fixing of the sublethal damage of one of the drugs by the other or may reflect enhancement of one of the drug targets by the other drug *(135)*. Exposure to irinotecan may increase the proportion of tumor cells in S phase, as has been shown on exposure of HL-60 cells to camptothecin in cell culture *(135)*, thus increasing the portion of tumor cells that are susceptible to the cytotoxic action of ALIMTA.

5. THE STEM-CELL SUPPORT MODEL

The search for malignant cell-selective therapeutics continues, but such agents are not currently available *(136–140)*. High-dose intensification regimens with stem-cell support by definition acknowledge that these highly cytoreductive regimens result in essentially lethal damage to hematological function necessitating rescue with autologous bone marrow cells, autologous peripheral blood progenitor cells, or a combination of these. The addition of the administration of hematopoietic growth factors along with reinfusion of hematopoietic stem cells has been shown to hasten hematological recovery in patients treated with high-dose intensification regimens *(141–145)*.

In 1986, Neta and Oppenheim *(146)* reported that administration of human recombinant interleukin-1 administered prior to total body radiation (950 Gy; 0.4 Gy/min) pro-

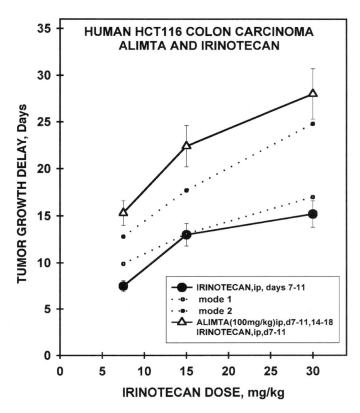

Fig. 6. Growth delay of human HCT116 colon carcinoma growth as a xenograft in nude mice after treatment with irinotecan (7.5, 15, or 30 mg/kg) intraperitoneally on d 7–11 after tumor cell implantation alone or along with ALIMTA (100 mg/kg) intraperitoneally on d 7–11 and d 14–18. The points are the mean values of two experiments with five animals per group per experiment; bars indicate the SEM. The dotted area represents the envelope of additivity by isobologram analysis. (Adapted from ref. *131*.)

tected mice from this lethal treatment. Later, Neta et al. *(147)* showed that human recombinant interleukin-1 and human recombinant tumor necrosis factor-α (TNF-α) protected lethally irradiated mice from death, whereas murine recombinant GM-CSF did not confer similar protection. Several studies have shown that pretreatment with human recombinant interleukin-1 can protect mice from lethal doses of several chemotherapeutic agents, including:

1. 5-Fluorouracil (150–400 mg/kg);
2. Cyclophosphamide (390 mg/kg);
3. Carboplatin (140–180 mg/kg);
4. Cisplatin (12–14 mg/kg);
5. Doxorubicin (12–16 mg/kg);
6. BCNU (50–70 mg/kg) *(148–152)*.

Interleukin-1 was not very effective as a protector against the lethality of high-dose cisplatin, was variably effective as a protector against the lethality of high-dose carboplatin, and was variably effective as a protector against the lethality of doxorubicin

(151,152). Naparstek et al. *(153)* found that continuous infusion of recombinant murine GM-CSF (1 μg/d in 3 mL 0.9% saline) by Harvard syringe pump for 4 d (d 3 through 6 post treatment) enhanced hematopoietic reconstitution of lethally irradiated (6 Gy; 70 cGy/min) Balb/c mice that received syngeneic bone marrow immediately after radiation treatment. The animals receiving stem-cell support also had improved survival (62 vs 30% on d 30) compared with those receiving no stem-cell support. Moore and Warren *(148)* found that human recombinant G-CSF (2 μg × 2/d for 14 d on d 1–14) enhanced recovery of neutrophils in mice treated with 5-fluorouracil (150 mg/kg on d 0).

The content of primitive and late stem cells in human peripheral blood, before or after mobilization, remains an area of investigation. Only limited work has been performed in the mouse. Molineux et al. *(154)* have determined that following administration of G-CSF, the blood of mice contains increased numbers on d 11 of spleen CFUs, and after transplantation into lethally irradiated mice can provide improved engraftment, survival, and recovery of long-term hematopoiesis compared with blood cells from unstimulated animals. This suggests that the numbers of both primitive stem cells and late progenitor cells increase in the blood after administration of G-CSF.

Neben et al. *(155)* further characterized the marrow and blood stem-cell compartments after treatment with cyclophosphamide *(156)*, G-CSF, and cyclophosphamide followed by G-CSF in a murine model. They demonstrated that the blood of unstimulated animals is deficient in primitive stem-cell content (cells capable of long-term hematopoietic repopulation) and that administration of cyclophosphmaide, G-CSF, and cyclophosphamide followed by G-CSF (cyclophosphamide + G-CSF) mobilizes both primitive and late hematopoietic stem cells from the marrow to the blood and spleen. With cyclophosphamide + G-CSF, there appears to be a true shift of hematopoietic stem cells from one compartment (marrow) to another (blood). Differences in the extent of mobilization also appeared to be dependent on prior exposure of the marrow to cytotoxic agents *(155,156)*. A protocol for the preparation of donor animals based primarily on the work of Neben et al. *(155)* is shown in Tables 1 and 2.

As preparation for a model for selection of agents appropriate for high-dose intensification stem-cell support regimens, the ability of G-CSF + mobilized peripheral blood to enhance hematopoietic recovery in female Balb/c mice after treatment with single high doses of several agents currently used in clinical high-dose regimens were tested. The animals, in groups of five, were monitored for weight loss, survival, and daily white blood cell and granulocyte counts over the first 2 wk post treatment (Figs. 7 and 8). The patterns of white cell and granulocyte depletion and recovery were similar to those observed in patients. Stem-cell support by G-CSF and peripheral blood cells was effective. For many treatments, there was severe rapid weight loss in the animals. In these groups, Lomotil® was added to the drinking water on d 1, and Gatorade was administered by gavage until recovery was apparent.

To validate the model system, several anticancer therapies currently used in the clinic at high doses were dose-escalated in the mouse and then compared with the dose escalation achievable with the same agent in the clinic. Literature values *(138,139)* for human conventional and bone marrow transplant or stem-cell support doses of each agent were used to calculate ratios of dose increase under stem-cell support conditions. Similar ratios were calculated for mice based on standard murine treatment regimens. It appears that in humans, dose ratio increases greater than those achieved in mice are possible. This

Table 1
Protocol for Preparation and Harvesting
of Donors for Collection of Peripheral Blood Stem Cells

Day	Procedure
0	Cyclophosphamide (200 mg/kg), ip
2–6	rhG-CSF (250 µg/kg)2x/d, sc
7	Heparin (50 U)iv → wait → 20–30 min →

Collect whole blood by cardiac puncture. Approx 1 mL/
mouse, then dilute into an equal volume of Hanks' balanced
salt solution → inject iv into recipients.

ABBREVIATIONS: rhG-CSR, recombinant human granulocyte
colony-stimulating factor.

Table 2
Recipients

Day	Procedure
0	Single dose test agent, ip, iv or TBI
0–5	Lomotil (1.5 mg/100 mL) in drinking water
1	1×10^7 peripheral blood cells iv
1–12	rhG-CSF (250 mg/kg) 2x/d, ip
1–as needed	Gatorade, po

Monitor Body weight, survival, and blood parameters (smear
from 1 animal/group d 1–14) count WBCs, granulocytes, and
lymphocytes

ABBREVIATIONS: rhG-CSF, recombinant human granulocyte colony-
stimulating factor; TBI, total body irradiation; WBCs, white blood cells.

difference may be owing to the somewhat more rapid changes in sensitive tissue damage
in mice and because supportive care in patients is better than that achieved in mice.

As an initial therapeutic high-dose study, the EMT-6/Parent tumor was implanted
subcutaneously in the hind leg of female Balb/c mice. Treatment was begun on d 7 when
the tumors were about 150 mm^3 in volume (Table 3). One group of animals was treated
with a standard cyclophosphamide regimen of 150 mg/kg, ip, on d 7, 9, and 11. Another
group received a single dose of cyclophosphamide of 450 mg/kg, ip, on d 7 and peripheral
blood stem cells (10^7) on d 8 as well as G-CSF on d 1–12 *(136,137)*. The standard
treatment regimen produced a tumor growth delay of 6.2 d, but no significant period of
tumor regression. The single high-dose regimen, on the other hand, resulted in a tumor
growth delay of 31.5 d and tumor regression duration of 9.5 d. Thus, a murine high-dose/
stem-cell support model has been developed that can be used to "discover" new drugs
suitable for stem-cell support regimens, by demonstrating dose escalation potential in the
presence of hematopoietic stem-cell infusion. This model system could also be very
useful in identifying potential protectors of sensitive normal tissues, such as the gut.

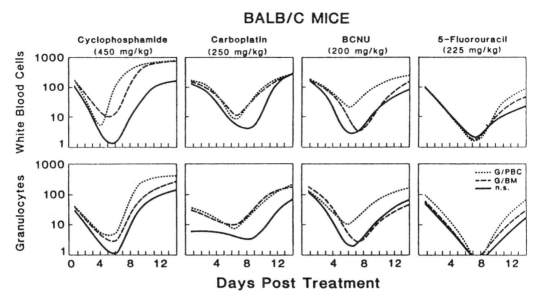

Fig. 7. Time-course of white blood cell and granulocyte depletion and recovery in female Balb/c mice treated with single doses of cyclophosphamide (450 mg/kg), carboplatin (300 mg/kg), BCNU (60 mg/kg), or 5-fluorouracil (200 mg/kg). The curves were derived from blood smears collected daily, stained with Giemsa, and counted manually (2 fields at 16×). n.s., no support; G/BM, granulocyte colony-stimulating factor (G-CSF; 2 µg/kg, ip, 2× daily on d 1–12) and bone marrow (10^7 cells, iv); G/PBC, G-CSF (2 µg/kg, ip, 2× daily on d 1–12) and peripheral blood (10^7 cells, iv).

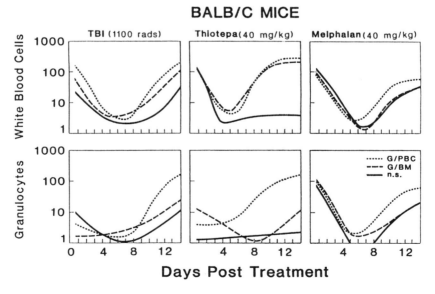

Fig. 8. Time-course of white blood cell and granulocyte depletion and recovery in female Balb/c mice treated with single doses of total body radiation (TBI; 650 rd), thiotepa (40 mg/kg), or melphalan (30 mg/kg). The curves were derived from blood smears collected daily, stained with Giemsa, and counted manually (2 fields at 16×). n.s., no support; G/BM, granulocyte colony-stimulating factor (G-CSF; 2 µg/kg, ip, 2× daily on d 1–12) and bone marrow (10^7 cells, iv); G/PBC, G-CSF (2 µg/kg, ip, 2× daily on d 1–12) and peripheral blood (10^7 cells, iv).

Table 3
Growth Delay of the EMT-6/Parent Tumor After Treatment
of Tumor-Bearing Animals With Cyclophosphamide to a Total Dose of 450 mg/kg

Treatment group	Tumor growth delay (d)	Regression duration (d)
Cyclophosphamide (150 mg/kg, d 7, 9, 11)	6.2 ± 0.5	< 1
Cyclophosphamide (450 mg/kg, d 7) stem cells	31.5 ± 2.8	9.5

6. SCHEDULING AND SEQUENCING OF HIGH-DOSE THERAPIES

As the knowledge of anticancer drug-drug and drug-target interactions has increased, as well as the realization that measurable drug resistance can be induced in tumor cells after, in some cases, only one exposure to the agent, the appreciation for the importance of drug scheduling both for individual agents and relative to other agents in a regimen has grown. In the development of maximally cytotoxic combinations of antitumor alkylating agents, pharmacokinetic and drug metabolism issues may be important. In previous studies (157–159), the two drug combinations of thiotepa or melphalan with cyclophosphamide were examined in 24 schedules administered over an 8-h period to the same total dose. Of these, six schedules resulted in greater-than-additive cell killing, and 15 schedules resulted in subadditve tumor cell killing. The generalizations that emerged from these studies were that dividing a total dose into fractions over an 8-h period resulted in less tumor cell killing and administering cyclophosphamide first in the sequence resulted in less tumor cell killing.

Three immediate sequences in which drugs were delivered as single injections were examined over a cyclophosphamide dose range (Fig. 9). Initial administration of cyclophosphamide followed 4 h later by either thiotepa or melphalan substantially negated the effect of the second drug, resulting in less-than-additive tumor cell killing over the dose range with both thiotepa and melphalan. Simulataneous administration of either cyclophosphamide and thiotepa or cyclophosphamide and melphalan produced essentially additive cell killing over the cyclophosphamide dose range examined. When either thiotepa or melphalan preceded the administration of cyclophosphamide, greater-than-additive tumor cell killing was observed over the cyclophosphamide dose range. With thiotepa, the degree of supra-additivity decreased with increasing cyclophosphamide dose, such that at the highest cyclophosphamide dose, there was no difference in tumor cell kill between the simultaneous drug schedule and the thiotepa $\rightarrow$ cyclophosphamide sequential schedule. The melphalan $\rightarrow$ cyclophosphamide sequential schedule resulted in a significant increase in more cell kill relative to that achieved with simultaneous drug administration; this increase persisted over the cyclophosphamide range tested.

Intensification regimens often employ antitumor alkylating agents, because bone marrow or peripheral blood stem-cell reinfusion has allowed previously lethal doses of these drugs to be administered to patients safely (160,161). Each of the antitumor alkylating agents, when administered to tumor-bearing animals, killed FSaIIC tumor cells in a log-linear manner with increasing dose of each drug. The tumor cell killing obtained when melphalan was administered first followed 3 d or 7 d later by a dose of cyclophosphamide is shown in Fig. 10.

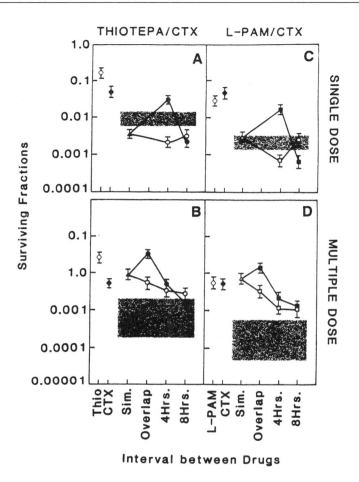

Fig. 9. Survival curves for EMT-6 tumor cells treated in vivo with various doses of cyclophosphamide (CTX) on different schedules. The symbols ◇ and ◆ represent the survival of EMT-6 tumors exposed to a single dose of thiotepa or cyclophosphamide, respectively. Survival after simultaneous exposure to single doses of cyclophosphamide and thiotepa or melphalan is shown as (●); cyclophosphamide followed 4 h later by thiotepa or melphalan is shown as (■); thiotepa or melphalan followed 4 h later by cyclophosphamide is shown as (○). Shaded areas indicate the envelopes of additivity determined by isobologram analysis of the survival curves for each drug combination. Data points represent the mean of three independent determinations; bars represent the SEM.

When a dose of 10 mg/kg of melphalan was followed 3 d later by various doses of cyclophosphamide, greater-than-additive tumor cell killing was obtained with 300 mg/kg of cyclophosphamide. If the interval between the drugs was extended to 7 d, the treatment combination resulted in subadditive-to-additive tumor cell killing. The FSaIIC fibrosarcoma is not very sensitive to the cytotoxicity of doxorubicin (Fig. 11). A dose of 10 mg/kg of doxorubicin kills 64% of the tumor cells (surviving fraction = 0.36). Administration of 10 mg/kg of doxorubicin 3 d prior to various doses of cyclophosphamide did not alter the tumor cell killing from that obtained with the antitumor alkylating agent alone.

In the design of sequential high-dose chemotherapy regimens, the selection of antitumor alkylating agents to be included in each intensification and the interval between the

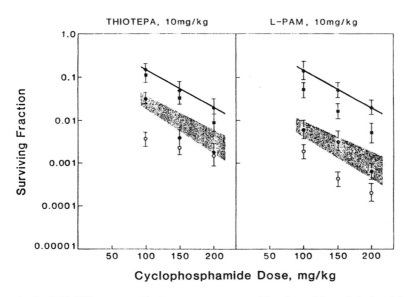

Fig. 10. Survival of FSaIIC tumor cells from tumors treated in vivo with melphalan 10 mg/kg (●) followed 3 d later (■) or 7 d later (○) by various doses of cyclophosphamide. The shaded areas are the envelopes of additivity by isobologram analysis. The second alkylating agent alone is shown as (□). Each experiment was repeated three times. Points are the means; bars are SEM.

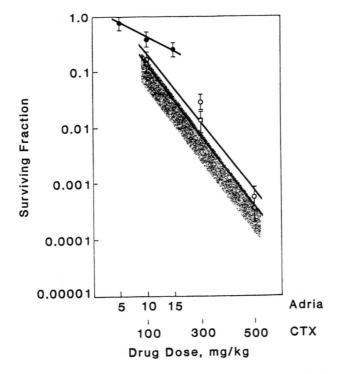

Fig. 11. Survival of FSaIIC tumor cells from tumors treated in vivo with doxorubicin (Adria) 10 mg/kg (●) followed 3 d later (○) by various doses of cyclophosphamide (CTX). The shaded areas are the envelopes of additivity by isobologram analysis. The alkylating agent alone is shown as (□). Each experiment was repeated three times. Points are the means; bars are SEM.

Table 4
Growth Delay of the EMT-6 Murine Mammary Carcinoma
After Two High-Dose Chemotherapy Treatments With Stem Cell Support

Treatment group	Tumor growth delay[a] (d)
Melphalan (30 mg/kg), d 5[b]	5.1 ± 0.4
Melphalan (30 mg/kg), d 5 → melphalan (30 mg/kg), d 12	7.2 ± 0.7
Melphalan (30 mg/kg), d 5 → cyclophosphamide (400 mg/kg), d 12	11.3 ± 1.4
Melphalan (30 mg/kg), d 5 → thiotepa (30 mg/kg), d 12	7.6 ± 0.5
Melphalan (30 mg/kg), d 5 → carboplatin (250 mg/kg, d 12	6.9 ± 0.8
Cyclophosphamide (400 mg/kg), d 5	19.6 ± 1.4
Cyclophosphamide (400 mg/kg), d 5 → melphalan (30 mg/kg), d 12	42.8 ± 2.3
Cyclophosphamide (400 mg/kg), d 5 → cyclophosphamide (400 mg/kg), d 12	46.4 ± 2.0
Cyclophosphamide (400 mg/kg), d 5 → thiotepa (30 mg/kg), d 12	29.8 ± 1.5
Cyclophosphamide (400 mg/kg), d 5 → carboplatin (250 mg/kg, d 12	30.8 ± 1.3

[a]Tumor growth delay is the difference in days for treated vs control tumors to reach 500 mm³. Control tumors reach 500 mm³ in 12.2 + 0.7 d after subcutaneous implantation.

[b]The tumor growth delays for the single-drug treatments were: melphalan (30 mg/kg), 5.1 ± 0.4 d; cyclophosphamide (400 mg/kg), 19.6 ± 1.4 d; thiotepa (30 mg/kg), 4.2 + 0.5 d; and carboplatin (250 mg/kg), 9.0 + 1.1 d.

intensifications are critical to the design of the therapy. The tumor cell survival assay and tumor growth delay assay using the murine EMT-6 mammary carcinoma were used as a solid tumor model in which to address these issues. Tumor-bearing mice were treated with high-dose melphalan or cyclophosphamide followed 7 or 12 d later by melphalan, cyclophosphamide, thiotepa, or carboplatin. After treatment with melphalan both 7 and 12 d later, the tumor was resistant to each of the four drugs studied. After treatment with cyclophosphamide both 7 and 12 d later, the tumor was resistant to melphalan and thiotepa but was not resistant to cyclophosphamide or carboplatin. To extend the interval between high-dose treatments to 14 and 21 d, after the first intensification the tumor was trans-ferred to second hosts that were either drug-treated or not drug treated. When high-dose melphalan-treated tumors were treated with a second high dose of melphalan, the tumors were very resistant with the 14-d interval and less resistant with the 21-d interval. This small effect was evident in the bone marrow colony-forming unit, GM-CFU, except in the hosts pretreated with melphalan. When high-dose cyclophosphamide-treated tumors were treated with a second high dose of cyclophosphamide, drug resistance was observed both with the 14-d and the 21-d intervals if the host was non-pretreated or was pretreated with melphalan, but not if the host was pretreated with cyclophosphamide. The same was true in the bone marrow GM-CFU.

Tumor growth delay studies supported these findings in that treatment with high-dose cyclophosphamide, melphalan, thiotepa, and carboplatin resulted in less-than-additive tumor growth delay, whereas treatment with high-dose cyclophosphamide prior to treat-ment with high-dose melphalan, cyclophosphamide, thiotepa, or carboplatin resulted in additivity to greater-than-additive tumor growth delay (Tables 4 and 5). High-dose com-bination regimens required dose reduction of the drugs, which resulted in decreased tumor growth delays. Allowing an interval between drug treatments produces a biologi-cally complex situation involving lysis and removal of dead cells as well as stasis or

Table 5
Growth Delay of the EMT-6 Mammary Carcinoma
and Dose Intensity After High-Dose Chemotherapy With Stem Cell Support

Treatment group	Dose intensity[a]	Tumor growth delay[b] (d)
Cyclophosphamide (400 mg/kg), d 7	1	19.2 ± 1.2
Thiotepa (30 mg/kg), d 7	1	4.2 ± 0.5
Carboplatin (250 mg/kg), d 7	1	9.0 ± 1.1
Cyclophosphamide (400 mg/kg) + thiotepa (30 mg/kg), d 7	2	6.3 ± 0.6 Toxic
Cyclophosphamide (400 mg/kg) + carboplatin (250 mg/kg), d 7	2	Toxic
Cyclophosphamide (225 mg/kg) + thiotepa (20 mg/kg), d 7	1.2	5.8 ± 0.4
Cyclophosphamide (225 mg/kg) + carboplatin (125 mg/kg), d 7	1.1	8.8 ± 0.7
Thiotepa (30 mg/kg), d 7 + carboplatin (225 mg/kg), d 7	2	5.0 ± 0.4
Thiotepa (20 mg/kg), d 7 + carboplatin (125 mg/kg), d 7	1.2	4.4 ± 0.4

[a]Dose intensity indicates the relative summation of the dose of each regimen in which the dose intensity of each single high-dose drug is equal to 1.
[b]Tumor growth delay is the difference in days for treated vs control tumors to reach 500 mm^3. Control tumors reach 500 mm^3 in 12.2 + 0.7 d after subcutaneous implantation.

proliferation of surviving cells. Survival may be facilitated by pre-existing biochemical factors conferring resistance or induction of biochemical changes conferring resistance. The current best solution may be to treat with the most effective agents early and to develop treatment sequences whereby overlapping anticancer mechanisms and/or overlapping resistance mechanisms do not occur.

7. CONCLUSIONS

Preclinical studies from the earliest murine leukemia model systems to the present range of syngeneic, xenograft, and transgenic leukemia, lymphoma, and solid tumor models have provided both cancer scientists and physicians with the awareness that tumor cure requires the eradication by exogenous treatments of nearly all tumor cells to be curative. High-dose chemotherapy regimens are based on the premise that undertreatment is the reason for failure to achieve cure in many cases. Exposures to cytotoxic therapy and especially to high-dose cytotoxic therapy produces major metabolic responses in the host and in the tumor (159). Some of these responses are acute and short-lived, but others may persist for weeks or longer. These metabolic changes, although not permanent genetic alterations, clearly affect the response of the host and the tumor to subsequent treatment. In the design of sequential and combination therapeutic treatment regimens, the response of the host and the tumor should be taken into account.

REFERENCES

1. Hill RP. Excision assays. In: Kallman RF, ed. *Rodent Tumor Models in Experimental Cancer Therapy.* New York: Pergamon. 1987:67–75.
2. Rockwell SC. Tumor-cell survival. In: Teicher BA, ed. *Tumor Models in Cancer Research.* Totowa, NJ: Humana. 2002:617–632.
3. Teicher BA. In vitro tumor response end points. In: Teicher BA, ed. *Tumor Models in Cancer Research.* Totowa, NJ: Humana. 2002:593–616.
4. Hewitt HB, Wilson CW. A survival curve for mammalian leukemia cells irradiated in vivo. *Br J Cancer* 1959; 13:69–75.
5. Rockwell SC, Kallman RF, Fajardo LF. Characteristics of serially transplanted mouse mammary tumor and its tissue-culture-adapted derivative. *J Natl Cancer Inst* 1972; 49:735–747.
6. Courtenay VD. A soft agar colony assay for Lewis lung tumor and B16 melanoma taken directly from the mouse. *Br J Cancer* 1976; 34:39–45.
7. Hill RP. An appraisal of in vivo assays of excised tumors. *Br J Cancer* 1980; 41(suppl IV):230–239, 1980.
8. Courtenay VD, Smith IE, Peckham MJ, Steel GG. In vitro and in vivo radiosensitivity of human tumor cells obtained from a pancreatic carcinoma xenograft. *Nature* 1976; 263:771–772.
9. Jung H. Radiation effects on tumors. In: Broerse JJ, Barendsen GW, Kal HB, van der Kogel AJ, eds. *Radiation Research.* Amsterdam: M. Nijhoff. 1983:427–434.
10. Kelley SD, Kallman RF, Rapacchietta D, Franko AJ. The effect of x-irradiation on cell loss in five solid murine tumors, as determined by the 125IudR method. *Cell Tissue Kinetics* 1981; 14:611–624.
11. Twentyman PR, Brown JM, Gray JW, Franko AJ, Scoles MA, Kallman RF. A new mouse tumor model (RIF-1) for a comparison of endpoint studies. *J Natl Cancer Inst* 1980; 64:595–604.
12. Teicher BA, Rose CM. Perfluorochemical emulsions can increase tumor radiosensitivity. *Science* 1984; 223:934–936.
13. Teicher BA, Herman TS, Holden SA, et al. Tumor resistance to alkylating agents conferred by mechanisms operative only in vivo. *Science* 1990; 247:1457–1461.
14. Teicher BA, Chatterjee D, Liu J-T, Holden SA, Ara G. Protection of bone marrow CFU-GM in mice-bearing in vivo alkylating agent resistant murine EMT-6 tumors. *Cancer Chemother Pharmacol* 1993; 32:315–319.
15. Chatterjee D, Liu CT-T, Northey D, Teicher BA. Molecular characterization of the in vivo alkylating agent resistant murine EMT-6 mammary carcinoma tumors. *Cancer Chemother Pharmacol* 1995; 35:423–431.
16. Holden SA, Emi Y, Kakeji Y, Northey D, Teicher BA. Host distribution and response to antitumor alkylating agents of EMT-6 tumor cells from subcutaneous tumor implants. *Cancer Chemother Pharmacol* 1997; 40:87–93.
17. Veroski V, De Ridder M, Van Den Berge D, Monsaert C, Wauters N, Storme G. Inhibition of NF-kappaB may impair tumor cell radioresponse: a possible complication for proteasome-targeting strategies. *Proc Am Assoc Cancer Res* 2002; 43:abstr 3217.
18. Perry WL, Jin S, Menon KE, Dantzig AH, Teicher BA. Microarray analysis of EMT-6 murine mammary tumors and sublines selected for drug resistance in vivo. *Proc Am Assoc Cancer Res* 2002; 43:abstr 5461.
19. Brandes LM, Hadjisavva IS, Peterson K, Patierno SR, Stephan DA, Kennedy KA. Expression analysis reveals a role for TGF-β and the PDGFR/MAPK signaling pathway in the development of both chemical- and physiologic-induced drug resistance of breast cancer cells. *Proc Am Assoc Cancer Res* 2002; 43:abstr 5371.
20. Teicher BA, Herman TS, Holden SA, Eder JP. Chemotherapeutic potentiation through interaction at the level of DNA. In: Chou T-C, Rideout DC, eds. *Synergism and Antagonism in Chemotherapy.* Orlando, FL: Academic. 1991:541–583.
21. Teicher BA and Frei E III. Laboratory models to evaluate new agents for the systemic treatment of lung cancer. In: Skarin AT, ed. *Multimodality Treatment of Lung Cancer.* New York: Marcel Dekker. 2000:301–336.
22. Chou TC, Talalay P. A simple generalized equation for the analysis of multiple inhibitions of Michaelis-Menten kinetic systems. *J Biol Chem* 1977; 252:6438–6442.
23. Chou TC, Talalay P. Generalized equations for the analysis of inhibitors of Michaelis-Menten and higher order kinetic systems with two or more mutually exclusive and nonexclusive inhibitors. *Eur J Biochem* 1981; 115:207–216.

24. Chou TC, Talalay P. Analysis of combined drug effects: A new look at a very old problem. *Trends Pharmacol Sci* 1983; 4:450–454.
25. Chou TC, Talalay P. Quantitative analysis of dose-effect relationships: the combined effects of multiple drugs or enzyme inhibitors. *Adv Enzyme Regul* 1984; 22:27–55.
26. Chou TC, Talalay P. Application of the median-effect principle for the assessment of low-dose risk of carcinogens and for the quantitation of synergism and antagonism of chemotherapeutic agents. In: Harrap K, Connors TA, eds. *New Avenues in Developmental Cancer Chemotherapy*. Bristol-Myers Symp 8. Orlando, FL: Academic. 1987:37–64.
27. Chou J, Chou TC. Dose-effect analysis with microcomputers: quantitation of ED_{50}, ID_{50}, synergism, antagonism, low-risk receptor ligand binding and enzyme kinetics. Software for Apple II microcomputers. Cambridge, England: Elsevier-Biosoft. 1985.
28. Chou J, Chou TC. Dose-effect analysis with microcomputers: Quantitiation of ED_{50}, ID_{50}, synergism, antagonism, low-risk receptor ligand binding and enzyme kinetics. Software for IBM-PC microcomputers. Cambridge, England: Elsevier-Biosoft. 1987.
29. Chou J, Chou TC. Computerized simulation of dose reduction index (DRI) in synergistic drug combinations. Pharmacologist 30: A231, 1988.
30. Chou T-C. The median-effect principle and the combination index for quantiation of synergism and antagonism. In: Chou T-C, Rideout DC, eds. *Synergism and Antagonism in Chemotherapy*. Orlando, FL: Academic. 1991:61–102.
31. Chou JH. Quantitation of synergism and antagonism of two or more drugs by computerized analysis. In: Chou T-C, Rideout DC, eds. *Synergism and Antagonism in Chemotherapy*. Orlando, FL: Academic. 1991: 223–241.
32. Berenbaum MC. What is synergy? *Pharmacol Rev* 1989; 41:93–141.
33. Berenbaum MC. Synergy, additivism and antagonism in immunosupression. *Clin Exp Immunol* 1977; 28: 1–18.
34. Gemcitabine HCl (LY188011 HCl) clinical investigational brochure. Indianapolis, IN: Eli Lilly. October, 1993.
35. Huang P, Chubb S, Hertel L, Plunkett W. Mechanism of action of 2',2'-difluorodeoxycytidine. triphosphate on DNA synthesis (abstr 2530). *Proc Am Assoc Cancer Res* 1990; 31:426.
36. Hertel L, Boder G, Kroin J. Evaluation of the antitumor activity of gemcitabine 2',2'-difluoro-2'-deoxycytidine. *Cancer Res* 1990; 50:4417–4422.
37. Bouffard D, Fomparlwer L, Momparler R. Comparison of the antineoplastic activity of 2',2'-difluorodeoxycytidine and cytosine arabinoside against human myeloid and lymphoid leukemia cells. *Anticancer Drugs* 1991; 2:49–55.
38. Heinemann V, Hertel L, Grindey G, Plunkett W. Comparison of the cellular pharmacokinetics and toxicity of 2',2'-difluorodeoxycytidine and 1-beta-D-arabinofuranosyl cytosine. *Cancer Res* 1988; 48:4024–4031.
39. Eckhardt I, Von Hoff D. New drugs in clinical development in the United States. *Hematol Oncol Clin North Am* 1994; 8: 300–332.
40. Anderson H, Lund B, Bach F, Thatcher N, Walling J, Hansen HH. Single-agent activity of weekly gemcitabine in advanced non-small cell lung cancer: a Phase 2 study. *J Clin Oncol* 1994; 12:1821–1826.
41. Gatzemeier U, Shapard F, LeChevalier T, et al. Activity of gemcitabine in patients with non-small cell lung cancer: a multicentre, extended phase II study. *Eur J Cancer* 1996; 32A:243–248.
42. Veweij J, Sparreboom A, Nooter K. Mitomycins. *Cancer Chemother Biol Response Mod* 1999; 18:46–58.
43. Yang XL, Wang AH. Structural studies of atom-specific anticancer drugs acting on DNA. *Pharmacol Ther* 1999; 83:181–215.
44. Spanswick VJ, Cummings J, Smyth JF. Current issues in the enzymology of mitomycin C metabolic activation. *Gen Pharmacol* 1998; 31:539–544.
45. Cummings J, Spanswick VJ, Tomasz M, Smyth JF. Enzymology of mitomycin C metabolic activation in tumor tissue: implications for enzyme-directed bioreductive drug development. *Biochem Pharm* 1998; 56:405–414.
46. Tomasz M, Palom Y. The mitomycin bioreductive antitumor agents: cross-linking and alkylation of DNA as the molecular basis of their activity. *Pharm Ther* 1997; 76:73–87.
47. Boyer MJ. Bioreductive agents: a clinical update. *Oncol Res* 1997; 9:391–395.
48. van Moorse CJ, Veerman G, Bergman AM, et al. Combination chemotherapy studies with gemcitabine. *Semin Oncol* 1997; 24(suppl 7):17–23.
49. Aung TT, Davis MA, Ensminger WD, Lawrence TS. Interaction between gemcitabine and mitomycin C in vitro. *Cancer Chemother Pharmacol* 2000; 45:38–42.

50. Highley MS, Calvert AH. Clinical experience with cisplatin and carboplatin. In: Kelland LR and Farrell NP, eds. *Platinum-Based Drugs in Cancer Therapy.* Totowa, NJ: Humana. 2000:171–194.

51. Perez RP, Cellular and molecular determinants of cisplatin resistance. *Eur J Cancer* 1998; 34: 1535–1542.

52. Eastman A. The formation, isolation and characterization of DNA adducts produced by anticancer platinum complexes. *Pharmacol Ther* 1987; 34:155–166.

53. Fink DZH, Nebel S, Norris S, et al. In vitro and in vivo resistance to cisplatin in cell that have lost DNA mismatch repair. *Cancer Res* 1997; 57:1841–1845.

54. van Moorsel CJ, Veerman G, Bergman AM, et al. Combination chemotherapy studies with gemcitabine. *Semin Oncol* 1997; 24:S717–S723.

55. Peters GJ, Ruiz van Haperen VW, Bergman AM, et al. Preclinical combination therapy with gemcitabine and mechanisms of resistance. *Semin Oncol* 1996; 23:16–24.

56. Braakhuis BJ, Ruiz van Haperen VW, Welters MJ, Peters GJ. Schedule-dependent therapeutic efficacy of the combination of gemcitabine and cisplatin in head and neck cancer xenografts. *Eur J Cancer* 1995; 31:2335–2340.

57. Bergman AM, Ruiz van Haperen VW, Veerman G, Kuiper CM, Peters GJ. Synergistic interaction between cisplatin and gemcitabine in vitro. *Clin Cancer Res* 1996; 2:521–530.

58. Tsai CM, Chang KT, Chen JY, Chen YM, Chen MH, Perng RP. Cytotoxic effects of gemcitabine-containing regimens against human non-small cell lung cancer cell lines which express different levels of p185neu. *Cancer Res* 1996; 56:794–801.

59. Voigt W, Bulankin AQ, Muller T, Schoeber C, Grothey A, Hoang-Vu C, Schmoll H-J. Schedule-dependent antagonism of gemcitabine and cisplatin in human anaplastic thyroid cancer cell lines. *Clin Cancer Res* 2000; 6:2087–2093.

60. Van Moorsel CJA, Pinedo HM, Veerman G, et al. Mechanisms of synergism between cisplatin and gemcitabine in ovarian and non-small cell lung cancer cell lines. *Br J Cancer* 1999; 80:981–990.

61. Kunimoto T, Nitta K, Tanaka T, et al. Antitumor activity of 7-ethyl-10-[4-(1-piperidino)-1-piperidino]-carbonyloxy-camptothecin, a novel water soluble derivative of camptothecin, against murine tumors. *Cancer Res* 1987; 47:5944–5947.

62. Kawato Y, Aonuma M, Hirota Y, Kuga H, Sato K. Intracellular roles of SN-38, a metabolite of the camptothecin derivative CPT-11, in the antitumor effect of CPT-11. *Cancer Res* 1991; 51:4187–4191.

63. Shimada Y, Rothenberg ML, Hilsenbeck SG, Burris HA, Degen D, Von Hoff DD. Activity of CPT-11 (irinotecan hydrochloride), a topoisomerase I inhibitor, against human tumor colony-forming units. *Anticancer Drugs* 1994; 5:202–206.

64. Kawato Y, Furuta T, Aonuma M, Yasuoka T, Matsumotot K. Antitumor activity of a camptothecin derivative, CPT-11, against human tumor xenografts in nude mice. *Cancer Chemother Pharmacol* 1991; 28:192–198.

65. Tsuruo T, Matsuzaki T, Matsushita M, Saito H, Yokokura T. Antitumor effect of CPT-11, a new derivative of camptothecin, against pleiotropic drug-resistant tumors in vitro and in vivo. *Cancer Chemother Pharmacol* 1988; 21:71–74.

66. Bahadori HR, Lima CMSR, Green MR, Safa AR. Synergistic effect of gemcitabine and irinotecan (CPT-11) on breast and small cell lung cancer cell lines. *Anticancer Res* 1999; 19:5423–5428.

67. Robinson MI, Osheroff N. Stabilization of the toposiomerase II-DNA cleavage complex by antineoplastic drugs: inhibition of enzyme-mediated DNA religation by 4'-(9-acridinylamino)methane-sulfon-m-anisidide. *Biochemistry* 1990; 29:2511–2515.

68. Dombernosky P, Nissen I. Combination chemotherapy with 4'-demethyl-epipodophyllotoxin 9-(4,6-O-ethylidene-β-D-glucopyranoside) VP-16-213 (NCS 141540) in L1210 leukemia. *Eur J Cancer* 1976; 12:181–188.

69. Pommier Y. DNA topoisomerase II inhibitors. In: Teicher BA, ed. *Cancer Therapeutics: Experimental and Clinical Aspects.* Totowa, NJ: Humana. 1997:153–174.

70. van Moorsel CJA, Pinedo HM, Veerman G, et al. Combination chemotherapy studies with gemcitabine and etoposide in non-small cell lung and ovarian cancer cell lines. *Biochem Pharmacol* 1999; 57: 407–415.

71. Rowinsky EK, Donehower RC. Paclitaxel (Taxol). *N Engl J Med* 1995; 332:1004–1014.

72. Hortobagyi GN, Holmes FA, Ibrahim N, Champlin R, Buzdar AU. The University of Texas M. D. Anderson Cancer Center experience with paclitaxel in breast cancer. *Semin Oncol* 1997; 1(suppl 3): S30–S33.

73. McGuire WP, Ozols RF. Chemotherapy of advanced ovarian cancer. *Semin Oncol* 1998; 3:340–348.

74. Schiff PB, Fant J, Horwitz SB. Promotion of microtubule assembly in vitro by paclitaxel. *Nature* 1979; 277:665–667.
75. Schiff PB, Horwtiz S. Paclitaxel stabilizes microtubules in mouse fibroblast cells. *Proc Natl Acad Sci USA* 1980; 77:1561–1565.
76. Kumar N. Paclitaxel-induced polymerization of purified tubulin. Mechanism of action. *J Biol Chem* 1981; 256:10,435–10,441.
77. Cos J, Bellmunt J, Soler C, Ribas A, Lluis JM, Murio JE, Margarit C. Comparative study of sequential combinations of paclitaxel and methotrexate on a human bladder cancer cell line. *Cancer Invest* 2000; 18:429–435.
78. McDaid HM, Johnston PG. Synergistic interaction between paclitaxel and 8-chloro-adenosine 3',5'-monophosphate in human ovarian carcinoma cell lines. *Clin Cancer Res* 1999; 5:215–220.
79. Perez EA, Buckwalter CA. Sequence-dependent cytotoxicity of etoposide and paclitaxel in human breast and lung cancer cell lines. *Cancer Chemother Pharmacol* 1998; 41:448–452.
80. Hamel E. Antimitotic natural products and their interactions with tubulin. *Med Res Rev* 1996; 16: 207–231.
81. Sackett DI. Vinca site agents induce structural changes in tubulin different from and antagonistic to changes induced by cholchicine site agents. *Biochemistry* 1995; 34:7010–7019.
82. Giannakakou P, Villalba L, Li H, Poruchynsky M, Fojo T. Combinations of paclitaxel and vinblastine and their effects on tubulin polymerization and cellular cytotoxicity: characterization of a synergistic schedule. *Int J Cancer* 1998; 75:57–63.
83. Beran M, McCredie KB, Keating MJ, Gutterman JU. Antileukemic effect of recombinant tumor necrosis factor α in vitro and its modulation by α and {g} interferons. *Blood* 1988; 72:728–738.
84. Berenbaum MC. Dose-response curves for agents that impair cell reproductive integrity. A fundamental difference between dose-response curves for antimetabolites and those for radiation and alkylating agents. *Br J Cancer* 1969; 23:426–433.
85. Harsthorn KL, Sandstrom EG, Neumeyer D, et al. Synergistic inhibition of human T-cell lymphotropic virus type III replication in vitro by phosphonoformate and recombinant alpha-A interferon. *Antibiot Agents Chemother* 1986; 30:189–191.
86. Hartshorn KL, Vogt MW, Chou T-C, et al. Synergistic inhibition of human immunodeficiency virus in vitro by azidothymidine and recombinant alpha A interferon. *Antibiot Agents Chemother* 1987; 31: 168–172.
87. Hubbell HR. Synergistic antiproliferative effect of human interferons in combination with mismatched double-stranded RNA on human tumor cells. *Int J Cancer* 1988; 37:359–365.
88. King TC, Krogstad DJ. Spectrophotometric assessment of dose-response curves for single antimicrobial agents and antimicrobial combinations. *J Infect Dis* 1983; 147:758–764.
89. Murohashi, I, Nagata K, Suzuki T, Maruyama Y, Nara N. Effects of recombinant G- CSF and GM-CSF on the growth in methylcellulose and suspension of the blast cells in acute myeloblastic leukemia. *Leuk Res* 1988; 12:433–440.
90. Sobrero AF, Bertino JR. Sequence-dependent synergism between dichloromethotrexate and 5-fluorouracil in a human colon carcinoma line. *Cancer Res* 1983; 43:4011–4013.
91. Tallarida RJ, Stone DJ, Raffa RB. Efficient deigns for studying synergistic drug combinations. *Life Sci* 1997; 61:417–425.
92. Steel GG, Peckham MJ. Exploitable mechanisms in combined radiotherapy-chemotherapy: the concept of additivity. *Int J Radiat Oncol Biol Phys* 1979; 5:85–91.
93. Dewey WC, Stone LE, Miller HH, Giblak RE. Radiosensitization with 5-bromodeoxyuridine of Chinese hamster cells x-irradiated during different phases of the cell cycle. *Radiat Res* 1977; 47: 672–688.
94. Deen DF, Williams MW. Isobologram analysis of x-ray-BCNU interactions in vitro. *Radiat Res* 1979; 79:483–491.
95. Schabel FM, Trader MW, Laster WR, Wheeler GP, Witt MH. Patterns of resistance and therapeutic synergism among alkylating agents. *Antibiot Chemother (Basel)* 1978; 23:200–215.
96. Schabel FM, Griswold DP, Corbett TH, Laster WR, Mayo JG, Lloyd HH. Testing therapeutic hypotheses in mice treated with anticancer drugs that have demonstrated or potential clinical utility for treatment of advanced solid tumors of man. *Methods Cancer Res* 1979; 17:3–51.
97. Schabel FM Jr. Concepts for systemic treatment of micrometastases. *Cancer* 1975, 35:15–24.
98. Schabel FM Jr, Griswold DP Jr, Corbett TH, Laster WR Jr. Increasing the therapeutic response rates to anticancer drugs by applying the basic principles of pharmacology. *Cancer* 1984, 54:1160–1167.

99. Schabel FM Jr, Simpson-Herren L. Some variables in experimental tumor systems which complicate interpretation of data from in vivo kinetic and pharmacologic studies with anticancer drugs. *Antibiot Chemother* 1978, 23:113–127.

100. Schabel FM Jr, Griswold DP Jr, Corbett TH, Laster WR. Increasing therapeutic response rates to anticancer drugs by applying the basic principles of pharmacology. *Pharm Ther* 1983, 20: 283–305.

101. Corbett TH, Griswold DP Jr, Roberts BJ, Peckham JC, Schabel FM Jr. Evaluation of single agents and combinations of chemotherapeutic agents in mouse colon carcinomas. *Cancer* 1977, 40:2660–2680.

102. Corbett TH, Griswold DP Jr, Wolpert MK, Venditti JM, Schabel FM Jr. Design and evaluation of combination chemotherapy trials in experimental animal tumor systems. *Cancer Treat Rep* 1979, 63:799–801.

103. Griswold DP Jr, Corbett TH, Schabel FM Jr. Cell kinetics and the chemotherapy of murine solid tumors. *Antibiot Chemother* 1980; 28:28–34.

104. Griswold DP, Corbett TH, Schabel FM Jr. Clonogenicity and growth of experimental tumors in relation to developing resistance and therapeutic failure. *Cancer Treat Rep* 1981; 65(suppl 2):51–54.

105. Teicher BA, Herman TS, Holden SA, et al. Tumor resistance to alkylating agents conferred by mechanisms operative only in vivo. *Science* 1990, 247:1457–1461.

106. Teicher BA, Holden SA, Cucchi CA, et al. Combination of N,N',N''-triethylenethiophosphoramide and cyclophosphamide in vitro and in vivo. *Cancer Res* 1988, 48:94–100.

107. Teicher BA, Holden SA, Eder JP, Brann TW, Jones SM, Frei E III. Preclinical studies relating to the use of thiotepa in the high-dose setting alone and in combination. *Semin Oncol* 1990, 17:18–32.

108. Teicher BA, Holden SA, Jones SM, Eder JP, Herman TS. Influence of scheduling on two-drug combinations of alkylating agents in vivo. *Cancer Chemother Pharmacol* 1989, 25:161–166.

109. Teicher BA, Waxman DJ, Holden SA, Wang Y, Clarke L, Alvarez Sotomayor E, Jones SM, Frei E III. Evidence for enzymatic activation and oxygen involvement in cytotoxicity and antitumor activity of N,N',N''-triethylenethiophosphoramide. *Cancer Res* 1989; 49:4996–5001.

110. Sugiura K, Stock C. Studies in a tumor spectrum. III. The effect of phosphoramides on the growth of a variety of mouse and rat tumors. *Cancer Res* 1955; 15:38–51.

111. Sugiura K, Stock C. Studies in a tumor spectrum. I. Comparison of the action of methylbis (2-chloroethyl)amine and 3-bis(2-chloroethyl) aqminomethyl-4-methoxymethyl-5-hydroxy-6-methylpyridine on the growth of a variety of mouse and rat tumors. *Cancer* 1952; 5:282–315.

112. Sugiura K, Stock C. Studies in a tumor spectrum. II. The effect of 2,4,6-triethyleneimino-s-triazine on the growth of a variety of mouse and rat tumors. *Cancer* 1952; 5:979–991.

113. DeWys W. A quantitative model for the study of the growth and treatment of a tumor and its metastases with correlation between proliferative state and sensitivity to cyclophosphamide. *Cancer Res* 1972; 32:367–373.

114. DeWys W. Studies correlating the growth rate of a tumor and its metastases and providing evidence for tumor-related systemic growth-retarding factors. *Cancer Res* 1972; 32:374–379.

115. Steel GG, Adams K. Stem-cell survival and tumor control in the Lewis lung carcinoma. *Cancer Res* 1975; 35:1530–1535.

116. Steel GG, Nill RP, Peckham MJ. Combined radiotherapy-chemotherapy of Lewis lung carcinoma. *Int J Radiat Oncol Biol Phys* 1978; 4:49–52.

117. Bertelli P, Mantica C, Farina G, et al. Treatment of non-small cell lung cancer with vinorelbine. *Proc Am Soc Clin Oncol* 1994; 13:362.

118. Bore P, Rahmani R, VanCamfort J. Pharmacokinetics of a new anticancer drug, navelbine, in patients. *Cancer Chemother Pharmacol* 1989; 23:247–251.

119. Cros S, Wright M, Morimoto M. Experimental antitumor activity of navelbine. *Semin Oncol* 1989; 16(suppl):15–20.

120. Cvitkovic E. The current and future place of vinorelbine in cancer therapy. *Drugs* 1992; 44(suppl 4): 36–45.

121. Marquet P, Lachatre G, Debord J. Pharmacokinetics of vinorelbine in man. *Eur J Clin Pharmacol* 1992; 42:545–547.

122. Navelbine (vinorelbine tartrate) clinical investigational brochure. Burroughs Wellcome. October, 1995.

123. Fumoleau P, Delgado F, Delozier T, et al. Phase II trial of weekly intravenous vinorelbine in first line advanced breast cancer chemotherapy. *J Clin Oncol* 1993; 11: 1245–1252.

124. Jehl F, Quoix E, Leveque D. Pharmacokinetics and preliminary metabolite fate of vinorelbine in human as determined by high performance liquid chromatography. *Cancer Res* 1991; 51: 2073–2076.

125. Lepierre A, Lemarie E, Dabouis G, Garnier G. A phase 2 study of navelbine in the treatment of non-small cell lung cancer. *Am J Clin Oncol* 1991; 14: 115–119.

126. Shih C, Thornton DE. Preclinical pharmacology studies and the clinical development of a novel multitargeted antifolate, MTA (LY231514). In: Jackman AL, ed. *Anticancer Drug Development Guide: Antifolate Drugs in Cancer Therapy.* Totowa, NJ: Humana. 1998:183–201.

127. Jones RJ, Tweleves CJ. Pemetrexed: a multitargeted antifolate (ALIMTA), LY231514. *Exp Rev Anticancer Ther* 2002; 2:13–22.

128. Bunn PA Jr. Incorporation of pemetrexed (Alimta) into the treatment of non-small cell lung cancer (thoracic tumors). *Semin Oncol* 2002; 29(3 suppl 9):17–22.

129. Novello S, le Chevalier T. ALIMTA (pemetrexed disodium, Ly231514, MTA): clinical experience in non-small cell lung cancer. *Lung Cancer* 2001; 34(suppl 4):S107–S109.

130. Shepherd FA, Dancey J, Arnold A, et al. Phase II study of pemetrexed disodium, a multitargeted antifolate and cisplatin as first-line therapy in patients with advanced nonsmall cell lung carcinomas: a study of the National Cancer Institute of Canada Clinical Trials Group. *Cancer* 2001; 92:595–600.

131. Teicher BA, Alvarez E, Liu P, et al. MTA (LY231514) in combination treatment regimens using human tumor xenografts and the EMT6 murine mammary carcinoma. *Semin Oncol* 1999; 26(suppl 6):55–62.

132. Giovanella BC. Topoisomerase I inhibitors. In: Teicher BA, ed. *Cancer Therapeutics: Experimental and Clinical Agents.* Totowa, NJ: Humana. 1997:137–152.

133. Chabot GC. Clinical pharmacokinetics of irinotecan. *Clin Pharmacokinet* 1997; 33:245–259.

134. Aschele C, Baldo C, Sobrero AF, et al. Schedule-dependent synergism between ZD1694 (ralititrexed) and CPT-11 (irinotecan) in human colon cancer in vitro. *Clin Cancer Res* 1998; 4:1323–1330.

135. O'Reilly S, Rowinsky EC. The clinical status of irinotecan (CPT-11), a novel water soluble camptothecin analogue: *Crit Rev Oncol Hematol* 1996; 24:47–70.

136. Teicher BA, Chatterjee D, Liu J-T, Holden SA, Ara G. Protection of bone marrow CFU-GM in mice-bearing in vivo alkylating agent resistant murine EMT-6 tumors. *Cancer Chemother Pharmacol* 1993; 32:315–319.

137. Chatterjee D, Liu CT-T, Northey D, Teicher BA. Molecular characterization of the in vivo alkylating agent resistant murine EMT-6 mammary carcinoma tumors. *Cancer Chemother Pharmacol* 1995; 35:423–431.

138. Chao NJ, Blume KG. Bone marrow transplantation Part II—Autologous. *West J Med* 1990; 152: 46–51.

139. Gulati S, Yahalow J, Portlock C. Autologous bone marrow transplantation. *Curr Prob Cancer* 1991; 15:5–56.

140. Williams SF. Application of peripheral blood progenitors to dose-intensive therapy of breast cancer. *Breast Cancer Res Treat* 1993; 26:25–29.

141. Crown J, Wassherheit C, Hakes T, et al. Rapid delivery of multiple high-dose chemotherapy courses with granulocyte colony-stimulating factor and peripheral blood-derived hematopoietic progenitor cells. *J Natl Cancer Inst* 1992; 84:1935–1936.

142. Koenigsmann M, Topp MS, Thiel E, Berdel WW. Recombinant human granulocyte colony-stimulating factor (rhG-CSF) does not stimulate in vivo tumor growth of the human colon cancer cell line HTB 38 which is responsive in vitro. *Int J Oncol* 1993; 3:1057–1059.

143. Knox SJ, Fowler S, Marquez C, Hoppe RT. Effect of filgrastim (G-CSF) in Hodgkin's disease patients treated with radiation therapy. *Int J Radiat Oncol Biol Phys* 1993; 28:445–450.

144. Johnson CS. Interleukin-1: therapeutic potential for solid tumors. *Cancer Invest* 1993; 11:600–608.

145. Kennedy MJ, David J, Passos-Coelho J, et al. Administration of human recombinant granulocyte colony-stimulating factor (Filgrastim) accelerates granulocyte recovery following high-dose chemotherapy and autologous marrow transplantation with 4-hydroperoxycyclophosphamide-purged marrow in women with metastatic breast cancer. *Cancer Res* 1993; 53:5424–5428.

146. Neta R, Oppenheim JJ. Interleukin 1 is a radioprotector. *J Immunol* 1986; 136:24,983–24,985.

147. Neta R, Oppenheim JJ, Douches SD. Interdependence of the radioprotective effects of human recombinant interleukin 1α, tumor necrosis factor α, granulocyte colony-stimulating factor and murine recombinant granulocyte-macrophage colony-stimulating factor. *J Immunol* 140: 108–111, 1988.

148. Moore MAS, Warren DJ. Synergy of interleukin 1 and granulocyte colony-stimulating factor: in vivo stimulation of stem-cell recovery and hematopoietic regeneration following 5-fluorouracil treatment of mice *Proc Natl Acad Sci USA* 1987; 84:7134–7138.

149. Moreb J, Zucali JR, Gross MA, Weiner RS. Protective effects of IL-1 in rodent models. *J Immunol* 1989; 142:1937–1942.

150. Castelli MP, Black PL, Schneider M, Pennington R, Abe F, Talmadge JE. Protective, restorative and therapeutic properties of recombinant human IL-1 in rodent models. *J Immunol* 1988; 140:3830–3837.

151. Damia G, Komschlies KL, Futami H, et al. Prevention of acute chemotherapy-induced death in mice by recombinant human interleukin-1: protection from hematological and nonhematological toxicities. *Cancer Res* 1992; 52:4082–4089.

152. Lynch DH, Rubin AS, Miller RE, Williams DE. Protective effects of recombinant human interleukin-1a in doxorubicin-treated normal and tumor-bearing mice. *Cancer Res* 1993; 53:1565–1570.

153. Naparstek E, Ohana M, Greenberger JS, Slavin S. Continuous intravenous administration of rmGM-CSF enhances immune as well as hematopoietic reconstitution following syngeneic bone marrow transplantation in mice. *Exp Hematol* 1993; 21:131–137.

154. Molineux G, Pojda Z, Hampson IN, Lord BI, Dexter TM. Transplantation potential of peripheral blood stem cells induced by granulocyte colony-stimulating factor. *Blood* 1990; 65:2153–2158.

155. Neben S, Marcus K, Mauch P. Mobilization of hematopoietic stem and progenitor cell subpopulations from the marrow to the blood of mice following cyclophosphamide and/or granulocyte colony-stimulating factor. *Blood* 1993; 81:1960–1967.

156. Craddock CF, Apperley JF, Wright EG, et al. Circulating stem cells in mice treated with cyclophosphamide. *Blood* 1992; 80:264–269.

157. Teicher BA, Holden SA, Jones SM, Eder JP, Herman TS. Influence of scheduling of two-drug combinations of alkylating agents in vivo. *Cancer Chemother Pharmacol* 1989; 25:161–166.

158. Teicher BA, Holden SA, Eder JP, Herman TS, Antman KH, Frei E III. Preclinical studies relating to the use of thiotepa in the high-dose setting alone and in combination. *Semin Oncol* 1990; 17:18–32.

159. Teicher BA, Ara G, Keyes SR, Herbst RS, Frei E III. Acute in vivo resistance in high-dose therapy. *Clin Cancer Res* 1998; 4:483–491.

160. Jones RB, Matthes S, Cagnoni PJ. Pharmacokinetics. In: Armitage JO, Antman KH, eds. *High-Dose Cancer Therapy: Pharmacology, Hematopoietins, Stem Cells.* Baltimore: Lippincott Williams & Wilkins. 1999:49–69.

161. Colvin OM, Petros W. Pharmacologic strategies for high-dose therapy. In: Armitage JO, Antman KH, eds. *High-Dose Cancer Therapy: Pharmacology, Hematopoietins, Stem Cells.* Baltimore: Lippincott Williams & Wilkins. 1999:3–14.

11 Models for Biomarkers and Minimal Residual Tumor

Beverly A. Teicher, PhD

CONTENTS

INTRODUCTION
HISTORY
ACUTE MYELOCYTIC LEUKEMIA IN THE BROWN NORWAY RAT
MURINE B-CELL LEUKEMIA/LYMPHOMA (BCL1)
MODERN DETECTION METHODS
CONCLUSION

1. INTRODUCTION

Systemic treatment of malignant disease now has a modern history of over 50 yr. Over that time, the successes of chemotherapy in curing cancer have been in leukemia, lymphoma, and selected solid tumors such as testis cancer. The administration of very high doses of chemotherapy requiring hematopoietic stem cell support has had more than a 10-yr history *(1–5)*. Even with this heroic treatment, cure of solid tumors, such as breast cancer and small-cell lung cancer, remains elusive *(6–8)*. High-dose chemotherapy regimens with hematopoietic stem cell support allowed the frequency of complete clinical response to be markedly increased; however, over the first 1–2 yr after therapy, tumors in most patients recur. These results, as well as the predictable times and patterns of recurrence of many solid tumors after standard courses of chemotherapy or standard regimens of radiation therapy, have led to the hypothesis that a few viable malignant cells with proliferative capacity remain after therapy and eventually repopulate the primary tumor and/or grow into metastatic lesions. These minimal residual tumor cells exist at levels below detectability by standard techniques. Dendritic cell (DC)-based cancers are currently being evaluated for the treatment of minimal residual disease *(9)*.

Biomarkers, especially those measurable in serum, are being developed for more and more cancers *(10,11)*. Biomarkers in malignant disease may serve as molecular targets, as well as detectors for minimal residual disease, recurrent disease, and early disease *(12–14)*. Circulating tumor DNA reflects the biological characteristics of the tumor and can allow the detection of minimal residual disease in patients *(15)*. Methods have been developed for the detection of individual micrometastatic cancer cells in patients with

From: *Cancer Drug Discovery and Development:*
Anticancer Drug Development Guide: Preclinical Screening, Clinical Trials, and Approval, 2nd Ed.
Edited by: B. A. Teicher and P. A. Andrews © Humana Press Inc., Totowa, NJ

epithelial tumors *(16)*. Molecular pathologic methods have allowed a revolution in diagonostic histopathology, improving detection of tumor, tumor classification, and identification of rare tumors *(17)*. Proteomics offers a new approach to identify and detect biomarkers that can be of prognostic, diagnostic, and therapeutic value *(18)*. Translational research from preclinical models offers an increasing opportunity to apply these techniques in clinical trials *(19)*. The multidrug resistance genes, P-glycoprotein, and other resistance proteins are useful markers in several major tumors such as lung and breast cancer and can be detected by gene amplification, mRNA, and protein expression *(20)*.

Thus, the two major issues being addressed by preclinical models in this area are (1) detection of very rare tumor cells in large populations of normal cells and (2) the significance and characterization of these tumor cells that have survived exposure to high doses of chemotherapeutic agents (and/or radiation therapy or immunotherapy). Both in vitro (cell culture) and in vivo (animal tumor) models are being used to address scientific issues related to the minimal residual tumor.

2. HISTORY

Preclinically, the scientific study of minimal tumor and minimal residual tumor became an active endeavor with the advent of the transplantable murine leukemia models, primarily L1210 and P388 leukemia *(21)*. It has been recognized since the 19th century that cancer cells could be carried in the circulating blood to form metastases at sites distant from the primary tumor *(22)*. From the mid-1950s to the early 1970s, many clinical studies confirmed the presence of malignant cells in the circulating blood of cancer patients, but correlation between the numbers of these cells and time to relapse or extent of metastatic disease was very difficult *(22)*. The significance of circulating cancer cells in patients remains controversial. In several animal studies, however, it was clear that the injection of blood from animals bearing a primary tumor into fresh syngeneic hosts could produce tumors in these animals *(23–26)*. In a quantitative study, Fidler *(27)* injected 2×10^5 radiolabeled B16 melanoma cells into the tail veins of mice. He found that most of the cells were lysed within 24 h, but that after 14 d, about 400 melanoma cells were present in the lungs of the animals, resulting in about 80 metastatic colonies. Working at Southern Research Institute, Skipper and coworkers *(28)* took a different tack in modeling minimal tumor. Using murine leukemia L1210, as well as other tumor models, known numbers of malignant cells from 1, 10, or 100 up to 10^4 were implanted in host animals, and the animals were scored for the presence of tumor and survival over time.

Several conclusions were possible from these studies. First, all single viable tumor cells from a given population do not behave identically. The median single tumor cell gives rise to progeny that proliferate about as would be expected in relation to larger inocula. However, if enough single-cell implantations are made with a micromanipulator or by dilution techniques (or by chemotherapy or radiation or surgery) some such single cells (<50%) will take slightly longer to much longer than the median to give rise to a detectable number or a lethal number of progeny. Thus, one "fast" tumor cell that gives rise to progeny with a high growth fraction will rather quickly overgrow many "slow" tumor cells *(28)*. Second, the median rate of growth (or regrowth) of animal tumor cell populations is often essentially exponential over the range of one or a few viable cells to about 10^8. Above this range, tumor growth curves become progressively asymptotic, particularly in solid tumor masses. Thus, animal tumors do not seem to grow (or regrow)

Table 1
Lethal Tumors From Implant of One Tumor Cell

Tumor	Host	References
Leukemias and plasma cell tumors		
AKF5 leukemia and S2 leukemia	Mouse	101
L1210 leukemia	Mouse	29
L1210 leukemia resistant to 6-mercaptopurine, 6-methyl mercaptopurine, 8-azaguanine, or methyl-GAG	Mouse	102
Plasmacytoma no. 1	Hamster	102
Solid tumors		
Yoshida sarcoma	Rat	103
Jensen sarcoma	Rat	104
Sarcoma 37	Mouse	105
Hepatoma AH-66F, AH-272, and AH-130	Rat	29
Walker carcinosarcoma 256	Rat	102
Sarcoma	Mouse	102

precisely in a gompertzian fashion, although they may come rather close (28). Finally, the growth or repopulation rates of a given tumor cell population in different animals are not highly variable over the range of one or a few to about 10^8, except when a single or several viable cells comprise the implant (28).

Theoretically, cancer arises when one normal cell transforms into a malignant neoplastic cell, either by natural mutation or following chemical, viral, or radiation induction. That a single cancer cell can establish fatal disease in several mammalian species with a number of different neoplastic cell types had been repeatedly demonstrated in the laboratory by 1970 (Table 1) (21).

Following parental implant (intraperitoneal [ip], intravenous [iv], or intracerebral [ic]) of L1210 (29) or P388 into BDF1 mice, life span is directly related to the number of leukemic cells implanted, and this relationship is consistent down to one cell. With L1210, the population doubling time of tumor cells surviving therapy with cyclophosphamide, selected nitrosoureas, methotrexate, 6-mercaptopurine, 5-fluorouracil, or 1-β-D-arabinofuranosyl-cytosine was not significantly different from the previously untreated tumor cell population from which they were selected (29,30). Therefore, the number of L1210 or P388 cells surviving drug treatment could be estimated reliably by determining the mean or median life span of drug-treated mice and the size of the tumor cell population that will give that life span for each tumor and implant site derived from the large historical experience at Southern Research Institute.

As quantitative methods for estimation of the number of viable tumor cells required for development of disease or survival of cytotoxic therapy were developed, other investigators were examining the relationship between primary and metastatic disease (31–33). Metastasis is a common occurrence in patients with cancer and is directly responsible for the death of many of them. However, in terms of cancer cells themselves, metastasis is a comparatively rare event in that of the millions of cells per day thought to be released from solid tumors, only a few give rise to metastases by successfully passing through a complex sequence of potentially traumatic events. If the basis for cell loss is selective, then, regardless of mechanisms, the populations of cancer cells in metastases might well be different from the populations in the primary lesions from which they arose *(31)*. Metastasis-specific work in this area is best exemplified by the experiments of Fidler and his colleagues. Fidler *(34)* argued that metastatic subpopulations of cancer cells might be preferentially involved and made attempts to isolate such metastatic lines of cells by cyclic pulmonary transplantation via tail vein injection. Fidler *(35–37)* observed clear-cut increases in the numbers of pulmonary tumors per animal following injection of B16 melanoma cells, when progressing from B16 line F1 through B16 line F6 (five selection cycles) to B16 line F10 (10 selection cycles) *(38)*.

Currently it is believed that differences between cells in primary cancers and their metastases may be owing to interactions between organ components and the cancer cells after the latter have reached the site of presumptive metastases—in other words, that the genes expressed by cells depend in part on the environment in which the cells are located *(31–33)*. Site or environmentally induced changes in cell populations are well recognized in other areas of biology, and reversible changes resulting from interactions of this type are known *(39)*. The evidence for heterogeneity among cancer cells in tumors is compelling. The concept that genetic instability of evolving cancer cell populations is the basis for the heterogeneity must be viewed against the background of physiologic change associated with proliferation and degeneration, which may be manifest on a topographic basis. The evidence for consistent genetic differences between the cancer cells in primary cancers and their metastases is rather sparse *(31)*.

3. ACUTE MYELOCYTIC LEUKEMIA IN THE BROWN NORWAY RAT

The acute myelocytic leukemia in the Brown Norway rat (BNML) has served as a model for comparative studies with human acute myelocytic leukemia for a number of years and has contributed considerably toward our understanding of the biologic characteristics of minimal residual tumor in acute leukemia *(40–43)*. In 1985, Martens and Hagenbeek *(44)* described the results of a study using a monoclonal antibody, MCA-Rm124, raised against BN acute myelocytic leukemia cells to detect disease in the bone marrow of rats. After intravenous injection of 10^7 BN leukemic cells, the growth of the leukemic cell population in the bone marrow, the liver, and the spleen was monitored using MCA-Rm124 and flow cytometry. For the bone marrow and the liver, a clonogenic assay for leukemic cells was used to quantify the cell content in these organs. A good correlation was found between the bioassay-derived data and the flow cytometry-derived data. The doubling times of the leukemic cell population were not equal for the two organs studied, indicating that a number of different processes contribute to the net cell production per organ *(44)*.

In a second study, rats were studied before chemotherapy as well as thereafter, i.e., in the minimal residual tumor phase. Bone marrow from different types of bones was analyzed from each animal. Before treatment, the ratio of the measured extreme values (i.e., highest/lowest value) for leukemic cell frequencies in bones from individual rats ranged from 3.7 to 11.7. During the minimal residual disease phase, the ratios of the extremes ranged from a factor of 36 to more than 13,000 from one rat to another. The variability between bones of comparable size was estimated by studying the ribs from each individual animal. Within individuals, the extremes differed by a factor of 1.2–4.0 before chemotherapy and from 2.4 to more than 320 after chemotherapy. The variability within the marrow cavity of a single bone was determined by analyzing multiple samples from femoral bones cut into slices. The leukemic cell frequency appeared to vary considerably, i.e., before treatment from 1.7 to 7.3 and during minimal residual tumor from 4 to 28,000. The conclusion from this study must be that the reliability of diagnoses based on the analysis of single bone marrow aspirates appears to be highly questionable (45).

Most recently, these investigators (46) transferred the *Escherichia coli* gene encoding β-galactosidase (lacZ) and the neomycin resistance gene (neo[r]) into the subline LT12 of the BN acute myelocytic leukemia, employing the retroviral BAG vector. In this way, leukemic cells were genetically marked. Ten independent cell lines were characterized during in vitro growth as well as during two subsequent in vivo passages for expression of neo[r], for which the neomycin analog G418 was used as the selection agent, and for lacZ expression, for which the substrate 5-bromo-4-chloro-3-indolyl-β-D-galactopyranoside (X-gal) was used as the selction agent. Out of 10 clonal lines, four had permanent high expression of lacZ in all cells. In four other lines, greatly varying lacZ expression between the individual cells was observed. In the remaining two lines, lacZ expression was gradually lost. In contrast, neo[r] expression was gradually lost in 8 of the 10 lines, particularly rapidly during in vivo passaging. In the remaining two lines, neo[r] expression was retained. The genetic modification did not alter the in vitro leukemogenicity of the cells.

Long-term in vivo expression of neo[r] and lacZ was followed in two selected lines up to 12 sequential passages, i.e., one from the group of homogeneous high lacZ expression and one from the group of heterogeneous lacZ expression. In both lines, lacZ expression was retained, whereas neo[r] expression was rapidly lost after the third passage. The feasibility of using genetically marked leukemic cells for studies of minimal residual tumor was explored by injecting rats with leukemic cells, treating them with chemotherapy at full-blown leukemia development to reduce the tumor load, mimicking the induction of a state of minimal residual tumor, and studying lacZ expression at relapse. LacZ expression was evident in 100% of the cells, whereas neor expression was lost in a considerable fraction. These results indicate that the viral vector BAG can be used to mark leukemia cells genetically, although a selection of clones with the desired stability of long-term expression is required (46).

The BN acute myelocytic leukemia model has also been used to study drug resistance (47–49). The efficacy of acetyldinaline (4-acetylamino-N-[2'-aminophenyl]-benzamide) for eradication of minimal residual tumor, which is left after bone marrow transplantation, and the risk of a bone marrow graft being jeopardized by this treatment were studied in the BN acute myelocytic leukemia model (50). To mimic the clinical situation, minimal residual tumor induction treatment was given to rats showing clinical signs of leukemia. The treatment consisted of 80 mg/kg cyclophosphamide and 7.0 Gy X-rays total body irradiation, resulting in a 6–8 log leukemic cell kill leaving 10–1000 leukemic cells in the animals. Treatment was completed with a syngeneic bone marrow transplant. A high-dose level treatment of 23.7 mg acetyldinaline/kg/d and a low-dose level treatment of 11.85 mg/kg/d, each given orally for 5 consecutive d, were compared.

The increase in the survival time, the cure rate, and the toxic death rate were evaluated. One 5-d course of low-dose treatment, started at a time interval of 10, 17, or 24 d following minimal residual disease induction, resulted in 44, 11, or 0% cures. With two 5-d courses of low-dose treatment, 89, 22, or 0% cures were achieved. With low-dose treatment, maximally an 8-log leukemic cell kill was obtained, and no toxicity-related deaths were observed (only <1 log kill of normal hematopoeitic stem cells). In contrast, a single course of high-dose treatment resulted in 56% of the rats (10/18) dying from intestinal tract toxicity, whereas from the remaining eight rats at risk for relapse, three (36%) showed a very late relapse and five were cured (63%). It was evident that the leukemic cell load at the start of the acetyldinaline treatment determined the probability of relapse. An important finding was that acetyldinaline did not interfere with bone marrow regeneration. The highly curative potential of acetyldinaline treatment in the BN acute myelocytic leukemia model during the phase of minimal residual disease suggests that this type of treatment strategy may warrant clinical investigation (50).

4. MURINE B-CELL LEUKEMIA/LYMPHOMA (BCL1)

Clinical data have suggested that allogenic interactions of donor immune cells with residual host leukemia cells that may differ from donor-derived effector cells by minor histocompatibility loci alone are sufficient to cause graft-vs-host disease, as well as desirable graft-vs-leukemia effects (51–53). It has not yet been established whether graft vs leukemia and graft-vs-host disease are mediated by an identical set of effector cells and mechanisms, or whether the two phemonena may be distinguishable by different effector cells, tumor-associated cell surface targets, or both.

The BCL1 tumor model originally described by Slavin and Strober (54,55) is a useful experimental model for studying graft-vs-leukemia effects in a non-immunogenic lymphoblastic/lymphoma (56,57). The BCL1 disease is characterized by marked splenomegaly (50 × normal spleen size, with up to $5–10 × 10^9$ cells/spleen) accompanied by extreme peripheral blood lymphocytosis (up to $500 × 10^6$ lymphocytes/mL) followed by death of 100% of all recipients of as few as 10–100 tumor cells (55). Studies have demonstrated that about 75% of Balb/c mice inoculated with a high number (10^7) of BCL1 cells were operationally cured after allogenic bone marrow transplantation using histoincompatible non-T-lymphocyte-depleted C57BL/6 grafts, following conditioning of the recipients with total lymphoid irradiation and cyclophosphamide 200 mg/kg (56). Some of the apparently "cured" chimeras (>18 mo with no evidence of disease) were shown to bear dormant tumor cells. An adoptive transfer of spleen cells from chimeras with no evidence of disease to secondary Balb/c recipients led to rapid development of typical leukemia in 50% of the mice (56).

Immunotherapy with recombinant human interleukin-2 (IL-2) and allogenic spleen cells has led to significant antitumor effects in BCL1-bearing mice following transplantation with T-lymphocyte-depleted allogenic bone marrow cells (58). Graft-vs-leukemia effects were studied in a model mimicking minimal residual disease following bone marrow transplantation. Lethally irradiated (Balb/c × C57BL/6)F1 recipients were reconstituted with $20 × 10^6$ T-lymphocyte-depleted C57BL/6 bone marrow cells mixed with $10^4–10^6$ BCL1 cells followed by administration of sequential increments of allogenic C57BL/6 spleen cells: 10^6 cells on d 1, 10^7 cells on d 5, and $5 × 10^7$ cells on d 9, with or without concomitant IL-2 treatment (ip injections of 20,000 U twice daily for 3 d) together with each spleen cell administration.

All mice receiving $10^4–10^6$ BCL1 cells developed marked splenomegaly by d 21, and all adoptive recipients of 105 spleen cells obtained from these mice developed leukemia within 21–36 d. Treatment of mice that received 10^4 BCL1 cells by either three courses of low-dose IL-2 or three increments of allogenic spleen cells alone, and certainly by a combination of both, resulted in normalization of splenomegaly on d 21. Only adoptive recipients of 10^5 spleen cells obtained from mice treated by both allogeneic spleen cells and IL-2 (10/10) or allogenic spleen cells alone (8/10) were disease-free (>100 d). Mice inoculated with 105 BCL1 cells developed mild splenomegaly on d 21 after IL-2 treatment alone but showed no clinical evidence of disease following administration of allogenic spleen cells and IL-2 (10/10), whereas a partial effect was observed in mice treated by allogenic spleen cell only (4/10). Mice inoculated with a high dose of BCL1 cells (10^6) showed some delay in onset of splenomegaly, but no curative antileukemic effects could be observed even following a synergistic combination of IL-2 and allogenic spleen cells.

These results suggest that immunocompetent allogenic lymphocyctes may play an important role against leukemic relapse, and thus cell therapy may be used therapeutically to treat minimal residual disease after bone marrow transplantation, even following initial reconstitution with T-cell-depleted bone marrow cells. Moreover, graft-vs-leukemia effects mediated by allogenic lymphocytes may be further augmented by concomitant administration of suboptimal doses of IL-2. A similar approach may prove beneficial in conjunction with autologous and allogenic bone marrow transplantation in humans as long as graft-vs-host disease can be prevented or controlled (58).

Severe combined immunodeficiency (SCID) mice can serve as a host for human leukemias (59). These models have been used to investigate whether in vivo engraftment and proliferation of primary leukemia cells in mice can predict outcome and identify patients who might benefit from more or less intensive or alternative therapy. Among the most studied lines established, NALM-6 human B-cell leukemia, HL-60 human leukemia, and U937 human myeloid leukemia have been useful in survival determinations.

5. MODERN DETECTION METHODS

5.1. Fluorescence In Situ Hybridization (FISH)

Fluorescence *in situ* hybridization (FISH) has been applied to chromosomal gene mapping and molecular cytogenetics (60–63). Most studies have used biotin- or haptene (e.g., digoxigenin and 2,4-dinitrophenol) labeled probes that require secondary detection reagents (e.g., avidin conjugated to fluorescein or rhodamine). However, fluorescently labeled nucleoside triphosphates that can be enzymatically incorporated into DNA by nick translation or random primer synthesis have also been examined. Chemically synthesized oligonucleotides (ribo or deoxy) can also be directly labeled with activated fluorophore molecules (64).

Directly fluorophorated probes can be visualized immediately after the post-hybridization wash (to remove excess probe), thereby eliminating the secondary incubations and washes required to provide the visualization of haptene-labeled probes. This is an important advantage, since it reduces the time and effort needed to complete an assay by several hours. However, the signal strength obtained with fluorophore-labeled probes is commonly only 10–15% of that produced by an equivalent haptene-labeled probe detected by secondary reagents (60). Fluorophore-labeled probes also are prone to photobleaching during preparation and hybridization, so care must be taken to avoid prolonged exposure to strong light. The fluorescence of direct-labeled probes is also quenched by many of the routinely used counterstains. Therefore, for many conventional histochemical applications, biotin- or digoxigenin-labeled probes may be preferable. Nevertheless, directly fluorophorated probes do offer specific advantages, e.g., very low background fluorescences, increased potential for multiplex analysis of target sequences *(65,66)*, and quantitative analysis of nucleic acid content of cell structures *(67)*.

Ward's group *(68)* has demonstrated the feasibility of combinatorial labeling of probes (i.e., with two or more different reporters) to increase the number of target sequences that can be detected simultaneously by FISH. They used an epifluorescence microscope equipped with a digital imaging cameras and computer software for pseudocoloring and merging images to distinguish up to seven different probes using only three fluorochromes. Chromosome-specific centromere repeat clones and chromosome-specific "composite" probe sets were generated by polymerase chain reaction (PCR) in which different mixtures of modified nucleotides, including fluorescein-conjugated dUTP, were incorporated. Cosmid clones were labeled similarly by nick translation. The technique has been used to delineate the centromeres of seven different human chromosomes, on both 4',6'-diamidino-2-phenylindole-stained metaphase spreads and interphase nuclei, to map six cosmid clones in a single hybridization experiment and to detect chromosome translocations by chromosome painting. Multiparameter hybridization analysis should faciltitate molecular cytogenetics, probe-based pathogen diagnosis, and gene mapping studies *(68)*.

5.2. Immunostaining

The protein products of oncogenes can sometimes be detected in extracellular fluids such as blood and can be useful markers for minimal residual disease, recurrent disease, and early cancer *(69)*. Carcinoembryonic antigen, human β-chorionic gonadotropin, and α_1-fetoprotein are a well-known examples of useful serum markers *(70,71)*. With monoclonal antibodies, it is possible to identify single tumor cells on a contrasting background of histogenetically different cells using differentiation markers *(72–74)*. The bone marrow is an exemplary anatomical site, where single metastasizing carcinoma cells with carcinomas of breast and large bowel using various monoclonal antibodies specific for epithelial antigens were examined *(75)*. The underlying hypothesis that, under normal circumstances, epithelial cells are barred from the marrow was tested by screening control aspirates from numerous patients without cancer.

Using a panel of monoclonal antibodies against cytokeratin and the 17-A epithelial antigen, Schlimok et al. *(75)* identified immunocytochemically tumor cells in bone marrow of patients with breast cancer ($n = 155$) and colorectal cancer ($n = 57$) at the time of surgery of the primary tumor. Monoclonal CK2, recognizing the human cytokeratin component 18 in simple epithelia, appeared to be the most suitable reagent because of its negative reaction with bone marrow samples of the noncarcinoma patients ($n = 75$). Its specificity was further demonstrated in a double-marker staining procedure using an antileukocyte common antigen monoclonal antibody (T200) as counterstain. A comparative analysis showed that immunocytology was clearly superior to conventional cytology ($n = 212$) and histology ($n = 39$). In 9.5–20.5% of patients without distant metastasis, tumor cells could be detected in bone marrow. They found a significant correlation between tumor cells in bone marrow and conventional risk factors, such as distant metastasis or lymph node involvement. In a first approach to immunotherapy, they demonstrated in three patients that infused monoclonal antibody 17-1A can label single tumor cells in bone marrow in vivo *(75)*.

One advantage of immunocytochemical staining is that it allows for visualization of the cell morphology, thus reducing the risk of false-positive resutls. Johnston et al. *(76)* developed a technique that uses an alkaline phosphatase-antialkaline phosphatase immunostaining procedure to detect tumor in normal donor marrow seeded with cultured breast cancer cells, as well as marrow samples from breast cancer patients at staging, harvest, and post transplant. This staining method was found to be extremely sensitive, consistently detecting as little as one breast cancer cell in 10^6 marrow cells. Since initial staging, therapeutic decisions, and response evaluations are to a large degree dependent on the extent of metastatic disease, this procedure may provide a valuable clinical aid in the treatment of breast cancer. Magnetic spectral analysis, a refinement of magnetic imaging (MR) imaging, can be used for detection and assessment of response to therapy of minimal residual disease *(77)*.

5.3. PCR

Clonal genetic alterations such as tumor suppressors, gene mutations, or microsatellite instability can be detected in clinical samples using DNA amplification techniques and used for detection of minimal residual disease or early cancer *(13,78)*. These techniques to detect genetic alterations are being used early to assess the status of individuals at high risk of developing specific inherited forms of cancer *(79)*. The National Cancer Institute is using DNA array technology to characterize genetically the NCI 60-cell human tumor line panel and to identify pharmacogenomic markers *(80)*. Animal models have been used to study minimal residual tumor after allogenic bone marrow transplantation and to support the concept that clinical relapse can evolve from residual malignant cells in transplant recipients *(81,82)*. However, these models have been limited by the fact that demonstration of minimal residual tumor in individual animals has generally required use of a bioassay system that necessitates killing the primary host. Consequently, the clinical fate of individual animals cannot be determined. The clinical relevance of these models may be questioned, because individualized therapeutic interventions cannot be made in animals in whom minimal residual tumor is detected.

Drobyski et al. *(83)* characterized a novel murine model for the study of minimal residual tumor after allogenic bone marrow transplantation. This model was designed to simulate high-risk bone marrow transplantation in humans; patients receive transplants in relapse, and disease recurrence is the major cause of treatment failure. The H-2-compatible, mixed lymphocyte culture nonreactive murine strains AKR (H-2k) and CBA (H-2k) were chosen to parallel marrow transplants from HLA-matched siblings, which represent the majority of allotransplants in humans. Male AKR leukemia cells were used in female donor/host chimeras, permitting the Y chromosome to serve as a leukemia-specific marker for minimal residual tumor. Detection of residual male leukemia cells in the peripheral blood of the primary host was facilitated by use of the PCR and sequence-specific oligonucleotide probe hybridization (SSOPH). Use of PCR/SSOPH was highly predictive of clinical outcome (relapse or cure) in animals receiving transplants ($p < 0.00002$) and detected disease recurrence earlier than comparative flow cytometric analysis studies. This murine model will be useful in evaluating the efficacy of therapeutic strategies aimed at reducing disease relapse post transplant and can be adapted to other transplant murine tumor systems for the study of minimal residual disease *(83)*.

Pugatsch et al. *(84)* used PCR to detect the minimal residual BCL1 leukemia originally described by Slavin and Strober *(54)*. Balb/c mice inoculated with as few as 10 BCL1 cells developed massive splenomegaly, and marked B-lymphocytosis, and died shortly after implantation of tumor *(55)*. Treatment of afflicted mice carrying a large tumor load with high-dose chemoradiotherapy followed by bone marrow transplantation or treatment of mice having a small tumor load with high-dose recombinant interleukin-2 can lead to operational cure; nevertheless, the animals might still harbor dormant leukemic cells *(85,86)*. The standard assay in animals for the detection of minimal residual tumor is adoptive transfer of 10^5 spleen cells from experimental mice into naïve Balb/c mice *(85)*. Clinical signs of BCL1 can be detected in the secondary recipients 3 wk to 3 mo after transfer. Pugatsch et al. *(84)* described the detection of minimal residual tumor in BCL1-carrying Balb/c mice using PCR. A BCL1-specific sequence from the rearranged Vh-region was amplified, yielding a 456-bp-long fragment. PCR products hybridized to the cloned BCL1 sequence allowed the detection of a single BCL1 cell. This assay, therefore, was able to reveal the presence of very small numbers of leukemic cells without sacrificing experimental animals *(84)*.

Genetic alterations in clinical cancer speciemen can be detected using DNA amplification techniques, and thus can be used for early detection of cancer *(78,87)*. PCR can detect tumor marker-expressing cells that are otherwise undetectable by other means in patients with localized or metastatic cancer *(88)*.

5.4. Colony Formation

The murine pre-B-cell lymphoma BCL1 is generally confined in vivo to the spleen and does not grow in culture *(54,89–91)*. Prindull et al. *(92)* have employed this system as a model of in vitro minimal residual tumor and have asked questions about the quality of the stroma of BCL1 spleen in terms of formation of fibroblastoid colonies and confluent layers, and of the survival of clonogenic BCL1 lymphoma cells in culture. Prindull et al. *(92)* have found quantitative deficiencies, such as reduced surface adherence of stromal cells, impaired colony-forming units-fibroblasts (CFU-F), and pre-CFU-F colony and layer formation in stromal cultures of lymphoma bearing spleen compared with cultures from normal spleen. There are two populations of clonogenic BCL1 lymphoma cells surviving in culture: one population is surface-adherent, and the other is nonadherent. Both populations transmit the lymphoma to healthy indicator mice *(92)*.

5.5. The Clinical Problem and Methods

In the past 5 yr, new methods with significantly higher sensitivity than light microscopy have been developed with the potential of detecting residual tumor cells *(93)*. The most sensitive and specific molecular biologic method is the amplification of chromosomal breakpoints using PCR. This technique also detects clone-specific nucleotide sequences in the joining region of T-cell receptor and immunoglobulin genes. The optimal sensitivity of PCR is 10^{-4}–10^{-6}. Immunologic methods, using monoclonal antibodies alone or in combination, are based on the detection of lineage- and stage-specific antigens and are analyzed by microscopy or automated flow cytometry. The sensitivity for detection of minimal residual tumor is limited by the percentage of normal cells carrying the same immunophenotype. In patients with acute myelogenous leukemia or acute lympho-cytic leukemia, leukemic cells can be distinguished from normal hematopoietic progeni-tors by their different aberrant antigen expression. This technique has an optimal sensitivity of 10^{-2}–10^{-4} and can also be used to identify leukemia blast colonies in vitro. Other techniques for sensitive or specific detection of minimal residual tumor or both include in vitro colony assays and cytogenetics. These methods continue to be investi-gated in larger patient groups with longer follow-up periods *(93)*.

In lymphoma, PCR amplification of tumor-specific chromosomal translocations such as t(14;18) provides a reproducible and highly sensitive technique for the detection of minimal residual tumor *(94)*. Therefore, PCR has largely superseded other methods, although it is, of course, applicable only to patients who have a PCR-amplifiable trans-location. In a series of 88 patients with advanced-stage low-grade lymphoma who were evaluated for evidence of bone marrow infiltration, PCR identification of minimal tumor added little to the morphologic assessment at the time of initial evaluation *(95)*. Bone marrow infiltration was detected morphologically in 73 of the 88 patients (83%). Bone marrow infiltration by PCR-detectable cells was found in 74 patients (84%), although the groups were not totally overlapping. Of interest, all patients with advanced-stage low-grade lymphoma and a PCR-amplifiable *bcl-2* translocation had evidence of bone mar-row involvement by PCR alone *(96)*.

In breast cancer, Cote et al. *(97)* used a monoclonal antibody to identify occult micrometastases in the bone marrow of 49 patients with operable (stage I and II) breast carcinoma. Follow-up (mean, 29 mo; median, 30 mo) revealed that disease recurred in 12 patients. The presence of bone marrow micrometastases (BMM) was significantly associated with early recurrence ($p < 0.04$). The estimated 2-yr recurrence rate for patients with no bone marrow micrometastases detected (BMM–) was 3%; in patients with BMMS, the 2-yr recurrence rate was 33%. When BMM and axillary lymph node (LN) status were combined, groups of patients at low risk (LN–, BMM–; 2-yr recurrence rate, 0%) and high risk (LN+, BMM+; 2-yr recurrence rate, 42%) for early recurrence were identified. Bone marrow tumor burden was related to early recurrence. Among patients with BMM, those whose disease did not recur had on average fewer extrinsic cells in their marrow than those whose disease recurred (15 vs 43 cells, respectively). Multivariate analysis comparing BMM, LN+ vs LN–, and tumor size (≤ 2 cm vs >2 cm) revealed that no factor was independently associated with early recurrence. Peripheral tumor burden of BMM (0 or <10 extrinsic cells vs >10 extrinsic cells) was the only independent predictor of early recurrence ($p < 0.003$). In conjunction with conventional prognostic factors, particularly axillary LN status, evaluation for BMM might be used to stratify patients for adjuvant treatment programs. Because this pilot study involved few patients with short-term follow-up, the results should be interpreted with caution. The examina-tion of BMM remains an experimental procedure; the clinical usefulness of the test remains to be established through larger studies with long-term follow-up *(97)*.

Combination chemotherapy can place most acute leukemia patients into remission; however, many of these patients will relapse *(98,99)*. At presentation, a patient may harbor up to 10^{12} leukemic cells, and after a 3-log kill from induction therapy, up to 10^9 leukemia cells may be present despite the appearance of morphologic remission. The limit of detection of cytogenetics is 10^8 leukemia cells for FISH is 10^7 leukemia cells, for flow cytometry it is 10^6 leukemia cells, and for PCR it is 10^4 leukemia cells *(98)*. Data concerning the clinical value of minimal residual disease detection is most highly developed in pediatric acute lymphoblastic leukemia. The most commonly used genetic markers in acute lymphoblastic leukemia are IgH, V-D-J, or T-cell receptor gene rearrangements. Nonetheless, progress in using this information to influence treatment options has been slow. Studies in pediatric acute lymphoblastic leukemia have shown that minimal residual disease after complete response is correlated with relapse *(100)*.

Chronic myelogenous leukemia is a clonal hematopoietic stem cell disorder characterized by the (9:22) translocation and resultant production of activated bcr-abl tyrosine kinase *(99)*. Assays using reverse transcriptase (RT) PCR to detect levels of bcr-abl transcripts are available to assess and differentiate response to therapy, to predict which patients will relapse, and to allow early detection. After allogenic stem cell transplantation, increasing levels of bcr-abl clearly predict relapse *(100)*. However, the persistence of bcr-abl does not necessarily predict relapse, provided that transcripts remain below a threshold level. Gleevec (STI 571), a bcr-abl tyrosine kinase inhibitor, has emerged as targeted therapy offering a hopeful new treatment for patients with chronic myelogenous leukemia *(99)*.

6. CONCLUSION

The importance of a minimal number of viable malignant cells to long-term survival has been recognized as a critically important issue by preclinical investigators from the outset of such studies. Preclinical studies have confirmed that very few malignant cells can survive treatment and proliferate to lethality *(101–105)*. Preclinical studies have also demonstrated that minimal tumor can be distributed very heterogeneously within the host. Preclinical models will continue to be of value in providing leads to detecting and testing new treatments to eradicate minimal malignant disease. Pepe et al. *(106)* have proposed a five-phase structure for the development of biomarkers for early detection and minimal residual disease detection of cancer *(106)*.

REFERENCES

1. Frei E III, Canellos GP. Dose, a critical factor in cancer chemotherapy. *Am J Med* 1980; 69:585–594.
2. Herzig G. Autologous marrow transplantation in cancer therapy. *Prog Hematol* 1981; 12:1–23.
3. Santos G, Tutschka P, Brookmeyer R. Marrow transplantation for acute nonlymphocytic leukemia after treatment with busulfan and cyclophosphamide. *N Engl J Med* 1983; 309:1347–1353.
4. Frei E III. Combined intensive alkylating agents with autologous bone marrow transplantation for metastatic solid tumors. In: Dicke K, Spitzer G, Zander A, eds. *Autologous Bone Marrow Transplantation: Proceedings of the First International Symposium.* Houston: The University of Texas M.D. Anderson Hospital and Tumor Institute at Houston. 1985:509–511.
5. Peters WP, Eder JP, Henner WD, et al. High-dose combination alkylating agents with autologous bone marrow support: a phase I trial. *J Clin Oncol* 1986; 4:646–654.
6. Antman K, Gale P. High dose chemotherapy and autotransplants for breast cancer. *Ann Inst Med* 1988; 108:570–574.
7. Frei E III, Antman K, Teicher B. Bone marrow autotransplantation for solid tumors—prospects. *J Clin Oncol* 1989; 7:515–526.
8. Frei E III. Curative cancer chemotherapy. *Cancer Res* 1985; 45:6523–6537.
9. Brugger W, Brossart P, Scheding S, et al. Approaches to dendritic cell-based immunotherapy after peripheral blood stem cell transplantation. *Ann NY Acad Sci* 1999; 872:363–371.
10. Thomas CM, Sweep CG. Serum tumor markers: past, state of the art, and future. *Int J Biol Markers* 2001; 16:73–86.

11. Zusman I, Ben-Hur H. Serological markers for detection of cancer. *Int J Mol Med* 2001; 7:547–556.

12. Hawk E, Viner JL, Lawrence JA. Biomarkers as surrogates for cancer development. *Curr Oncol Rep* 2000; 2:242–250.

13. Meyskens FL. Cancer population genetics and tumor prevention: an unfulfilled paradigm. *Eur J Cancer* 2000; 36:1189–1192.

14. Duffy MJ. Clinical uses of tumor markers: a critical review. *Crit Rev Clin Lab Sci* 2001; 38:225–262.

15. Wong IH, Lo YM, Johnson PJ. Epigenetic tumor markers in plasma and serum: biology and applications to molecular diagnosis and disease monitoring. *Ann NY Acad Sci* 2001; 945:36–50.

16. Von Knebel Doebertiz M, Weitz J, Koch M, Lacroix J, Schrodel A, Herfarth C. Molecular tools in the detection of micrometastatic cancer cells—technical aspects and clinical relevance. *Recent Results Cancer Res* 2001; 158:181–186.

17. Jones D, Fletcher CD. How shall we apply the new biology to diagnostics in surgical pathology? *J Pathol* 1999; 187:147–154.

18. Chambers G, Lawrie L, Cash P, Murray GI. Proteomics: a new approach to the study of disease. *J Pathol* 2000; 192:280–288.

19. Bartelink H, Begg AC, Martin JC, van Dijk M, Moonen L, Van't Veer LJ. Translational research offers individually tailored treatments for cancer patients. *Cancer J (Sci Am)* 2000; 6:2–10.

20. Ramachandran C, Melnick SJ. Multidrug resistance in human tumors—molecular diagnosis and clinical significance. *Mol Diagn* 1999; 4:81–94.

21. Schabel FM, Griswold DP, Laster WR, Corbett TH, Lloyd HH. Quantitative evaluation of anticancer agent activity in experimental animals. In: Satorelli AC, Creasey WA, Bertino JR, eds. *Pharmacology Therapy*. London: Pergamon. 1977:411–435.

22. Salsbury AJ. The significance of the circulating cancer cell. *Cancer Treat Rev* 1975; 2:55–72.

23. Crile G Jr, Isbister W, Deodhar SD. Lack of correlation between the presence of circulating tumor cells and the development of pulmonary metastases. *Cancer NY* 1971; 28:655–656.

24. Crile G Jr, Isbister W, Deodhar SD. Demonstration that large metastases in lymph nodes disseminate cancer cells to blood and lungs. *Cancer NY* 1971; 28:657.

25. Ketcham AS, Ryan JR, Wexler H. The shredding of viable circulating tumor cells by pulmonary metastases in mice. *Ann Surg* 1969; 169:297–299.

26. Wexler H, Ryan JR, Ketcham AS. The study of circulating tumor cells by the formation of pulmonary embolic tumor growths in a secondary host. *Cancer NY* 1969; 23:946–951.

27. Fidler IJ. Metastasis: quantiative analysis of distribution and fate of tumor emboli labeled with ^{125}I-5-Iodo-2'-deoxyuridine. *J Natl Cancer Inst* 1970; 45:773–782.

28. Skipper HE. The Ernst W. Bertner Memorial Award Lecture—some thoughts on rates and other things. In: Derwinko B, Humphrey RM, eds. *Growth Kinetics and Biochemical Regulation of Normal and Malignant Cells*. Baltimore, MD: Williams & Wilkins. 1977:11–19.

29. Skipper HE, Schabel FM Jr, Wilcox WS. Experimental evaluation of potential anticancer agents—XIII. On the criteria and kinetics associated with curability of experimental leukemia. *Cancer Chemother Rep* 1964; 15:1–111.

30. Schabel FM Jr. In vivo leukemic cell kill kinetics and "curability" in experimental systems. In: McCay J, Heideman C, eds. *Twenty-First Annual Symposium on Fundamental Cancer Research*. The University of Texas, M.D. Anderson Hospital and Tumor Institute at Houston. Baltimore: Williams & Wilkins. 1968:397–408.

31. Weiss L. Metastasis: differences between cancer cells in primary and secondary tumors. In: Ioachim HL, ed. *Pathobiology Annual 1980*. New York: Raven. 1980:51–81.

32. Weiss L, Holmes JC, Ward PM. Do metastases arise from pre-existing subpopulations of cancer cells? *Br J Cancer* 1983; 47:81–89.

33. Weiss L, Haydock K, Pickren JW, Lane WW. Organ vascularity and metastatic frequency. *Am J Pathol* 1980; 101:101–114.

34. Fidler IJ. Selection of successive tumor lines for metastasis. *Nature (New Biol)* 1973; 242:148–150.

35. Fidler IJ. The relationship of embolic homogeneity, number, size and viability to the incidence of experimental metastasis. *Eur J Cancer* 1973; 9:223–227.

36. Fidler IJ. Patterns of tumor cell arrest and development. In: Weiss L, Gilbert HA, eds. *Fundamental Aspects of Metastasis*. Amsterdam: North Holland. 1976:275–289.

37. Fidler IJ. The heterogeneity of metastatic neoplasma. In: Weiss L, Gilbert HA, eds. *Pulmonary Metastasis*. Boston: GK Hall.1978: 43–61.

38. Fidler IJ, Kripke ML. Metastasis results from pre-existing vacant cells within a malignant tumor. *Science* 1977; 197:893–895.

39. Weiss P. Some introductory remarks on the cellular basis of differentiation. *J Embryol Exp Morphol* 1953; 1:181–211.

40. Van Bekkum DW, Hagenbeek A. The relevance of the BN leukemia as a model for acute myelocytic leukemia. *Blood Cells* 1977; 3:565–579.

41. Hagenbeek A, Van Bekkum DW. Proceedings of an International Workshop on "Comparative evaluation of the L5222 and the BNML rat leukemia." *Leuk Res* 1977; 1:75–256.

42. Martens ACM, Van Bekkum DW, Hagenbeek A. The BN acute myelocytic leukemia (BNML). A rat model for acute myelocytic leukemia (AML). *Leukemia* 1990; 4:241–257.

43. Martens ACM, Van Bekkum DW, Hagenbeek A. Minimal residual disease in leukemia: studies in an animal model for acute myelocytic leukemia (AML). *Int J Cell Cloning* 1990; 8:27–38.

44. Martens ACM, Hagenbeek A. Detection of minimal disease in acute leukemia using flow cytometry: studies in a rat model for human acute leukemia. *Cytometry* 1985; 6:342–347.

45. Martens ACM, Schultz FW, Hagenbeek A. Nonhomogeneous distribution of leukemia in the bone marrow during minimal residual disease. *Blood* 1987; 70:1073–1078.

46. Yan Y, Marten ACM, de Groot CJ, Hendrik PJ, Valerio D, van Bekkum DW, Hagenbeek A. Retrovirus-mediated transfer and expression of marker genes in the BN rat acute myelocytic leukemia model for the study of minimal residual disease (MRD). *Leukemia* 1993; 7:131–139.

47. Martens ACM, de Groot CJ, Hagenbeek A. Development and characterization of a cyclophosphamide resistant variant of the BNML rat model for acute myelocytic leukemia. *Eur J Cancer* 191; 27:161–166.

48. El-Beltagi HM, Martens ACM, Haroun EA, Hagenbeek A. In vivo development of an acetyldinaline resistant subline of the BN rat acute myelocytic leukemia (BNML). *Leukemia* 1993; 7:1275–1280.

49. El-Beltagi HM, Martens ACM, Lelieveld P, Haroun EA, Hagenbeek A. Acetyldinaline: a new oral cytostatic drug with impressive differential activity against leukemic cells and normal stem cells—preclinical studies in a relevant rat model for human myelocytic leukemia. *Cancer Res* 1993; 53: 3008–3014.

50. El-Beltagi HM, Martens ACM, Dahab GM, Hagenbeek A. Efficacy of acetyldinaline for treatment of minimal residual disease (MRD): preclinical studies in the BNML rat model for human acute myelocytic leukemia. Leukemia 1993; 7:1795–1800.

51. Weiden PL, Flournoy N, Thomas ED. Antileukemic effect of graft-versus-host disease in human recipients of allogeneic-marrow grafts. *N Engl J Med* 1979; 800:1068.

52. Weiden PL, Sullivan KM, Flournoy N, Storb R, Thomas ED. Antileukemic effect of chronic graft-versus-host disease: contributions to improved survival after allogeneic marrow transplantation. *N Engl J Med* 1981; 304:1529.

53. Horowitz MM, Gale RP, Sondel PM. Graft-versus-leukemia reactions after bone marrow transplantation. *Blood* 1990; 75:555.

54. Slavin S, Strober S. Spontaneous murine B-cell leukemia. *Nature* 1978; 272:624–626.

55. Slavin S, Weiss L, Morrecki S, et al. B-cell leukemia (BCL1), a murine model of chronic lymphocytic leukemia. Ultra-structural, cell emmbrane and cytogenetic characteristics. *Cancer Res* 1981; 41: 4162–4166.

56. Slavin S, Weiss L, Morecki S, Weigensberg M. Eradication of murine leukemia with histoincompatible marrow grafts in mice conditioned with total lymphoid irradiation (TLI). *Cancer Immunol Immunother* 1918; 11:155.

57. Weiss L, Morecki S, Vitetta ES, Slavin S. Supression and elimination of BCL1 leukemia by allogeneic bone marrow transplantation. *J Immunol* 1981; 130:2452.

58. Weiss L, Reich S, Slavin S. Use of recombinant human interleukin-2 in conjunction with bone marrow transplantation as a model for control of minimal residual disease in malignant hematological disorders: treatment of murine leukemia in conjunction with allogeneic bone marrow transplantation and IL-2-activated cell-mediated immunotherapy. *Cancer Invest* 1992; 10:19–26.

59. Uckun FM, Sensel MG. SCID mouse model of human leukemia and lymphoma as tools for new agent development. In: Teicher BA, ed. *Tumor Models in Cancer Research.* Totowa, NJ: Humana. 2001: 521–540.

60. Ballard SG, Ward DC. Fluorescence in situ hybridization using digital imaging microscopy. *J Histochem Cytochem* 1993; 41:1755–1759.

61. Lichter P, Boyle AL, Cremer T, Ward DC. Analyses of genes and chromosomes by non-iso-topic in situ hybridization. *Genet Anal Technol Appl* 191; 8:24.

62. Poddighe PJR, Ramaekers ECS, Hopman ANH. Interphase cytogenetics of tumors. *J Pathol* 1992; 166:215.

63. Gray JW, Pinkel D. Molecular cytogenetics in human cancer diagnosis. *Cancer* 1992; 69(suppl):1536.

64. Matera AG, Ward DC. Oligonucleotide probes for the analysis of specific DNA sequences by fluorescence in situ hybridization. *Hum Mol Genet* 1992; 1:535.

65. Ried T, Baldini A, Rand T, Ward DC. Simultaneous visualization of seven different DNA probes by in situ hybridization using combinatorial fluorescence and digital imaging microscopy. *Proc Natl Acad Sci USA* 1992; 89:1388.

66. Ried T, Landes G, Dackowski W, Klinger K, Ward DC. Multicolor fluorescence in situ hybridization for the simultaneous detection of probe sets for chromosome 13, 18, 21 X and Y in uncultured amniotic fluid cells. *Hum Mol Genet* 1992; 1:307.

67. Matera AG, Ward DC. Nucleoplasmic organization of small nuclear ribonucleoproteins in cultured human cells. *J Cell Biol* 1993; 121:715.

68. Ried T, Baldini A, Rand TC, Ward DC. Simultaneous visualization of seven different DNA probes by in situ hybridization using combinatorial fluorescence and digital imaging microscopy. *Proc Natl Acad Sci USA* 1992; 89:1388–1392.

69. Brandt-Rauf PW, Pincus MR. Molecular markers of carcinogenesis. *Pharmacol Ther* 1998; 77:135–148.

70. Maxwell P. Carcinoembryonic antigen: cell adhesion molecule and useful diagnostic marker. *Br J Biomed Sci* 1999; 56:209–214.

71. Schneider DT, Calaminus G, Gobel U. Diagnostic value of alpha 1-fetoprotein and beta-human chorionic gonadotropin in infancy and childhood. *Pediatr Hematol Oncol* 2001; 18:11–26.

72. Wells CA, Heryet A, Brochier J, Gatter KC, Mason DY. The immunocytochemical detection of axillary micrometastases in breast cancer. *Br J Cancer* 1984; 50:193–197.

73. Ghosh AK, Mason DY, Spriggs AJ. Immunocytochemical staining with monoclonal antibodies in cytologically 'negative' serous effusions from patients with malignant disease. *J Clin Pathol* 1983; 36:1150–1153.

74. Ghosh AK, Erben WN, Hatton CS, et al. Detection of metastatic tumour cells in routine bone marrow smears by immuno-alkaline phosphatase labeling with monoclonal antibodies. *Br J Hematology* 1985; 61:21–30.

75. Schlimok G, Funke I, Holzmann B, et al. Micrometastatic cancer cells in bone marrow: in vitro detection with anti-cytokeratin and in vivo labeling with anti-17-1A monoclonal antibodies. *Proc Natl Acad Sci USA* 1987; 84:8672–8676.

76. Johnston CS, Shpall EJ, Williams S, et al. Detection of minimal residual breast cancer in bone marrow. In: Worthington-White D, Gee A, Gross S, eds. *Advances in Bone Marrow Purging and Processing*. New York: Wiley-Liss. 1992:637–642.

77. Calvo BF, Semelka RC. Beyond anatomy: MR imaging as a molecular diagnostic tool. *Surg Oncol Clin N Am* 1999; 8:171–183.

78. Ahrendt SA, Sidransky D. The potential of molecular screening. *Surg Oncol Clin N Am* 1999; 8:641–656.

79. Russo A, Zanna I, Tubiolo C, et al. Hereditary common cancers: molecular and clinical genetics. *Anticancer Res* 2000; 20:4841–4851.

80. Weinstein JN. Searching for pharmacogenomic markers: the synergy between omic and hypothesis-driven research. *Dis Markers* 2001; 17:77–88,.

81. Truitt RL, Atasoylu AA. Impact of pretransplant conditioning and donor T cells on chimerism, graft-versus-host disease, graft-versus-leukemia reactivity and tolerance after bone marrow transplantation. *Blood* 1991; 77:2515.

82. Weiss L, Morecki S, Viettta ES, Slavin S. Suppression and elimination of BCL1 leukemia by allogeneic bone marrow transplnatation. *J Immunol* 1983; 130:2452.

83. Drobyski WR, Baxter-Lowe LA, Truitt RL. Detection of residual leukemia by the polymerase chain rection and sequence-specific oligonucelotide probe hybridization after allogeneic bone marrow transplantation for AKR leukemia: a murine model for minimal residual disease. *Blood* 1993; 81: 551–559.

84. Pugatsch T, Weiss L, Slavin S. Minimal residual disease in murine B-cell leukemia (BCL1) detected by PCR. *Leuk Res* 1993; 17:999–1002.

85. Slavin S, Eckerstein A, Weiss L. Adoptive immunotherapy in conjunction with bone marrow transplantation—amplification of natural host defense mechanisms against cancer by recombinant IL-2. *Nat Immun Cell Growth Regul* 1988; 7:180–184.

86. Slavin S, Ackerstein A, Kedar E, Weiss L. IL-2 activated cell mediated immunotherapy: control of minimal residual disease in malignant disorders by allogeneic lymphocytes and IL-2. *Bone Marrow Transplant* 1990; 6:86–90.

87. Fleischhacker M, Beinert T. Tumor markers—new aspects of an old discussion? *Eur J Med Res* 1999; 4:144–148.

88. Raj GV, Moreno JG, Gomella LG. Utilization of polymerase chain reaction technology in the detection of solid tumors. *Cancer* 1998; 82:1419–1442.

89. Knapp MR, Jones PP, Black J, Vitteta ES, Slavin S, Strober S. Characterization of a spontaneous murine B cell luekemia (BCL-1). Cell surface expression of IgM, IgD, Ia and FeR. *J Immunol* 1979; 123:992.

90. Strober S, Gronowicz ES, Knapp MR, et al. Immunobiology of a spontaneous murine B cell leukemia (BCL-1) *Immun Rev* 1979; 48:169.

91. Wranke RA, Slavin S, Cofman RL, et al. The pathology and homing of a transplantable murine B cell leukemia (BCL-1). *Immunology* 1979; 123:1181.

92. Prindull G, Ben-Ishay Z, Bergholz M, Prindull B. Minimal residual disease in vitro for a pre-B-lymphoma. *Leuk Res* 1993; 17:579–584.

93. Wormann B. Implications of detection of minimal residual disease. *Curr Opin Oncol* 1993; 5:3–12.

94. Gribben JG, Nadler LM. Monitoring minimal residual disease. *Semin Oncol* 1993; 20:143–155.

95. Gribben JG, Freedman AF, Woo SD. All advanced stage non-Hodgkin's lymphomas with a polymerase chain reaction amplifiable bcl-2 translocation have residual cells containing the bcl-2 rearrangement at evaluation and following treatment. *Blood* 1991; 78:3275–3280.

96. Favrot MC, Herve P. Detection of minimal malignant cell infiltration in the bone marrow of patients with solid tumors, non-Hodgkin's lymphomas and leukemias. *Bone Marrow Transplant* 1987; 2:117–122.

97. Cote RJ, Rosen PP, Lesser ML, Old LJ, Osborne MP. Prediction of early relapse in patients with operable breast cancer by detection of occult bone marrow micrometastases. *J Clin Oncol* 1991; 9:1749–1756.

98. Radich JD. Clinical applicability of the evaluation of minimal residual disease in acute leukemia. *Curr Opin Oncol* 2000; 12:36–40.

99. Mauro MJ, Druker BJ. Chronic myelogenous leukemia. *Curr Opin Oncol* 2001; 13:3–7.

100. Radich JP, Gehly G, Gooley T, et al. Polymerase chain reaction detection of the BCR-ABL fusion transcript after allogeneic marrow transplantation for chronic myeloid leukemia: results and implications in 346 patients. *Blood* 1995; 85:224–228.

101. Furth J, Kahn MC. The transmission of leukemia of mice with a single cell. *Am J Cancer* 1937; 31:276–282.

102. Schabel FM Jr. Concept and practice of total tumor cell kill. In: Clark RL, Cumley RW, McCay JE, Copeland MM, eds. *Oncology 1970, Proceedings of the Tenth International Cancer Congress.* Chicago: Yearbook Medical Publishers. 1970:35–45.

103. Ishibashi K. Studies on the number of cells necessary for the transplantation of Yoshida sarcoma. *Gann* 1950; 41:1–14.

104. Sharlikova LF, Min U. Preparation of clonal (tumor derived from single cell) Jensen's sarcoma. *Bull Eksp Biol Med* 1961; 3:85–88.

105. Sharlikova LF, Min U. Preparation of clonal ascitical sarcoma 37 in mice. *Vop Onkol* 1964; 10:110–111.

106. Pepe MS, Etzioni R, Feng Z, et al. Phases of biomarker development for early detection of cancer. *J Natl Cancer Inst* 2001; 93:1054–1061.

12 Spontaneously Occurring Tumors in Companion Animals As Models for Drug Development

David M. Vail, DVM
and Douglas H. Thamm, VMD

CONTENTS

INTRODUCTION
ADVANTAGES OF COMPANION ANIMAL MODELS
INCIDENCE OF TUMORS IN COMPANION ANIMALS
RESOURCES FOR PRECLINICAL STUDY
CANINE NHL
FELINE NHL
SOFT TISSUE SARCOMAS
HEMANGIOSARCOMA
CANINE OSTEOSARCOMA
CANINE MAMMARY TUMORS
FELINE MAMMARY CARCINOMA
CANINE ORAL MELANOMA
CANINE URINARY BLADDER CARCINOMA

1. INTRODUCTION

The use of animals for the preclinical study of cancer therapeutics has a long history, and important information has been gained regarding new and innovative therapies. Most of this work has been performed on inbred rodent models and laboratory-derived canine populations. Working with inbred populations in controlled, artificial laboratory environments raises some degree of concern over the applicability of information as it relates to naturally occurring tumors in people. Many of these concerns may be allayed through the study of naturally occurring tumors in our companion animal population, (i.e., dog and cat pet population). Companion animals with naturally occurring tumors, although

From: *Cancer Drug Discovery and Development:*
Anticancer Drug Development Guide: Preclinical Screening, Clinical Trials, and Approval, 2nd Ed.
Edited by: B. A. Teicher and P. A. Andrews © Humana Press Inc., Totowa, NJ

presently underutilized, have and should continue to provide an excellent opportunity to investigate many aspects of malignancy from etiology to treatment.

2. ADVANTAGES OF COMPANION ANIMAL MODELS

Several aspects of companion animal disease make for attractive comparative models. Companion animals share a common environment with people and represent a more natural outbred population. Exposure to environmental carcinogens should, therefore, be similar to that in people. In support of this, evidence exists that environmental factors may play a role in the development of canine nasal tumors (1), bladder tumors (2), and lymphoma (3–5), and asbestos exposure has been associated with the development of canine mesothelioma (6). Malignancies in companion animals develop spontaneously, whereas experimental laboratory models utilize induced tumors either through exposure to known carcinogens or from transplantation, often in the presence of artificially induced immunologic modification.

Incidence rates for certain malignancies in companion animals (e.g., canine osteosarcoma, non-Hodgkin's lymphoma [NHL]) are higher than those observed in people, providing a large population for study. Conversely, certain other neoplasms, such as hemangiosarcoma (angiosarcoma) and mast cell neoplasia, are extremely rare in humans but abundant in companion animals, allowing meaningful clinical data to be generated in tumor types with "orphan" status in humans (7–9). Tumors in companion animals generally progress at a more rapid rate than their human counterparts. This time-course is both long enough to allow comparison of response durations, but short enough to ensure rapid accrual of data. Companion animal cancers more closely resemble human cancers than rodent models in terms of size, cell kinetics, and biologic variables such as hypoxia and clonal variation (10–12). By virtue of their body size, sample collection (i.e., serum, urine, cerebrospinal fluid, multiple tissue samples), surgical interventions, imaging, and novel drug delivery systems are more readily applied than in rodent models. This is illustrated by our recent work with inhalational drug delivery development using dogs with spontaneous primary and metastatic tumors (13,14).

In addition, an expanding animal rights movement is making investigations with laboratory animals more difficult. Provided that well-designed, humane guidelines are adhered to, clinical trials involving companion animals may be more acceptable. Because the standard of care is not established for many tumors encountered in the veterinary profession, more latitude in prospective clinical trials is allowable, and it is easier and morally acceptable to attempt new and innovative treatment strategies. Importantly, such latitude should not be abused, and present-day veterinary institutions consistently use informed client consent and institutional review boards to ensure that study design and ethical standards are maintained.

In general, clinical trials using veterinary patients can be completed at significantly less expense than similar human clinical trials. Professional services, clinical pathology, and diagnostic imaging, although of the highest quality, are of lower cost in comparison.

Finally, experience with veterinary clientele provides further evidence for the companion animal as a model. Most companion animal caregivers are highly committed and are actively seeking innovative and promising new therapies for their companion's cancer. As a whole, either through personal experience with family members and friends, or media coverage of available and leading-edge therapy, they demand the highest quality

Table 1
Comparative Annual Incidence Rates (per 100,000)
for Common Sites or Types of Cancer
in Dogs, Cats, and Humans

Site/type	Dog	Cat	Human
Oral	20.4	—	11.6
Skin	90.4	34.7	5.2
Connective tissue	35.8	17.0	2.5
Testes	33.9	—	4.7
Melanoma	25	—	12.6
Mammary	198.8	25.4	108.8
Bone	7.9	4.9	1.0
Non-Hodgkin's lymphoma	25	125	16.6
Leukemia	—	35.6	13.3

Data from ref. 9.

of care. Most are gratified by honest and aggressive attempts at cure or palliation, and the potential for improving our ability to treat cancer in other companion animals and people is seen as an additional benefit by many. Compliance with treatment and recheck visits is exceptional, and autopsy compliance approaches 85%, significantly better than most human clinical trials.

3. INCIDENCE OF TUMORS IN COMPANION ANIMALS

Over half of all households in the United States include a companion animal, representing about 55 million dogs and 60 million cats at risk for developing cancers (15). Being resistant to atherosclerosis-associated cardiovascular disease, cancer is the number one cause of death overall in dogs. In a necropsy series of 2000 dogs, 23% of all dogs, regardless of age, and 45% of dogs 10 yr of age or older died of cancer. Estimates of age-adjusted overall cancer incidence rates per 100,000 individuals/years at risk range from 243 to 381 for dogs and 156 to 264 for cats (16). These rates are comparable to those reported by the National Cancer Institute Surveillance, Epidemiology, and End Results (SEER) program for human beings (approx 300 per 100,000).

Cancer rates for dogs and cats based on site are illustrated In Table 1 (7–9,17). Rates for some tumor types such as canine osteosarcoma, canine soft tissue sarcomas, and feline NHL are significantly higher than those of humans, and their relative abundance increases their model potential.

4. RESOURCES FOR PRECLINICAL STUDY

4.1. Cell Lines

Myriad canine and feline tumor cell lines are available for preclinical in vitro and xenograft studies in preparation for clinical investigations. Although relatively few are available through commercial suppliers such as the American Type Culture Collection (ATCC), many are available through individual investigators. Canine lines include B-cell and T-cell lymphoma/leukemia (18–20), hemangiosarcoma (21), osteosarcoma (22,23), mammary carcinoma *(24,25)*, melanoma *(26–28)*, and bladder carcinoma *(29)*, among many others. Available feline lines include squamous cell carcinoma *(30)*, mammary carcinoma *(25)*, soft tissue sarcoma *(31)*, and lymphoma *(32,33)*.

4.2. In Vivo Assessment

Although canine- and feline-specific reagents are not as abundant as those for humans and rodents, a variety of tools are available for the in vivo assessment of therapeutic response in companion animal tumors. Studies evaluating tumor hypoxia *(11,34–39)*, perfusion *(39–41)*, angiogenesis *(42–46)*, apoptosis *(43,45,47–51)*, and immune cell immunophenotype *(52,53)* have all been performed successfully in tumor-bearing dogs and cats.

4.3. Etiopathogenesis/Biology

Companion animal and human tumors share a great deal in terms of etiopathogenesis and biology. Mutations in many oncogenes and tumor suppressor genes commonly mutated in human cancer, such as *p53 (51,54–62)*, *rB (56)*, *Ras (27,63–65)*, *Myc (27,54)*, and *bcl-2 (48,49)* have been detected in a variety of canine and feline tumors *(66,67)*. Likewise, overexpression of telomerase *(47,68–70)* and matrix metalloproteinases *(23,71–73)* have been detected in various canine tumors.

A variety of tyrosine kinase growth factors and receptors have been detected in canine and feline tumors, and thus they may serve as excellent models for the preclinical development of small-molecule inhibitors of these growth factors. For example, human growth factor (HGF), insulin-like growth factor-1 (IGF-1), and their respective receptors have been detected in the majority of canine osteosarcomas *(74–76)*. Expression of *c-erbB2* has been detected in canine melanoma and mammary tumors *(24,27,59,77)*. A large number of canine malignant mast cell tumors (MCTs) display aberrant expression of *c-kit*, the receptor for stem cell factor, and many canine MCTs have mutations in *c-kit* that confer constitutive activation of the receptor in the absence of ligand binding *(78–80)*. Indeed, in vitro ligand activation and tumor cell growth can be inhibited in canine MCT cell lines using novel split-tyrosine kinase inhibitors *(81)*. Expression of platelet-derived growth factor (PDGF) receptor has been detected in the majority of feline vaccine-associated sarcomas (VAS), and our laboratory has shown that the drug Gleevec® (STI571: Novartis) is capable of potently inhibiting the PDGF-stimulated growth of feline VAS cells in vitro and of inhibiting VAS xenograft growth as well *(31)*.

Analogs of most major angiogenic growth factors and their receptors exist in dogs and cats, and elevations in serum or urine vascular endothelial growth factor (VEGF) and/or basic fibroblast growth factor (bFGF) have been detected in canine hemangiosarcoma (HSA) *(82,83)*, transitional cell carcinoma of the urinary bladder *(43,84)*, and osteosarcoma *(85)*. Finally, canine and feline tumors may share important tumor-associated antigens with human tumors. For example, our laboratory and others have detected the expression of canine analogs of gp100, melanoma common tumor antigen MART-1, and tyrosinase in the majority of canine melanomas *(28,86,87)*, and immunotherapeutic strategies designed to target canine gp100 have shown promise in early clinical trials in dogs *(86)*.

The intent of the remainder of this chapter is to provide the reader with a basic understanding of the biology of tumor types occurring most frequently in companion animal

Table 2
World Health Organization Clinical Staging
for Domestic Animals With Lymphoma

Stage	Involvement
I	Single lymph node
II	Multiple lymph nodes in a regional area
III	Generalized lymphadenopathy
IV	Liver and/or spleen (with or without stage II)
V	Bone marrow or blood
Substage	
a	Without clinical signs of disease
b	With clinical signs of disease

species and their perceived model potential. Examples of individual tumor types currently utilized as models for therapy development are presented where applicable.

5. CANINE NHL

5.1. Incidence, Signalment, and Etiology

NHL in the dog is commonly encountered in veterinary practice. It has an annual incidence rate of 25/100,000 and accounts for 5% of all malignant neoplasms and 83% of all hematopoietic malignancies in the species (88–90). Middle-aged to older dogs are affected, with no sex predilection known. Although it may occur in any breed, it may be more prevalent in German shepherds, boxers, poodles, basset hounds, golden retrievers and Saint Bernards. The etiology of canine lymphoma is unknown. A retroviral etiology for certain forms of NHL has been documented in cats, chickens, cattle, and humans. However, it has not been confirmed in the dog.

5.2. Classification and Prognosis

Canine NHL can be classified clinically according to anatomic site and the World Health Organization clinical staging system for domestic animals (91) (Table 2), and histologically according to the Working Formulation (92). Relative frequencies of histologic types for canine NHL are presented in Table 3. In general, canine NHL equates to intermediate and high-grade, advanced-stage (III or higher) NHL in people (93–96). Approximately 80–85% of NHL in dogs is of B-cell origin, and the T-cell (CD3+) immunophenotype is associated with a significantly worse prognosis (95,96). Null (neither B or T) cell lineage lymphoma also occurs in low frequency in dogs. Other known negative prognostic factors in dogs with NHL include clinical stage V, anatomic location, presence of symptoms (substage b), aneuploidy, and possibly male sex (93–99). We have evaluated tumor cell proliferation indices, including potential doubling time (T_{pot}), argyrophilic nucleolar organizing region (AgNOR) frequency, and proliferating cell nuclear antigen labeling index (PCNA-LI) as prognostic factors in canine NHL (12). Both T_{pot} and AgNOR frequency were found to be predictors of chemotherapy response in the canine NHL model. T_{pot} values ranging from 0.84 to 28.05 d with a mean of 5.01 and median of 3.3 d for canine NHL are similar to those reported for high-grade NHL from

Table 3
Canine Lymphomas Classified by the Working Formulation

		Percent		
Grade	Category	Greenlee et al. (95) (n = 176)	Carter et al. (94) (n = 285)	Teske et al. (96) (n = 116)
Low	Small lymphocytic	11.0	5.3	16.3
	Follicular small cleaved	10.0	49.	—
	Follicular small cleaved	—	—	12.0
	Follicular mixed small cleaved	1.0	0.4	4.3
Immediate	Follicular large cell	59.9	28.4	74.6
	Diffuse small cleaved cell	3.4	0.4	31.0
	Diffuse mixed small and large	3.4	5.9	8.6
	Diffuse mixed small and large	5.1	2.1	5.0
	Diffuse large cell	48.0	20.0	30.0
High	Diffuse immunoblastic	29.4	66.3	6.0
	Diffuse lymphoblastic	25.6	24.9	6.0
	Diffuse lymphoblastic	0.6	17.2	—
	Diffuse small noncleaved	3.2	24.2	—

264

humans *(100)*. PCNA-LI and AgNOR frequencies found in the canine NHL population were also similar to levels reported for intermediate and high-grade NHL in humans *(54,101–105)*. This serves to reinforce the application of human histologic categories to the dog and strengthens the model potential of this species for intermediate- and high-grade NHL.

5.3. Treatment

Without therapy, most dogs with lymphoma succumb to their disease within 4–6 wk following diagnosis *(106)*. Canine NHL is similar to human NHL with respect to chemo-therapeutic drug sensitivity. The most effective chemotherapeutics to date against canine NHL include doxorubicin, cyclophosphamide, the vinca alkaloids, L-asparaginase, and corticosteroids. Most veterinary protocols involve the use of multiple drugs used in alternating combinations and result in reported response rates of 86–91%, with median first remission duration and survival times of approx 200 and 300 d respectively *(98,107,108)*. Most dogs eventually succumb to recurrence of increasingly chemotherapy-resistant NHL. Multidrug resistance (MDR) induction has been reported in canine lymphoma following exposure to chemotherapy *(109–111)*. Recently, a study of expression levels of mRNA encoding the canine *MDR1* gene was performed in canine cell lines and lymphomas *(111)*. Additionally, apoptosis (programmed cell death) can be altered in tumor cells, leading to resistance. Indeed, alterations in *p53*, a gene intimately involved in the regulation of apoptosis, has been shown to occur in various canine tumors, including lymphoma *(60,112)*.

5.4. Model Relevance

Several advantages exist for the use of a canine model of NHL. It is a common spon-taneous tumor not associated with viral infection and is, therefore, similar to most human NHLs. It is one of the most chemoresponsive neoplasms in the dog, with remission and survival times long enough to allow comparison of response times, but short enough to ensure rapid accrual of data. It represents a relatively homogenous population with respect to histologic type (i.e., 85% are medium- to high-grade B-cell NHLs). However, as in humans, there is wide prognostic heterogeneity within the group. Canine NHL appears to be a relevant model for preclinical testing of new chemotherapeutics, either for initial induction or rescue of multiple drug resistance *(113,114)*. Canine NHL has been used successfully as a model for development of hypoxic cell markers as well as the effect of whole-body hyperthermia on the pharmacokinetics of systemic chemotherapy *(35,115)*. Canine NHL has also been a particularly good model for the study of autologous bone marrow transplantation *(116,117)*.

6. FELINE NHL

6.1. Incidence, Signalment, and Etiology

NHL is the most common malignancy in the cat, accounting for approx one-third of all tumors in this species, with an incidence rate of 125/100,000 *(118)*. Feline NHL is unlike its canine counterpart in that approx 25% are composed of T cells transformed by the retrovirus feline leukemia virus (FeLV) *(119,120)*. Prior to the routine availability of commercially available FeLV vaccines, FeLV was causally associated with 70% of lymphomas in this species *(121,122)*. Since the mid-1980s, however, FeLV has been causally associated with only approx 10–20% of lymphomas, presumably owing to the availability of the vaccine *(123,124)*. There is mounting evidence that the feline immunodeficiency virus (FIV) infection increases the incidence of lymphomas. FIV has been associated with lymphoma in the kidney, liver, and intestinal tract *(125,126)*.

6.2. Classification

Approximately 90% of NHLs in cats are classified as intermediate- or high-grade by the Working Formulation *(127)*. Prevalence of anatomic forms in cats varies with geographic location, but overall, the alimentary form is the most common, followed by multicentric, thymic, nasal, renal, leukemic, and miscellaneous extranodal forms *(128)*.

6.3. Treatment

As in the dog, feline NHL is initially quite chemoresponsive. In 103 cats treated with sequential combination chemotherapy, initial complete remission rates of 62% were observed, with a median survival time (MST) of 7 mo and one-third of cats surviving for 1 yr or more *(123,129)*. Although FeLV status does not appear to affect initial response rates, active viremia is associated with significantly shorter survival.

6.4. Model Relevance

The prevalence of NHL in cats and its documented retroviral association suggest that feline NHL may have relevant potential as a model for HIV-associated lymphoma in people.

7. SOFT TISSUE SARCOMAS

7.1. Incidence, Signalment, and Etiology

Soft tissue sarcomas (STS) comprise 15% of all subcutaneous cancers in the dog and 7% in the cat *(130)*. Annual incidence rates are 35 and 17/100,000 dogs and cats at risk, respectively *(8)*. With few exceptions, the etiology is unknown for the more common STS. A multicentric form of fibrosarcoma (FSA) has been associated in young cats with the feline sarcoma virus (FeSV) *(118)*. This replication-defective acute transforming virus requires cotransfection with FeLV in order to acquire, through recombination, replication ability. A possible vaccine-induced STS has also been reported in the cat and is referred to as feline vaccine-associated sarcoma (VAS) *(131–134)*. Most of these postvaccinal sarcomas are fibrosarcomas, and the annual incidence rate is estimated to be 2/10,000 vaccinated cats. An association with aluminum hydroxide or aluminum phosphate vaccine adjuvants has been suggested in their pathogenesis *(132)*. In a sampling of 40 VAS, immunohistochemical detection of *p53* mutations were detected in about 60% of samples *(57)*. In the dog, STS have been associated with radiation, trauma, and parasitic infiltration (*Spirocerca lupi*) *(135,136)*.

7.2. Classification

STS represent a diverse group of tumors derived from a variety of mesenchymal tissues (Table 4). With the exception of hemangiosarcoma (covered in the next section),

Table 4
Soft Tissue Sarcomas Identified in Dogs and Cats

Tissue of origin[a]	Benign	Malignant[a]	Metastatic potential[b]
Fibrous and histiocyte		Fibrous histiocytoma	+
Fibrous tissue	Fibroma	Fibrosarcoma	+/++
Myxomatous tissue	Myxoma	Myxosarcoma+/++	
Pericyte of blood vessel (unproven)		Hemangiopericytoma	+
Vessels	Lymphangioma	Lymphangiosarcoma	++
	Hemangioma	Hemangiosarcoma	+++
Adipose tissue	Lipoma	Liposarcoma	++
Nerve		Neurofibrosarcoma	+
		Malignant schwannoma	+
Smooth muscle	Leiomyoma	Leiomyosarcoma	+
Synovial cell	Synovial cyst/synovioma	Synovial cell sarcoma	++
Skeletal muscle	Rhabdomyoma	Rhabdomyosarcoma	++
Miscellaneous	—	Granular cell tumor	+
		Mesenchymoma	+

[a]Some neoplasms are so primitive and anaplastic that they can only be classified as undifferentiated sarcoma or undifferentiated spindle cell sarcoma.
[b]+, low; ++, moderate; +++, high.

267

the STS are locally aggressive tumors with low to moderate metastatic potential. Local recurrence, therefore, is the most clinically significant obstacle to overcome.

7.3. Treatment

STS in companion animals can serve as relevant models for therapeutic approaches, since these tumors tend to respond to radiation and/or chemotherapy in a way that is similar to that of human STS. The majority of STS in companion animals are treated with local surgical resection (137–139). If surgical margins are incomplete, adjuvant radiotherapy often provides long-term control (140–142). STS in companion animals, as in people, are only moderately responsive to available chemotherapeutics.

7.4. Model Relevance

The model relevance of spontaneously arising canine STS has not escaped cancer researchers. They have served as models for development of local and whole-body hyperthermia techniques, as well as pharmacologic manipulation of hyperthermia with vasoactive drugs (e.g., hydralazine, nitroprusside) (143–147). Canine STS have also served as models for the study of the effects of hyperthermia on the pharmacokinetics of chemotherapy (148), development of hypoxic cell markers (11,34–36,38) and cancer imaging techniques (149,150). Additionally, feline VAS has potential to provide information regarding carcinogenesis and genetic susceptibility (131).

8. HEMANGIOSARCOMA

8.1. Overview

Also known as malignant hemangioendothelioma or angiosarcoma (AS), hemangiosarcoma (HAS), a highly aggressive tumor, occurs much more frequently in dogs than in other species. The infrequency of AS in humans makes meaningful clinical trials impossible; however, novel treatments with direct relevance to human AS can be evaluated readily in a large population of dogs with disease that strongly resembles its human homolog. The German shepherd breed is reported to have the highest risk (9). In the dog, as in humans, common primary sites include the spleen, liver, right atrium, skin, and subcutaneous sites (151–154). As in humans, an actinic etiology is proposed for HSA arising in the cutis of light, short-haired breeds (155). HSA tends to metastasize rapidly (except from the primary dermal site), to liver, lung, omentum, kidney, and brain. The MST with surgery alone in dogs with visceral HSA is 2–3 mo, with less than 10% surviving for 1 yr (152,156).

8.2. Treatment and Experimental Therapeutics

Treatment of canine HSA with surgery and adjuvant doxorubicin (DOX)-based chemotherapy (DOX-cyclophosphamide [CTX] or DOX-CTX-vincristine) yields MSTs of 4–6 mo, with less than 10% 1-yr survival (157,158). We recently completed a placebo-controlled study in 32 dogs with splenic HSA without detectable metastatic disease, treated with splenectomy and DOX-CTX chemotherapy and randomized to receive liposome muramyl tripeptide-phosphatidylethanolamine (L-MTP-PE) or placebo liposomes (159). Liposome MTP-PE is a potent monocyte/macrophage activator that has demonstrated antitumor activity in a number of rodent models (160,161). Liposome encapsulation facilitates delivery of MTP to monocytes and macrophages, enhances their activation, and prolongs circulating half-life. The MST in the L-placebo group was 4.7 mo, and the L-MTP-PE group had an MST of 9.3 mo ($p < 0.03$), with 40% of dogs alive at 1 yr. This study confirms the activity of L-MTP-PE in another relevant tumor type and shows that it can be administered concurrently with chemotherapy without a loss of therapeutic activity. Canine HSA is thus a tumor type amenable to immunotherapeutic approaches, as it appears to be in humans (162).

Recently, we completed a randomized trial in dogs with splenic HSA evaluating the efficacy of DOX delivered by a pulmonary route, in conjunction with systemic DOX-based chemotherapy. Dogs with micrometastatic splenic HSA receiving DOX-CTX intravenously plus inhaled DOX once every 3 wk had median survivals of 8 mo compared with 4 mo for dogs receiving DOX-CTX by the intravenous route alone (163).

As a tumor derived from vascular endothelium, HSA may represent the most extreme example of dysregulated angiogenesis. Strategies designed to target angiogenesis may have an exceptional role in diseases such as HSA and other vascular neoplasms, targeting not only the blood supply but the tumor cells as well (82). Canine HSA may serve as an excellent preclinical model for the evaluation of such strategies. Our laboratory has demonstrated the expression of mRNA and/or protein for canine bFGF, VEGF, angiopoietin-2, and their respective receptors in most canine HSA (21). The coexpression of these angiogenic growth factors and their receptors suggests putative autocrine stimulation, as is proposed in many human vascular malignancies, and thus canine HSA may be a useful model for the study of inhibitors of angiogenic growth factor signaling. A recent trial evaluated the efficacy of minocycline, an inhibitor of matrix metalloproteinase activity, used in conjunction with DOX-CTX chemotherapy, in dogs with HSA. No meaningful survival advantage was obvious in this single-arm study (164).

9. CANINE OSTEOSARCOMA

9.1. Overview

Osteosarcoma (OSA) in dogs closely resembles OSA in people (15,165,166). A comparison of human OSA and canine OSA is presented in Table 5. Canine OSA is a spontaneous tumor of outbred large breed dogs. These tumors are histologically indistinguishable from those in people. The vast majority are high-grade tumors and present with extracompartmental (stage IIB) disease. The only known prognostic factor identified for dogs with OSA is the presence of elevated serum alkaline phosphatase at diagnosis and the absence of normalization of alkaline phosphatase following amputation (167–169). Although there is a difference in incidence based on breed, there is no evidence that the biologic behavior is altered with regard to breed (166).

Dogs treated with amputation alone survive for a median of 3–4 mo, with death commonly caused by lung metastasis. Only 10% of the dogs treated with surgery alone survive for 1 yr (170,171). Adjuvant chemotherapy using cisplatin, doxorubicin, or carboplatin results in MSTs of 9–11 mo (172–174). However, 80% are dead of metastasis by 24 mo following chemotherapy.

9.2. L-MTP-PE Immunotherapy

Over 150 dogs with OSA have been entered into various studies using the immunotherapy drug L-MTP-PE (175–178). We have performed a randomized, double-blind study in dogs with spontaneous long-bone OSA treated with amputation. Following

Table 5
Comparative Aspects of Human and Canine Osteosarcoma

Variable	Dog	Humans
Incidence in U.S.	>8000/yr	2000/yr
Mean age	7	14
Race/breed	Large purebreds	None
Gender	1.5:1 male	1.5:1 male
Body weight	99% >20 kg	Heavy
Site	77% long bones	90% long bones
	Metaphyseal	Metaphyseal
	Distal radius > proximal humerus	Distal femur > proximal tibia
	Distal femur > tibia	Proximal humerus
Etiology	Generally unknown	Generally unknown
Percent clinically confined to limb at presentation	80–90%	80–90%
Percent high grade	95%	85–90%
Percent aneuploid	75%	75%
Metastatic rate without chemotherapy	90% before 1 yr	80% before 2 yr
Metastatic sites	Lung > bone > soft tissue	Lung > bone > soft tissue
Improved survival with chemotherapy	Yes	Yes
Radiosensitivity	Generally poor	Generally poor

amputation, dogs were randomized either to L-MTP-PE or empty liposomes (placebo) *(176)*. The dogs receiving the L-MTP-PE had an MST of 7 mo, comparing favorably with those dogs treated by placebo, which had an MST of 3 mo ($p < 0.002$). L-MTP-PE did not produce toxicity and was well tolerated. The MST for the dogs receiving empty liposomes was no different from that reported for surgery alone (3 mo). This trial clearly demonstrated that L-MTP-PE has significant activity for the treatment of canine OSA metastasis. However, since 70% of the dogs still died of metastases, we have further expanded this study using amputation combined with cisplatin (CDDP) chemotherapy *(175,178)*. Briefly, dogs with spontaneous OSA of the extremities, without evidence of distant metastases, were treated with amputation, followed by four courses of CDDP. One month following the completion of chemotherapy, dogs were randomized to either saline liposomes (placebo) or L-MTP-PE. This was a double-blind study in which 40 dogs were entered. Thirteen dogs developed lung metastases during the chemotherapy period, 2 died of unrelated cause prior to liposome therapy, and 25 were randomized and completed all phases of therapy. Dogs receiving L-MTP-PE had a significantly longer MST (median 14.4 mo) than those dogs receiving empty liposomes (median 9.7 mo; $p < 0.021$). In another randomized trial in dogs with OSA, administration of the L-MTP-PE concurrently with CDDP resulted in a complete loss of antitumor activity of the L-MTF-PE *(178)*. Because of this study, we advise that L-MTP-PE should not be administered simultaneously with CDDP.

9.3. Cisplatin Drug Delivery Systems

Recently, studies have been conducted to evaluate a new drug delivery system that can release a very high dose of chemotherapy into a surgical wound and cause slow release of relatively low concentrations of chemotherapy systemically *(179)*. The system is a biodegradable polymer called open cell lactic acid containing cisplatin (OPLA-PT). Studies are being conducted to prevent local recurrence of OSA in dogs undergoing limb-sparing procedures as well as combined with amputation to treat microscopic metastatic disease. When OPLA-PT was implanted in normal dogs, no systemic toxicity and no retardation of bone allograft healing were identified at doses of up to 80.6 mg/m^2. Surprisingly, serum pharmacokinetic data following OPLA-PT implantation revealed a roughly 30-fold increase in the area under the curve (AUC) for systemic platinum concentration compared with similar doses given intravenously. In a clinical study, 39 dogs with OSA of the extremities treated with amputation and one dose of OPLA-PT implanted at the surgical amputation site had a survival time of 8 mo, with a 1-yr survival rate of 41.2%. These results compare favorably with treatment with multiple courses of iv CDDP.

A second example of canine OSA in pets being utilized to model cisplatin drug delivery systems was recently completed *(167)*. The efficacy of adjuvant STEALTH® liposome-encapsulated cisplatin (SPI-77) compared with standard-of-care carboplatin therapy was evaluated in dogs with OSA in the context of a randomized study design. Although STEALTH liposome encapsulation of cisplatin allowed the safe administration of five times the maximally tolerated dose (MTD) of free cisplatin to dogs without concurrent hydration protocols, this did not translate into significantly prolonged disease-free survival. However, a larger proportion of dogs receiving SPI-77 enjoyed long-term disease free survival compared with dogs receiving carboplatin.

10. CANINE MAMMARY TUMORS

10.1. Overview

In North America, breast cancer is the most common malignancy among women and accounts for 27% of their cancers *(180)*. In dogs, mammary neoplasms account for 52% of all neoplasms detected in the female *(7)*. Canine mammary tumors are hormonally dependent, as evidenced by the fact early ovariohysterectomy will reduce the incidence to 0.05% *(181)* and may also be an effective adjunct to tumor removal *(182)*. Most studies indicate that between 50 and 60% of all malignant canine mammary tumors express either estrogen or, to a lesser extent, progesterone receptors *(183–187)*. However, studies evaluating the antiestrogen tamoxifen in dogs have not demonstrated significant antitumor activity *(188)*.

Most malignant mammary tumors will be classified as epithelial tumors or carcinomas *(189–192)*. Mammary gland sarcomas make up a smaller proportion of tumor types seen in both dogs and humans *(193,194)*. Significant prognostic factors identified for canine mammary tumors are histologic subtype, degree of invasion, nuclear differentiation, evidence of lymphoid reaction near the tumor, tumor size, lymph node involvement, hormone receptor activity, ulceration, and fixation *(195,196)*. Factors that do not influence prognosis are tumor location, extent of surgery (conservative vs radical), ovariohysterectomy at surgery, age at diagnosis, and number of tumors present *(197)*. Table 6 presents the significant prognostic factors in a series of 233 dogs treated with surgery. Recently, *p53* gene mutations in mammary carcinoma from dogs were found to be an independent risk factor for recurrence and early death in a way comparable to that of human tumors *(62)*.

10.2. Treatment

No chemotherapeutic agent has been shown to be consistently effective in the dog. Few studies have been reported, but some responses have been noted in dogs with adenocarcinoma using combinations of doxorubicin and cyclophosphamide or cisplatin as a single agent. Studies with nonspecific immunomodulation using *Corynebacterium parvum* with bacillus Calmette-Guérin (BCG) showed little effectiveness over surgery alone *(198)*. In a randomized, double-blind trial using levamisole combined with surgery, no antitumor activity was found *(197)*. Another study reported that iv BCG following mastectomy increased MST from 24 wk (control) to 100 wk in the BCG group *(199)*.

10.3. Model Relevance

Canine mammary carcinoma is similar to human breast cancer because of its hormonal dependence, spontaneous development in middle-aged to older animals, and metastatic behavior to regional lymph nodes and lungs. Dissimilarities to human breast cancer are the lack of responsiveness to tamoxifen treatment and chemotherapy, although large clinical trials evaluating their effectiveness in the species are lacking.

11. FELINE MAMMARY CARCINOMA

Mammary tumors are the third most common neoplasm in cats and are primarily observed at 10–12 yr of age. These tumors are not as hormonally dependent as in people and dogs. Early ovariohysterectomy may have some protective effect *(200)*. Both estrogen receptors and progesterone receptors have been identified but at very low levels *(201–203)*.

Table 6
Prognosis Related to Clinical and Histologic Features in Canine Mammary Tumors

| | % Local or distant recurrence at | |
Feature	12 mo	24 mo
Tumor size		
< 3 cm	30	40
>3 cm	70	80
Histologic grade		
Grade 0	10	19
Grade I	40	60
Well differentiated	NR	24
Moderately differentiated	NR	68
Poorly differentiated	NR	70
Grade II	85	97
Lymph node status		
Negative	20	30
Positive	90	100
Lymphoid cellular reactivity (histologic grade I)		
Positive	NR	45
Negative	NR	83

ABBREVIATION: NR, not reported

The histology of mammary tumors is more homogeneous than in dogs. Eighty-five percent of the tumors are carcinomas *(204)*. Their biologic behavior is more aggressive than in dogs. Metastases to regional lymph nodes and lungs can occur rapidly after diagnosis, depending on the stage of disease *(204)*. The most significant prognostic factor is tumor size *(204,205)*. Cats with a tumor size >3 cm in diameter have an MST of 4–6 mo. Cats with tumors 2–3 cm have an MST of 2 yr, and those with tumors < 2 cm can have an MST of 3 yr. Radical mastectomy will improve disease-free survival, but does not influence overall survival *(205)*.

In contrast to canine mammary carcinoma, feline mammary carcinomas appear more responsive to chemotherapy (doxorubicin and cyclophosphamide) *(206,207)*. Studies evaluating biologic response modifiers such as levamisole *(208)*, *C. parvum (209)*, or L-MTP-PE combined with radical mastectomy *(210)* have failed to show any beneficial effects.

12. CANINE ORAL MELANOMA

12.1. Overview

The oral cavity of the dog is a common site for a variety of malignant and benign tumors. It is estimated that oral tumors account for 5–6% of all canine malignancies *(211)*. Malignant melanoma is the most common canine oral malignancy. Canine oral melanomas are highly malignant tumors, with metastasis occurring via lymphatics or blood vessels to regional lymph nodes, lungs, liver, brain, and kidney.

As previously mentioned, our laboratory and others have detected the expression of canine analogs of the human melanoma antigens gp100, MART-1, and tyrosinase in the majority of canine melanomas *(28,86,87)*. These provide potential common targets for the development of immunotherapeutic approaches for both human and canine melanoma.

12.2. Treatment and Prognosis

Following complete surgical removal, approx 25% of dogs with oral melanoma will survive for 1 yr or more *(212)*. The only recognized prognostic factors are size (<2 cm maximal diameter), lymph node metastasis, and the ability of the first surgery to afford local control *(212,213)*.

Treatment of oral melanomas with single-agent melphalan or carboplatin yields objective response rates of approx 20–25% *(214,215)*. Local coarsely fractionated radiotherapy (800–900 cGy for 3–4 weekly treatments) induces an 83–94% objective response rate; however, the rapid development of metastatic disease remains problematic *(216–218)*.

12.3. Experimental Therapeutics

Adjuvant immunotherapy using killed *Corynebacterium parvum* was superior to surgery alone in dogs with advanced stage (>2 cm or node-positive) oral melanoma *(213)*. More recently, 98 dogs stratified by stage were randomized to receive placebo liposomes, L-MTP-PE, or L-MTP-PE plus recombinant canine granulocyte-macrophage colony-stimulating factor (GM-CSF) *(219)*. Dogs with stage I disease receiving L-MTP-PE had a significantly improved outcome vs dogs receiving placebo. No survival benefit was reported in dogs receiving GM-CSF in addition to L-MTP-PE, but a significant increase in in vitro pulmonary alveolar macrophage cytotoxicity was demonstrated in dogs receiving the combination therapy.

Our group has recently evaluated the efficacy of human GM-CSF-transfected autologous tumor cell vaccines for the treatment of advanced canine oral melanoma *(220)*. Vaccines were uniformly well tolerated, and objective responses were seen in 19% of dogs. Response was often associated with a T-cell infiltrate, and delayed-type hypersensitivity conversion was observed in several cases. This approach is currently the subject of a randomized, placebo-controlled surgical adjuvant trial.

A recent study investigated the efficacy of intralesional injection of cationic liposome-DNA complexes encoding *Staphylococcus* enterotoxin B and human GM-CSF or interleukin-2 in dogs with oral malignant melanoma. A 46% overall response rate was reported, with significant prolongation of survival in patients with WHO stage III tumors compared with historical controls treated with surgery alone. Clinical response was associated with a profound lymphocytic infiltrate and increased autologous tumor-directed peripheral blood mononuclear cell cytotoxicity *(53)*. This approach is the subject of an ongoing human clinical trial *(221)*.

These studies demonstrate the potential of canine oral melanoma to serve as a model for the investigation of a variety of immunotherapeutic approaches.

13. CANINE URINARY BLADDER CARCINOMA

13.1. Overview

Transitional cell carcinoma (TCC) is the most common form of canine urinary bladder cancer. Canine TCC closely resembles invasive human TCC with regard to histologic appearance, biologic behavior, and response to therapy. Most canine TCCs are infiltrative, intermediate or high-grade tumors, and they usually involve the trigone. Scottish terriers have an 18-fold increased risk, compared with mixed-breed dogs, for the development of TCC *(222)*. An increased risk of TCC development has been identified in dogs exposed to topical insecticide dips, and this risk is further increased in overweight or obese female dogs *(2)*.

13.2. Treatment and Experimental Therapeutics

Surgical excision of canine TCC is usually not feasible owing to its invasive nature and trigonal location. Platinum- and anthracycline-based protocols are the standard treatments, with objective response rates in the 20% range and MSTs of 4–8 mo *(42,223–225)*.

The dog bladder is a useful model for the preclinical investigation of novel photodynamic therapy technologies *(226–228)*, and it would be expected that clinical evaluation of photodynamic approaches could be conducted successfully in dogs with TCC.

Recent clinical investigations have focused on the use of the cyclooxygenase inhibitor piroxicam for the treatment of canine TCC. Most TCC-bearing dogs treated with piroxicam experience subjective improvement in clinical signs (pollakuria, hematuria, stranguria), and an objective response rate of 18% has been reported *(229)*. Response to piroxicam therapy in dogs with bladder TCC is associated with an increase in tumor cell apoptosis and a decrease in urinary bFGF production *(43)*. Combination therapy with cisplatin and piroxicam has been evaluated: although the objective response rate is significantly improved, the combination is associated with unacceptable nephrotoxicity *(230)*. Other piroxicam chemotherapy combinations are being investigated currently.

REFERENCES

1. Reif JS, Bruns C, Lower KS. Cancer of the nasal cavity and paranasal sinuses and exposure to environmental tobacco smoke in pet dogs. *Am J Epidemiol* 1998; 147:488–492.
2. Glickman LS, Shofer FS, McKee IJ. Epidemiologic study of insecticide exposure, obesity, and risk of bladder cancer in household dogs. *J Toxicol Environ Health* 1989; 28:407–414.
3. Gavazza A, Presciuttini S, Barale R, Lubas G, Gugliucci B. Association between canine malignant lymphoma, living in industrial areas, and use of chemicals by dog owners. *J Vet Intern Med* 2001; 15:190–195.
4. Hayes HM, Tarone RE, Cantor KP, Jessen CR, McCurnin DM, Richardson RC. Case-control study of canine malignant lymphoma: positive association with dog owner's use of 2,4-dichlorophenoxyacetic acid herbicides. *J Natl Cancer Inst* 1991; 83:1226–1231.
5. Reif JS, Lower KS, Ogilvie GK. Residential exposure to magnetic fields and risk of canine lymphoma. *Am J Epidemiol* 1995; 141:352–359.
6. Glickman LT, Domanski LM, Maguire TG, Dubielzig RR, Churg A. Mesothelioma in pet dogs associated with exposure of their owners to asbestos. *Environ Res* 1983; 32:305–313.
7. Dorn CR, Taylor DON, Schneider R, Hibbard HH, Klauber MR. Survey of animal neoplasms in Alameda and Contra Costa Counties. Cancer morbidity in dogs and cats from Alameda County. *J Natl Cancer Inst* 1968; 40:307–318.
8. Dorn CR. Epidemiology of canine and feline tumors. *Comp Cont Ed Pract Vet* 1976; 12:307–312.
9. Priester WA, McKay FW. The occurrence of tumors in domestic animals. *Natl Cancer Inst Monogr No. 54.* Washington, DC: US Government Printing Office. 1980:152.
10. LaRue SM, Fox MH, Withrow SJ, ddd, smdl. Impact of heterogeneity in the predictive value of kinetic parameters in canine osteosarcoma. *Cancer Res* 1994; 54:3916–3921.
11. Zeman EM, Calkins DP, Cline JM, Thrall DE. The relationship between proliferative and oxygenation status in spontaneous canine tumors. *Int J Radiat Oncol Biol Phys* 1993; 27:891–898.
12. Vail DM, Kisseberth WC, Obradovich JE, et al. Assessment of potential doubling time (Tpot), argyrophilic nucleolar organizer regions (AgNOR), and proliferating cell nuclear antigen (PCNA) as predictors of therapy response in canine non-Hodgkin's lymphoma. *Exp Hematol* 1996; 24:807–815.

13. Hershey AE, Kurzman ID, Forrest LJ, et al. Inhalation chemotherapy for macroscopic primary or metastatic lung tumors: proof of principle using dogs with spontaneously occurring tumors as a model. *Clin Cancer Res* 1999; 5:2653–2659.

14. Sharma S, White D, Imondi AR, Placke ME, Vail DM, Kris MG. Development of inhalational agents for oncologic use. *J Clin Oncol* 2001; 19:1839–1847.

15. Vail DM, MacEwen EG. Spontaneously occurring tumors of companion animals as models for human cancer. *Cancer Invest* 2000; 18:781–792.

16. Bronson RT. Variation in age at death of dogs of different sexes and breeds. *Am J Vet Res* 1982; 43:2057–2059.

17. Teclaw R, Mendlein J, Garbe P, Mariolis P. Characteristics of pet populations and households in the Purdue Comparative Oncology Program catchment area. *J Am Vet Med Assoc* 1988; 201:1725–1729.

18. Steplewski Z, Rosales C, Jeglum KA, McDonald-Smith J. In vivo destruction of canine lymphoma mediated by murine monoclonal antibodies. *In Vivo* 1990; 4:231–234.

19. Ghernati I, Auger C, Chabanne L, et al. Characterization of a canine long-term T cell line (DLC 01) established from a dog with Sezary syndrome and producing retroviral particles. *Leukemia* 1999; 13:1281–1290.

20. Nakaichi M, Taura Y, Kanki M, et al. Establishment and characterization of a new canine B-cell leukemia cell line. *J Vet Med Sci* 1996; 58:469–471.

21. Thamm DH, Dickerson EB, Helfand SC, MacEwen EG. Expression of angiogenic growth factors and receptors in canine angiosarcoma. In: *Proceedings of the American Association of Cancer Research*, New Orleans, LA, 2001.

22. Shoieb AM, Hahn KA, Barnhill MA. An in vivo/in vitro experimental model system for the study of human osteosarcoma: canine osteosarcoma cells (COS31) which retain osteoblastic and metastatic properties in nude mice. *In Vivo* 1998; 12:463–472.

23. Cakir Y, Hahn KA. Direct action by doxycycline against canine osteosarcoma cell proliferation and collagenase (MMP-1) activity in vitro. *In Vivo* 1999; 13:327–331.

24. Ahern TE, Bird RC, Bird AE, Wolfe LG. Expression of the oncogene c-erbB-2 in canine mammary cancers and tumor-derived cell lines. *Am J Vet Res* 1996; 57:693–696.

25. Muleya JS, Nakaichi M, Sugahara J, Taura Y, Murata T, Nakama S. Establishment and characterization of a new cell line derived from feline mammary tumor. *J Vet Med Sci* 1998; 60:931–935.

26. Hogge GS, Burkholder JK, Culp J, et al. Preclinical development of hGM-CSF transfected melanoma cell vaccines using established canine cell lines and normal canines. *Cancer Gene Ther* 1998; 6:26–36.

27. Ahern TE, Bird RC, Bird AE, Wolfe LG. Overexpression of c-erbB-2 and c-myc but not c-ras, in canine melanoma cell lines, is associated with metastatic potential in nude mice. *Anticancer Res* 1993; 13: 1365–1371.

28. Koenig A, Wojcieszyn J, Weeks BR, Modiano JF. Expression of S100a, vimentin, NSE, and melan A/MART-1 in seven canine melanoma cell lines and twenty-nine retrospective cases of canine melanoma. *Vet Pathol* 2001; 38:427–435.

29. Knapp DW, Chan TC, Kuczek T, Reagan WJ, Park B. Evaluation of in vitro cytotoxicity of nonsteroidal anti-inflammatory drugs against canine tumor cells. *Am J Vet Res* 1995; 56:801–805.

30. Tannehill-Gregg S, Kergosien E, Rosol TJ. Feline head and neck squamous cell carcinoma cell line: characterization, production of parathyroid hormone-related protein, and regulation by transforming growth factor-beta. *In Vitro Cell Dev Biol Anim* 2001; 37:676–683.

31. Katayama R, Huelsmeyer MK, Vail DM, Kurzman ID, MacEwen EG. Selective inhibition of platelet-derived growth factor receptor activity in feline vaccine-associated sarcoma. In: *Proceedings of the American Association Cancer Research*, San Francisco, April 6–10, 2002.

32. Ma Z, Khatlani TS, Li L, et al. Molecular cloning and expression analysis of feline melanoma antigen (MAGE) obtained from a lymphoma cell line. *Vet Immunol Immunopathol* 2001; 83:241–252.

33. Okai Y, Nakamura N, Matsushiro H, et al. Molecular analysis of multidrug resistance in feline lymphoma cells. *Am J Vet Res* 2000; 61:1122–1127.

34. Cline JM, Thrall DE, Page RL, et al. Immunohistochemical detection of a hypoxia marker in spontaneous canine tumours. *Br J Cancer* 1990; 62:925–931.

35. Cline JM, Thrall DE, Rosner GL, Raleigh JA. Distribution of the hypoxic marker CCI-103F in canine tumors. *Int J Radiat Oncol Biol Phys* 1994; 28:921–933.

36. Raleigh JA, Zeman EM, Rathman M, et al. Development of an ELISA for the detection of 2-nitroimidazole hypoxia markers bound to tumor tissue. *Int J Radiat Oncol Biol Phys* 1992; 22:403–405.

37. Raleigh JA, Zeman EM, Calkins DP, McEntee MC, Thrall DE. Distribution of hypoxia and proliferation associated markers in spontaneous canine tumors. *Acta Oncol* 1995; 34:345–349.

38. Thrall DE, McEntee MC, Cline JM, Raleigh JA. ELISA quantification of CCI-103F binding in canine tumors prior to and during irradiation. *Int J Radiat Oncol Biol Phys* 1994; 28:649–659.

39. Vujaskovic Z, Poulson JM, Gaskin AA, et al. Temperature-dependent changes in physiologic parameters of spontaneous canine soft tissue sarcomas after combined radiotherapy and hyperthermia treatment. *Int J Radiat Oncol Biol Phys* 2000; 46:179–185.

40. Mathias CJ, Green MA, Morrison WB, Knapp DW. Evaluation of Cu-PTSM as a tracer of tumor perfusion: comparison with labeled microspheres in spontaneous canine neoplasms. *Nucl Med Biol* 1994; 21:83–87.

41. Van Camp S, Fisher P, Thrall DE. Dynamic CT measurement of contrast medium washin kinetics in canine nasal tumors. *Vet Radiol Ultrasound* 2000; 41:403–408.

42. Rocha TA, Mauldin GN, Patnaik AK, Bergman PJ. Prognostic factors in dogs with urinary bladder carcinoma. *J Vet Intern Med* 2000; 14:486–490.

43. Mohammed SI, Bennett PF, Craig BA, et al. Effects of the cyclooxygenase inhibitor, piroxicam, on tumor response, apoptosis, and angiogenesis in a canine model of human invasive urinary bladder cancer. *Cancer Res* 2002; 62:356–358.

44. Coomber BL, Denton J, Sylvestre A, Kruth S. Blood vessel density in canine osteosarcoma. *Can J Vet Res* 1998; 62:199–204.

45. Gonzalez CM, Griffey SM, Naydan DK, et al. Canine transmissible venereal tumour: a morphological and immunohistochemical study of 11 tumours in growth phase and during regression after chemotherapy. *J Comp Pathol* 2000; 122:241–248.

46. Griffey SM, Verstraete FJ, Kraegel SA, Lucroy MD, Madewell BR. Computer-assisted image analysis of intratumoral vessel density in mammary tumors from dogs. *Am J Vet Res* 1998; 59:1238–1242.

47. Fukanoshi Y, Nakayama H, Uetsuka K, Nishimura R, Sasaki N, Doi K. Cellular proliferative and telomerase activtiy in canine mammary gland tumors. *Vet Pathol* 2000; 37:177–183.

48. Madewell BR, Gandour-Edwards R, Edwards BF, Walls JE, Griffey SM. Topographic distribution of bcl-2 protein in feline tissues in health and neoplasia. *Vet Pathol* 1999; 36:565–573.

49. Madewell BR, Gandour-Edwards R, Edwards BF, Matthews KR, Griffey SM. Bax/bcl-2: cellular modulator of apoptosis in feline skin and basal cell tumours. *J Comp Pathol* 2001; 124:115–121.

50. Phillips BS, Kass PH, Naydan DK, Winthrop MD, Griffey SM, Madewell BR. Apoptotic and proliferation indexes in canine lymphoma. *J Vet Diagn Invest* 1999; 12:111–117.

51. Roels S, Tilmant K, Ducatelle R. p53 expression and apoptosis in melanomas of dogs and cats. *Res Vet Sci* 2001; 70:19–25.

52. Nicholls PK, Moore PF, Anderson DM, et al. Regression of canine oral papillomas is associated with infiltration of CD4+ and CD8+ lymphocytes. *Virology* 2001; 283:31–39.

53. Dow SW, Elmslie RE, Wilson AP, Gorman C, Potter TA. *In vivo* tumor transfection with superantigen plus cytokine genes induces tumor regression and prolongs survival in dogs with malignant melanoma. *J Clin Invest* 1998; 101:2406–2414.

54. Korkolopoulou P, Oates J, Kittos C, Crocker J. p53, c-myc, p62 and proliferating cell nuclear antigen (PCNA) expression in non-Hodgkin's lymphomas. *J Clin Pathol* 1994; 47:9–14.

55. Levine RA, Fleischli MA. Inactivation of p53 and retinoblastoma family pathways in canine osteosarcoma cell lines. *Vet Pathol* 2000; 37:54–61.

56. Mendoza S, Konishi T, Dernell WS, Withrow SJ, Miller CW. Status of the p53, Rb and MDM2 genes in canine osteosarcoma. *Anticancer Res* 1998; 18:4449–4453.

57. Nambiar PR, Jackson ML, Ellis JA, Chelack BJ, Kidney BA, Haines DM. Immunohistochemical detection of tumor suppressor gene p53 protein in feline injection site-associated sarcomas. *Vet Pathol* 2001; 38:236–238.

58. Nasir L, Rutteman GR, Reid SW, Schulze C, Argyle DJ. Analysis of p53 mutational events and MDM2 amplification in canine soft-tissue sarcomas. *Cancer Lett* 2001; 174:83–89.

59. Rungsipipat A, Tateyama S, Yamaguchi R, Uchida K, Miyoshi N, Hayashi T. Immunohistochemical analysis of c-yes and c-erbB-2 oncogene products and p53 tumor suppressor protein in canine mammary tumors. *J Vet Med Sci* 1999; 61:27–32.

60. Veldhoen N, Stewart J, Brown R, Milner J. Mutations of the p53 gene in canine lymphoma and evidence for germ line p53 mutations in the dog. *Oncogene* 1998; 16:249–255.

61. Veldhoen N, Watterson J, Brash M, Milner J. Identification of tumour-associated and germ line p53 mutations in canine mammary cancer. *Br J Cancer* 1999; 81:409–415.

62. Wakui S, Muto T, Yokoo K, et al. Prognostic status of p53 gene mutation in canine mammary carcinoma. *Anticancer Res* 2001; 21:611–616.

63. Griffey SM, Kraegel SA, Madewell BR. Rapid detection of K-ras gene mutations in canine lung cancer using single-strand conformational polymorphism analysis. *Carcinogenesis* 1998; 19:959–963.

64. Merryman JI, Buckles EL, Bowers G, Neilsen NR. Overexpression of c-Ras in hyperplasia and adenomas of the feline thyroid gland: an immunohistochemical analysis of 34 cases. *Vet Pathol* 1999; 36:117–124.

65. Watzinger F, Mayr B, Gamerith R, Vetter C, Lion T. Comparative analysis of ras proto-oncogene mutations in selected mammalian tumors. *Mol Carcinog* 2001; 30:190–198.

66. Mayr B. Cytogenetic and tumour suppressor gene studies on feline soft tissue tumours. *Vet Med Czech* 2000; 45:327–330.

67. Kolb E. Patho-biochemical aspects of the development of tumors in the dog. *Tierarztliche Umschau* 2001; 56:128–134.

68. Nasir L, Devlin P, Mckevitt T, Rutteman G, Argyle DJ. Telomere lengths and telomerase activity in dog tissues: a potential model system to study human telomere and telomerase biology. *Neoplasia* 2001; 3:351–359.

69. Yazawa M, Okuda M, Setoguchi A, et al. Measurement of telomerase activity in dog tumors. *J Vet Med Sci* 1999; 61:1125–1229.

70. Yazawa M, Okuda M, Setoguchi A, et al. Telomere length and telomerase activity in canine mammary gland tumors. *Am J Vet Res* 2001; 62:1539–1543.

71. Lana SE, Ogilvie GK, Hansen RA, Powers BE, Dernell WS, Withrow SJ. Identification of matrix metalloproteinases in canine neoplastic tissue. *Am J Vet Res* 2000; 61:111–114.

72. Leibman NF, Lana SE, Hansen RA, et al. Identification of matrix metalloproteinases in canine cutaneous mast cell tumors. *J Vet Intern Med* 2000; 14:583–586.

73. Yokota H, Kumata T, Taketaba S, et al. High expression of 92 kDa type IV collagenase (matrix metalloproteinase-9) in canine mammary adenocarcinoma. *Biochim Biophys Acta* 2001; 1568:7–12.

74. MacEwen EG, Kutzke J, Carew J, et al. C-Met tyrosine kinase receptor expression and function in human and canine osteosarcoma cells. *Clin Exp Metastasis* 2003; 20:421–430.

75. MacEwen EG, Pastor J, Kutzke J, et al. IGF-1 receptor expression and function contribute to the malignant phenotype in human and canine osteosarcoma. *J Cell Biochem* 2002; submitted.

76. Ferracini R, Angelini P, Cagliero E, et al. MET oncogene aberrant expression in canine osteosarcoma. *J Orthop Res* 2000; 18:253–256.

77. Matsuyama S, Nakamura M, Yonezawa K, et al. Expression patterns of the erbB subfamily mRNA in canine benign and malignant mammary tumors. *J Vet Med Sci* 2001; 63:949–954.

78. London CA, Kisseberth WC, Galli SJ, Geissler EN, Helfand SC. Expression of stem cell factor receptor (c-kit) by the malignant mast cells from spontaneous canine mast cell tumors. *J Comp Pathol* 1996; 115:399–414.

79. Ma Y, Longley BJ, Wang X, Blount JL, Langley K, Caughey GH. Clustering of activating mutations in c-KIT's juxtamembrane coding region in canine mast cell neoplasms. *J Invest Dermatol* 1999; 112:165–170.

80. Reguera MJ, Rabanal RM, Puigdemont A, Ferrer L. Canine mast cell tumors express stem cell factor receptor. *Am J Dermatopathol* 2000; 22:49–54.

81. Liao AT, Chien MB, Shenoy N, et al. Inhibition of constitutively active forms of mutant kit by multitargeted indolinone tyrosine kinase inhibitors. *Blood* 2002; 100:585–593.

82. Clifford CA, Mackin AJ, Henry CJ. Treatment of canine hemangiosarcoma: 2000 and beyond. *J Vet Intern Med* 2000; 14:479–485.

83. Clifford CA, Hughes D, Beal MW, et al. Plasma vascular endothelial growth factor concentrations in healthy dogs and dogs with hemangiosarcoma. *J Vet Intern Med* 2001; 15:131–135.

84. Allen DK, Waters DJ, Knapp DJ, Kuczek T. High urine concentrations of basic fibroblast growth factor in dogs with bladder cancer. *J Vet Intern Med* 1996; 10:231–234.

85. Wetterman C, Chun R, Winter B, Ross C. RT-PCR cloning and sequencing of vascular endothelial growth factor in canine osteosarcoma. *Proc Vet Cancer Soc* 1999; 19:30.

86. Alexander AN, Huelsmeyer MK, Vail DM, Kurzman ID. Phase I/II clinical trial utilizing a tumor cell vaccine encoding xenogeneic gp100 in canine patients with metastatic melanoma: immunological and clinical outcomes. In: *Proceedings of the American Association Cancer Research*, San Francisco, April 6–10, 2002.

87. Huelsmeyer MK, Alexander AN, Thamm DH, Vail DM, MacEwen EG. Development of a genetically modified allogeneic tumor cell vaccine targeting canine melanoma. In: *Proceedings of the Americna Association Cancer Research*, San Francisco, CA, April 6–10, 2002.

88. Crow SE. Lymphosarcoma in the dog: diagnosis and treatment. *Comp Cont Ed Pract Vet* 1982; 4: 283–289.

89. Leifer CE, Matus RE. Canine lymphoma: clinical considerations. *Semin Vet Med Surg* 1986; 1:43–51.

90. Rosenthal RC. Epidemiology of canine lymphosarcoma. *Comp Cont Ed Pract Vet* 1982; 4:855–859.

91. Owen LN, ed. *World Health Organization TNM Classification of Tumors in Domestic Animals*. Geneva,: WHO. 1980.

92. Anonymous. The non-Hodgkin's lymphoma pathologic classification project: National Cancer Institute sponsored study of classifications of non-Hodgkin's lymphomas. Summary and description of a Working Formulation for Clinical Usage. *Cancer* 1982; 49:2112.

93. Teske E, Rutteman GR, Kuipers-Dijkshoorn NJ, et, al. DNA ploidy and cell kinetics in canine non-Hodgkin's lymphoma. *Exp Hematol* 1993; 21:579–584.

94. Carter RF, Valli VEO, Lumsden JH. The cytology, histology and prevalence of cell types in canine lymphoma classified according to the National Cancer Institute Working Formulation. *Can J Vet Res* 1986; 50:154–164.

95. Greenlee PG, Fillipps DA, Quimby FW. Lymphomas in dogs. *Cancer* 1990; 66:480–490.

96. Teske E, van Heerde P, Rutteman GR, Kurzman ID, Moore PF, MacEwen EG. Prognostic factors for treatment of malignant lymphoma in dogs. *J Am Vet Med Assoc* 1994; 205:1722–1728.

97. Hahn KA, Richardson RC, Hahn EA, Chrisman CL. Diagnostic and progostic importance of chromosomal aberrations identified in 61 dogs with lymphosarcoma. *Vet Pathol* 1994; 31:528–540.

98. Keller ET, MacEwen EG, Rosenthal RC, Helfand SC, Fox LE. Evaluation of prognostic factors and sequential combination chemotherapy with doxorubicin for canine lymphoma. *J Vet Intern Med* 1993; 7:289–295.

99. Baskin CR, Couto CG, Wittum TE. Factors influencing first remission and survival in 145 dogs with lymphoma: a retrospective study. *J Am Hosp Assoc* 2000; 36:404–409.

100. Brons PPT, Raemaekers JMM, Bogman MJJT. Cell cycle kinetics in malignant lymphoma studied with in vivo iodeoxyuridine administration, nuclear Ki-67 staining, and flow cytometry. *Blood* 1992; 80:2336–2343.

101. Mikou P, Kanavaros P, Aninos D. Nucleolar organizer regions (NORs) staining and proliferating cell nuclear antigen (PCNA) immunostaining in mucosa-associated lymphoid tissue (MALT) gastric lymphomas. *Pathol Res Pract* 1993; 189:1004–1009.

102. Jakic-Razumovic J, Tentor D, Petrovecki M, Radman I. Nuclear organizer regions and survival in patients with non-Hodgkin's lymphoma classified by the working formulation. *J Clin Pathol* 1993; 46:943–947.

103. Crocker J, Nar P. Nucleolar organizer regions in lymphomas. *J Pathol* 1987; 151:111–118.

104. Crocker J, McCartney JC, Smith PJ. Correlation between DNA flow cytometric and nucleolar organizer region data in non-Hodgkin's lymphomas. *J Pathol* 1988; 154:151–156.

105. Gorczyca W, Kram A, Tuziak T. Proliferating cell nuclear antigen in archival surgical specimens of malignant lymphoma and metastatic carcinoma: immunohistochemical and flow cytometric analysis. *Pathol Polska* 1993; 44:121–128.

106. Brick JO, Roenigk WJ, Wilson GP. Chemotherapy of malignant lymphoma in dogs and cats. *J Am Vet Med Assoc* 1968; 153:47–52.

107. Vail DM. Recent advances in chemotherapy for lymphoma of dogs and cats. *Comp Cont Ed Pract Vet* 1993; 15:1031–1037.

108. Garrett LD, Thamm DH, Chun R, Dudley R, Vail DM. Evaluation of a six-month chemotherapy protocol with no maintenance therapy for dogs with lymphoma. *J Vet Intern Med* 2002; 16:704–709.

109. Bergman PJ, Ogilvie GK, Powers BE. Monoclonal antibody C219 immunohistochemistry against P-glycoprotein: sequential analysis and predictive ability in dogs with lymphoma. *J Vet Intern Med* 1996; 10:354–359.

110. Lee JJ, Hughes CS, Fine RL, Page RL. P-glycoprotein expression in canine lymphoma. *Cancer* 1986; 77:1892–1898.

111. Steingold SF, Sharp NJ, McGahan MC, Hughes CS, Dunn SE, Page RL. Characterization of canine MDR1 mRNA: its abundance in drug resistant cell lines and *in vivo*. *Anticancer Res* 1998; 18: 393–400.

112. Gamblin RM, Sagartz JE, Couto CG. Overexpression of p53 tumor suppressor protein in spontaneously arising neoplasms of dogs. *Am J Vet Res* 1997; 58:857–863.
113. Vail DM, Kravis LD, Cooley AJ, Chun R, MacEwen EG. Preclinical trial of doxorubicin entrapped in sterically stabilized liposomes in dogs with spontaneously arising malignant tumors. *Cancer Chemother Pharmacol* 1997; 39:410–416.
114. Thamm DH, MacEwen EG, Phillips BS, et al. Preclinical study of dolastatin-10 in dogs with spontaneous neoplasia. *Cancer Chemother Pharmacol* 2002; 49:251–255.
115. Page RL, Macy DW, Ogilvie GK. Phase III evaluation of doxorubicin and whole-body hyperthermia in dogs with lymphoma. *Int J Hyperthermia* 1992; 8:187–197.
116. Applebaum FR, Deeg HJ, Storb R. Marrow transplant studies in dogs with malignant lymphoma. *Transplantation* 1985; 39:499–504.
117. Weiden PL, Storb R, Deeg HJ, et al. Prolonged disease-free interval in dogs with lymphoma after total-body irradiation and autologous marrow transplantation consolidation of combination-chemotherapy-induced remissions. *Blood* 1979; 54:1039–1049.
118. Hardy Jr WD. The feline leukemia virus. *J Am Anim Hosp Assoc* 1981; 17:951–957.
119. Hardy Jr WD, Zuckerman EE, MacEwen EG, et al. A feline leukemia and sarcoma virus-induced tumor specific antigen. *Nature* 1977; 270:249–251.
120. Cockerell GL, Krakowa S, Hoover EA. Characterization of feline T- and B-lymphocytes and identification of an experimentally induced T-cell neoplasm in the cat. *J Natl Cancer Inst* 1976; 57:907–913.
121. Hardy Jr WD, McClelland AJ, Zuckerman EE, et al. Development of virus nonproducer lymphosarcomas in pet cats exposed to FeLV. *Nature* 1980; 288:90–92.
122. Rojko JL, Kociba GJ, Abkowitz JL, et al. Feline lymphomas: immunological and cytochemical characterization. *Cancer Res* 1989; 49:345–351.
123. Vail DM, Moore AS, Ogilvie GK, Volk LM. Feline lymphoma (145 cases): proliferation indices, CD3 immunoreactivity, and their associateion with prognosis in 90 cats. *J Vet Intern Med* 1998; 12:349–354.
124. Mauldin GE, Mooney SC, Meleo KA, et al. Chemotherapy in 132 cats with lymphoma: 1988–1994. In: *Proceedings of the 15th Annual Conference of Veterinary Cancer Society*, Tuscon, AZ, 1995. Vol. 15.
125. Poli A, Abramo F, Baldinotti F, Pistello M, Da Prato L, Bendinelli M. Malignant lymphoma associated with experimentally induced feline immunodeficiency virus infection. *J Comp Pathol* 1994; 110: 319–328.
126. Shelton GH, Grant CK, Cotter SM, Gardner MB, Hardy WD Jr, DiGiacomo RF. Feline immunodeficiency virus and feline leukemia virus infections and their relationships to lymphoid malignancies in cats: a retrospective study (1968–1988). *J Acquir Immunodef Syndr* 1990; 3:623–630.
127. Valli VE, Jacobs RM, Norris A, et al. The histologic classification of 602 cases of feline lymphoproliferative disease using the National Cancer Institute working formulation. *J Vet Diagn Invest* 2000; 12:295–306.
128. Hardy WD Jr. Hematopoietic tumors of cats. *J Am Anim Hosp Assoc* 1981; 17:921–940.
129. Mooney SC, Hayes AA, MacEwen EG, Matus RE, Geary A, Shurgot BA. Treatment and prognostic factors in lymphoma in cats: 103 cases (1977–1981). *J Am Vet Med Assoc* 1989; 194:696–702.
130. Theilen GH, Madewell BR. Tumors of the skin and subcutaneous tissues. In: Theilen GN, Madewell BR, eds. *Veterinary Cancer Medicine.* Philadelphia: Lea & Febinger, 1979:123–191.
131. McNiel EA. Vaccine-associated sarcomas in cats: a unique cancer model. *Clin Orthop* 2001; 382:21–27.
132. Hendrick MJ, Goldschmidt MH, Shofer FS, Wang YY, Somlyo AP. Postvaccinal sarcomas in the cat: epidemiology and electron probe microanalytical identification of aluminum. *Cancer Res* 1992; 52:5391–5394.
133. Hendrick MJ, Kass PH, McGill LD, Tizard IR. Postvaccinal sarcomas in cats. *J Natl Cancer Inst* 1994; 86:341–343.
134. Kass PH, Barnes WGJ, Spangler WL, Chomel BB, Culbertson MR. Epidemiologic evidence for a causal relation between vaccination and fibrosarcoma tumorigenesis in cats. *J Am Vet Med Assoc* 1993; 203:396–405.
135. Hardy WD Jr. The etiology of canine and feline tumors. *J Am Anim Hosp Assoc* 1976; 12:313–334.
136. Madewell BR, Theilen GN. Etiology of cancer in animals. In: Theilen GN, Madewell BR, eds. *Veterinary Cancer Medicine.* Philadelphia: Lea & Febinger. 1979:13–25.
137. McEntee MC, Page RL. Feline vaccine-associated sarcomas. *J Vet Intern Med* 2001; 15:176–182.
138. Kuntz CA, Dernell WS, Powers BE, Devitt C, Straw RC, Withrow SJ. Prognostic factors for surgical treatment of soft-tissue sarcomas in dogs: 75 cases (1986–1996). *J Am Vet Med Assoc* 1997; 211:1147–1151.

139. Cohen M, Wright JC, Brawner WR, Smith AN, Henderson R, Behrend EN. Use of surgery and electron beam irradiation, with or without chemotherapy, for treatment of vaccine-associated sarcomas in cats: 78 cases (1996–2000). *J Am Vet Med Assoc* 2001; 219:1582–1589.

140. Atwater SW, LaRue SW, Powers BE, Withrow SJ. Adjuvant radiotherapy of soft-tissue sarcomas in dogs. In: *Proceedings of the 12th Annual Conference of the Veterinary Cancer Society*, Pacific Grove, CA, Oct 18–21, 1992.

141. McKnight JA, Mauldin GN, McEntee MC, Meleo KA, Patnaik AK. Radiation treatment for incompletely resected soft-tissue sarcomas in dogs. *J Am Vet Med Assoc* 2000; 17:205–210.

142. Forrest LJ, Chun R, Adams WM, Cooley AJ, Vail DM. Postoperative radiotherapy for canine soft tissue sarcoma. *J Vet Intern Med* 2000; 14:578–582.

143. Prescott DM, Charles HC, Sostman HD, et al. Manipulation of intra- and extracellular pH in spontaneous canine tumors by use of hyperglycemia. *Int J Hyperthermia* 1993; 9:745–754.

144. Prescott DM, Samulski TV, Dewhirst MW, et al. Use of nitroprusside to increase tissue temperature during local hyperthermia in normal and tumor-bearing dogs. *Int J Radiat Oncol Biol Phys* 1992; 23:377–385.

145. Thrall DE, Dewhirst MW, Page RL, et al. A comparison of temperatures in canine solid tumors during local and whole-body hyperthermia administered alone and simultaneously. *Int J Hyperthermia* 1990; 6:305–317.

146. Dewhirst MW, Prescott DM, Clegg S, et al. The use of hydralazine to manipulate tumor temperatures during hyperthermia. *Int J Hyperthermia* 1990; 6:971–983.

147. Gillette SM, Dewhirst MW, Gillette EL, et al. Response of canine soft tissue sarcomas to radiation or radiation plus hyperthermia: a randomized phase II study. *Int J Hyperthermia* 1992; 8:309–329.

148. Page RL, Thrall DE, George SL, et al. Quantitative estimation of the thermal dose-modifying factor for cis-diamminedichloroplatinum (CDDP) in tumor-bearing dogs. *Int J Hyperthermia* 1992; 8:761–769.

149. Sostman HD, Prescott DM, Dewhirst MW, et al. MR imaging and spectroscopy for prognostic evaluation in soft-tissue sarcomas. *Radiology* 1994; 190:269–275.

150. Prescott DM, Charles HC, Sostman HD, et al. Therapy monitoring in human and canine soft tissue sarcomas using magnetic resonance imaging and spectroscopy. *Int J Radiat Oncol Biol Phys* 1994; 28:415–423.

151. Oksanen A. Hemangiosarcoma in dogs. *J Comp Pathol* 1978; 88:585–595.

152. Brown NO, Patnaik AK, MacEwen EG. Canine hemangiosarcoma: retrospective analysis of 104 cases. *J Am Vet Med Assoc* 1985; 186:56–58.

153. Kline LJ, Zook BC, Munson TO. Primary cardiac hemangiosarcoma in dogs. *J Am Vet Med Assoc* 1970; 157:326–337.

154. Spangler WL, Culbertson MR. Prevalence, type, and importance of splenic diseases in dogs: 1,480 cases (1985–1989). *J Am Vet Med Assoc* 1992; 200:829–834.

155. Nikula KJ, Benjamin SA, Angleton GM, Saunders WJ, Lee AC. Ultraviolet radiation, solar dermatosis, and cutaneous neoplasia in beagle dogs. *Radiat Res* 1992; 129:11–18.

156. Johnson KA, Powers BE, Withrow SJ, et al. Splenomegaly in dogs. *J Vet Intern Med* 1989; 3:160–166.

157. Hammer AS, Couto CG, Filppi J, et al. Efficacy and toxicity of VAC chemotherapy (vincristine, doxorubicin, and cyclophosphamide) in dogs with hemangiosarcoma. *J Vet Intern Med* 1991; 5: 160–166.

158. Sorenmo KU, Jeglum KA, Helfand SC. Chemotherapy of canine splenic hemangiosarcoma with doxorubicin and cyclophosphamide. *J Vet Intern Med* 1993; 7:370–376.

159. Vail DM, MacEwen EG, Kurzman ID, et al. Liposome-encapsulated muramyl tripeptide phosphatidylethanolamine adjuvant immunotherapy for splenic hemangiosarcoma in the dog: a randomized multi-institutional clinical trial. *Clin Cancer Res* 1995; 1:1165–1170.

160. Fidler IJ. Macrophages and metastasis—a biological approach to cancer therapy. *Cancer Res* 1985; 45:4714–4726.

161. Kleinerman ES, Fidler IJ. Systemic activation of macrophages by liposomes containing immunomodulators. In: DeVita VT, Hellman S, Rosenberg SA, eds. *Biologic Therapy of Cancer*. Philadelphia: Lippincott. 1995:829–839.

162. Inadomi T, Fujioka A, Suzuki H. A case of malignant hemangioendothelioma showing response to interkeukin-2 therapy. *Br J Dermatol* 1992; 127:442–449.

163. Hershey AE, Kurzman ID, Moore AS, et al. Efficacy of combined inhalational doxorubicin and systemic doxorubicin/cytoxan for adjuvant treatment of canine splenic hemangiosarcoma. In: *Proceedings of the 18th Annual ACVIM Forum*, Seattle, WA, 2000.

164. Sorenmo K, Duda L, Barber L, et al. Canine hemangiosarcoma treated with standard chemotherapy and minocycline. *J Vet Intern Med* 2000; 14:395–398.

165. Brodey RS. The use of naturally occurring cancer in domestic animals for research into human cancer: general information and a review of canine skeletal osteosarcoma. *Yale J Biol Med* 1979; 52:345–361.

166. Withrow SJ, Powers BE, Straw RC, Wilkins RM. Comparative aspects of osteosarcoma. *Clin Orthop* 1991; 270:159–168.

167. Vail DM, Kurzman ID, Glawe PC, et al. STEALTH liposome-encapsulated cisplatin (SPI-77) versus carboplatin as adjuvant therapy for spontaneously arising osteosarcoma (OSA) in the dog: a randomized multicenter clinical trial. *Cancer Chemother Pharmacol* 2002; 50:131–136.

168. Garzotto CK, Berg J, Hoffmann WE, Rand WM. Prognostic significance of serum alkaline phosphatase activity in canine appendicular osteosarcoma. *J Vet Intern Med* 2000; 14:587–592.

169. Ehrhart N, Dernell WS, Hoffmann WE, Weigel RM, Powers BE, Withrow SJ. Prognostic importance of alkaline phosphatase activity in serum from dogs with appendicular osteosarcoma: 75 cases (1990–1996). *J Am Vet Med Assoc* 1998; 213:1002–1006.

170. Spodnick GJ, Berg RJ, Rand WM, et al. Prognosis for dogs with appendicular osteosarcoma treated by amputation alone: 162 cases (1978–1988). *J Am Vet Med Assoc* 1992; 200:995–999.

171. Brodey RS, Abt DA. Results of surgical treatment in 65 dogs with osteosarcoma. *J Am Vet Med Assoc* 1976; 168:1032–1035.

172. Berg J, Weinstein MJ, Springfield DS, Rand WM. Results of surgery and doxorubicin chemotherapy in dogs with osteosarcoma. *J Am Vet Med Assoc* 1995; 206:1555–1560.

173. Bergman PJ, MacEwen EG, Kurzman ID, et al. Amputation and carboplatin for treatment of dogs with osteosarcoma: 48 cases (1991–1993). *J Vet Intern Med* 1995; 10:76–81.

174. Straw RC, Withrow SJ, Richter SL, et al. Amputation and cisplatin for treatment of canine osteosarcoma. *J Vet Intern Med* 1991; 5:205–210.

175. MacEwen EG, Kurzman ID, Rosenthal RC, et al. MLV-MTP-PE with cisplatin in canine osteosarcoma model. A randomized trial. In: Novak JF, MacMaster JH, eds. *Frontiers in Osteosarcoma Research.* Toronto: Hogrefer and Huber. 1993:117–119.

176. MacEwen EG, Kurzman ID, Rosenthal RC, et al. Therapy for osteosarcoma in dogs with intravenous injection of liposome encapsulated muramyl tripeptide. *J Natl Cancer Inst* 1989; 81:935–938.

177. MacEwen EG, Kurzman ID, Helfand S, et al. Current studies of liposome muramyl tripeptide (CGP 19835A Lipid) therapy for metastasis in spontaneous tumors: a progress review. *J Drug Target* 1994; 2:391–396.

178. Kurzman ID, MacEwen EG, Rosenthal RC. Therapy for osteosarcoma in dogs with combined liposome-encapsulated muramyl tripeptide and cisplatin. *Clin Cancer Res* 1995; 1:1595–1601.

179. Straw RC, Withrow SJ, Brekke JH, et, al. The effects of cis-diammine-dichloroplatinum II released from D,L-polylactic acid implants adjacent to cortical allografts in dogs. *J Orthop Res* 1994; 12: 871–877.

180. Sliverberg E, Lubera J. Cancer statistics. *CA* 1987; 37:2–19.

181. Schneider R, Dorn CR, Taylor DON. Factors influencing canine mammary cancer development and postsurgical survival. *J Natl Cancer Inst* 1969; 43:1249–1261.

182. Sorenmo KU, Shofer FS, Goldschmidt MH. Effect of spaying and timing of spaying on survival of dogs with mammary carcinoma. *J Vet Intern Med* 2000; 14:266–270.

183. Nieto A, Pena L, Perez-Alenza MD, Sanchez MA, Flores JM, Castano M. Immunohistologic detection of estrogen receptor alpha in canine mammary tumors: clinical and pathologic associations and prognostic significance. *Vet Pathol* 2000; 37:239–247.

184. Sartin EA, Barnes S, Kwapien RP, et al. Estrogen and progesterone receptor status of mammary carcinomas and correlation with clinical outcome. *Am J Vet Res* 1992; 53:2196–2200.

185. Rutteman GR, Misdorp W, Blankenstein MA, et al. Oestrogen (ER) and progestin receptors (PR) in mammary tissue of the female dog: different receptor profile in malignant and nonmalignant states. *Br J Cancer* 1988; 58:594–599.

186. MacEwen EG, Patnaik AK, Harvey HJ, et al. Estrogen receptors in canine mammary tumors. *Cancer Res* 1982; 42:2255–2259.

187. Martin PM, Cotard M, Mialot JP, et al. Animal models for hormone-dependent human breast cancer. *Cancer Chemother Pharmacol* 1984; 2:13–17.

188. Morris JS, Dobson JM, Bostock DE. Use of tamoxifen in the control of mammary neoplasia. *Vet Rec* 1993; 133:539–542.

189. Gilbertson SR, Kurzman ID, Zachrau RE, Hurvitz AI, Black MM. Canine mammary epithelial neoplasms: biologic implications of morphologic characteristics assessed in 232 dogs. *Vet Pathol* 1983; 20:127–142.
190. Misdorp W, Cotchin E, Hampe JF, Jabara AG, von Sandersleben J. Canine malignant mammary tumours. I. Sarcomas. *Vet Pathol* 1971; 8:99–117.
191. Misdorp W, Cotchin E, Hampe JF, et, al. Canine malignant mammary tumors. II. Adenocarcinomas, solid carcinomas, and spindle cell carcinomas. *Vet Pathol* 1972; 9:447–470.
192. Misdorp W, Cotchin E, Hampe JF, Jabara AG, von Sandersleben J. Canine malignant mammary tumors. III. Special types of carcinomas, malignant mixed tumors. *Vet Pathol* 1973; 10:241–256.
193. Hellmen E, Moller M, Blankenstein MA, Andersson L, Westermark B. Expression of different phenotypes in cell lines from canine mammary spindle-cell tumours and osteosarcomas indicating a pluripotent mammary stem cell origin. *Breast Cancer Res Treat* 2000; 61:197–210.
194. Silver SA, Tavassoli FA. Primary osteogenic sarcoma of the breast: a clinicopathologic analysis of 50 cases. *Am J Surg Pathol* 1998; 22:925–933.
195. Kurzman ID, Gilbertson SR. Prognostic factors in canine mammary tumors. *Semin Vet Med Surg (Small Anim)* 1986; 1:25–32.
196. Hellmen E, Bergstrom R, Holmberg L, Spangberg IB, Hansson K, Lindgren A. Prognostic factors in canine mammary tumors: a multivariate study of 202 consecutive cases. *Vet Pathol* 1993; 30:20–27.
197. MacEwen EG, Harvey HJ, Patnaik AK, et al. Evaluation of effects of levamisole and surgery on canine mammary cancer. *J Biol Response Mod* 1985; 4:418–426.
198. Parodi AL, Misdorp W, Mialot JP, et al. Intratumoral BCG and Corynebacterium parvum therapy of canine mammary tumours before radical mastectomy. *Cancer Immunol Immunother* 1983; 15:172–177.
199. Bostock DE, Gorman NT. Intravenous BCG therapy of mammary carcinoma in bitches after surgical excision of the primary tumour. *Eur J Cancer* 1978; 14:8789–883.
200. Hayes HMJ, Milne K, Mandell CP. Epidemiological features of feline mammary carcinoma. *Vet Rec* 1981; 108:476–479.
201. Elling H, Ungemach FR. Progesterone receptors in feline mammary cancer cytosol. *J Cancer Res Clin Oncol* 1981; 100:325–327.
202. Johnston SD, Hayden DW, Kiang DT, Handschin B, Johnson KH. Progesterone receptors in feline mammary adenocarcinomas. *Am J Vet Res* 1984; 45:397–382.
203. Rutteman GR, Blankenstein MA, Minke J, Misdorp W. Steroid receptors in mammary tumours of the cat. *Acta Endocrinol (Copenh)* 1991; 125(suppl):32–37.
204. Weijer K, Hart AA. Prognostic factors in feline mammary carcinoma. *J Natl Cancer Inst* 1983; 70: 709–716.
205. MacEwen EG, Hayes AA, Harvey HJ, Patnaik AK, Mooney S, Passe S. Prognostic factors for feline mammary tumors. *J Am Vet Med Assoc* 1984; 185:201–204.
206. Jeglum K, A, deGuzman E, Young KM. Chemotherapy of advanced mammary adenocarcinoma in 14 cats. *J Am Vet Med Assoc* 1985; 187:157–1650.
207. Mauldin G, Matus R, Patnaik A. Efficacy and toxicity of doxorubicin and cyclophosphamide used in the treatment of selected malignant tumors in 23 cats. *J Vet Intern Med* 1988; 2:60–65.
208. MacEwen EG, Hayes AA, Mooney S, et al. Evaluation of effect of levamisole on feline mammary cancer. *J Biol Response Mod* 1984; 3:541–546.
209. Rutten VP, Misdorp W, Gauthier A, et al. Immunological aspects of mammary tumors in dogs and cats: a survey including own studies and pertinent literature. *Vet Immunol Immunopathol* 1990; 26:211–225.
210. Fox LE, MacEwen EG, Kurzman ID, et al. Liposome-encapsulated muramyl tripeptide phosphatidylethanolamine for the treatment of feline mammary adenocarcinoma—a multicenter randomized double-blind study. *Cancer Biother* 1995; 10:125–130.
211. Hoyt RF, Withrow SJ. Oral malignancy in the dog. *J Am An Hosp Assoc* 1982; 20:83–92.
212. Harvey HJ, MacEwen EG, Braun D, Patnaik AK, Withrow SJ, Jongeward S. Prognostic criteria for dogs with oral melanoma. *J Am Vet Med Assoc* 1981; 178:580–582.
213. MacEwen EG, Patnaik AK, Harvey HJ, Hayes AA, Matus R. Canine oral melanoma: comparison of surgery versus surgery plus Corynebacterium parvum. *Cancer Invest* 1986; 4:397–402.
214. Page RL, Thrall DE, Dewhirst MW, et, al. Phase I study of melphalan alone and melphalan plus whole body hyperthermia in dogs with malignant melanoma. *Int J Hyperthermia* 1991; 7:559–566.
215. Rassnick KM, Ruslander DM, Cotter SM, et al. Use of carboplatin for treatment of dogs with malignant melanoma: 27 cases (1989–2000). *J Am Vet Med Assoc* 2001; 218:1444–1448.

216. Blackwood L, Dobson JM. Radiotherapy of oral malignant melanomas in dogs. *J Am Vet Med Assoc* 1996; 209:98–102.
217. Bateman KE, Catton PA, Pennock PM, Kruth SA. 0-7-21 radiation therapy for the palliation of advanced cancer in dogs. *J Vet Intern Med* 1994; 8:394–-399.
218. Proulx DR, Ruslander DM, Dodge RK, et al. A retrospective analysis of 140 dogs with oral melanoma treated with external beam radiation. *Vet Radiol Ultrasound* 2003; 44:352–359.
219. MacEwen EG, Kurzman ID, Vail DM, et al. Adjuvant therapy for melanoma in dogs: results of randomized clinical trials using surgery, liposome-encapsulated muramyl tripeptide, and GM-CSF. *Clin Cancer Res* 1999; 5:4249–4258.
220. Hogge GS, Burkholder JK, Culp J, et al. Development of hGM-CSF transfected tumor cell vaccines in spontaneous canine cancer. *Human Gene Ther* 1998; 9:1851–1861.
221. Walsh P, Gonzalez R, Dow S, et al. A phase I study using direct combination DNA injections for the immunotherapy of metastatic melanoma. University of Colorado Cancer Center Clinical Trial. *Hum Gene Ther* 2000; 11:1355–1368.
222. Knapp DW, Glickman NW, DeNicola DB, et al. Naturally occurring canine transitional cell carcinoma of the urinary bladder: a relevant model of human invasive bladder cancer. *Urol Oncol* 2000; 5:47–59.
223. Helfand SC, Hamilton TA, Hungerford LL, et al. Comparison of three treatments for transitional cell carcinoma of the bladder in the dog. *J Am An Hosp Assoc* 1994; 30:270–275.
224. Chun R, Knapp DW, Widmer WR, et al. Cisplatin treatment of transitional cell carcinoma of the urinary bladder in dogs: 18 cases (1983–1993). *J Am Vet Med Assoc* 1996; 209:1588–1591.
225. Moore AS, Cardona A, Shapiro W, et al. Cisplatin (cisdiamminedichloroplatinum) for treatment of transitional call carcinoma of the urinary bladder or urethra: a retrospective study of 15 dogs. *J Vet Intern Med* 1990; 4:148–152.
226. Marynissen JP, Jansen H, Star WM. Treatment system for whole bladder wall photodynamic therapy with in vivo monitoring and control of light dose rate and dose. *J Urol* 1989; 142:1351–1355.
227. Nseyo UO, Dougherty TJ, Boyle DG, Potter WR. Study of factors mediating effect of photodynamic therapy on bladder in canine bladder model. *Urology* 1988; 32:41–45.
228. Nseyo UO, Whalen RK, Lundahl SL. Canine bladder response to red and green light whole bladder photodynamic therapy. *Urology* 1993; 41:392–396.
229. Knapp DW, Richardson RC, Chan TC, et al. Piroxicam therapy in 34 dogs with transitional cell carcinoma of the urinary bladder. *J Vet Intern Med* 1994; 8:273–278.
230. Knapp DW, Glickman NW, Widmer WR, et al. Cisplatin versus cisplatin combined with piroxicam in a canine model of human invasive urinary bladder cancer. *Cancer Chemother Pharmacol* 2000; 46:221–226.

III

NONCLINICAL TESTING TO SUPPORT HUMAN TRIALS

13 Nonclinical Testing

From Theory to Practice

Denis Roy, PhD and Paul A. Andrews, PhD

CONTENTS

INTRODUCTION
DESIGNING THE NONCLINICAL SAFETY DEVELOPMENT PROGRAM:
   MAPPING YOUR SUCCESS
DESIGNING TOXICOLOGY STUDIES
OUTSOURCING SAFETY STUDIES
COMMON ISSUES IN TOXICOLOGY TESTING
CONCLUSIONS

1. INTRODUCTION

Plans are only good intentions unless they immediately degenerate into hard work.
—Peter F. Drucker

In the pharmaceutical development arena, Drucker's quotation represents one of the biggest challenges to be faced. One can set up many great plans and strategies, but until they are set in motion they remain abstract. Planning is one of the key steps for efficiently leading a project to a successful completion and its importance has long been recognized in many disciplines besides pharmaceutical development. Although the plan itself does not constitute a guarantee for a successful outcome, it maximizes the chances of success while attempting to minimize unexpected and unnecessary detours. Success in the pharmaceutical development process is often measured by the ability of a company to discover compounds with promising therapeutic effects and, through efficient testing in animals and humans, learn enough about their properties so they can be used in a manner such that the observed benefits outweigh the potential risks to the patient. From a business perspective, with efficiency being the key to survival, success is most often measured by the company's ability to reach its destination in the most expeditious manner while using

From: *Cancer Drug Discovery and Development:*
Anticancer Drug Development Guide: Preclinical Screening, Clinical Trials, and Approval, 2nd Ed.
Edited by: B. A. Teicher and P. A. Andrews © Humana Press Inc., Totowa, NJ

the fewest resources and without compromising the quality of the essential information gathered along the process.

Currently, there is an abundance of scientists from research, biotechnology, pharmaceutical, and government organizations with extensive knowledge, expertise, and training in regulatory toxicology. Additionally, the recent availability of numerous guidance documents and more open lines of communications between these organizations make today's drug development industry a much more accessible field. Nonetheless, few publications are available that provide tangible practical information and guidance on how to execute a toxicology program for an oncology product. The purpose of this chapter is therefore to provide readers with useful tools, key information, and practical guidance that will allow them not only to design a nonclinical safety development plan, but also to execute the toxicology plan efficiently and successfully to achieve the targeted scientific, regulatory, and corporate goals.

2. DESIGNING THE NONCLINICAL SAFETY DEVELOPMENT PROGRAM: MAPPING YOUR SUCCESS

The famous French quotation from Alain de Lille "Tout les chemins mènent à Rome" ("All roads lead to Rome") originating from his Latin medieval publication, the *Liber parabolatum* in 1175, describes the drug development process very well. Indeed, if one would ask five toxicologists to design a nonclinical safety development plan for a given compound, they would probably come up with five different strategies even if they all had the same goal of supporting the safety of a specific phase I trial. Interestingly, the same phenomenon would probably be observed if one would ask five toxicologists to design a specific toxicology study. Even though some of those plans would probably be much less efficient than others (e.g., using more resources or time), it is likely that most of them would nonetheless be successful. Therefore, it is critical to understand that in the drug development process there are many ways to develop an investigational product successfully, but only a few ways to do it in the most efficient manner.

2.1. The Fine Balance Among Sound Science, Regulatory Expectations, and Corporate Objectives

Toxicology testing involves many steps and calls for a complete integration of multiple disciplines, including chemistry, manufacturing, and controls (CMC), as well as clinical, regulatory, corporate, and project management in order to be successful. One of the most common misconceptions about toxicology testing is that one needs to conduct the full range of studies listed in guidance documents in the belief that they will undoubtedly be required by regulatory agencies. In addition, some nonclinical planners also rely heavily on toxicology programs of previously approved products in the same or a similar therapeutic class, inappropriately assuming that what was good for others must be good for them. Although it may sound like a reasonably safe approach, it often leads to one of the most common mistakes made by sponsors: toxicology programs are designed and even executed without a clear understanding and integration of the different key components involved. Indeed, multiple factors (e.g., the clinical plan, the physicochemical properties, pharmacokinetic and pharmacodynamic profiles) will require careful considerations when one is designing a nonclinical plan. Each of these factors may be very different from those associated with the already approved product, and therefore a previously successful plan may not be suitable for the contemplated investigational new drug or biologic product.

Overall, the toxicology program needs to support the proposed clinical trials from phase I to a marketing application. Indeed, it is critical to understand that the toxicology program will probably not be efficient or successful if the clinical approach contemplated has not been clearly defined (i.e., targeted population, indication, route of administration, dosing regimen, treatment duration, phase of development). As an example, dermal toxicology studies are not likely to be adequate for supporting an initial clinical trial using the intravenous route in humans. Similarly, single-dose toxicology studies will generally not support a 3-mo daily dosing clinical trial. This does not mean that a fully defined clinical protocol needs to be in place before initiating the toxicology program but rather that the critical components (particularly the population[s] to be exposed, route of administration, dosing regimen, and treatment duration) are known or at least estimated so that the toxicology program is tailor-made for the clinical approach. A good rule of thumb in toxicology testing, and drug development in general, is that you always plan backward and execute forward. Indeed, this is also true for many aspects of the drug development process, including CMC, in which the clinical use (e.g., route of administration, treatment duration, dose range) will significantly drive the CMC development plan decisions. Sponsors failing to meet their corporate objectives often realize, after the fact, that a clear understanding of the clinical objectives along with the proper integration of all the disciplines involved was neglected or underestimated.

Another component that needs to be considered when designing a toxicology program is the corporate objectives of the company. Nonclinical program strategists often hear that even though they have provided the most scientifically sound toxicology program for their product, the project will not be viable for the company if it takes that long and costs that much. Obviously, from a corporate perspective, the toxicology program should be short and inexpensive but of sufficient quality and informational content so that safety can be thoroughly addressed and so that no major questions are raised either internally or by the regulatory agencies. Therefore, one of the biggest challenges for the toxicologist is trying to find the right balance between corporate needs and sound science while satisfying current regulatory agencies' expectations.

This quest for the best compromise often leads to a series of unwise decisions, which eventually results in serious problems during the toxicology program. The serious problem may look to the untrained spectator like a complete failure in planning owing to severe strategic or scientific deficiencies. In reality, the problem is often the culmination of many small, apparently insignificant risks taken at different times during the development process for the wrong reasons rather than an inadequate plan to start with.

2.2. Toxicology Program for Oncology Products

For most young biotechnology and small pharmaceutical companies, the biggest challenge is successfully filing an initial Investigational New Drug (IND) application in the Unites States, or a Clinical Trial Application (CTA) in Canada. As discussed in other chapters of this book, the type and nature of toxicology studies required for an oncology product depend on multiple factors. On numerous occasions, the first question that consultants address is what would be a typical toxicology program for an oncology product.

Unfortunately, the true answer is that there is no typical toxicology program, especially when considering biologic products. However, even if the toxicology program needs to be customized to fulfill precise and unique needs of the product being developed, there are a number of components that are consistently present in most toxicology programs. For example, per ICH M3 and S6 guidance documents (1,2), toxicology studies should be conducted in at least two animal species, one being a non-rodent species, unless it can be scientifically justified that only one appropriate species exists. In addition, the studies should use the intended route of administration and be of sufficient duration to cover the intended clinical trial.

Detailed information on the type and nature of the toxicology studies required for different types and classes of oncology product are provided in other chapters of this book. It is important to understand that each program needs to be adapted based on the technology being developed, the targeted population, the clinical stage of development, the route of administration, and the treatment duration.

The need for conducting range-finding studies will be driven by the available safety data from animals studies conducted to explore pharmacology and pharmacokinetic properties, from experience with the class, and from the level of risk determined to be acceptable for the program. Range-finding studies are usually conducted to provide preliminary identification of the target organs of toxicity as well as to select doses for the definitive study intended to support the clinical trials. Many oncology drug products being developed today are intended to be given chronically, and initial trials can usually be supported with 28-d studies, as described in other chapters. There are many approaches available for identifying appropriate doses for the essential 28-d studies for these investigational agents, but the two most common are discussed. The first approach usually consists of conducting acute (single-dose) studies in rodents and non-rodents followed by 7-, 10-, or 14-d range finding studies, and then definitive 28-d studies. This approach has the advantage of providing much valuable information on the safety profile of the product while minimizing the chances of selecting the wrong dose levels for the pivotal repeated dose toxicology studies. However, such an approach is longer, as it involves running multiple studies consecutively and may therefore not be compatible with the corporate objectives. This approach is also more costly.

A second approach is to conduct combined single and repeated dose range-finding studies. These studies usually attempt to define the maximally tolerated dose (or maximal feasible dose) given as a single administration; once the findings from the acute portion of the study are available, they are used to project the appropriate high dose for the pivotal study. A separate set of animals is typically then used to establish whether the dose selected is relatively tolerable when administered over 7–14 consecutive d. This combined approach usually shortens the range-finding phase of the program by approx 2–3 mo without adding a significant amount of risk to the program. Costs and animal usage are also greatly reduced. The type of range-finding studies selected will be highly driven by the nature of the product being developed, the corporate tolerance for risk, and timeline constraints.

Although it is not required to conduct range-finding studies according to Good Laboratory Practice (GLP) regulations for regulatory submissions of oncology products, conducting those studies according to U.S. GLP regulations (3) is recommended, as it usually does not significantly increase the costs of the overall program. In addition, based on our experience, the quality of the study conduct and the data generated is usually higher for GLP studies compared with non-GLP studies. In addition, GLP-compliant range-finding studies can sometimes offer a fallback strategy to enter a drug into the clinic with a more attenuated schedule than planned, if the subsequent definitive studies fail (e.g., because of early termination owing to excessive toxicity).

Toxicokinetic assessments, although not required, are strongly recommended for inclusion into all single-dose and repeated-dose toxicology studies. Toxicokinetic analyses should be included whenever possible because these data will assist in interspecies comparisons, help establish appropriate doses and dosing schedules in humans, and aid in the selection of appropriate doses for subsequent repeated-dose toxicology studies.

2.3. Typical Cost Estimates and Standard Timelines

The toxicology program usually consumes most of the initial financial resources allocated for nonclinical development of a product candidate. Most companies therefore have a great interest in obtaining precise external cost estimates for their toxicology program. In this chapter, the term *external cost estimates* will be used to refer to the costs associated with subcontracting the toxicology study to a specialized GLP laboratory, often referred to as a toxicology Contract Research Organization (CRO). External cost estimates typically include costs associated with the conduct of the entire study, i.e., animal costs, technical activities, standard safety evaluations and analyses, results reporting, and overheads. Study costs can vary greatly depending on the animal species, the route of administration, the duration of treatment, the laboratory selected, and the economic situation of the laboratory or the CRO market. Differences in study costs between toxicology CROs should be expected even for an identical study design. Reputation, experience, quality, timeliness, professionalism, financial status, sophistication of instrumentation, and company organization are all contributing factors that will lead to appreciable cost variations between CROs. Additional costs should also be expected when specific or specialized analyses like special stains, histopathologic examinations, or clinical chemistry parameters; specific cardiovascular assessments; or toxicokinetic analyses and modeling are requested.

With amounts typically ranging from $500,000 to $1,000,000 U.S., the initial toxicology program quickly becomes the center of attention and scrutiny from the different management and financial levels of the company. Indeed, underestimation of the expected IND-enabling toxicology program cost in a business plan can be devastating to any company, especially smaller ones. On many occasions, we have encountered companies that realized they had significantly underestimated the costs associated with their toxicology program (often by 2–10 times the actual costs). Unfortunately, many of them try to fill the money gap by minimizing expenses, which often means modifying the toxicology program (deleting some important studies) or even altering study designs (sizing down the type and number of safety endpoints, decreasing the number of animals, shortening the duration of the study). Therefore, getting accurate cost estimates so that appropriate resources can be budgeted becomes a critical step for ensuring a strong and scientifically sound toxicology program.

We recognize that providing cost estimates for toxicology studies is always questionable, as they can become outdated in a relatively short period, depending on the nuances of the marketplace. The cost estimates outlined in this chapter nonetheless provide a good reflection of the actual market and can be used to estimate better the projected toxicology program costs. Table 1 presents cost estimates and typical durations for report generation for most toxicology studies generally conducted for most products. These estimates may vary greatly depending on the study design, the species selected, the type and nature of the analyses conducted during the study, and the toxicology CRO selected.

In addition, the cost estimates provided do not include test article costs, analytical method development, validation and analyses, toxicokinetic sample assessment and modeling, special histopathology assessment and/or tissue collection, special clinical pathology, satellite groups for toxicokinetics, recovery groups, or modified study designs.

2.3.1. TIME AND RESOURCES: GETTING BEYOND THE FIRST IMPRESSION

Overall toxicology program costs are often the first and foremost criteria used in the corporate strategic decision-making process when it comes to toxicology testing. Although minimizing the study costs may not always be in the best interests of science, it is definitely a major consideration for corporate finance departments and strategic investors.

In many cases, toxicologists need to design a scientifically sound toxicology program while satisfying both regulatory expectations and corporate needs. A good strategy that can be used to achieve cost-saving objectives is to select the minimal study duration required for supporting the initial clinical trial. For example, a company may choose to conduct pivotal 14-d toxicology studies rather than 28-d studies to support an initial clinical trial in which patients will be treated for no more than 14 consecutive days per cycle. In addition to fulfilling regulatory expectations in accordance with the current oncology division practices and the ICH M3 guidance document, this approach would also decrease associated costs by approx $85,000 U.S. and the overall timeline by approx 2 wk (Table 2).

Although in many cases it does provide a significant advantage to the company for an initial IND, it is important to realize that this approach often leads to a more expensive toxicology program later during the development process. For example, the company that conducted 14-d pivotal toxicology studies to support the initial clinical trial with 14 d of treatment per cycle may subsequently desire to treat patients for 28 consecutive days per cycle (e.g., amended schedule in the phase I trial or phase II study) to explore a new potential for efficacy. The available nonclinical safety information from the 14-d toxicology program (option 1) would not support, in most cases, the intended 28 d of dose administration. Accordingly, the company would need to conduct additional 28-d toxicology studies in order to support the new phase I or phase II clinical trials, which would lead to additional costs and require additional time.

As shown in Table 2, although the initial 14-d strategy was beneficial to the company, it may well become an obstacle for initiating subsequent phase I or phase II clinical trials of longer duration (i.e., 28 d). Consequently, the overall costs for the toxicology program (option 1) would be increased by approx $245,000 U.S. and would require an additional 4 mo compared with option 2.

Ultimately, the selection of the appropriate toxicology studies should be guided by the planned clinical trial duration. Indeed, 14-d toxicology studies will generally support clinical trials of up to 14 d, whereas 28-d toxicology studies will support trials of up to 28 d. On many occasions, the 28-d option provides the advantage of supporting clinical

Table 1
Estimated External Costs for Representative Nonclinical Safety Studies

Study type	Approximate external costs[a] (U.S. $)			Approximate duration[b] (wk)
	Rats	*Dogs*	*Monkeys*	
Single-dose and range-finding				
Single dose	6000–25,000	20,000–50,000	20,000–70,000	10–12
Combined Single and 7-d repeat dose	20,000–80,000	40,000–90,000	80,000–120,000	10–12
Combined single and 10-d repeat dose	35,000–67,000	45,000–75,000	85,000–125,000	10–12
Repeat dose toxicology				
7-d	20,000–35,000	34,000–70,000	55,000–75,000	14–16
14-d	40,000–115,000	90,000–130,000	100,000–190,000	14–16
28-d	70,000–150,000	80,000–195,000	150,000–300,000	16–18
3-mo	110,000–270,000	165,000–200,000	240,000–500,000	30–34
6-mo	215,000–350,000	190,000–300,000	350,000–500,000	40–44
9-mo	275,000–375,000	250,000–500,000	400,000–620,000	52–56
12-mo	320,000–490,000	320,000–470,000	500,000–840,000	68–74
Genetic toxicity				
Ames test		5000–10,000		8–12
In vitro chromosomal aberration assay		10,000–35,000		12–16
In vivo micronucleus test (mice/rats)		10,000–30,000		12–16
	Mice/rats		*Rabbits*	
Reproductive toxicology				
Fertility study: rats	75,000–160,000		—	20–24
Range-finding developmental toxicity	30,000–50,000		40,000–60,000	12–16
Developmental Toxicity	60,000–145,000		125,000–175,000	16–24
Peri- and Postnatal/multigeneration	155,000–250,000		—	22–42

[a]Cost may vary greatly depending on study design, the species selected, and the Contract Research Organization. Costs do not include test article costs, analytical method development and validation, toxicokinetic sample assessment and modeling, special histopathology assessment and/or tissue collection, or special clinical pathology.

[b]Approximate duration represents the total duration starting from the initiation of treatment up to the completion of an audited draft report.

Table 2
Estimated Costs and Timeline Comparisons for a 14-Day (Option 1) or 28-Day (Option 2)
Pivotal Toxicology Program to Support up to 28 Days of Treatment in Clinical Trials[a]

Studies	Species	Option 1 Costs[b] (U.S. $)	Option 2 Costs[b] (U.S. $)
To support initial phase I and II clinical trials of up to 14 d of treatment (initial IND)			
14-d	Rats	115,000	—
	Dogs	130,000	—
28-d	Rats	—	135,000
	Dogs	—	195,000
Total costs		245,000	330,000
Total duration		16 wk	18 wk
To support phase II clinical trials of up to 28 d of treatment or longer			
28-d	Rats[c]	135,000	Not applicable
	Dogs[c]	195,000	Not applicable
Additional costs		330,000	0
Additional timeline		18 wk	0 wk
Overall costs		575,000	330,000
Overall timeline		34 wk	18 wk

[a] Costs and timelines are only represented for the repeated-dose toxicology studies and do not account for other studies or activities involved as they would be expected to be the same for both options.
[b] Only maximal costs represented for comparison purposes.
[c] Additional studies required for option 1.

trials of longer duration with minimal additional costs and time compared with a 14-d program. Additionally, the overall costs for the nonclinical safety program to support treatment for up to 28 consecutive days in clinical trials would be much less and would save time. Of course there will always be exceptions, especially in the biologic product arena, but this approach would be applicable to most investigational products.

The estimated timelines for a standard toxicology program is normally from 9 to 12 mo, depending on the actual initial clinical trial study design, the availability of the test article, the safety profile of the investigational new drug, and the sponsor's corporate objectives. The toxicology program timeline should allow for conducting appropriate range-finding studies in a timely manner to gather appropriate information for the subsequent studies. It is also generally recommended that early rodent studies be initiated before non-rodent studies, as this approach will usually provide very useful information on the safety profile of the product, especially those that have not been administered at high doses before or those that represent a new therapeutic class. In addition, rodent studies are generally less expensive than non-rodent studies and therefore provide an additional cost-saving strategy in cases in which unexpected or severe toxicity occurs. Another typical mistake made when planning the toxicology program timeline is not accounting for pre-in-life (e.g., animal ordering and acclimation) and post-in-life activities (e.g., histopathology processing, quality assurance activities, report writing). Typical timelines from the initiation of dosing up until the issuance of an audited (quality-assured) draft report are presented in Table 1.

As with any plan, optimized strategies can be developed to allow for an accelerated development of the investigational new product while minimizing the associated costs. However, the potential benefits associated with a more optimized or aggressive approach are generally proportional to the risks involved. In our experience, nonclinical development plans can be optimized to bring down the overall timeline by approx 2–4 mo and the nonclinical study costs by approx $50,000–$400,000. This optimization is usually achieved through strategic combination of some key studies or safety assessments while maximizing the safety information gathered. However, the strategy used should always be carefully selected, especially when project leaders have limited experience or when little or no information is available on the product.

3. DESIGNING TOXICOLOGY STUDIES

Once the toxicology program has been established, the toxicologist will then be confronted with the conceptualization and conduct of each study protocol that need to generate adequate data to support the safety of the intended clinical trial(s). Properly designing a toxicology study requires appropriate training; a thorough understanding of the regulatory requirements and expectations, and standard good industry practices, as well as hands-on experience in the field of toxicology. The transition from a theoretical plan to a practical protocol is typically one of the major obstacles for most companies, as many scientists involved in outlining the toxicology program are lacking experience and knowledge in toxicology testing. Understanding the difference between toxicology and toxicology testing is critical as both terms are often used interchangeably. The educated toxicologist needs an intensive practical training before being able to transition from a theoretical development plan to the actual successful completion of the program.

Most toxicology CROs have extensive experience in conducting different types of nonclinical studies and are undoubtedly a very good source of information and guidance. Experienced study directors with proper toxicology training are exposed to a wide variety of complex and unusual problems, findings, and challenges and should therefore always be involved in the discussions regarding the design of a study protocol. A good toxicology CRO should provide sponsors with draft study protocols, which are often designed in accordance with current industry practice standards and most regulatory requirements. However, the toxicology study design should always be tailor-made for the product being developed in order to meet scientific, regulatory, and corporate objectives.

3.1. Route of Administration

The route of administration for oncology products must be carefully selected based on multiple considerations (e.g., physicochemical properties, pharmacokinetics, pharmacodynamics, intended therapeutic use, technical practicality, marketability, and patient compliance). The implications and limitations of the selected route of administration in animal toxicology studies is often underestimated and taken for granted.

Indeed, failure to consider the route of administration carefully in a toxicology program can lead to serious problems as the program progresses. For example, the route of administration will significantly impact on the amount of test article that is required. The best example is the typical two- to fourfold increase in test article requirements for a product to be given by inhalation compared with the intravenous route, assuming that toxicity will occur at similar doses. Although the example may seem scientifically questionable, it is mainly owing to the "inefficient" nature of the exposure system used for inhalation studies in which a large amount of material is lost in the system. Similarly, continuous intravenous infusion studies require substantially more test article than when administering the same dose by intravenous bolus owing to the dead volumes in the pumps, reservoirs, and tubing.

3.1.1. DOSE VOLUMES AND GOOD PRACTICES

The most common mistake in toxicology testing is the use of an inappropriate dose volume to administer the product in animals. Even with the availability of excellent publications *(4–6)* on the subject, many sponsors are still facing major complications in their toxicology program owing to inappropriate dose volumes being used. This may in part be explained by the general lack of awareness of the effects of excessive volume loading in mammals and the lack of knowledge about recommended good industry and veterinary practices.

Another reason that often explains why such problems occur is the misunderstanding of current regulatory toxicology expectations. Indeed, toxicologists at regulatory agencies generally expect that the highest dose tested in any pivotal animal toxicology study induce significant toxicity to define the toxicity profile of a test article adequately. Therefore, it is generally believed that failure to do so would warrant repeating the study. Although this principle is endorsed by most regulatory toxicologists and is generally applicable to most products being developed, except for certain biologics, it should never compromise the scientific integrity of the study. For example, in cases in which the physicochemical properties of a test article dictate that the maximum feasible or achievable dose (i.e., maximal biocompatible concentration given at the maximal recommended dose volume) does not elicit any adverse effects in animals, this dose would represent an adequate high dose for the study. Increasing the dose volume in ranges that are not recommended may leave the impression that one has achieved the ultimate goal, but in reality the study may have just compromised the test system and may consequently lead to the confounding of study results. A summary of some recommended dose volumes extracted from different key literature sources *(4–6)* is presented in Table 3. The reader is strongly encouraged to consult those publications for more details and information.

3.2. Species Selection

One of the important factors to consider when designing a toxicology program is the selection of appropriate animal species, often referred to as the test system. Indeed, selection of proper animal species will optimize the usefulness of the safety data generated and improve its predictiveness for effects in humans. Historically, animal species were typically selected based on little or no considerations other than practicality and availability. However, the selection process was often based on a default system approach with little or no considerations for the technology being tested. Indeed, rats and mice were definitely the most popular rodent species, whereas dogs ruled as the preferred nonrodent species. Accordingly, it was generally recognized and granted that rats and dogs were the best animal species for safety testing purposes, and unless some unexpected toxicities were observed when the investigational product was administered to these species, they were automatically assumed to be adequate. The experience gained by many

Table 3
Summary of Recommended Dose Volumes for Toxicology Studies[a]

Route of administration

Species	iv Bolus (mL/kg)		iv Short infusion (mL/kg/h)		24-h infusion (mL/kg/h)		po (mL/kg)		sc (mL/site)		ip (mL/kg)		im (mL/site)		Dermal (mL/kg)		Intranasal (mL/nostrils)	
	Optim	Max	Optim	Max	Optim	Max	Optim	Max	Optim	Max	Optim	Max	Optim	Max	Optim	Max	Optim	Max
Mouse	5	10–25	—	25	4	8	10	20–50	1–10	10–40	5–20	20–80	0.05–1	—	—	—	0.05	—
Rat	1–5	5–20	5	20	2.5	4	10	20–50	1–5	5–20	5–10	10–20	0.1–10	—	2	6	0.1	0.2
Hamster	—	5	—	—	—	—	—	20	—	5	—	10	0.1	—	—	—	0.1	—
Guinea pig	—	5	—	—	—	—	—	20	—	5	—	10	0.1	—	—	—	0.2	—
Rabbit	1–3	2–10	—	10	1	3	10	10–20	1–2.5	1–10	5	4–20	0.25–1	—	2	8	0.5	—
Dog	1–2.5	2.5–10	5	5	1	4	5–10	10–20	0.5–1	1–2	1–3	1–20	—	—	—	—	0.5	—
Macaque	1–2	2–10	2.5	—	—	—	5–10	10–15	0.5–2	1–5	3	5–10	—	—	—	—	0.5	—
Marmoset	1–2.5	2.5–10	2.5	10	—	—	10	10–15	0.5–2	1–5	3	5–20	—	—	—	—	0.2	—
Mini pig	2.5	—	1.0	5	—	—	10	15	1	2	1	20	—	—	—	—	—	—

[a]Values extracted from refs. 4–6.

ABBREVIATIONS: Optim, optimal; Max, maximum under any circumstance; iv, intravenous; po, oral gavage; sc, subcutaneous; ip, intraperitoneal; im, intramuscular.

Table 4
Species Selection Considerations

Criteria	Comments or examples
Phamacodynamics, biological activity	Receptor presence, homology and distribution; mechanism of action
Pharmacokinetic, ADME	Comparable kinetics or adequate kinetics vs humans; metabolic and detoxification pathways
Biology, anatomy, and physiology	Absence of gallbladder and higher endogenous folate levels in rats; deficient glucuronidation in cats; deficient N-acetylation in dogs; longevity in rodents is shorter than in non-rodents and they are therefore most suitable for carcinogenicity testing
Historical databases	Background biologic variability in normal animals must be known; most GLP toxicology laboratories have significant databases for most standard species
Regulatory requirements	Specific species requirements as per guidance documents and regulatory expectations; class effects
Economical considerations	Rodents are fairly inexpensive compared with dogs and primates; primates are approx 10 times more expensive than dogs
Timelines	The time to get animals to the toxicology laboratory is significantly longer for monkeys than dogs; generally not an issue for rodents
Route of administration	Continuous intravenous administration is more challenging in small rodents like mice and is difficult to perform for very long duration
Test article availability	More test article is required for bigger species assuming that there are no major interspecies differences in sensitivity

ABBREVIATIONS: ADME, absorption, distribution, metabolism, and excretion; GLP, Good Laboratory Practice.

toxicologists over the years has shown on many occasions that such an approach is no longer sufficient.

The selection of species for any toxicology program requires multiple careful and meticulous considerations before initiating a very expensive safety program. Indeed, regulatory agencies are now more stringent on the justifications provided to support the choice of any species used in a toxicology program, and sponsors are now expected to provide a scientifically sound rationale supporting the relevancy of the species used. A list of some key criteria that should be considered is presented in Table 4.

One of the key factors that will determine the relevance of a species is the presence (or absence) of the intended biological effects of the investigational product. In cases in which one particular species does not have the targeted receptor or has a very different distribution or sequence homology compared with other species, including humans, careful considerations should be given regarding the use of such species for safety testing, as the relevance to humans may be low or questionable. Additionally, species that are well known to be insensitive to some therapeutic agents or to display a very unique toxicity profile compared with other species should not be used, as they may not provide useful data on the potential safety profile in humans.

Dogs have historically been used for most pharmaceutical products including oncology products. However, the recent increases in biologic product development and primate availability have changed the industry quite drastically. Indeed, the use of non-human primates has increased substantially over the past years, even to the extent that the worldwide supplies have probably reached their limit. The recent expansion of primate use in toxicology testing is not only owing to the closer phylogenetic links with humans, but also to the substantial decrease in the amount of test material required for the toxicology program. Indeed, rhesus, cynomolgus, and marmoset monkeys are approx 2.5, 3, and 12 times smaller than a dog, which leads to significant savings on test article. Another factor that should be considered, however, is the rapidity with which primate and dog studies can be scheduled and initiated at contracting facilities, excluding those that retain breeding colonies where animals are readily available. If timing is a more critical issue than the supply of test material, then dogs may be a more suitable choice, provided that it is still a relevant species based on the other considerations.

3.3. Number of Animals

One area of debate regards the number of animals that should be used in toxicology testing. Although animal welfare, scientific, regulatory, statistical, technical, practical, and financial considerations need to be considered, the study design should nonetheless optimize the reliability of the safety information generated. Multiple scientific organizations meet on a regular basis to refine further animal use in scientific research, and publications can be found in the literature. A number of excellent publications also provides very useful information on study designs and safety endpoints. Tables 5 through 9 summarize the number of animals typically used for different studies by different groups.

3.4. Dose Level Selection

A scientifically valid toxicology study should ideally establish a high dose level at which toxicity is observed and characterized so that toxicity may be carefully monitored or avoided in clinical trials. Establishing a low dose at which no toxicity is observed is typically required for nononcology indications and is usually desirable but not essential for oncology products. As discussed previously, doses should be high enough to induce toxicity unless limitations restrict the achievable doses in these studies (e.g., dose volume, solubility).

Dose levels for pivotal repeated-dose toxicology studies are usually selected based on the results of acute and dose range-finding toxicology studies. The study design should ideally include at least one control group and three treated groups. Accordingly, the initial toxicology program should be designed to provide the required key information on the safety profile of the investigational product so that appropriate dose levels for the IND-enabling, repeated-dose toxicology studies can be selected.

3.5. Toxicity Endpoints

A scientifically sound toxicology study should assess appropriate safety endpoints to establish the safety profile of a product. There are some fairly standard endpoints in the

Table 5
Typical Number of Animals Used in Single-Dose Nonclinical Toxicology Studies[a]

Group no. and identification	No. of animals/sex				
	Rodents[b]			Nonrodents[b]	
	Main	TK	Recovery[c]	Main	Recovery[c]
1. Control	3–5	—[d]	3–5	1–2	1–2
2. Low dose	3–5	—[d]	0–5	1–2	0–2
3. Mid dose	3–5	—[d]	0–5	1–2	0–2
4. High dose	3–5	—[d]	3–5	1–2	1–2

[a]For rodents, different sets of animals are typically used for escalating the doses. For non-rodents, different approaches are available. A single group of animals can be used for acute toxicity testing and treated in a dose-escalation fashion until the maximum tolerated dose (MTD) or maximum feasible dose (MFD) has been reached.

[b]For expanded acute toxicology studies the number of animals used would be increased as the study would support single-dose administration in humans. Accordingly, the number of animals used would be similar to a repeated dose study (up to 1-mo duration).

[c]Recovery groups are typically not included in single-dose studies; however, for some therapeutic agents (e.g., cytotoxic drugs), it is generally a key component of the study design to detect any delayed toxicity or recovery from the toxicity observed.

[d]Generally not conducted in rodents.

Table 6
Typical Number of Animals Used in Range-Finding Repeated Dose
(Less Than 1 Month) Nonclinical Toxicology Studies

Group no. and identification	No. of animals/sex				
	Rodents			Nonrodents	
	Main	TK[a]	Recovery[b]	Main	Recovery[b]
1. Control	5–10	0 (0)	3–5	2–3	1–3
2. Low dose	5–10	6–12 (36)	0–5	2–3	0–3
3. Mid dose	5–10	6–12 (36)	0–5	2–3	0–3
4. High dose	5–10	6–12 (36)	3–5	2–3	1–3

[a]Rat data shown for a typical six-timepoint toxicokinetic (TK) profile; number of animals required is dependent on the number of timepoints needed and the amount of blood required for analysis. Number of mice for the TK analysis in parentheses is typically 1 mouse per timepoint. Therefore, the total number is for two occasions.

[b]Recovery groups are typically not included; however, for some therapeutic agents (e.g., cytotoxic drugs), it is generally a key component of the study design to detect any delayed toxicity or recovery from the toxicity observed.

drug development industry that are typically assessed in toxicology studies, and these are presented in the following sections.

3.5.1. CLINICAL SIGNS, BODY WEIGHT, FOOD CONSUMPTION

One of the best but often underestimated indicators of toxicity in animals is the clinical signs or reactions to treatment that can be easily assessed in any toxicology study. Early

Table 7
Typical Number of Animals Used
in Repeated-Dose Nonclinical Toxicology Studies (Up to 1 Month)

Group no. and identification	No. of animals/sex				
	Rodents			Nonrodents	
	Main	TK^a	$Recovery^b$	Main	$Recovery^b$
1. Control	10–15	0 (0)	5–10	3–4	2–3
2. Low dose	10–15	6–12 (36)	0–10	3–4	0–3
3. Mid dose	10–15	6–12 (36)	0–10	3–4	0–3
4. High dose	10–15	6–12 (36)	5–10	3–4	2–3

[a]Rat data shown for a typical six-timepoint toxicokinetic (TK) profile; number of animals required is dependent on the number of timepoints needed and the amount of blood required for analysis. Number of mice for the TK analysis in parentheses is typically 1 mouse per timepoint; therefore total number is for two occasions.

[b]Recovery groups are typically not included for low- and mid-dose groups; however, for some therapeutic agents (e.g., cytotoxic drugs), it is generally a key component of the study design to detect any delayed toxicity or recovery from the toxicity observed.

Table 8
Typical Number of Animals Used
in Repeated-Dose Nonclinical Toxicology Studies (3 Months or Longer)

Group no. and identification	No. of animals/sex				
	Rodents			Nonrodents	
	$Main^a$	TK^b	$Recovery^c$	Main	$Recovery^c$
1. Control	20–70	0 (0)	10–20	4	2–3
2. Low dose	20–70	6–12 (36)	0–20	4	0–3
3. Mid dose	20–70	6–12 (36)	0–20	4	0–3
4. High dose	20–70	6–12 (36)	10–20	4	2–3

[a]Higher number provided for carcinogenicity study.

[b]Rat data shown for a typical six-timepoint toxicokinetic (TK) profile; number of animals required is dependent on the number of timepoints needed and the amount of blood required for analysis. Number of mice for the TK analysis in parentheses is typically 1 mouse per timepoint; therefore total number is for two occasions.

[c]Recovery groups are typically not included for low- and mid-dose groups; however, for some therapeutic agents (e.g., cytotoxic drugs), it is generally a key component of the study design to detect any delayed toxicity or recovery from the toxicity observed.

and even subtle changes can often be identified solely by clinical observations of the animals after treatment. For example, animals that vocalize significantly during an intravenous injection in a dose-related fashion are often indicating significant local irritation at the injection site. Body weight loss along with decreased food consumption will indicate that the animal well-being or homeostasis has been compromised and can provide useful clues on the toxicity profile of the investigational new product.

Toxicology CROs use different terminologies to describe different types of clinical observations that are typically done in a toxicology study, and this is often the source of

Table 9
Typical Number of Animals Used in Reproductive Toxicology Studies

Group no. and identification	No. of animals/sex			
	Range-finding[a]		Main study	
	Mice/rats	Rabbits	Mice/rats[b]	Rabbits
1. Control	6–12	6–8	22–30	16–25
2. Low dose	6–12	6–8	22–30	16–25
3. Mid dose	6–12	6–8	22–30	16–25
4. High dose	6–12	6–8	22–30	16–25

[a]Numbers shown for range-finding teratology studies.
[b]Thirty represents maximum numbers for pre- and postnatal studies.

confusion or misunderstanding in the industry. There are typically three types of clinical observations described in a toxicology protocol. The first one is a general daily clinical observation, often called a mortality check, daily visual check, or room check. It is generally done twice a day and involves looking at the animals from outside the cage (i.e., animals are not manipulated) to establish the general state of the animals and identify any potential major clinical manifestations related to treatment (e.g., mortality, activity, obvious behavioral changes, food consumption, secretions). Such activity usually takes a few seconds per animal, and documentation typically consists of a positive entry type of system (i.e., if signs are recorded for a particular animal, they are documented to its file; otherwise a simple check mark or note is made about all animals). The second type of observation is called a detailed examination or detailed clinical observations. This type of examination involves a more thorough assessment of the animal by the technician, and the animal needs to be manipulated or taken out of its cage. The animal's body surface and orifices are closely examined and palpated for the presence of any abnormalities or masses. Injection or infusion sites are also closely monitored during those examinations to ensure that no severe problems or reactions are present. Body temperature measurements (non-rodents) and cardiovascular assessments can be conducted when needed. The cages are also typically closely verified for the presence or absence of feces, any biologic fluids, or material.

The third type is the veterinary examination that is usually conducted on demand by a certified veterinarian and is similar to a detailed examination except that it may also include clinical veterinary assessments (e.g., clinical pathology, cardiovascular, and functional examinations). The frequency of the detailed clinical examinations is typically once a week for most studies, and veterinary examinations are typically conducted during the acclimation period and as needed during the study. It is therefore important to differentiate between these different types of examinations.

The frequency and timing of these different types of observations are therefore a critical component of the toxicology study protocol. Ideally, for acute or early range-finding studies in which little or no information on the toxicity profile of the test article is available, clinical observations should be done more frequently. In addition, when signs of toxicity are seen, they should be conducted at regular intervals and up until the animal has completely recovered. Some laboratories typically examine animals at least

Table 10
Standard Hematology Parameters Assessed in Toxicology Studies

Parameter	Typical abbreviation
Hematocrit	Hct
Red blood cell counts	RBC
Hemoglobin	Hgb
Mean corpuscular volume	MCV
Mean corpuscular hemoglobin	MCH
Mean corpuscular hemoglobin concentration	MCHC
Red cell distribution width	RDW
Leukocyte counts	WBC
Differential leukocyte counts	
Neutrophil counts	NEUT
Lymphocyte counts	LYMPH
Monocyte counts	MONO
Eosinophil counts	EOS
Basophil counts	BASO
Platelet counts	PLT
Mean platelet volume	MPV
Prothrombin time	PT
Activated partial thromboplastin time	APTT

every 30 min for the first 4 h immediately following treatment, unless signs of toxicity warrant more frequent observations. The documentation of the time-course and severity of the observed clinical signs will provide valuable information on the safety profile of the product and should therefore be rigorously followed.

3.5.2. CLINICAL PATHOLOGY

Clinical pathology assessments allow toxicologists to assess potential test article-related adverse effects on major organ systems that may not be readily visible upon physical examination. Hematology (including coagulation), clinical chemistry, and uri-nalysis assessments constitute the standard clinical pathology panel that should be inte-grated in all toxicology studies. Typical parameters measured in these panels are presented in Tables 10, 11, and 12. Note that additional specific assessments may be required from the European and Japanese agencies. Clinical pathology assessments should also be carefully scheduled and modified based on the technology being tested. For example, early and late assessments after treatment with a cytotoxic agent should be conducted to determine early changes and potential recovery from the insult. In addition, it would be valuable to add troponin T, lactate dehydrogenase, and creatine kinase en-zyme measurements if the product being tested is expected to elicit cardiotoxicity.

As it is outside the scope of this chapter, the reader is highly encouraged to consult available references on the scientific interpretation of clinical pathology results and special parameters that may be needed for specific effects or technology.

3.5.3. SAMPLING VOLUMES AND GOOD PRACTICES

Clinical pathology assessments are typically done at different timepoints during the conduct of the toxicology study and are used to determine the potential toxicity induced

Table 11
Standard Clinical Chemistry Parameters
Assessed in Toxicology Studies

Parameter	Abbreviation
Alanine aminotransferase	ALT
Albumin	Alb
Albumin-to-globulin ratio	A/G
Alkaline phosphatase	ALP
Aspartate aminotransferase	AST
Bilirubin	Bil
Blood urea nitrogen	BUN
Calcium	Ca
Chloride	Cl
Cholesterol	Chol
Creatinine	Creat, Cr
γ-Glutamyl transferase	GGT
Globulin	Glob, Gb
Glucose	Gluc
Lactate dehydrogenase	LDH
Phosphorus	P, Phos
Potassium	K
Protein	Prot, TP
Sodium	Na
Triglycerides	Trig, TG

by an investigational product. When planning clinical pathology assessments in a toxicology study, careful consideration should be given to the type, number, and timing of the assessments, as excessive blood volume collection can lead to profound effects on the test system. Therefore, standard guidelines have been established in the industry for limiting blood volumes that should be taken in different animal species. As a rule of thumb, no more than 7.5% of the total blood volume (TBV) should be taken on a weekly basis, no more than 10% TBV on a biweekly basis, and no more than 15% TBV on a monthly basis (variations can be found in the literature). Collecting volumes that exceed the recommended amounts are generally considered to impact on the test system negatively, although this does not necessarily mean that death will occur. These values do not include the volume that may be obtained when animals are sacrificed for necropsy. The total blood volume of the different animal species used in toxicology studies is presented in Table 13.

3.5.4. Macroscopic and Microscopic Pathology

Excellent textbooks providing a detailed assessment and description of all the potential findings or toxicities that can be described in animals are available, and this section is not intended to provide such information. Since most oncology products are inherently cytotoxic, the typical manifestations that are expected are generally more severe than other classes of products. Indeed, the hematopoietic, digestive, immune, and reproduc-

Table 12
Standard Urinalysis Parameters Assessed in Toxicology Studies

Semiquantitative	Analytical
Color	Calcium
Appearance	Chloride
pH	Creatinine
Protein	Phosphorus
Glucose	Potassium
Ketones	Sodium
Bilirubin	Specific gravity
Urobilinogen	Volume
Leukocytes	γ-Glutamyl transferase[a]
Blood	N-acetyl-β-D-glucosaminidase (NAG)[a]
Nitrite	Microscopic sediments analysis

[a]Not standard assessments but sometimes included.

Table 13
Typical Blood Volumes (mL) Allowable for Sampling in Different Animal Species

Species	BW (kg)	TBV (mL/kg)	TBV (mL)	Weekly 7.5% (mL)	Biweekly 10% (mL)	Monthly 15% (mL)	Terminal (mL)
Mouse	0.025	72	1.8	0.1	0.2	0.3	1
Rat	0.25	64	16	1.2	1.6	2.4	10
Hamster	0.3	65	20	1.5	2.0	3.0	10
Guinea pig	0.6	65	40	3.0	4.0	6.0	20
Rabbit	4	56	225	16	23	32	100
Dog	12	83	1000	75	100	150	500
Mini-pig	15	65	975	70	100	140	500
Pig	60	65	4000	300	400	600	2500
Small macaque	3	67	200	15	20	30	100
Large macaque	8	65	520	40	50	80	260
Marmoset	0.4	70	28	2.1	2.8	4.2	15

ABBREVIATIONS: TBV, Total blood volume; BW, body weight.

tive systems are the typical target organs of toxicity. Accordingly, the adequate safety assessment of an oncology product in a toxicology study depends on a complete macroscopic and microscopic assessment. The typical tissues generally weighed, collected, fixed, and examined are presented in Tables 14 and 15. Note that additional tissues may be required from the European and Japanese agencies.

One of the most popular approaches often taken by sponsors is to perform only limited histopathologic examinations on a limited number of animals or groups, typically control and high-dose group animals. Although such an approach definitely provides a cost-saving advantage (histopathology can represent from 25 to 40% of the total study cost),

Table 14
Standard Tissues/Organs Weighed
in Toxicology Studies

Adrenal glands	Prostate
Brain	Salivary glands
Epididymis	Seminal vesicles
Heart	Spleen
Kidneys	Testes
Liver	Thymus or remnant
Lungs	Thyroid and parathyroid glands
Ovaries	Uterus with cervix
Pituitary gland	Vagina

Table 15
Standard Tissues/Organs Examined Histopathologically in Toxicology Studies

Adrenal glands	Skeletal muscle
Animal identification	Nerve (sciatic)
Aorta (thoracic)	Ovaries
Bone (femur, rib, sternum, vertebra)	Pancreas
Bone Marrow (femur, rib, sternum, vertebra)	Pituitary gland
Brain (cortex, midbrain, cerebellum, and medulla oblongata)	Prostate
Cecum	Rectum
Colon	Salivary gland (mandibular and sublingual)
Duodenum	Seminal vesicles (with coagulating glands)
Epididymis	Skin (dorsal)
Esophagus	Spinal cord (cervical, thoracolumbar)
Eyes-optic nerve-harderian glands	Spleen
Gallbladder	Stomach
Heart	Testes
Ileum	Thymus or remnant
Jejunum (with Peyer's patches if visible)	Thyroid glands (with parathyroid)
Kidneys	Tongue
Liver	Trachea
Lungs with main stem bronchi	Urinary bladder
Lymph nodes (representative)	Uterus (horns and cervix)
Mammary gland (inguinal)	Vagina

it can nonetheless become a rate-limiting factor for regulatory submissions. Indeed, when severe toxicities or even a high mortality rate is observed in the high-dose group animals, histopathologic data from other dose groups may be necessary to establish properly the safety profile of the product. The additional time required to perform the additional histopathology examinations may range from a few days to many weeks, depending on the study design and the CRO capabilities. The overall study costs including the required additional histopathology in this scenario are more or less the same as if it was initially integrated into the design, but it can vary between different CROs. When pivotal nonclinical study data are key for the regulatory submission, significant delays for additional histopathological examinations can sometimes have devastating consequences, and one should always evaluate the risks associated with such an approach.

Similar consequences can be expected from range-finding studies in which limited numbers of tissues are usually collected and rarely examined histopathologically. A discrete and significant irreversible finding in a critical organ or a tissue could definitely raise major safety concerns in humans, even in the oncology setting, in which risks are often offset by the potential benefits. The histopathologic data from range-finding studies may therefore be the determining factor for not moving the product into more expensive nonclinical development work or for monitoring special functions or systems that are not typically conducted in a toxicology study. The initial higher expenses associated with additional histopathologic assessments in early nonclinical studies may become a cost-saving option later during the development program by preventing or minimizing the risks of repeating expensive pivotal toxicology studies.

4. OUTSOURCING SAFETY STUDIES

For many companies, the technical and regulatory requirements relating to the conduct of nonclinical safety studies will require the use of external laboratories. Such laboratories will allow a sponsor to produce valid nonclinical safety information to support the eventual regulatory submission to agencies. As with any subcontracted work, the selection of the appropriate partner is a critical component that should be carefully evaluated.

4.1. Selecting a Toxicology CRO

The selection of a laboratory that will ultimately be responsible for conducting an entire toxicology program initially necessitates much meticulous work and is often an area that is rapidly neglected, especially when staff is overburdened with other tasks. On many occasions, people confronted with a very busy schedule will tend to take short cuts when it comes to toxicology laboratory selection and therefore end up making decisions based on questionable criteria.

A list of the most common criteria that should be evaluated when selecting a laboratory is presented in Table 16. The order in which they are presented does not necessarily correspond with their order of importance, as it would definitely be different for different companies. However, it is important to note that one of the most famous criteria, and often the sole one, cost, is not listed first in the list. Indeed, many people make decisions strictly or mainly based on costs without any serious considerations of other factors such as expertise, experience, responsiveness, compliance, and reliability.

On many occasions we have encountered sponsors that were having serious problems with their nonclinical program and quickly realized that they had not dedicated much effort toward selecting the appropriate laboratory to conduct the work. Some selected the laboratories based mainly on the costs but realized too late that the laboratory did not have the expertise to conduct the study (e.g., dermal and inhalation studies). Some others had considered other criteria in their decision process but never realized that the costs were lower because some of the assessments were not incorporated in the quotation. It is important to note that everyone understands the sensitive nature of the costs associated with executing a toxicology program, and some toxicology laboratories will even use that to attract new sponsors. It is therefore critical to ensure that when one is comparing costs

Table 16
Criteria for Selecting a Toxicology CRO

Criteria	Comments
Expertise	Make sure the laboratory has the experience to conduct the type of studies requested. Relying solely on corporate brochures or assurances is not a reliable method.
Responsiveness	The laboratory should be able to respond to your requests and be reachable when needed. Important delays in returning calls or for providing information on a study are good indicators of potential responsiveness problems.
Organization	The level of organization in a toxicology laboratory usually greatly reflects the level of organization in your study.
Staff qualification and experience	Study directors, technical staff, and experts involved in the conduct of the study should be qualified (training records, education). Unqualified personnel invariably lead to problems in studies. At an initial visit, the people that you meet are most likely not going to be the people conducting your study.
Localization/accessibility	The laboratory should be accessible. Time zone differences complicate communication and require more intensive management and traveling.
Costs/timelines	Costs vary greatly between different laboratories for the same design. Decisions made strictly based on costs are discouraged, as it is not by itself a reliable decision-making criterion.
Species Availability	The laboratory should not only have access to the appropriate species selected for your program but should also have significant experience working with them.
Reliability	One of the key determinants in filing a regulatory submission within the established timeline.
GLP compliance	Conducting qualification audit prior to making final decision should be done to ensure current GLP status. Laboratory status changes over time and they may be experiencing some major GLP compliance issues.
Capacity	Overworked employees and overloaded animal facilities will almost certainly lead to multiple mistakes or problems during the study conduct.
Reputation	Good laboratories will strive to maintain their reputation by meeting sponsor's demands. Time in the business is also a good indicator. Scientific meeting attendance is a good way to learn about the different laboratories.

Abbreviations: CRO, Contract Research Organization; GLP, Good Laboratory Practice.

between different laboratories, the same basis (i.e., study design) is used. Indeed, some differences that may seem minor to the untrained eye could have a significant impact on the overall study cost. For example, a full histopathologic examination of a 28-d toxicology study could account for a 30–40% difference in costs compared with a study design in which only limited histopathology (fewer tissues or only in control and high-dose animals) is conducted.

4.2. Requests for Quotations

As with any project, a clear understanding of the nonclinical development plan is critical before initiating requests for quotations to toxicology laboratories. Anyone who has been engaged in requesting quotations from safety laboratories will tell you that it is far from being a simple and short-lived task. In contrast to the common misconception, it involves much time, energy, and resources, and therefore it is critical that the nonclinical plan be clearly laid out before the bidding process is initiated.

Once a nonclinical plan has clearly been established, the identification of potential laboratories that could do the work based on the multiple criteria listed in Table 16 can take place. Once a list of potential laboratories has been created, the competitive selection process can be initiated.

A typical mistake in outsourcing is requesting quotes from different laboratories without clearly specifying what is needed. Indeed, many sponsors will often rely on the laboratory's expertise to provide them with suggested study designs that will most likely not be adapted to their investigational new drug or biologic product. Although it may provide the sponsor with some general idea of what is involved in the different types of studies, it inevitably results in confusion and inefficiency. Providing toxicology laboratories with a clear and concise description of each study design, which has been adapted to the technology developed, is therefore critical. A single protocol outline should be prepared for each study. When the exact study design is not known yet, at least a standard study outline should be sent to the toxicology laboratories so quotes will still be comparable. Toxicology laboratories are actually very collaborative with sponsors, and although it does not create more work on their side, it allows sponsors to gather valuable quotes that are going to have the same comparison basis. Failure of a toxicology laboratory to comply with your request of providing a quote strictly based on your outline is a potential indicator of some compliance or communication problems within the laboratory and should therefore raise some suspicion that should be explored further with the laboratory. In addition, significantly out-of-range costs should raise suspicion as to whether or not the laboratory quoted on the right study design or has enough experience at conducting such a study to evaluate the costs properly. Remember that, like other business areas, what looks like the best deal of the day generally indicates some potential risks, unless the laboratory clearly indicated that the costs were greatly reduced to attract new business.

4.3. Monitoring Toxicology Studies

Another major misconception is that once the studies have been awarded to a laboratory, the biggest part of the job has been completed. Actually, selecting a toxicology CRO and requesting quotations accounts for about 5–15% of the total work involved. To have a successful nonclinical safety program, one must make sure that the program is closely followed to ensure that proper actions are taken when necessary. The typical activities involved in the conduct of a nonclinical safety program are outlined below:

1. Contact the nonclinical study sites, request price quotations, and set up details for the contractual agreement.

2. Review and implement each study protocol to ensure that it fulfills the company's needs and regulatory requirements.
3. Act as the primary contact for critical toxicology issues raised during the conduct of each study. This includes extensive, unanticipated work that might be needed to remedy major problems such as severe toxicity, technical complications, or formulation issues that threaten the validity of the study.
4. Monitor critical steps (e.g., dose formulation preparation, treatment, toxicokinetic sampling, necropsy) in each study to ensure compliance to study protocol, GLP regulations, and the toxicology laboratory standard operating procedures.
5. Review each audited draft report and ensure its finalization in a timely fashion for inclusion into the regulatory submission(s) where applicable.

As shown above, every study requires a number of activities that may become time-consuming, especially when many studies are being conducted at the same time. A significant error in nonclinical program oversight is neglect of any of these activities for multiple reasons, like project leaders are too busy or that the toxicology laboratory should know what they are doing and have the proper expertise to conduct the study. Although it may be true that the laboratory is competent, it can nonetheless lead to serious delays or problems if some of the activities listed above are overlooked or neglected during the program.

5. COMMON ISSUES IN TOXICOLOGY TESTING

Although it would be impossible to list or discuss all the potential problems that may arise during the conduct of a nonclinical safety development program, we've come across some common issues that occur frequently.

Interestingly, the most common issues in nonclinical testing are related to another challenging area of the drug development process, namely, manufacturing and supplying the test article. Indeed, on many occasions, sponsors initiate major development activities, including securing contracts with toxicology laboratories and initiating studies, without a clear understanding of the amount of test article that is required for the entire program. On many occasions, sponsors realize just before shipping the material to the toxicology laboratory that the amount of test article suddenly appears insufficient not only for completing the program, but also often for even completing a single study. Many factors could actually explain such a problem, and some have been mentioned here, but it could also relate to unexpected problems during the manufacturing. Of course, when the toxicology studies have already been scheduled and animals are being acclimated at the facility, this will have a tremendous impact not only on the scheduling but also on the budget. Indeed, most toxicology CROs will charge extra housing fees (typically a cost per animal or per day) for any delays in study initiation. When the delay is one of many weeks, the animals may even have to be euthanized (rodents only), and therefore additional costs are involved as a new set of animal needs to be ordered.

Another major issue we have often seen is inadequate formulation development leading to serious problems. Indeed, some test articles can present some physicochemical, solubility, and/or stability issues that create many problems in animal studies. For example, a limit solubility that did not appear to represent a significant problem based on pharmacologic concentrations may indeed become a major issue in animal toxicology studies in which higher concentrations are contemplated. Indeed, dosing animals with a poorly soluble product will ultimately greatly limit the achievable dose in animals and consequently may limit the starting dose in humans if the product is administered parenterally. Preparation of different solutions by diluting a stock solution with a given solvent may also modulate the solubility of the product and would therefore represent a concern for preparing dosing solution of different strengths.

Dosing animals via the intravenous route with highly concentrated product and/or nonbiocompatible solutions may lead to serious toxicity, including local irritation that may jeopardize the conduct or completion of the study. In addition, such reactions could be delayed and may not be seen in short-term or range-finding toxicology studies.

Finally, dose formulations with unknown stability (i.e., at the concentrations used and in the presence of the needed excipients for the study) could compromise the validity of the data generated if it is retrospectively revealed that the dose formulations were unstable.

6. CONCLUSIONS

Designing a toxicology program to support clinical trials of oncology products is only the beginning of this critical component of overall nonclinical development. Poor financial planning, inadequate design of studies, inappropriate species selection, nonoptimized scheduling, haphazard CRO selection, and inadequate monitoring activities can all introduce significant delays and risks of failure into the nonclinical safety development program. A cost-effective, time-efficient, scientifically sound, and information-rich nonclinical safety program should be the goal of all who endeavor to bring new oncology therapeutics into clinical testing. The seriousness of the disease and the great need for more effective therapies make it critical that those charged with these tasks have the proper training, experience, and time commitment to implement a successful program so that unnecessary delays are avoided. Careful attention to the issues presented in this chapter should minimize the potential for major problems and expedite the availability of new therapies in clinical trials.

ACKNOWLEDGMENTS

The authors thank Ms. Janet Hanna for her help in compiling the toxicology study costs table and Dr. Carolyn Laurençot for her critical review of the chapter.

REFERENCES

1. Guidance for Industry: ICH M3 Non-Clinical Safety Studies for the Conduct of Human Clinical Trials for Pharmaceuticals, U.S. Department of Health and Human Services, Food and Drug Administration, Center for Drug Evaluation and Research, Center for Biologics Evaluation and Research, November, 2000.
2. Guidance for Industry: ICH S6 Preclinical Evaluation of Biotechnology-Derived Pharmaceuticals, U.S. Department of Health and Human Services, Food and Drug Administration, Center for Drug Evaluation and Research, Center for Biologics Evaluation and Research, July, 1997.
3. United States Good Laboratory Practices Regulation. Title 21 of the Code of Federal Regulations, Part 58 (21 CFR part 58).
4. Derelanko MJ, Hollinger MA. *Handbook of Toxicology*, 2nd ed. New York: CRC Press. 2001.
5. Hull RM. Guidelines limit volumes for dosing animals in the preclinical stage of safety evaluation. *Hum Exp Toxicol* 1995; 14:305–307.
6. Diehl KH, Hull R, Morton D, et al. A good practice guide to the administration of substances and removal of blood, including routes and volumes. *J Appl Toxicol* 2001; 21:15–23.

14 Nonclinical Testing for Oncology Drug Products

Paul A. Andrews, *PhD* and Denis Roy, *PhD*

Contents

Introduction
Cytotoxic Drugs
Chronically Administered, Molecularly Targeted Drugs
Drug Combinations
Trials of Oncology Drugs in Normal Volunteers
Integration of New Guidances Into Nonclinical Programs
Interspecies Dose Conversions and Starting Dose Selection
Conclusions

1. INTRODUCTION

Cancers that cannot be eliminated by surgical resection are life-threatening, and aggressive approaches are used in treating the primary tumor and metastatic disease. Antineoplastic therapies designed to induce necrosis, apoptosis, or cytostasis of the malignant tissue are frequently toxic to normal tissues. Even with the serious adverse effects of many anticancer drugs, careful dosing, clinical monitoring, and prompt treatment of toxicity usually make the side effects less threatening to a patient than their disease. Because the serious side effects in patients are considered acceptable risks when weighed against the potential benefits in patients with advanced neoplasias, the nonclinical testing of oncology drugs differs from testing of nononcology drugs. For oncology drugs, all potential risks do not have to be thoroughly evaluated nonclinically, no observed adverse effect levels (NOAELs) do not have to be defined, and only minimal nonclinical proof-of-concept studies need to be provided. Nonetheless, the difficulty and importance of providing a relevant nonclinical safety assessment program is greatly increased because the first patients treated with a new oncology drug are most often in poor health and have been heavily pretreated with other toxic therapies *(1)*. The reality of desiring to administer doses that might offer clinical benefit and that will probably be associated with toxicity to patients in poor health poses a great challenge for the

From: *Cancer Drug Discovery and Development:*
Anticancer Drug Development Guide: Preclinical Screening, Clinical Trials, and Approval, 2nd Ed.
Edited by: B. A. Teicher and P. A. Andrews © Humana Press Inc., Totowa, NJ

nonclinical testing plan, as the data provided must be accurate, reasonably thorough, and conducted in appropriate models.

The Division of Oncology Drug Products (DODP) within the Center for Drug Evaluation and Research (CDER) at the U.S. Food and Drug Administration (FDA) recognizes the urgency of developing new anticancer drugs and the need to move promising agents into clinical trials rapidly. DODP pharmacologists have published detailed recommendations regarding the nonclinical studies they expect to support the clinical development of various classes of oncology drugs *(2)*. Drug development in oncology has changed significantly in the few years since that manuscript was published. This chapter reiterates the critical features of those published instructions and offers an update on the regulatory considerations for the nonclinical development of a variety of drugs intended to be administered chronically such as angiogenesis inhibitors and molecularly targeted anticancer drugs.

2. CYTOTOXIC DRUGS

Until recently, the oncology drug development arena was dominated by cytotoxic drugs such as alkylating agents, platinating agents, topoisomerase I and II inhibitors, microtubule inhibitors, and antimetabolites. Initial clinical trials of these agents typically administer the drug as a single dose that is repeated every 3–4 wk to allow patients to recover from the toxicities (typically myelosuppression and gastrointestinal toxicity). To support this clinical trial design, single-dose nonclinical studies are generally considered adequate. Although toxicology studies with full safety assessments (four dose groups with a standard battery of safety parameters) in both rodents and non-rodents are typically preferred to support phase I trials, a minimal approach would often be adequate, particularly if the cytotoxic drug was from a well-known class. A rodent toxicology study to define severely toxic doses and a non-rodent study (usually dogs) to ensure that a safe starting dose had been selected were considered the minimum set of studies needed to support the safety of a new cytotoxic drug as long as one of those studies included histopathology assessments at a toxic dose level *(2–4)*.

Current DODP recommendations indicate that sponsors are now strongly encouraged to provide either "expanded acute" studies or multiple cycles of treatment to support the safety of cytotoxic therapies. The expanded acute study design is described in an FDA guidance document *(5)*. These studies should be designed to assess dose-response relationships, and toxicokinetic assessments are strongly encouraged. The primary feature of an expanded acute study is the monitoring of clinical pathology and histopathology at both an early time and at termination to assess the maximum acute effect (typically study d 3) and the potential for recovery, progression, or delayed appearance of toxicities over a period of time following treatment (typically 14 d). As this design requires additional animals and analyses (e.g., clinical pathology and histopathology) for early euthanasia (interim groups), costs are significantly increased compared with a regular single-dose study. Although expanded acute or multicycle studies are not strictly required to support initial trials of cytotoxic agents, the sponsor must supply convincing evidence that the safety of the investigational new drug has been adequately addressed nonclinically if such studies are not provided.

Regardless of the approach taken for establishing the safety of cytotoxic oncology drugs for early clinical trials, repeat cycle studies in rodents and non-rodents are now requested as development proceeds. In such studies, the drug is administered once every 3 or 4 wk (matching the intended clinical schedule of the marketed product) up to approx six to eight cycles or a total of 6 mo. Repeat cycle toxicology studies are now expected by the DODP to support a New Drug Application (NDA) for cytotoxic drugs. The intent of these studies is to reveal cumulative toxicities in animals that, when seen in humans, may have a significant impact on the clinical development of the drug.

3. CHRONICALLY ADMINISTERED, MOLECULARLY TARGETED DRUGS

As described by DeGeorge et al. *(2)*, the DODP has generally allowed indefinite chronic dosing for hormonal and immunomodulating drugs in advanced cancer patients based on 28-d toxicology studies. Longer duration studies are usually expected for supporting larger trials of these agents in patients likely to have extended survival. The acceptable approach for addressing the safety of other drugs probably needing chronic daily administration to demonstrate clinical benefit was not specifically discussed *(2)*. These types of therapeutics are difficult to define with an all-encompassing term such as "noncytotoxic" or "molecularly targeted" drugs, but all share the common feature that, based on the perceived mechanism, they will probably need frequent, long-duration dosing to demonstrate clinical benefit. These are often drugs that inhibit steps involved in key signaling pathways or inhibit enzymes critical for tumor progression and include farnesyl transferase inhibitors, angiogenesis inhibitors, receptor tyrosine kinase inhibitors, matrix metalloprotease inhibitors, apoptosis modulators, cyclin-dependent kinase inhibitors, tumor suppressor protein mimics, and histone deacetylase inhibitors. The DODP has generally applied the same published principles used for developing hormonal and immunomodulatory drugs to other chronically administered, molecularly targeted drugs. This approach is consistent with the DODP's philosophy that greater risks are tolerable in the oncology setting and that new drugs for treating cancer need to enter phase I and II testing as soon as possible so that clinical activity can be determined. Mandating that the duration of administration in nonclinical testing needs to exceed the duration in clinical trials (as expected for non-life-threatening indications according to the ICH M3 guidance *[6]*) would add significant financial and time burdens to the early development process. The following sections describe in more detail the expected nonclinical development program for these types of agents.

3.1. Nonclinical Program to Support Phase I and II Trials

Generally, the repeated-dose toxicology studies need to meet or exceed the duration of treatment planned in one cycle in the phase I trial of an oncology drug. At a minimum, to support chronic administration of an oncology drug in early clinical development, 28-d repeated-dose studies in relevant rodent and non-rodent species should be conducted according to Good Laboratory Practice (GLP) regulations using the intended clinical route of administration, dosing regimen, and schedule (Table 1). This proposed approach has typically supported a phase I trial with 28 d of dosing per cycle. In addition,

Table 1
Toxicology Studies Typically Needed for Supporting Phase I and II Trials
of Chronically Administered Drug Products in Cancer Patients

Study type	Currently required for an initial IND
28-d repeated dose: rodents[a]	Yes
28-d repeated dose: non-rodents[a]	Yes
Single-dose and range-finding studies: rodents	As needed
Single-dose and range-finding studies: non-rodents	As needed
Safety pharmacology	No
Pharmacokinetic/toxicokinetic, ADME studies	No
Genetic toxicity studies	No

[a]Schedule should match intended human schedule, e.g., twice per day dosing or every other day dosing in the clinic should be mimicked in the nonclinical studies. Species selection should be justified.

ABBREVIATIONS: ADME, absorption, distribution, metabolism, and excretion; IND, Investigational New Drug application.

the DODP has generally allowed indefinite chronic dosing (multiple 28-d cycles) for hormonal, immunomodulating, molecularly targeted, and noncytotoxic drugs (e.g., antiangiogenesis inhibitors) in advanced cancer patients based on 28-d toxicology studies. The more robust the nonclinical package, the more likely this will be allowed. Factors that would contribute to making the package robust include the following: survival or toxicity data from nonclinical efficacy models; safety pharmacology screens; absorption, distribution, metabolism, and excretion data; acute toxicology studies; 7–14 d repeated-dose toxicology studies; use of the clinical formulation and lot in toxicology studies; mechanistic data; main toxicities that can be attributed to exaggerated pharmacologic effects; anticipated toxicities that can be readily monitored; recovery groups to determine reversibility or progressive toxicity; and full toxicology in rodents rather than just lethality. Depending on the breadth of the toxicology program and the toxicity profile, the DODP often prefers a short break in dosing between cycles to allow the human safety profile to become apparent before chronic daily dosing is allowed. The preferred phase I approach for a particular drug should be discussed with the DODP review team in a pre-Investigational New Drug (IND) meeting when sufficient nonclinical information is available to make an informed decision.

Key design features of the definitive toxicology studies are described in detail in Chapter 13. The studies should comply with GLP regulations as specified in the Code of Federal Regulations (7). The studies should establish a high dose level at which significant toxicity is observed and should characterize those toxicities so that they may be carefully monitored or avoided in clinical trials. The repeated-dose toxicity studies should include toxicokinetic analyses [e.g., C_{max}, areas under the curve (AUCs), half-life, volume of distribution, clearance], ophthalmology, full clinical pathology, cardiovascular (electrocardiographic, blood pressure, heart rate) measurements in the non-rodent studies, and complete histopathology. Recovery groups should be included to investigate the reversibility of the toxicities observed, if any. As long as the standard safety assessments are not compromised, measurements of pharmacodynamic effects can also be included in toxicology studies and are becoming increasingly important. Confirmation of an effect on the intended target in an easily accessible tissue or quantitation of a biomarker that is believed to indicate the intended activity can provide useful information regarding the exposure needed for activity, the appropriateness of the animal model for assessing human safety, and the practicality of incorporating such assessments in human trials. Although the fields are in their infancy, toxicogenomic and metabonomic assessments may see increasing incorporation in toxicology studies, as these data may provide some predictions of possible long-term toxicity liabilities and mechanisms of toxicity.

3.2. Nonclinical Chronic Toxicology Studies to Support Phase III Trials and Marketing Applications

Twenty-eight-day toxicology studies can support repeat cycles or repeated daily dosing through phase I and limited phase II testing as long as the route, schedule, and formulation are not changed significantly. Longer duration studies are usually needed to support phase III trials of chronically administered oncology drugs and will be essential for supporting an NDA. The maximum duration needed is 6 mo in rodents, and the default duration is 9 mo in non-rodents, as specified in the ICH M3 and ICH S4A guidances *(6,8)*. However, a study duration of 6 mo may be acceptable in non-rodents, and this issue should be discussed with the DODP when the results of the 28-d toxicology studies are available and when the toxicities and pharmacokinetics in humans have been clearly identified *(9)*. Three-month studies can be included in the nonclinical plan, but these are optional. A primary utility of these studies is to project the appropriate doses for the essential 6-mo rodent and 6- or 9-mo non-rodent studies, as projecting the appropriate doses for these studies solely from the 28-d data can sometimes be difficult. Bypassing the 3-mo studies carries the risk of choosing doses that lead to premature study termination (doses too high) or studies that do not adequately assess the potential hazards of chronic therapy (doses too low). The decision to proceed with the 3-mo studies can be addressed when the 28-d studies are completed and the timelines and urgency of clinical development are better defined. The chronic studies must also comply with GLP regulations.

3.3. Nonclinical Program for Marketing Applications

3.3.1. GENETIC TOXICITY

Genetic toxicity testing is not needed to support clinical trials of investigational drugs in patients with cancer; however, a genetic toxicity assessment is needed to support an NDA *(2)*. The genetic toxicity testing battery includes a gene mutation assay in bacteria, an in vitro chromosomal damage test in mammalian cells, and an in vivo chromosomal damage test in a rodent species *(10)*. All these studies should be done according to GLP regulations. If plans for the drug evolve to include the conduct of studies in normal volunteers or in subjects without cancer (including preneoplastic conditions), then genetic toxicity studies would be needed earlier in development as specified in the ICH M3 guidance *(6)*.

3.3.2. CARCINOGENICITY

Carcinogenicity studies are not currently needed to support marketing applications for drug products indicated for the treatment of patients with cancer and are not often included in the nonclinical development plans *(2)*. However, if approval is eventually sought for adjuvant treatment (i.e., patients without detectable disease and a significant life expectancy), then a carcinogenicity assessment program would be needed.

3.3.3. Developmental and Reproductive Toxicology Studies

The practice of the DODP has been to request ICH stage C–D (segment II) developmental toxicity studies to support all NDAs. This expectation has historically been made regardless of whether the drug product is intended to be used only in populations that have no potential to become pregnant. The need for developmental toxicology studies in a rodent (usually rat) and a non-rodent (usually rabbit) should be addressed with the DODP at an appropriate point in development, typically an end-of-phase II meeting. Considering that most chronically administered or molecularly targeted drugs in clinical trials affect new therapeutic targets, two development toxicity studies should be included in the nonclinical development plan so that a thorough integrated assessment of the potential for adverse human developmental outcomes can be conducted *(11)*.

3.3.4. Targeted Toxicity Studies

The studies described above represent the default program of essential nonclinical studies needed for supporting development of a chronically administered oncology drug. Depending on the nature of toxicities seen in the clinic or with other drugs in the class in either animals or humans, targeted special toxicity studies to support the filing of an NDA may also be needed. For example, a specific study may be requested to define the exact nature, potential mechanism, reversibility, or preventability of a specific end-organ toxicity.

4. DRUG COMBINATIONS

4.1. Combinations of Cytotoxic Drugs

Combination chemotherapy is used to treat the majority of cancers. Although activity has usually been explored in nonclinical models, the toxicity of the combination was not often addressed prior to clinical trials. This empirical clinical approach has historically been adequate for combinations of cytotoxic drugs; however, nonclinical studies allow a thorough exploration of doses, dose ratios, and schedules to optimize benefit and minimize toxicity. Unless there is reason to believe that synergistic interactions occur that would substantially increase the toxicity of the combination, nonclinical safety testing has not been considered essential by the DODP *(2)*. This approach assumes that the toxicity of each drug has already been evaluated in humans. Nonclinical safety testing of the combination can be desirable when synergistic toxicities are suspected, such as when one agent modulates the metabolism or elimination of the other agent, when both cytotoxic agents are directed at the same target, when both cytotoxic agents target complementary metabolic pathways (e.g., *de novo* synthesis and salvage pathways for nucleosides), or when the drugs exhibit overlapping toxicity profiles.

4.2. Combinations of Molecularly Targeted Drugs With Cytotoxic Drugs

Combining cytotoxic drugs with modulators of signal transduction pathways may raise special concerns. These molecularly targeted agents may be selected for combination with specific cytotoxic drugs based on knowledge of critical pathways that confer resistance or lower the threshold for apoptosis. If clinical combinations are rationalized on synergistic in vitro biochemical interactions, then one must assume that such synergistic interactions will occur in normal tissues as well as tumor cells. If selectivity for tumor cells cannot be addressed with convincing data (i.e., with compelling evidence that the modulating drug only has activity against a mutant signaling pathway that is only activated in tumor cells, or with a well-designed, well-documented efficacy study that includes appropriate safety endpoints), then a nonclinical study assessing the safety of the proposed combination is generally warranted. Justifying safety based solely on in vitro data of the combination will be exceedingly difficult. A single study in rodents is usually sufficient. The study should determine whether the toxicity is enhanced by examining lethality (lethal dose for 10% of test animals [LD_{10}]) or other quantifiable endpoints (e.g., effects on clinical pathology endpoints) and the severity of the end-organ toxicities for each of the respective drugs. The study should ideally assess toxicity at both minimally and significantly toxic doses of the cytotoxic therapy. The dose ratio intended for clinical use should be examined in this study. The primary goal of nonclinical evaluation of combination chemotherapies is to allow selection of safe starting doses.

4.3. Combinations of Two Molecularly Targeted Drugs

Similarly to combinations of molecularly targeted drugs with cytotoxic drugs, proposed combinations of two molecularly targeted drugs in a clinical trial will often require a nonclinical assessment of safety in vivo prior to administration of the two drugs to humans. As for all combinations, the adverse event profile of each of these drugs will need to have been evaluated in humans. Since many of the new approaches for treating cancer modulate signal transduction pathways that are present in normal cells as well as transformed cells, one can reasonably assume that there is a significant potential for enhancing toxicity to normal tissues, as intended for the tumor target, when such agents are combined. The nonclinical study design for the combination must be relevant to the clinical trial design and needs to use appropriate routes, schedules, dose ratios, duration of treatment, and endpoint assessments in a relevant species.

5. TRIALS OF ONCOLOGY DRUGS IN NORMAL VOLUNTEERS

The first clinical studies of oncology drugs are occasionally proposed in normal volunteers. Such studies are usually driven by the desire to acquire pharmacokinetic data for novel structures prior to dosing in cancer patients or the belief that obtaining pharmacokinetic data in healthy subjects will expedite development. The nonclinical program needed to support studies in these populations differs in several substantial ways from the standard program for cancer patients. Besides the toxicology studies in a rodent and nonrodent species, genetic toxicity and safety pharmacology studies will have to be conducted according to the ICH M3, S2B, S7A, and draft S7B guidances (6,10,12,13). In addition, unlike the nonclinical studies used to support trials in cancer patients in which the focus is on defining a maximally tolerated or severely toxic dose, a NOAEL must be defined in the nonclinical studies used to support trials in subjects without cancer (assuming a nontoxic dose has not yet been defined in any human population). The default starting dose for administration of an oncology drug to a subject without cancer is usually one-tenth the NOAEL in the most sensitive species on a mg/m^2 basis, as described in the recently issued FDA guidance (14).

Genetic toxicity must be assessed in vitro prior to administration of investigational agents to normal volunteers *(6)*. Positive signals in genetic toxicity studies would not necessarily preclude single-dose studies in healthy volunteers. Administration of a positive genotoxicant would be allowed presuming (1) the genotoxicity signal(s) are not disconcerting, (2) the compound is not from a known carcinogenic structural class (e.g., alkylating agent), (3) the compound is not from a mechanistic class known to be carcinogenic class (e.g., topoisomerase II inhibitors), (4) the volunteer study is a single-dose trial, and (5) the positive findings are appropriately conveyed in the informed consent form. The ultimate decision will depend on the FDA review team's assessment on a case-by-case basis and also on the nature of the genetic toxicity findings, consideration of the full safety profile of the drug, and the perceived risks derived from knowledge of other drugs in the class.

To support initial trials in normal volunteers, safety pharmacology data must also be provided to identify physiologic effects that would not be detected through clinical observations, biochemical changes, or morphometric lesions in conventional toxicity studies. Although cardiac effects can usually be addressed with well-designed electrocardiographic and hemodynamic monitoring in the standard toxicology studies, effects on other major organ systems (e.g., the central nervous system and pulmonary function) will have to be addressed as described in the ICH 7A guidance *(12)*. Careful observation of clinical signs in the standard toxicology studies can be useful for identifying any potential effects on the central nervous system and pulmonary functions but may not be sufficient for justifying the safety of the drug product in normal healthy volunteers. In addition, adherence to the draft ICH 7B guidance, which specifies a panel of in vitro and in vivo studies to address the potential for causing QT prolongation, will be strongly encouraged *(13)*.

Regardless of toxicity profile, the DODP typically challenges a proposal for a normal volunteer trial in order to collect pharmacokinetic data. It is understood that accrual will be faster than a trial in cancer patients, but doses can be significantly lower than for cancer patients (based on the NOAEL rather than the severely toxic dose in animals), and one cannot usually escalate beyond the first evidence of toxicity in volunteers. The pharmacokinetic data at low doses may not be relevant to the pharmacokinetics at therapeutic doses, and the data from healthy volunteers are often significantly different than data from cancer patients. The pharmacokinetic data and toxicity profile will always have to be established in patients, so there is often no compelling strategic reason to put normal volunteers at risk by administration of a new oncology product.

6. INTEGRATION OF NEW GUIDANCES INTO NONCLINICAL PROGRAMS

6.1. Safety Pharmacology

Since the publication of the manuscript by DeGeorge et al. *(2)*, several new regulatory guidances have been issued and include recommendations that might pertain to oncology drug product development. The ICH S7A guidance (Safety Pharmacology for Human Pharmaceuticals) recommends that the core battery of safety pharmacology studies be provided for all drugs. However, the guidance states "Safety pharmacology studies prior to the first administration in humans may not be needed for cytotoxic agents for treatment of end-stage cancer patients. However, for cytotoxic agents with novel mechanisms of action, there may be value in conducting safety pharmacology studies." An unaddressed issue in that guidance document was whether safety pharmacology studies are required for noncytotoxic therapies. In practice, safety pharmacology studies have not been needed to support clinical trials of oncology drug products in cancer patients as long as appropriate cardiovascular assessments (electrocardiogram, blood pressure, and heart rate) are included in the non-rodent study, and detailed observations of clinical signs (to address central nervous system and pulmonary toxicity) are included in all studies. Likewise, considering the great need for expediting the entry of new oncology drugs into clinical testing, it is unlikely that the DODP will require the battery of proposed in vitro and in vivo tests for assessing the potential for delayed ventricular repolarization (as recommended in the draft ICH S7B guidance) to support clinical trials in cancer patients any time in the near future.

6.2. Immunotoxicology

An FDA Guidance for Industry suggests that follow-up immune function studies be conducted when there is evidence of immunosuppression in nonclinical studies *(15)*. Immunosuppression is a common occurrence with oncology drugs and causes no special concerns with clinical oncologists who administer investigational drugs. Although conducting follow-up studies to explore immune function is reasonable advice, these data are not a critical component of the nonclinical safety program for oncology drugs.

6.3. Phototoxicology

A few oncology drug products are developed that fulfill the criteria for needing photosafety testing, e.g., topical products or photodynamic agents. As described in an FDA guidance document, short-term photosensitivity testing in animals should be considered for drug products that absorb ultraviolet B or A, or visible radiation (290–700 nm) and are (1) directly applied to the skin or eyes, or persist or accumulate in one of these areas; or (2) known to affect the skin or eyes *(16)*. There are a number of choices for assessing the potential for photosensitivity of an investigational new drug. Animal models and several in vitro screens for photoirritation, such as the 3T3 NRU phototoxicity test, have been used *(16)*.

7. INTERSPECIES DOSE CONVERSIONS AND STARTING DOSE SELECTION

The starting dose for cytotoxic drugs in subjects with advanced refractory cancer is usually one-tenth the dose causing severe toxicity or lethality to 10% of rodents on a body surface area basis (mg/m^2) *(1–4,17)*. This starting dose is acceptable provided that it does not cause serious irreversible toxicity in a non-rodent species *(2–4)*. If irreversible toxicities are produced at the proposed starting dose in non-rodents (usually dogs) or if the non-rodent is known to be the more appropriate animal model, then the starting dose would generally be one-sixth of the highest dose tested in non-rodents that does not cause severe, irreversible toxicity. This approach has been highly successful in the development of cytotoxic drugs, but using the rodent as the default species for starting dose selection may not always be suitable for noncytotoxic or molecularly targeted drugs. For these drugs, careful attention needs to be applied to species selection so that the data generated have reasonably predictive value for humans. The many principles described in the ICH S6 guidance on nonclinical development of biologic products are germane to molecularly targeted drugs, and a particularly important point is the need to justify the relevance of the animal models that will be used for extrapolating starting doses in humans *(18)*. Chapter 13 includes a detailed presentation of the factors that should be considered when selecting species for a nonclinical safety assessment program. With some of these agents, basing starting doses on expected pharmacologically active doses rather than the maximal allowable dose extrapolated from toxicology studies may also be desirable.

8. CONCLUSIONS

Designing a toxicology program to support clinical trials of an oncology drug product is a critically important step in overall nonclinical development. Without a carefully formulated strategy, the toxicology studies that are implemented may fail to support the intended clinical plan, may fail to collect valuable information that can aid rational clinical development, and may need to be repeated at significant costs in time and money. The class of product, the anticipated dosing regimen needed for activity, the route of administration, and the intended subjects in clinical trials are all important factors to consider in designing individual toxicology studies and the overall program. Although the nonclinical safety studies needed for supporting clinical development are less intensive than for most other therapeutics, designing a nonclinical development plan that is relevant to cancer patients is nonetheless a challenge because of the desire to administer potentially therapeutic doses to patients in poor health early in development. The fundamental goals of nonclinical safety testing for oncology drug products are to allow determination of a reasonably safe starting dose and escalation scheme for use in humans by revealing the toxicity profile, the dose-response for toxicity, and the reversibility of the observed toxicities in appropriate animal models. The ever increasing development of oncology drugs that will probably need chronic administration to provide effective long-term management of malignancies presents additional challenges for nonclinical safety assessment. The selection of appropriate animal models is a critically important decision for these types of agents since they have been designed to target specific pathways that may not be equally important in normal cell functioning across all species. The incorporation of additional assessments into toxicology studies, such as pharmacodynamic endpoints, biomarkers, or gene expression changes, may provide valuable information that aids overall development *(1)*.

For cytotoxic oncology drugs, either expanded acute studies or multicycle studies are expected to support early clinical development. As is expected for hormonal drugs and immunomodulators, 28-d studies can usually support chronic dosing in phase I and limited phase II trials of molecularly targeted drugs. Plans to study drug combinations in the clinic will need to be supported by appropriate in vivo studies that address the safety of the combination. If initial clinical trials of oncology drugs are proposed in normal healthy volunteers, then the nonclinical program will need to include the full battery of studies recommended by ICH guidances, including safety pharmacology studies and genetic toxicity assays. Careful design of nonclinical studies can maximize the value of the data obtained for enhancing clinical development and minimize the potential for data deficiencies that delay development. The expectations for nonclinical safety development continue to evolve as science advances and consensus is reached on various approaches for addressing critical safety endpoints. To verify that the proposed nonclinical program will satisfy current DODP expectations, feedback from the DODP review team should be sought in a pre-IND interaction.

REFERENCES

1. Tomaszewski JE, Smith AC, Covey JM, Donohue SJ, Rhie JK, Schweikart KM. Relevance of preclinical pharmacology and toxicology to phase I trial extrapolation techniques: relevance of animal toxicology. In: Baguley BC, Kerr DJ, eds. *Anticancer Drug Development*. New York: Academic. 2002:301–328.
2. DeGeorge JJ, Ahn C-H, Andrews PA, et al. Regulatory considerations for preclinical development of anticancer drugs. *Cancer Chemother Pharmacol* 1998;41:173–185.
3. Grieshaber CK, Marsoni S. Relation of preclinical toxicology to findings in early clinical trials. *Cancer Treat Rep* 1986;70:65–72.
4. Lowe MC, Davis RD. The current toxicology protocol of the National Cancer Institute. In: Hellmann K, Carter SK, eds. *Fundamentals of Cancer Chemotherapy*. New York: McGraw-Hill. 1984:228–235.
5. Food and Drug Administration. Guidance for Industry: Single Dose Acute Toxicity Testing for Pharmaceuticals. 1996; http://www.fda.gov/cder/guidance/pt1.pdf.
6. International Conference on Harmonisation of Technical Requirements for Registration of Pharmaceuticals for Human Use. Guidance for Industry: ICH M3 Non-Clinical Safety Studies for the Conduct of Human Clinical Trials for Pharmaceuticals. 1997; http://www.fda.gov/cder/guidance/1855fnl.pdf.
7. Food and Drug Administration. Good laboratory practice for nonclinical laboratory studies (2003); (codeified at 21 CFR) 58. http://www.access.gpo.gov/nara/cfr/waisidx_03/21cfr58_03.html.
8. International Conference on Harmonisation of Technical Requirements for Registration of Pharmaceuticals for Human Use. ICH S4A. Duration of Chronic Toxicity Testing in Animals (Rodent and Non-Rodent Toxicity Testing). 1998. http://www.emea.eu.int/pdfs/human/ich/030095en.pdf.
9. Food and Drug Administration International Conference on Harmonisation. Guidance on the duration of chronic toxicity testing in animals (rodent and non rodent toxicity testing). 64 *Fed Register* 34259–34260 (1999). http://www.fda.gov/cder/guidance/62599.pdf.
10. International Conference on Harmonisation of Technical Requirements for Registration of Pharmaceuticals for Human Use. ICH S2B. A Standard Battery for Genotoxicity Testing of Pharmaceuticals. 1997; http://www.fda.gov/cder/guidance/1856fnl.pdf.
11. Food and Drug Administration. Draft Reviewer Guidance: Integration of study results to assess concerns about human reproductive and developmental toxicities. 2001; http://www.fda.gov/cder/guidance/4625dft.pdf.
12. International Conference on Harmonisation of Technical Requirements for Registration of Pharmaceuticals for Human Use. ICH S7A: Safety Pharmacology Studies for Human Pharmaceuticals. 2001; http://www.fda.gov/cder/guidance/4461fnl.pdf.
13. International Conference on Harmonisation of Technical Requirements for Registration of Pharmaceuticals for Human Use. Draft Consensus Guideline: Safety Pharmacology Studies for Assessing the Potential for Delayed Ventricular Repolarization (QT Interval Prolongation) by Human Pharmaceuticals. 2002; http://www.fda.gov/cder/guidance/4970dft.pdf.
14. Food and Drug Administration. Guidance for Industry and Reviewers: Estimating the Safe Starting Dose in Clinical Trials for Therapeutics in Adult Healthy Volunteers. 2002; http://www.fda.gov/cder/guidance/3814dft.pdf.
15. Food and Drug Administration. Guidance for Industry: Immunotoxicology Evaluation of Investigational New Drugs. 2002; http://www.fda.gov/cder/guidance/4945fnl.pdf.
16. Food and Drug Administration. Guidance for Industry: Photosafety Testing. 2003; http://www.fda.gov/cder/guidance/3640fnl.pdf.
17. Newell DR, Burtles SS, Fox BW, Jodrell DI, Connors TA. Evaluation of rodent-only toxicology for early clinical trials with novel cancer therapeutics. *Br J Cancer* 1999; 81:760–768.
18. International Conference on Harmonisation of Technical Requirements for Registration of Pharmaceuticals for Human Use. Guidance for Industry: ICH S6 Preclinical Evaluation of Biotechnology-Derived Pharmaceuticals. 1997; http://www.fda.gov/cder/guidance/1859fnl.pdf.

15 Nonclinical Testing for Oncology Biologic Products

Carolyn M. Laurençot, PhD, Denis Roy, PhD, and Paul A. Andrews, PhD

CONTENTS

INTRODUCTION
GENERAL NONCLINICAL SAFETY PRINCIPLES FOR BIOLOGICS
MONOCLONAL ANTIBODY PRODUCTS
SOMATIC CELL THERAPY AND GENE THERAPY
RECOMBINANT PROTEINS
THERAPEUTIC CANCER VACCINES
CONCLUSIONS

1. INTRODUCTION

Different statutes govern the regulation of drug and biologic products in the United States. Whereas both are subject to the Food, Drug, and Cosmetic Act of 1948, biologic products are mainly regulated by the Public Health Service Act of 1944. The differences in the regulation of drug and biologic products are mainly owing to the basic premise that most drug products have a known structure and are chemically synthesized, whereas biologic products are derived from living sources (such as humans, animals, plants, and micro-organisms), may not have a completely defined structure, tend to be heat-sensitive, and are prone to microbial contamination. According to the regulations, a biologic product is any virus, therapeutic serum, toxin, antitoxin, vaccine, blood, blood component or derivative, allergenic product, or analogous product applicable to the prevention, treatment, or cure of disease or injuries to humans (http://www.fda.gov/cber/faq.htm) *(1)*. Oncologic products classified as biologics include preventative and therapeutic vaccines, somatic cell and gene therapy, monoclonal antibodies, immunotoxins, radioimmunotherapy, recombinant proteins (e.g., cytokines, growth factors, and fusion proteins), and most other biotechnology-derived products.

From: *Cancer Drug Discovery and Development:*
Anticancer Drug Development Guide: Preclinical Screening, Clinical Trials, and Approval, 2nd Ed.
Edited by: B. A. Teicher and P. A. Andrews © Humana Press Inc., Totowa, NJ

The Center for Biologics Evaluation and Research (CBER) of the U.S. Food and Drug Administration (FDA) was previously responsible for ensuring the safety of all biologic products, but on September 6, 2002 the FDA announced that the responsibility for reviewing many new biologic therapeutics would be transferred to the Center for Drug Evaluation and Research (CDER). The FDA has indicated that consolidation of the review process for therapeutic drug and biologic products will enhance the efficiency and consistency of the FDA's regulatory process. Under this new initiative, the review of biologic products other than vaccines, blood cells, tissues, cellular and gene therapy, and related products will be transferred to CDER. Regulation of the following products will be transferred from CBER to CDER: monoclonal antibodies intended for therapeutic use; cytokines, growth factors, enzymes, and interferons (including recombinant versions) intended for therapeutic use, as well as proteins intended for therapeutic use that are extracted from animals or micro-organisms. The review of therapeutic cancer vaccines will remain in CBER. The CBER-CDER Product Consolidation Working Group has been implemented to address the timing of the transfer of review responsibilities to CDER during the 2003 calendar year. The FDA is advising sponsors of new pharmaceutical products to continue working with CBER and CDER according to current policies and practices until the FDA issues further guidance on any change in the review responsibilities for biologic products (available at http://www.fda.gov/cder/biologics/default.html).

2. GENERAL NONCLINICAL SAFETY PRINCIPLES FOR BIOLOGICS

The FDA has published numerous guidance documents and points-to-consider (PTC) documents to assist sponsors in the nonclinical and clinical development of biologic products (available at http://www.fda.gov/cber/guidelines.htm). In addition, the International Conference on Harmonisation of Technical Requirements for Registration of Pharmaceuticals for Humans (ICH) has issued several documents pertinent to the development of biologic products (available at http://www.ich.org/ich5.html). The ICH is an initiative that brings together government regulators and drug industry representatives from the United States, the European Union, and Japan to make the international drug regulatory process more efficient and uniform. The FDA and ICH guidance and PTC documents are not legally binding but do provide pertinent information on current FDA policies and usual practices. Even though it is prudent to review these documents prior to initiating any nonclinical studies, they should not be viewed as a guaranteed manual for an adequate nonclinical safety development program. Regulatory science is dynamic, with new issues and new approaches for addressing safety arising continually. In addition, virtually every biologic product has unique issues. Therefore, CBER encourages sponsors to request a pre-Investigational New Drug (pre-IND) meeting at which manufacturing issues, nonclinical study plans, and the proposed clinical trial can be discussed and, if necessary, revised according to the FDA reviewers' comments.

The ICH S6 Guidance "Preclinical Safety Evaluation of Biotechnology-Derived Pharmaceuticals" provides a general overview of issues relevant to nonclinical development of biologic products. Similar to new drugs, the main objectives for nonclinical safety studies for biologics are to determine the target tissues for toxicity (hazard identification), the dose response for toxicity, and the reversibility of toxicities so that a safe starting dose and dose escalation scheme can be selected for use in humans (risk assessment). The nonclinical studies should identify appropriate parameters for clinical monitoring of safety in the clinic, even if doses many-fold those anticipated clinically are needed to induce toxicity in animals. Nonclinical studies addressing these issues are conducted throughout the clinical development of the biologic product, not only prior to initiation of clinical studies. Safety concerns may arise from the presence of impurities or contaminants; therefore, it is essential that the biologic product meet specifications for purity, safety (free of adventitious agents), sterility, identity, and potency throughout nonclinical and clinical testing. Comparability testing for each lot of the biologic must be performed to ensure that the product used for pharmacology and toxicology studies meets the same specifications as the product used in the clinical trials.

The nonclinical studies of oncology biologic products recommended for supporting ongoing clinical development and eventually a Biologic License Application for marketing are conceptually similar to those discussed in the previous chapter for oncology drug products, with numerous caveats. For example, genetic toxicity studies are generally not applicable to most biologic products. Certain characteristics of biologic products, such as species specificity and immunogenicity, often preclude the conventional paradigms for toxicity testing of pharmaceuticals (i.e., testing in one rodent and one non-rodent species).

The following issues should be considered when designing and implementing nonclinical safety studies for biologics: selection of the relevant animal species, use of sexually mature healthy animals, dose and route of administration, schedule and duration of treatment, and stability of the test material under the conditions of use. Biologics for oncology should be tested for toxicity only in species in which the product is pharmacologically active owing to the expression of the target molecule. For example, when testing a monoclonal antibody, the animal model should express the epitope recognized by the antibody (although there are numerous exceptions such as antibodies designed to neutralize viral products associated with specific malignancies). In order to serve as a more predictive model for human toxicity, the animal model should also display similar tissue distribution patterns for the biologic target as observed in the human. If two relevant species exist, some studies may be required in both species. Conversely, if no relevant animal models exist, the use of relevant transgenic animals expressing the human target or the use of a homologous protein should be considered for safety testing. Dose selection for the nonclinical studies should take into account differences in receptor affinity between species. A scientifically valid and informative study is expected to identify a substantially toxic dose level as well as a no observed adverse effect level (NOAEL). However, it is not essential to identify a NOAEL in nonclinical studies for oncology products that will be administered to advanced cancer patients. In order to correctly interpret the toxicological findings observed in nontraditional but pharmacologically relevant animal models (if used), it is necessary to include positive and negative controls in the study design as well as to provide extensive baseline data *(2)*.

Biologic products can be immunogenic in some animal species. Even though, it is generally accepted that antibody formation in animals does not predict antibody formation in humans, the immunogenicity of biologic products should be evaluated in repeat-dose toxicology studies to aid in the interpretation of the toxicity observed in these studies. The scope and effect of the antibody response should be characterized. Antibodies or immune complexes could inherently cause new toxic events or affect the pharmacological parameters of the biologic resulting in an altered toxicity or efficacy profile. For example, immunogenic responses may reduce the bioactivity of the biologic by causing an increase in clearance, or the formation of neutralizing antibodies. In addition, the toxicity profile of the biologic may be compromised if systemic exposure is not maintained, or if toxicity is owing to a reaction to a foreign protein *(3)*. Immunotoxicity may also result from products that are intended to stimulate or suppress the immune system or that change the expression of surface antigens on target cells. In such cases, animal studies should be implemented to address the potential for autoimmunity.

3. MONOCLONAL ANTIBODY PRODUCTS

Monoclonal antibody (MAb) products include intact immunoglobulins produced by hybridomas; immunoconjugates; and immunoglobulin fragments and recombinant proteins derived from immunoglobulins, such as chimeric and humanized immunoglobulins, F(ab') and F(ab')$_2$ fragments, single-chain antibodies, and recombinant immunoglobulin variable regions. In 1997, CBER issued the document "Points to Consider in the Manufacturing and Testing of Monoclonal Antibody Products for Human Use" to facilitate development of MAbs. This PTC document is not legally binding but specifies the usual approach expected for the development of MAb products. This guidance should be used in conjunction with the regulations for biologics contained in 21 CFR Parts 200-299 and 600-680. As mentioned previously, safety issues related to impurities in the manufactured product are of paramount importance. It is essential that a reliable and continuous source of the antibody, such as a master cell bank and working cell banks, be established and determined to be free of adventitious agents (bacteria, fungi, mycoplasma, and viruses). Product safety testing must be incorporated in all stages of the antibody manufacturing, which generally includes all cell banks, end of production cells, unprocessed bulk, final purified bulk, and final biologic product. The actual tests required for product safety testing are dependent on the source and nature of the product and the method of manufacture.

Mechanism of action studies for MAbs should include in vitro and in vivo studies for antibody specificity, affinity, and efficacy. For example, during the preclinical development of trastuzumab, a humanized MAb specific for HER-2, the antiproliferative effect of trastuzumab was demonstrated in cell lines with increased levels of HER-2 and in a breast cancer xenograft model *(4)*. When designing a nonclinical development program, properties of MAb products such as immunogenicity, stability, tissue crossreactivity, and effector mechanisms should be carefully addressed. Prior to phase I testing in humans, the crossreactivity of a MAb product to a panel of normal human tissues or human cells in vitro must be evaluated to determine whether the antibody binds to nontarget organ tissue *(5)*. For bispecific antibodies, each parent antibody should be evaluated individually, in addition to testing the bispecific product. Conjugated, chemically modified antibodies or antibody fragments should be tested in the form to be used clinically. Conjugates of MAbs with cytotoxic drugs will be considered as drug products and must be developed according to the additional expectations for a drug product. The PTC document lists 32 normal human tissues that should be used to evaluate crossreactivity *(5)*. In addition, a comparison of antibody tissue crossreactivity in different species should preferably be evaluated so that the most relevant animal model can be selected for toxicology studies. Biodistribution, function, and structure of the antigen in the species selected for nonclinical testing should be comparable to the human. Identification of differences between the animal and human with regard to the abundance of the antigen, antibody affinity for the antigen, and the effector function of the antibody will aid in the prediction of the therapeutic index in humans.

Pharmacokinetic, pharmacodynamic, and toxicology studies of the MAb should all be conducted in a relevant animal model when feasible. If the product is an unconjugated MAb, and crossreactivity studies with human tissues are unequivocally negative, and if there is no relevant animal model, CBER should be consulted regarding the necessity for toxicity testing. However, if the product is an immunoconjugate, toxicity testing is required regardless of the presence of the antigen in an animal model owing to the nonspecific nature of the attached molecule. In addition, the stability of immuno-conjugates should be evaluated in vitro in pooled human serum at 37°C and in vivo in pharmacokinetic studies. Since manufacturing changes often occur in the development of MAb products, further in vitro or in vivo nonclinical studies may be required to demonstrate comparability between lots of product.

4. SOMATIC CELL THERAPY AND GENE THERAPY

Because of the increase in development activity and regulatory oversight in the areas of cellular and tissue-based products, gene therapies, and all forms of stem cell transplantation, CBER created the Office of Cellular, Tissue, and Gene Therapies (OCTGT) in October of 2002. Products pertinent to oncology, which will be reviewed and regulated by the OCTGT, include cellular and tissue-based products, gene therapies, and combination products containing living cells/tissues. The OCTGT plans to update guidance documents for somatic cell and gene therapy and conduct several public discussions at workshops and at the Biological Response Modifiers Advisory Committee meetings. To develop these types of products intelligently, it is essential that sponsors stay attuned to the evolving guidances in this arena.

4.1. Somatic Cell Therapy

In the 1998 CBER publication "Guidance for Human Somatic Cell Therapy and Gene Therapy," somatic cell therapy is defined as "the administration to humans of autologous, allogeneic, or xenogeneic living cells which have been manipulated or processed *ex vivo*." Examples of somatic cell therapies include immunotherapies, such as activated dendritic cells and tumor-infiltrating lymphocytes, and stem cell reconstitution therapies for use after myeloablative chemotherapy such as CD34+ hematopoietic stem cells. The numerous cellular therapy product safety issues are addressed in several CBER guidance documents, which should be consulted very early in product development. Addressing issues related to donor screening and testing, possible transmission of Creutzfeldt-Jakob disease (CJD) and variant Creutzfeldt-Jakob disease (vCJD), cell banking, and testing of materials used during in vitro manipulation for adventitious agents is of paramount importance in product safety testing. Release testing for cellular therapy products should include tests for cell identity, viability, potency, purity, and adventitious agents. If there is a possibility that the cellular therapy product may contain cancer cells (such as with tumor-infiltrating lymphocytes), the product must also be evaluated for the presence of tumor cells.

Because of the strict species specificity of many cellular therapy products, CBER staff should be consulted for concurrence on nonclinical study designs prior to initiating any studies. For proof-of-concept and pharmacologic studies, an animal model of disease can often be used to study the homologous animal cellular therapy product. These studies may provide information on in vivo function, survival time, and trafficking of the manipulated cells. Toxicology studies should be conducted in a relevant animal model and should evaluate distribution, trafficking, and persistence of the cells in addition to the standard toxicity parameters. Depending on the nature of the cellular therapy product, carcinogenicity testing may also be required.

4.2. Gene Therapy

Gene therapy is defined as any recombinant DNA product used to prevent, treat, diagnose or cure diseases in humans. Gene therapy products can be characterized as either "in vivo" or "ex vivo" products depending on whether they are directly administered to the patient or are administered as a component of a cellular therapy product. Research involving recombinant DNA molecules is regulated by several federal agencies including the National Institutes of Health (NIH) and the FDA. The NIH Guidelines for Research Involving Recombinant DNA Molecules should be consulted prior to initiating any gene therapy studies in animals or humans (available at http://www.nih.gov/od/oba/). The NIH Guidelines are applicable to all recombinant DNA research within the United States or its territories that is conducted at or sponsored by an institution that receives any support for recombinant DNA research from the NIH. The NIH guidelines are also applicable to research that involves testing in humans of materials containing recombinant DNA developed with NIH funds, if the institution that developed those materials sponsors or participates in those projects. Privately funded projects employing recombinant DNA must also adhere to the NIH Guidelines if these projects are being carried out at, or funded by, an organization that has any NIH contracts, grants, or other support for this kind of research. Numerous sponsors of privately funded recombinant DNA research who do not receive NIH support voluntarily follow the NIH Guidelines.

Nonclinical studies for nearly all types of recombinant DNA molecules will require submission of the protocols to the Institutional Biosafety Committee prior to initiation. Approval of the study design by the Committee may also be required depending on the type of recombinant DNA molecule. Appendix M of the NIH Guidelines "Points to Consider in the Design and Submission of Protocols for the Transfer of Recombinant DNA Molecules into One or More Human Research Participants" outlines the requirements for conducting human gene therapy clinical trials. The review process involves both the NIH Office of Biotechnology Activities (OBA) and the Recombinant DNA Advisory Committee (RAC).

The FDA guidance document "Guidance for Human Somatic Cell Therapy and Gene Therapy" addresses issues related to the production, characterization, release testing, and nonclinical testing of gene therapy products. This guidance does not cover issues of concern for preventative vaccines. Similar to other biologic products, gene therapy products must be fully characterized and tested for identity, potency, purity, and adventitious agents prior to release. Owing to the presence of unexpected genetic material commonly observed in vectors, tests for identity now include vector sequencing prior to the initiation of phase I clinical studies. This ensures that the manufactured vector has the appropriate

characteristics and that production did not alter the structure of the vector. For vectors
≤ 40 kb, a complete sequence of intermediates and vectors should be performed prior to
phase I clinical studies. For vectors ≥ 40 kb, intermediates introduced and flanking
regions should be sequenced prior to phase I clinical studies, and the complete vector
sequence should be determined before phase II clinical trials. The vector sequence should
be compared with the expected sequence, analyzed for open reading frames, and compared with nucleotide and protein databases. The cell and gene therapy guidance document should be consulted for issues related to the production and characterization of
specific classes of vectors. Of particular importance with retroviral, adenoviral, and
lentiviral products is the testing for replication competent virus. The FDA, in conjunction
with industry, has developed Adenovirus Type 5 Reference Material that would allow
useful comparison of experimental results from different studies with respect to measurements of viral particles and infectious titers.

The final formulated gene therapy product should be used in the nonclinical studies.
Changing the formulation, e.g., by adding liposomes, altering pH, or adjusting salt concentration, may change the biodistribution of the product and thereby affect bioactivity
or toxicity or both. When one is designing nonclinical studies for gene therapy products,
factors such as the species specificity of the transduced gene, permissiveness for infection by viral vectors, and comparative physiology should be considered. Bioactivity
studies provide the rationale for the introduction of the gene therapy product into human
clinical trials. These studies should be designed to determine the duration and level of
gene expression, the dose-response relationship, and the optimal route of administration
and dosing regimen to be used in the clinical trial. If there is previous clinical experience
with a comparable gene therapy product, OCTGT should be consulted to determine
whether less extensive nonclinical testing would be adequate for assessing safety.

A relevant animal model should be employed in which the biologic response to the
product is expected to be similar to the response observed in humans. Primates are not
necessarily the best animal model to study since less is known about primate immunology
and infectivity with gene transfer vectors than in rodents. If the human protein expressed
by the gene therapy vector does not bind with similar affinity, or elicits a suboptimal
biologic effect in the animal model, it may be prudent to investigate the same gene therapy
vector that will express the homologous protein in the animal model. For example, the
pharmacologic effects of some human cytokines in mice differs from the effects observed
in humans. However, the murine cytokine and the human cytokine elicit the same effects
in their respective species. Therefore, in the nonclinical studies for a vector encoding this
cytokine, in order to achieve the appropriate biologic activity in the animal model, it may
be more relevant to use a vector encoding the murine cytokine. Efficacy studies in animal
models for cancer can be used to support the safety of gene therapy products if the animal
is monitored for toxicity endpoints during the efficacy study.

Safety issues of great concern with gene therapy products include distribution of the
vector from the site of injection and genomic integration of vector sequences.
Biodistribution studies are necessary to determine the distribution and persistence of the
vector in nontarget organs. Of particular importance is the vector distribution to the germ
cells; testicular and ovarian tissues must therefore be analyzed for the presence of the
gene therapy product. Other tissues that should be evaluated in the biodistribution study
include peripheral blood, tissue at the injection site, highly perfused organs such as brain,

liver, kidneys, heart, and spleen, as well as tissues that would potentially be affected owing to the route of administration or the toxicity of the transgene. The presence of the vector sequence in tissues can be evaluated via DNA-polymerase chain reaction (PCR) methodology designed to detect a sequence unique to the product. If vector sequences are observed in nontarget tissues, studies should be conducted to determine whether the gene is expressed or associated with any toxicities *(6)*.

Biodistribution studies may not be needed prior to phase I clinical trials if the following criteria apply: there is previous clinical experience with the vector including a similar formulation, route of administration, and schedule; the transgene product is innocuous if expressed in nontarget organs; and the size of the vector (i.e., plasmid DNA) is not excessively different from the previously tested product. Even though biodistribution studies may not be required prior to phase I clinical trials for some gene therapy products, biodistribution studies will be required for these products at some point during the course of product development. Often the safety and biodistribution of vectors can be evaluated in the same toxicology study. Toxicology testing should obtain information regarding the toxicities related to the vector delivery system and the safety of the expressed gene. Vector persistence, in vivo expression of the transgene, identification of the target organs, and the reversibility of toxicities should be determined. Abbreviated toxicology studies may be appropriate for some vectors if there is previous experience with similar vectors, as indicated above.

A weight of evidence approach should be taken when evaluating the safety of gene therapy products for use in phase I clinical trials. This approach includes analysis of the pertinent data published in the literature in addition to evaluation of vector safety, safety of the transgene, and nonclinical and clinical experience with similar products (including dose and dose regimen). As clinical development of the gene therapy product progresses, nonclinical studies will need to address genetic toxicity, chronic toxicity, and reproductive toxicity to support licensure. The host immune response and development of antibodies to the gene therapy product should be considered when designing long-term toxicology studies.

A useful resource for the support of vector production and nonclinical studies for gene therapy clinical trials is The National Gene Vector Laboratories (NGVL). The NGVLs are NIH-funded academic production and pharmacology/toxicology laboratories that manufacture vectors for phase I/II clinical trials and provide support for pharmacology/toxicology studies used to support these clinical trials. The NGVL accepts requests for retrovirus, adenovirus, adeno-associated virus, DNA plasmid, herpesvirus, lentivirus, and other novel vectors. The NGVL coordinating center maintains a pharmacology/toxicology database for specific classes of vector. This information is accessible through the NGVL website (http://www.ngvl.org). Data will be comprised of summaries submitted by NGVL-supported investigators. The purpose of these data is to inform investigators of the type of pharmacology/toxicology information that is available. If an investigator determines that the data would support the nonclinical development of their product, a letter of cross-reference can be obtained to include in the IND submissions to the FDA.

4.3. Ancillary Products

Ancillary products are defined as products used in the manufacture of other products intended for in vivo use. Ancillary products include MAbs that are used for purification of other products (ex vivo purging of cells to remove tumor cells) and cytokines or growth factors used in the ex vivo culturing of cellular therapies such as dendritic cells. The primary concern with ancillary products is that they could potentially affect the safety, purity, and potency of the final therapeutic product. These products should be characterized in the same way as products intended for in vivo administration. Two main considerations for ancillary products are the identity and source (i.e., containing recombinant or animal-derived materials) and the role of the ancillary product in the manufacturing of the therapeutic product *(7)*. It is recommended that animal- or human-derived materials not be used if other alternatives are available. A qualification program should be established for ancillary products that consists of an analysis of the safety profile, purity, and potency in the manufacturing system intended for use. Safety testing should include tests for sterility, pyrogenicity, mycoplasma and other adventitious agents. Generally, reagent-grade ancillary products can be used for phase I and II clinical trials; however, this is contingent on adequately testing the product, as described above. For phase III clinical trials, ancillary products should be manufactured under Good Manufacturing Practices (GMPs).

5. RECOMBINANT PROTEINS

Recombinant proteins include such products as cytokines, growth factors, tumor suppressors, enzymes, angiogenesis inhibitors, and fusion proteins. As mentioned earlier in this chapter, testing for product safety, identity, purity, and potency as well as the selection of a relevant animal model for nonclinical testing is essential for successful product development. Because of the species specificity of certain recombinant protein products (i.e., cytokines), the most relevant model may include investigation of a homologous protein. Of particular concern for recombinant proteins is the immunogenicity of the product owing to foreign protein responses, or induction of autoimmunity if the protein crossreacts with normal tissues. Predictive models of immunogenicity such as peptide-MHC binding algorithms can aid in the determination of the potential immunogenic epitopes of recombinant proteins prior to patient administration. Immunogenicity assessment can often be included in the toxicology studies if the studies are adequately designed to focus on immunogenicity. For example, characterization of the antibody response (including titer, neutralizing or non-neutralizing status, and number of responding animals) would be required to determine the effect of antibody formation on pharmacologic or toxicologic parameters *(8)*. As mentioned earlier, immunogenicity observed in animal models is not predictive for humans; however, the assessment of immunogenicity is often essential for the interpretation of toxicologic results.

6. THERAPEUTIC CANCER VACCINES

Therapeutic cancer vaccines include peptides, recombinant proteins (e.g., cytokines, modified tumor-associated antigens), MAbs, idiotypic proteins, gene therapy products, and cellular therapy products. In addition to following the regulations and guidances specific to each separate class of biologic product mentioned previously in this chapter, properties associated with immunotherapeutic agents, such as the potential for immunotoxicity, should be evaluated in nonclinical studies. As with all biologic products, demonstration of the safety, identity, purity, and potency of cancer vaccine products is essential. However, testing for these parameters may be challenging for the immunotherapeutic agents since many aspects of the biology of the antitumor immune responses are often unknown. Issues to be considered during the development of cancer vaccines include generation of a consistent product from inconsistent starting material; qualification of the source and characterization of the cell substrate used to produce the vaccine; evaluation of the effect of cryopreservation on yield, viability, and activity of the vaccine; timing and methods of sterility testing; and lot release specifications for identity, purity, and potency *(9)*. Clinical trials may be initiated prior to establishing well-defined lot release assays (i.e., potency test, identity test); however, these assays must be established and validated prior to starting phase III clinical trials to ensure that a reproducible and consistent vaccine is available for assessing safety and efficacy *(10)*.

Most therapeutic cancer vaccines are designed to produce immunity to tumor-associated antigens. Tumor-associated antigens are either expressed solely in tumor tissue or have more prevalent expression in tumor tissue compared with normal tissue. Therefore, it is essential to determine whether a vaccine targeting a tumor-associated antigen has the potential to cause autoimmunity to normal tissues. The level of expression of the tumor-associated antigen in a panel of normal human tissues should be evaluated. Autoimmunity may arise if the antigen is expressed in normal tissue and the normal tissue is capable of presenting the antigenic epitope to T cells in the MHC-restricted fashion required for eliciting an immune response. The autoimmune potential of peptide vaccines should be further evaluated by performing a homology search in a protein database to assess the abundance of the peptide amino acid sequence in all known proteins. Depending on the immunogenic properties of the cancer vaccine, it may be prudent to evaluate further the potential for autoimmune-mediated toxicity in relevant animal models.

7. CONCLUSIONS

Nonclinical studies are performed at various stages of clinical development with the eventual goal of supporting market approval of the biologic product *(11)*. The purpose of nonclinical studies for oncology biologic products is similar to that for oncology drug products; however, the approach for obtaining relevant safety information may be more challenging for most biologic therapies. Nonclinical studies for all oncology products are designed to allow determination of a reasonably safe starting dose and escalation scheme for use in humans by revealing the toxicity profile, the dose-response for toxicity, and the reversibility of the observed toxicities in appropriate animal models. In addition, nonclinical data identify the safety parameters that need to be monitored in the clinical trials. For biologic products, nonclinical testing may also be required to demonstrate comparability since biologics are difficult to manufacture and characterize consistently *(12)*.

There are many correct approaches for assessing the safety of biologic products in nonclinical studies. Each product has unique properties that should be considered when designing the safety studies; therefore a "check the box" approach for nonclinical testing is strongly discouraged. The selection of a relevant animal model for safety studies and the incorporation of additional safety assessments in these studies, such as biodistribution or immunogenicity, are essential for obtaining the necessary pertinent data for the initiation of clinical trials. Relevant animal models must be chosen using a science-based approach for each product, and inappropriate models should not be studied. In addition, it is imperative to include the appropriate controls and baseline assessments in these studies to ensure proper interpretation of the toxicological findings. The FDA encourages sponsors to discuss their product with them early in development under a pre-IND program. Presentation and discussion of the nonclinical and clinical study plans with FDA scientists in a pre-IND meeting can facilitate the advancement of the product into clinical trials by identifying problematic areas prior to IND filing *(13)*. Open communication with the FDA should continue throughout product development to ensure that the proper strategy is being employed for achieving product licensure.

REFERENCES

1. Food and Drug Administration. 21 Code Federal Regulations 600.3(h).
2. Serabian M, Pilaro AM. Safety assessment of biotechnology-derived pharmaceuticals: ICH and beyond. *Toxicol Pathol* 1999; 27:27–31.
3. Green JD, Black LE. Overview status of preclinical safety assessment for immunomodulatory biopharmaceuticals. *Hum Exp Toxicol* 2000; 19:208–212.
4. Harries M, Smith I. The development and clinical use of trastuzumab (Herceptin). *Endocr Relat Cancer* 2002; 9:75–85.
5. Points to Consider in the Manufacture and Testing of Monoclonal Antibody Products for Human Use: U.S. Department of Health and Human Services, Food and Drug Administration, Center for Biologics Evaluation and Research, February, 1997.
6. Pilaro AM, Serabian MA. Preclinical development strategies for novel gene therapeutic products. *Toxicol Pathol* 1999; 27:4–7.
7. Martin A, Frey-Vasconcells J. A view on ancillary products for the emerging area of tissue engineered products. *Regul Affairs Focus* 1999; June:16–17.
8. Guidance for Industry: ICH S6 Preclinical Evaluation of Biotechnology-Derived Pharmaceuticals, U.S. Department of Health and Human Services, Food and Drug Administration, Center for Drug Evaluation and Research, Center for Biologics Evaluation and Research, July, 1997.
9. Keilholz U, Weber J, Finke JH, et al. Immunologic monitoring of cancer vaccine therapy: results of a workshop sponsored by the Society for Biological Therapy. *J Immunol* 2002; 25:97–138.
10. Razzaque A, Dye E, Puri RK. Characterization of tumor vaccines during product development. *Vaccine* 2000; 19:644–647.
11. Guidance for Industry: ICH M3 Non-Clinical Safety Studies for the Conduct of Human Clinical Trials for Pharmaceuticals, U.S. Department of Health and Human Services, Food and Drug Administration, Center for Drug Evaluation and Research, Center for Biologics Evaluation and Research, November, 2000.
12. FDA Guidance Concerning Demonstration of Comparability of Human Biolgcial Products, including Therapeutic Biotechnology-Derived Products, U.S. Department of Health and Human Services, Food and Drug Administration, Center for Drug Evaluation and Research, Center for Biologics Evaluation and Research, April, 1996.
13. Black LE, Bendele AM, Bendele RA, Zack PM, Hamilton M. Regulatory decision strategy for entry of a novel biological therapeutic with a clinically unmonitorable toxicity into clinical trials: pre-IND meetings and a case example. *Toxicol Pathol* 1999; 27:22–26.

IV CLINICAL TESTING

16

Working With the National Cancer Institute

Paul Thambi, MD
and Edward A. Sausville, MD, PhD

CONTENTS

INTRODUCTION
HISTORY OF THE NCI DRUG DEVELOPMENT PROGRAM
THE DRUG DISCOVERY AND DEVELOPMENT PROCESS AT THE NCI
PATHWAYS TO COLLABORATING WITH THE NCI
CONCLUSIONS

1. INTRODUCTION

This chapter outlines how the National Cancer Institute (NCI) can aid researchers in academia, industry, and elsewhere in the development of promising new compounds as antineoplastic drugs. The NCI has centered this task in the Division of Cancer Treatment and Diagnosis (DCTD). The NCI is unique among the caetgorical Institutes of the National Institutes of Health in having the capacity to engage in drug discovery and development operations from screening of natural product or synthetic compound mixtures all the way through the conduct of phase III trials. Preclinical work occurs in the Developmental Therapeutics Program (DTP); the Cancer Therapy Evaluation Program (CTEP) coordinates clinical study of compounds when the NCI holds Investigational New Drug (IND) applications or when the NCI cross-files on the INDs of collaborating institutions or commercial firms. The DTP focuses on generating the data needed to file an IND application with the Food and Drug Administration (FDA), whereas the CTEP is responsible not only for filing INDs with the FDA but also for providing guidance and oversight to funded grantee institutions throughout the country for the execution of clinical trials utilizing these agents.

Collaboration with the NCI can begin at almost any point in the drug development process. An interesting compound can enter the NCI development system with essentially no preclinical data through the NCI in vitro anticancer drug screen, or after the

From: *Cancer Drug Discovery and Development:*
Anticancer Drug Development Guide: Preclinical Screening, Clinical Trials, and Approval, 2nd Ed.
Edited by: B. A. Teicher and P. A. Andrews © Humana Press Inc., Totowa, NJ

originator has completed certain aspects of development, or even after the compound has already received IND status from the FDA. The originating organization retains intellectual property rights to the compound through confidentiality agreements including the Discreet Screening Agreement, by which compound data are treated as confidential ("discreet") and returned to the originator without the accrual of intellectual property to the U.S. government.

A relationship with the NCI can be beneficial to both parties. The originating organization is able to defray the costs of drug development substantially by using the resources available at the DTP and CTEP, whereas the NCI is better able to fulfill its congressionally mandated goal of promoting the emergence of novel therapies to fight cancer. A complete description of both programs is available on the Internet at http://dtp.nci.nih.gov and at http://ctep.cancer.gov.

2. HISTORY OF THE NCI DRUG DEVELOPMENT PROGRAM

The original federally funded initial anticancer drug screening program was formed by the U.S. Public Health Service Office of Cancer Investigations at Harvard University and involved testing bacterial extracts for their ability to induce hemorrhage and necrosis in the S37 tumor model. In 1937, by order of the National Cancer Institute Act, this office was combined with the U.S. Public Health Service Pharmacology Laboratory to form the National Cancer Institute, one of the first institutes of the then new National Institutes of Health. By the 1950s, over 3000 compounds were screened using this model; however, there was no systematic link to a clinical development program.

Access to both laboratory and clinical facilities were available only at the Sloan-Kettering Institute, the Children's Cancer Research Foundation, and the Columbia University College of Physicians and Surgeons. Of these, Sloan-Kettering was especially productive and screened over 20,000 compounds; however, the capacity of all these sites could not meet the demand of the increasing number of contributors of compounds.

In response to this situation, the NCI created the Cancer Chemotherapy National Service Center (CC-NSC) in 1955. The "NSC" derived from the name of this service center is still in use today as the prefix of a cataloging system for new compounds. The screening process changed from using the S37 tumor model to using three animal tumor models (S180, Ca 755, and L1210). Initially, the service center coordinated the screening, preclinical studies, and clinical evaluation of compounds submitted by various outside sources. To promote industry participation, the precursor to today's "Discreet Screening Agreement" was created to ensure contributors that they would retain proprietary rights to their compounds. By 1976, the CC-NSC evolved and eventually became the drug research and development program currently centered in the DTP *(1,2)*.

The goal of the drug development program of the NCI is to facilitate the availability of novel treatments to patients in a way that advances the best scientific and clinical leads. To achieve this goal, the DTP budget exceeds $60 million a year for research and development contracts directed by NCI staff to support procurement, screening, informatics, in vivo testing, formulation, and pharmacology and toxicology. In addition, over $200 million a year is awarded in a competitive process for grant support to extramural investigators with various degrees of cooperation with DTP. Over the last 45 yr, NCI has screened more than 400,000 compounds for antineoplastic activity and has played a role in the discovery and/or development of approx 60% of the small-molecule, nonhormonal chemotherapeutic agents approved for use in cancer treatment today in the United States.

Table 1
Drugs With NCI, DTP Involvement (1997–2001)

Small molecules	
Cordycepin/deoxycoformycin	Rapamycin analog
COL-3	2-Methoxyestradiol
Aminoflavone	R(+)XK469
Benxothiazole	6-MCDF
EF5	CDDO
MGI-114 (HMAF)	Zebularine
Gadolinium texaphyrin	Flavopiridol
SarCNU	17-DMAG
Paullones	Life compound
17-AAG	Cytochlor + tetrahydrouridine
Perifosine	Halichondrin B analog
PS-341	**Biologics**
UCN-01	E2.3 and A27.15 antitransferrin receptor
KRN 5500	Erb-38 immunotoxin
Dimethane sulfonates	Anti-Her2 immunoliposomes
Pyrrolobenzodiazepine	Saprin immunoconjugates
Clotrimazole analog	LMB-9 immunotoxin
Halofuginone	Angiostatin
Dimethyl benzylphenylurea	RFB4 onconase
F18-FMAU	BL-22
BNP7787	Endostatin
Adaphostin	G3139 antisense
Dithiophenes	Synerlip-p53
2-Methoxyantimycin	IL-2/IL-12
MS-275	E1A gene therapy
	HeFi-1 anti-CD30 monoclonal antibody

Table 1 lists the agents (biologics and small molecules) with which the DTP has been involved over the last 5 yr.

3. THE DRUG DISCOVERY AND DEVELOPMENT PROCESS AT THE NCI

The governance of the NCI drug development process described above was vested in a standing committee of NCI staff, the Decision Network, from the late 1960s until 2000. During 1997–1998, an in-depth review of DTP activities and prioritization process led to a revision of the DTP's mission and operating procedures. In particular, extramural participation in decision making and extramural access to NCI drug discovery and development resources was articulated as an important goal. Random screening in favor of devising strategies to link the actions of drugs to particular molecular targets was strongly endorsed (3). Accordingly, decision-making groups were reoriented to include the opportunity for participation by extramural experts, and this has resulted in new NCI efforts to fold these points of view into its process.

3.1. NCI Drug Development Group

No matter the source of the compound, if the clinical development of the agent is to take place under an NCI-held IND, the Drug Development Group (DDG) will be responsible for overseeing the development process (as detailed in Fig. 1) and for making key

I/IB: Acquisition and Screening

WHAT NCI IS LOOKING FOR:
Unique mechanism of action and/or unique chemical structure
Effect of the compound on the target is demonstrated *in vitro*
Preliminary hollow fiber *in vivo* activity studies

WHAT HAPPENS AT THIS STAGE:
Assurance of supply of compound by synthesis or extraction
Mechanism of action studies
Preliminary *in vivo* model activity studies
Pharmacology studies to define desired concentrations to affect the target
Pre-range finding toxicology studies
Solubility/stability studies

Stage II: Pre-Clinical Development
IIA:

WHAT NCI IS LOOKING FOR:
PK/PD studies showing the effect of the compound on the target *in vivo*
Clear evidence of activity in detailed *in vivo* model studies
Compound availability is assured
Compound is pharmaceutically tractable
Intellectual Property issues are clarified

WHAT HAPPENS AT THIS STAGE:
Range finding toxicology studies
Development of a formulation suitable for clinical use

IIB:

WHAT NCI IS LOOKING FOR:
Range finding toxicology results are acceptable and there is a tenable clinical formulation

WHAT HAPPENS AT THIS STAGE:
IND-directed toxicology on the clinically relevant schedule

Stage III: Clinical Development

NCI requires an acceptable toxicity profile
IND is filed by CTEP for NCI sponsored clinical trials to begin

Fig. 1. Stages of drug development (adapted from the DTP website at http://dtp.nci.nih.gov).

recommendations of whether to proceed to the next stage. Formerly known as the entirely in-house "Decision Network," the DDG now incorporates extramural guidance and review at various critical junctures in the drug development process. This process allows for a mechanism to prioritize the best use of resources by the NCI. An additional source of valued opinions from the extramural research community is the Biological Resources

Branch Oversight Committee, which advises on the relative prioritization of agents for production in the NCI's biologicals production facility. A detailed description of the how the review process is conducted is also obtainable through http://dtp.nci.nih.gov.

3.2. Drug Discovery and Screening (Stage I)

The NCI actively solicits various organizations in the United States and abroad to submit compounds to the screening process in an effort to identify novel therapeutic agents not studied previously. Following the execution of a confidentiality agreement (available from http://dtp.nci.nih.gov), NCI staff examine the compound structure. If the structure has not been studied previously or is new to the screening system, the compound may be accepted for screening. The Natural Product Branch of DTP also procures natural products (plant, marine, microbial) extracts from around the world (4).

The initial drug development stage involves stage I screening. The in vitro anticancer drug screen at NCI has been described in an earlier chapter and will only be commented on briefly here. In the mid-1980s the initial screening model changed from in vivo animal model activity as the primary screen to an in vitro process, allowing screening to be completed with less compound, and more information yielded through the use of computational techniques. The current version of the screen employs a prescreen, seeking evidence of cytotoxicity in three cell lines (MCF7 breast carcinoma, NCI-H460 lung carcinoma, and SF268 glioma). If a compound has significant activity in one or more of these cell lines, it will proceed to the full 60-cell line panel, derived from nine cancer types (5). The pattern of activity of the compound is analyzed and compared with an extensive database of compounds by a computational algorithm, COMPARE. This program can give insight into the mechanism of action of the compound and indicates whether the compound has similarity in sensitivity pattern or mechanism of action to classes of known agents (6). If the pattern appears to be unique, the compound will progress to the next step, in vivo testing. The screening data from >40,000 compounds, along with the capacity to perform web-based COMPARE analyses, is available through http://dtp.nci.nih.gov.

In addition to the COMPARE algorithm, DTP's screening resource has promoted numerous distinct bioinformatics-based approaches to reveal relations between compound action and structures of the agents. These include neural networks (7), cluster analysis (8), and integration of drug action with gene expression patterns in the cell line panel by microarray analysis (9). More recently, nonhierarchical self-organizing map (SOM) techniques (10) have been developed and are available through a web-accessible tool through http://spheroid.ncifcrf.gov. Other uses of the data extend to correlation of compound action with the expression of molecular targets in the cell line panel. This type of application proceeds from the hypothesis that targets relevant to a compound's action would be over- or underexpressed in cells with high or low degrees of sensitivity to the agent. This possibility has been borne out in several examples, including, for instance, the pgp multidrug resistance transporter (11).

If a compound has a known mechanism of action, the screening process can be tailored to address cell lines certain to contain or functionally depend on the target. In addition to the 60-cell line panel, efforts to put in place screening algorithms using defined molecular targets in response to opportunities arising with both extramural collaborators and in-house NCI scientists have been an emerging priority for the DTP (12). Screens have been implemented against defined oncogene targets, e.g., c-met (13), or mediators of physiologic processes such as hypoxia-inducible factor-1 *(14)*, with the goal of ultimately posting in the public domain the detailed results of these screens. Sets of compounds (Training, Diversity, and Open Repository sets) are potentially available from the NCI to promote these goals. The nature of these collections and how to access them is available from through http://dtp.nci.nih.gov.

3.3. Advanced Screening and Preclinical Development (Stages IB–IIB)

Compounds that advance to stage IB will have evidence of preliminary in vivo activity. This is accomplished in mice with 12 human tumor cell lines grown in hollow fibers placed subcutaneously and intraperitoneally *(15)*. Compounds that are active in the hollow fiber assay, or have a rationale for a molecular basis of activity, may be further studied as a stage IB candidate compound. Every attempt is made to discover the mechanism of action of the compound and to develop an appropriate in vivo model that contains the believed target of the drug lead. Initial formulation studies are conducted, and pharmacology studies in animals and in vitro convey information about the time and duration of drug concentration necessary for a useful effect. In vivo activity in mice with an established tumor model is key in advancing a compound further in the development process. If in vivo results are promising, the compound proceeds to the next step of preclinical development, stage IIA (Fig. 1) after consideration of the screening data by the DDG.

NCI's experience with testing agents in athymic mouse xenografts of human tumors has recently been addressed in detail *(16)*, comparing the activity of agents screened in the preclinical models with subsequent activity observed during phase II testing. This analysis revealed that the degree of correspondence between activity in a xenograft model of a particular histology and activity in the same disease in the clinic was poor. However, the greater the number of models in which a test compound (all cytotoxics undergoing testing in nonmolecularly characterized xenografts) showed activity, then the greater the likelihood that activity would be manifest in at least one human clinical disease. Whether more predictive value of xenograft or other animal model studies might emerge from alternative approaches using molecules targeted to a defined biologic process is a matter of great relevance to the field, and of interest to the DTP.

Stage IIA compounds are studied in detailed animal model studies to define a schedule of administration appropriate for clinical use. In addition, range-finding toxicology studies are performed in animals to define the initial basis for choosing doses for detailed safety evaluations. The choice of the schedule for toxicology studies mirrors the anticipated schedule to be used in clinical trials. Toxicity evaluations are correlated with plasma drug concentrations. Following the completion of stage IIA studies, the data are again reviewed by the DDG with at least two extramural reviewers to determine whether the compound will be taken to the next step, stage IIB. Approval to the stage IIB level results in full-scale IND-directed toxicology and production of a clinically viable dose formulation.

3.4. Clinical Development (Stage III)

Compounds entering the process at stage III have either completed NCI-sponsored stage IIB studies or come to the NCI from external organizations. If an organization enters a compound into the NCI development process at stage III, review by extramural reviewers for the DDG also occurs. At this point a Clinical Trials Agreement (CTA) is formulated whereby the supplier agrees to supply sufficient quantities of the drug for

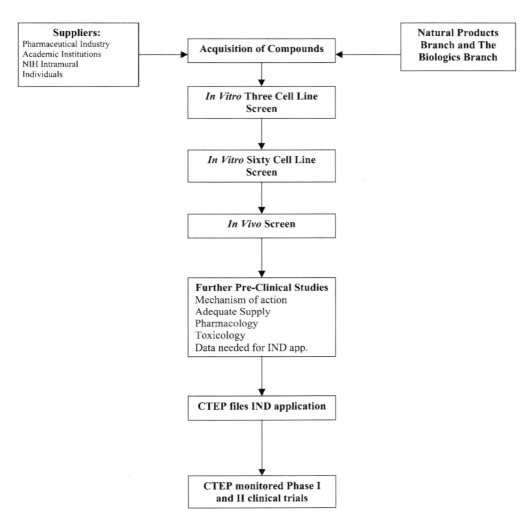

Fig. 2. Summary of NCI drug discovery and development process.

clinical trials, or the NCI manufactures its own supplies of the agent, usually under a Cooperative Research and Development Agreement (CRADA) with the originating supplier. Following successful completion of stage IIB toxicology studies for NCI-originated compounds or biologics, or successful review of agents originating with other organizations, the responsibility for further development passes to the CTEP. An IND application is prepared, or the CTEP cross-files on the IND of collaborating organizations. The CTEP then solicits from its peer-reviewed academic institutions letters of intent to conduct phase I clinical trials with the new agent. The CTEP then monitors and provides guidance in the writing and conduct of the protocol. In addition, the CTEP underwrites the cost of data collection, regulatory reporting, and monitoring. The data generated by the phase I trials may then be used to solicit further phase II clinical trials; if the results are promising, data needed to file a New Drug Application with the FDA for approval for standard clinical use will be generated. A summary of the development process is detailed in Fig. 2. The goal of the process is certainly not to compete with private industry, but to maximize the likelihood that promising agents can make the transition from preclinical discovery to clinical use. NCI activities are in all cases carefully coordinated to complement the activities of the private sector in bringing new agents to the clinic.

4. PATHWAYS TO COLLABORATING WITH THE NCI

The DTP/NCI has helped various types of organizations promote drugs through preclinical development, and the CTEP has helped with clinical development. Various mechanisms for establishing such collaborations have been formed and will be outlined in this section.

4.1. Drug Development Group

As described above, the DDG is comprised of NCI staff supplemented by *ad hoc* reviewers for particular compounds. The normal operations of this group result in compounds for where NCI holds the IND, or cross-files on a commercial firm's IND. Applications to enter compounds at any stage along the process are made to the DDG, and the applications are reviewed according to the strength of the preclinical data to date, the uniqueness of the compound, the anticipated costs for development, and the need for NCI involvement (i.e., whether or not the drug be developed if the NCI is not involved). In addition, the nature of the drug in addressing the goals of the NCI portfolio of investigator-initiated clinical studies is considered, which emphasize agents with novel mechanisms of action, and not analogs of existing agents. Smaller pharmaceutical companies tend to enter their compounds at earlier stages in the DDG process, whereas larger pharmaceutical companies typically use this process to enter their compounds at stage III in an effort to broaden the portfolio of phase I–II trials. Corporate sponsors tend to retain governance of the larger licensing-directed trials, while supporting NCI studies to address diseases that afflict smaller groups of patients or have scientific and pharmacological endpoints. Further information is available at http://dtp.nci.nih.gov/docs/ddg_descript.html.

4.2. Rapid Access to Intervention Development (RAID)

This program was developed to facilitate the development of novel agents arising from the academic community into therapeutic agents, with control of the initial clinical studies remaining the responsibility of the originating academic investigator. To achieve this goal, NCI preclinical development resources are made available to investigators on a competitive basis. The research and development tasks undertaken during this process are similar to the DDG process described earlier; however, the data and products of the research are returned to the applicant to allow for the filing of an investigator-held IND application. The purpose of RAID is to remove any rate-limiting steps and to allow investigators to file their own IND application for eventual testing in clinical trials. RAID applications are accepted by the DTP twice yearly; further information on the program and the application process can be found at the DTP website at http://dtp.nci.nih.gov/docs/raid.

4.3. RAID Clones: R*A*N*D and IIP

Following the successful implementation of the RAID initiative, efforts to bring this general approach (investigator-directed, peer-reviewed) to utilization of NCI contract research resources in relation to earlier preclinical tasks (such as library generation, production of large quantities of target protein for screening, medicinal chemistry in conjunction with pharmacology) stimulated the development of the Rapid Access to NCI Discovery (R*A*N*D) program. Likewise, the Inter-Institute Program (IIP) for Development of AIDS-Related Therapeutics is a joint effort between the NCI and the National Institute for Allergy and Infectious Diseases (NIAID) to provide contract research resources to investigators in the areas of non-protease inhibitor and non-reverse transcriptase inhibitor approaches to anti-retroviral therapy, novel approaches to opportunistic pathogen treatment, and treatment of AIDS-related malignancies. Both R*A*N*D and IIP use a review and application procedure similar to RAID. Information about these programs may be obtained through http://dtp.nci.nih.gov.

4.4. Grants and Contracts Programs

The Grants and Contract Operations Branch of the DTP administers a large number of grants and cooperative agreements with various investigators who have applied independently for grants and assistance. Various programs have been established for this purpose (*see* http://dtp.nci.nih.gov/branches/gcob/gcob_index.html for more information).

4.4.1. National Cooperative Drug Discovery Group Program

This program was established in the early 1980s to foster collaboration between talented researchers in academia and other centers with investigators in the pharmaceutical industry. The program is a cooperative agreement, awarded after a competitive process, whereby the NCI can advise the group on progress but does not direct the work. At least one industrial and typically three to four academic participants comprise each group. The NCI is able to supply such resources as databases, drug repositories, and the equipment and material needed for preclinical drug development. Three currently licensed drugs have emerged from the NCDDG program.

4.4.2. Small Business Innovation Research (SBIR) and Small Business Technology Transfer (STTR) Program

These programs are specifically designed to assist small companies (<500 employees) and to provide funding and other NCI resources for the development of new compounds. The STTR program was designed to support cooperative research between the NCI and small companies or nonprofit research organizations.

4.4.3. Molecular Target Drug Discovery Program

This program includes a variety of grant mechanisms including cooperative agreements (UO1s), pilot project grants (R21s), and small business innovation research (SBIR) grants that have as a primary focus the definition of how a novel molecular target defined as present in tumors might be "credentialed" as a viable drug target. Additional NCI resources can be awarded as supplements to these grants to promote the elucidation of molecular structure or the production of the target protein or agents directed at the target.

4.5. Repositories

The DTP maintains several compounds that are available at no cost to university-based researchers and small businesses through a Materials Transfer Agreement. The types of repositories include Synthetics, Natural Products, Radiolabeled Materials, Biologics, Tumor Repository, and the Angiogenesis Resource Center. Further information on the repositories can be obtained at http://dtp.nci.nih.gov.

4.6. Web-Accessible Databases and Tools

Access to various databases including screening results, chemical structures, characterizations of molecular targets in cell lines, and other data is available free of charge at the DTP website http://dtp.nci.nih.gov.

5. CONCLUSIONS

A primary goal of the NCI is to assist academic and industrial partners in bringing active therapeutic agents to the clinic in a timely manner. The DTP and CTEP have a number of programs designed to achieve this goal. By making data from over 45 yr of drug development at NCI available to investigators, and by applying the expertise and resources of the NCI drug development process to compounds supplied by outside sources, the NCI has been successful in achieving this goal. Active solicitation of new agents and continued collaboration with industry, academia, and others will ensure that exciting new agents will continue to be developed.

REFERENCES

1. Zubrod CG, Schepartz S, Leiter J, Endicott KM, Carrese LM. Baker CG. The chemotherapy program of the National Cancer Institute: history, analysis, plans. *Cancer Chemother Rep* 1966; 50:349–540.
2. Grever MR, Schepartz SA, Chabner BA. The National Cancer Institute drug discovery and development program. *Semin Oncol* 1992; 19:622–638.
3. Sausville EA, Feigal E. Evolving approaches to cancer drug discovery and development at the National Cancer Institute, USA. *Ann Oncol* 1999; 10:1287–1291.
4. Cragg GM, Boyd MR, Hallock YF, Newman DJ, Sausville EA, Wolpert MK. Natural product drug discovery at the National Cancer Institute: past achievements and new directions for the new millennium. In: Wrigley SK, Hayes MA, Thomas R, Chrystal EJT, Nicholson N, eds. *Biodiversity: New Leads for the Pharmaceutical and Agrochemical Industries*. Cambridge, UK: Royal Society of Chemistry. 2000:22–44.
5. Monks AP, Scudiero D, Skehan P, et al. Feasibility of a high-flux anti-cancer drug screen using a diverse panel of cultured human tumor cell lines. *J Natl Cancer Inst* 1991; 83:757–766.
6. Paull KD, Hamel E, Malspeis L. Prediction of biochemical mechanism of action from the in vitro antitumor screen of the National Cancer Institute. In: Foye WO, ed. *Cancer Chemotherapeutic Agents*. Washington, DC: American Chemical Society. 1995:9–45.
7. Weinstein J, Kohn KW, Grever MR, et al. Neural computing in cancer drug development: predicting mechanism of action. *Science* 1992; 258:447–451
8. Weinstein J, Myers TG, O'Connor PM, et al. An information-intensive approach to the molecular pharmacology of cancer. *Science* 1997; 275:343–349.
9. Scherf U, Ross DT, Waltham M, et al. A gene expression database for the molecular pharmacology of cancer. *Nat Genet* 2000; 24:236–244.
10. Rabow AA, Shoemaker RH, Sausville EA, Covell DG. Mining the National Cancer Institute's tumor-screening database: identification of compounds with similar cellular activities. *J Med Chem* 2002; 45:818–840.
11. Lee J, Paull K, Alvarez M, et al. Rhodamine efflux patterns predict p glycoprotein substrates in the National Cancer Institute drug screen. *J Pharmacol Exp Ther* 1994; 46:627–638.
12. Shoemaker RH, Scudiero DA, Melillo G, et al. Application of high-throughput, molecular-targeted screening to anticancer drug discovery. *Curr Top Med Chem* 2002; 2:229–246.
13. Webb CP, Hose CD, Koochekpour S, et al. The geldanamycins are potent inhibitors of the hepatocyte growth factor/scatter factor-met-urokinase plasminogen activator-plasmin proteolytic network. *Cancer Res* 2000; 60:342–349.
14. Rapisarda A, Uranchimeg B, Scudiero DA, et al. Identification of small molecule inhibitors of hypoxia-inducible factor 1 transcriptional ativation pathway. *Cancer Res* 2002; 62:4316–4324.

15. Hollingshead M, Plowman J, Alley M, Mayo J, Sausville E. The hollow fiber assay. In: Fiebig H, Burger AM, eds. *Contributions to Oncology*, vol 54: *Relevance of Tumor Models for Anticancer Drug Development*. Freiburg: Karger. 1999:109–120.
16. Johnson JI, Decker S, Zaharevitz D, et al. Relationships between drug activity in NCI preclinical in vitro and in vivo models and early clinical trials. *Br J Cancer* 2001; 84:1424–1431.

17 Phase I Trial Design and Methodology for Anticancer Drugs

Patrick V. Acevedo, MD,
Deborah L. Toppmeyer, MD,
and Eric H. Rubin, MD

CONTENTS

INTRODUCTION
OBJECTIVES OF A PHASE I STUDY
CHOICE OF SCHEDULE AND ROUTE OF ADMINISTRATION
DETERMINATION OF INITIAL DOSE LEVEL
DOSE ESCALATION STRATEGIES
PATIENT SELECTION
TOXICITY ASSESSMENT
PHARMACOLOGIC EVALUATIONS
ETHICAL CONSIDERATIONS IN PHASE I ONCOLOGY TRIALS

1. INTRODUCTION

Phase I trials play a pivotal role in the introduction of new anticancer drugs into the clinic, and there are important ethical differences between phase I oncology trials and phase I trials involving normal volunteers. In addition, recent advances in cancer biology have resulted in many new drug targets and have led to new approaches in phase I trial design. Although phase I oncology trials may involve Food and Drug Administration (FDA)-approved drugs (used in new schedules or combinations), this chapter reviews objectives, design, methodology, and ethics for trials involving a single investigational compound.

2. OBJECTIVES OF A PHASE I STUDY

The primary objective of a phase I trial is to determine an optimal dose for a given schedule and route of administration for a new drug. This dose is also known as the recommended phase II dose. The recommended phase II dose is typically defined as the maximum tolerated dose (MTD) for the given schedule and route of drug administration.

From: *Cancer Drug Discovery and Development:*
Anticancer Drug Development Guide: Preclinical Screening, Clinical Trials, and Approval, 2nd Ed.
Edited by: B. A. Teicher and P. A. Andrews © Humana Press Inc., Totowa, NJ

The MTD is defined according to toxicity criteria, and thus accurate assessment of drug-related toxicity is essential in the conduct of a phase I trial (*see* Subheading 7.). The underlying assumption of this strategy is that the dose-antitumor response relationship for the drug is at least linear within the studied dose ranges (Fig. 1). For many anticancer compounds this assumption may be true, since the difference between toxic and effective doses is probably small (i.e., small therapeutic index; Fig. 1, first example). However, for certain compounds the therapeutic index may be quite large (Fig. 1, second example), in which case alternate strategies for determining optimal dose need to be considered, such as pharmacokinetic or pharmacodynamic-based methods (*see* Subheading 8.).

Secondary objectives for phase I trials usually include evaluation of pharmacokinetic parameters associated with the compound, since understanding human pharmacology is critical in optimizing the use of a new anticancer drug. Modern phase I trials may also include pharmacodynamic and pharmacogenetic analyses that are designed to evaluate drug targets and to identify associations between genetic polymorphisms and clinical endpoints such as toxicity and response (*see* Subheadings 7. and 8.).

Assessment of antitumor activity is also included as a secondary objective in phase I trials. Antitumor activity is assessed using imaging studies such as computed tomography or magnetic resonance imaging, with response typically defined according to bidimensional *(1)* or unidimension *(2)* criteria. For certain types of cancer, serum protein evaluations are also used to evaluate response (e.g., prostate-specific antigen for prostate cancer patients). Although evaluation of antitumor response is not a primary objective for a phase I oncology trial, for an individual patient this is the most important aspect of the trial. This issue results in significant differences in trial design for phase I studies involving cancer patients vs normal volunteers. For example, in phase I trials involving normal patients there is no need for prolonged drug administration, whereas in trials involving cancer patients, a patient whose cancer is responding is allowed to continue to receive the investigational compound until cancer progression, which could involve months or even years of drug administration.

3. CHOICE OF SCHEDULE AND ROUTE OF ADMINISTRATION

For certain anticancer drugs (e.g., etoposide), it is clear that schedule of administration is a critical determinant of drug efficacy, and thus choosing a schedule of administration is an important consideration in phase I trial design. Typical variables that are considered in this decision include the following: (1) target biology, (2) whether the compound is cytotoxic for cells in a particular phase of the cell cycle, (3) animal pharmacokinetics, and (4) whether certain schedules appear to be superior in terms of efficacy and/or toxicity in animal models. For example, an every-3-wk administration schedule is a common choice for a compound whose target is present in both proliferating and nonproliferating cells, is cytotoxic for cells in all parts of the cell cycle, has a terminal half-life of 48 h, and produces a myelosuppression nadir 10 d after a single dose in animals. Contrastingly, multiday or prolonged infusions might be chosen for an agent that is only cytotoxic to cells in S phase, which has a short half-life, and for which prolonged administration schedules are more effective than bolus administrations in animal studies. Notably, since single-dose intermittent schedules are more convenient for patients when a drug is administered intravenously, these kinds of schedules are preferred if animal data suggest that the drug is active using a variety of schedules. In practice, since preclinical data are

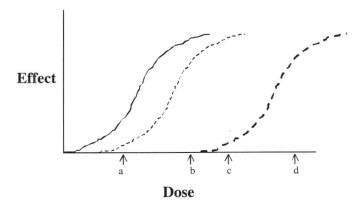

Fig. 1. Examples of dose-response relationships and their effects on determination of maximum tolerated dose (MTD). The solid curved line represents the relationship between dose and antitumor activity of a hypothetical anticancer compound, whereas the dotted curved lines represent two different examples of dose-toxicity relationships. In the first example (thin dotted line), escalation from *dose a* to the *MTD b* is associated with an increase in antitumor efficacy, and the MTD is also the most effective dose. By contrast, in the second example (thick dotted line), increase in *dose c* to the MTD *dose d* does not yield any increase in antitumor efficacy.

not always predictive of schedule-dependent efficacy and toxicity in humans, phase I trials of a new agent are often conducted simultaneously at different institutions using different schedules.

With regard to route of administration, intravenous delivery is preferred in early phase I trials, to avoid issues related to interpatient differences in oral absorption. However, it is important to note that when prolonged administration of a compound is critical for efficacy, an oral formulation may be preferred to allow for convenient prolonged dosing.

4. DETERMINATION OF INITIAL DOSE LEVEL

Selection of the initial dose level is also a critical parameter in an oncology phase I trial. Since many anticancer drugs have a narrow therapeutic index, selection of a high starting dose may result in toxic deaths, leading to discontinuation of development of a potentially useful compound. On the other hand, selection of a low starting dose may result in a prolonged trial and poor utilization of resources, as well as having ethical implications for patients enrolled at dose levels that are unlikely to be therapeutic (*see* Subheading 5.). For both normal volunteer and oncology phase I trials, selection of the initial dose level is based mostly on toxicity studies in animals, with these studies typically involving rodents, dogs, and, rarely, primates. Animal studies are performed to identify a no observed adverse effect level (NOAEL), with this dose then converted to a human equivalent dose using scaling factors *(3)*. However, unlike a trial involving normal volunteers, administration of a low and possibly ineffective dose to cancer patients may be "harmful" by allowing progression of the cancer. Thus, although the FDA recommends use of a safety factor of 10 for normal volunteer phase I trials (i.e., the starting dose level is 10-fold lower than the predicted human NOAEL), this is not required for phase I oncology trials. A common choice involves a starting dose level that is one-third of the NOAEL predicted from the most sensitive animal species.

It should also be noted that, depending on the target, specialized toxicity evaluations may be required to ensure an appropriate starting dose level. For example, since neurotoxicity is a common problem in patients receiving microtubule-targeting agents and may not be detected in routine animal toxicology studies, this toxicity should be evaluated in specific preclinical models for any new microtubule-targeting compound.

5. DOSE ESCALATION STRATEGIES

The dose escalation strategy is also an important parameter in phase I trial design. For both ethical and efficiency reasons, there should be few dose levels between the starting dose level and the MTD. A variety of phase I dose escalation strategies are now available (Table 1). Older, "up-and-down" dose escalation algorithms employ dose levels that are usually fixed prior to and during the trial and are based on mathematical series, whereas newer algorithms employ ongoing analyses of toxicity and flexible dose levels in an attempt to identify the MTD more rapidly. A commonly used up-and-down algorithm involves three patient cohorts and employs a modification of the Fibonacci mathematical series (in which the next number in the series is the sum of the previous two) to choose dose levels *(4)* (Table 2). This strategy involves initial dose increments that are larger than later dose increments (Table 2). Cohorts are expanded to include six patients if one patient has a dose-limiting toxicity (DLT; *see* Subheading 7.), and the MTD is defined as that dose level that is below a dose level at which two or more patients experience DLT. This classic dose escalation scheme has been criticized because patients entering early in the trial may be treated with doses far below the MTD, and it does not yield information regarding the probability of toxicity at the recommended MTD *(5)*.

Efforts to minimize the number of patients treated at low and possibly ineffective doses have resulted in modifications of the traditional three-patient Fibonacci-based dose escalation method. One method involves a two-stage, *accelerated titration* design whereby initial cohorts involve single patients and doses are increased by a factor of 2 until grade 2 toxicity occurs *(6)*. Subsequently, dose escalation proceeds using a traditional Fibonacci-based approach *(6)*. This approach also allows intrapatient dose escalation *(6)*. Another approach, the *biased coin method*, is also based on up-and-down dose escalations, uses a stochastic probability function to guide dose escalation decisions, and results in clustering of individual patient doses around the MTD *(7)*.

Other dose escalation methods employing Bayesian mathematical techniques allow calculation of toxicity probabilities at each dose level. These methods are designed so that each patient is treated at the currently estimated MTD, which is revised continually based on toxicity data. The Continual Reassessment Method (CRM) *(5)* and the Escalation with Overdose Control (EWOC) *(8)* method are examples of this kind of approach. The CRM method has also been modified to allow more rapid accrual for drugs that are expected to yield late-onset toxicities, which would result in a long trial duration using the original CRM algorithm *(9)*. Simulations indicate that, compared with traditional Fibonacci-based dose escalation designs, these methods reduce the number of patients who are treated at doses that are far from the MTD *(5)*. An approach with a similar goal was developed for drugs whose most prominent toxicity is likely to be myelosuppression *(10)*. In this method, dose escalation is based on a pharmacodynamic model that is fit to individual white blood cell nadirs that occur during the trial. Simulations indicate that this approach increases the precision of determination of MTD *(10)*.

Table 1
Common Phase I Trial Dose Escalation Schemes

	Method of dose escalation	Advantages	Disadvantages	Reference
Modified Fibonacci, three-patient cohort	Fixed increments, up-and-down	Simple to implement; PK/PD data available in each cohort	Conservative dose escalation, may require large number of patients	4
Accelerated titration	Fixed increments, up-and-down using a two-stage design	Rapid dose escalation, intrapatient dose escalation may be allowed	Small initial cohorts preclude meaningful PK/PD data	6
Continual Reassessment Method	Bayesian, uses a dose-response model	Rapid dose escalation, minimizes patients treated at dose levels far from MTD	Complex mathematics, small cohorts may preclude meaningful PK/PD data	5
Escalation with overdose control	Bayesian, uses a dose-response model	Rapid dose escalation, minimizes patients treated at dose levels far from MTD, decreased chance of treating patients above MTD compared with Continual Reassessment Method	Complex mathematics, small cohorts may preclude meaningful PK/PD data	8
Pharmacokinetically guided dose escalation	Escalation based on plasma drug levels	Rapid dose escalation and identification of MTD	Requires ongoing PK evaluations	11

ABBREVIATIONS: MTD, maximum tolerated dose; PK/PD, pharmacokinetics/pharmacodynamics.

Table 2
Modified Fibonacci Dose Escalation Scheme

Dose	% Increase above previous dose
N	—
2.0 N	100
3.3 N	67
5.0 N	50
7.0 N	40
9.0 N	30
12.0 N	33

As discussed above, for certain compounds an MTD-based approach to determining optimal dose may not be appropriate. Under these circumstances, pharmacology-based dose escalation is an attractive choice. Originally proposed by Collins and coworkers *(11)*, this method involves comparison of human pharmacokinetic data with that of animals. The idea is that drug exposures (measured by determining the area under the curve for plasma drug concentration vs time plots) associated with toxicity and efficacy are often similar in animals and humans. For trials designed to determine MTD, there is evidence that this approach can reduce the number of cohorts needed to identify MTD *(11)*. Despite the apparent usefulness of this approach, it is not commonly used, perhaps because of the requirement that pharmacokinetic analyses be performed on an ongoing basis during the trial, rather than batched at the end of the trial.

Concerns regarding the ethics of enrolling patients at low, but "safe," dose levels have also resulted in efforts to allow patients to be involved in dose selection. This concept was shown to be feasible in a phase I study of the combination of vinorelbine and paclitaxel *(12)*. In this study, the first patient was allowed to choose among three initial dose levels. Subsequently, patients were allowed to choose among dose levels that included the dose level just above a level at which at least one patient had enrolled and not experienced DLT. Patients underwent a three-step informed consent process that included written information regarding all previously enrolled patients. Patients who did not want to choose their dose level were enrolled at the highest dose level at which at least one patient had been enrolled and there were no DLTs. The results of this trial indicated that most patients (76%) chose their dose. Among 29 patients enrolled, 8 (28%) chose the highest available dose. Some patients (28%) felt either uncomfortable or very uncomfortable in being asked to choose their dose. Interestingly, many patients appeared to choose one particular dose level (which was below an MTD) because an earlier patient had experienced a complete response at this level. This finding indicates that this study design may delay identification of the MTD compared with other dose escalation methods.

6. PATIENT SELECTION

Selection of patients for enrollment in a phase I study is an important consideration and can greatly affect the primary objective, which is determination of the MTD/phase II dose. For example, patients with abnormal hepatic or renal function may be at risk for significant toxicity at relatively low dose levels, owing to alterations in drug clearance.

Table 3
ECOG Performance Status Scale

Score	Activity level
0	Fully active, able to carry out all predisease performance without restriction
1	Restricted in physically strenuous activity, but ambulatory and able to carry out work of a light or sedentary nature
2	Ambulatory and capable of self-care, but unable to carry any work activities; up and about more than 50% of waking hours
3	Capable of only limited self-care; confined to bed or chair more than 50% of waking hours
4	Completely disabled; cannot carry out any self-care; totally confined to bed or wheelchair
5	Deceased

Thus, unless the objective of trial is to define the MTD in patients with organ dysfunction, most trials exclude patients with elevated serum creatinine or liver enzymes. Similarly, if myelosuppression is likely to be a major toxicity for a new compound, enrollment of patients who were treated previously with regimens associated with bone marrow toxicity will probably yield a lower MTD than enrollment of chemotherapy-naïve patients. Performance status is also frequently used as a selection criterion. Two common measures are the Eastern Cooperative Oncology Group (ECOG) assessment and the Karnofsky assessment (Tables 3 and 4) *(13)*. Patients with a poor performance status are at higher risk for toxicity from chemotherapy *(14)*, and this is likely to be true for all drugs, owing to poor physiologic function in these patients. In addition, patients with a poor performance status are likely to experience symptoms caused by their disease that will confound evaluation of drug-related toxicity. Therefore, requirement of an ECOG performance status of ≤2 or a Karnofsky status of ≥60% are commonly used selection criteria. Similarly, patients with active medical problems, such as untreated brain metastases or infection, are usually excluded owing to concerns over interpretation of the causality of adverse events that occur during the trial.

For ethical reasons, age, ethnicity, and gender generally should not be used in the selection of patients for phase I trials. In particular, there is no scientific reason to exclude patients who are young adults under age 18. By contrast, because of differences in body surface area/weight ratio in children younger than 1 yr, use of body surface area-based dosing (which is common in phase I oncology trials) may result in inappropriately high doses in this age group *(15)*. In addition, children may tolerate higher doses of drugs than adults, and thus separate trials are often performed in pediatric populations. Indeed, for a variety of chemotherapy drugs, the ratio of the MTD for children/adults is 1.2 or higher *(15)*.

Elderly patients are often excluded from phase I trials despite evidence that age is not a good predictor for toxicity from chemotherapy *(16,17)*. Nevertheless, although age may not be an accurate surrogate for physiologic function, elderly patients may have reduced hepatic or renal function, and thus individual elderly patients may be excluded on this basis, rather than on the basis of age alone.

Table 4
Karnofsky Performance Status Scale

Score	Activity level
100	Normal, no complaints, no evidence of disease
90	Able to carry on normal activity, minor signs or symptoms of disease
80	Normal activity with effort, some signs or symptoms of disease
70	Cares for self; unable to carry on normal activity or to do active work
60	Requires occasional assistance, but is able to care for most self needs
50	Requires considerable assistance and frequent medical care
40	Disabled, requires special care and assistance
30	Severely disabled, hospitalization is indicated, death not imminent
20	Hospitalization necessary, very sick, active supportive treatment
10	Moribund, fatal processes progressing rapidly
0	Deceased

Another common exclusion criterion involves recent treatment with chemotherapy, since this may predispose a patient to toxicity owing to incomplete recovery from the previous treatment. Generally, a 4-wk interval from previous chemotherapy is preferred (6-wk if the patient received nitrosoureas). Similarly, many phase I studies require at least a 2-wk interval from exposure to drugs that may compete with the study drug for enzymatic metabolism.

7. TOXICITY ASSESSMENT

Toxicity assessment is the scientific measuring device in a phase I trial. Although abnormal laboratory values can be assessed objectively, much of the toxicity assessment in a phase I trial involves subjective evaluation of patient symptoms and thus is dependent on perceptions of both the patient and the evaluator of the patient. For assessment of patient symptoms, most phase I trials employ the National Cancer Institute (NCI) Common Toxicity Criteria (CTC), which was updated to version 2.0 in 1999 and can be found on the NCI website (http://ctep.info.nih.gov/). The CTC utilize a grading scale from 0 to 5 and include a detailed, categorized listing of possible adverse events for each organ system and various clinical settings. For example, diarrhea in patients without a colostomy is graded according to the number of stools per day, whereas this parameter is not used in grading diarrhea in patients with a colostomy. The CTC also include guidelines for assessing the relationship between an adverse event and the study drug, which involve the terms "clearly related," "likely related," "may be related," "doubtfully related," and "clearly not related." The term adverse event is defined as "any unfavorable symptom, sign, or disease (including an abnormal laboratory finding) temporally associated with the use of a medical treatment or procedure that may or may not be considered related to the medical treatment or procedure." This definition results in phase I oncology trials typically generating hundreds or even thousands of adverse events, since many patients will experience symptoms/adverse events owing to their cancer, rather than to the study drug. The common practice of involving multiple research centers in phase I oncology trials further increases the complexity and regulatory burden of toxicity assessment (18).

Although the CTC provide a standard for measuring toxicity, they do not define DLT, which must be included in a phase I trial protocol. The definition of DLT usually includes the occurrence of a grade 3 or higher adverse event that is attributable to the study drug. However, the definition of DLT may vary depending on the selection of patients for the trial. For example, prolonged grade 4 neutropenia is often defined as a DLT for patients with nonhematologic malignancies, but not for patients with leukemia. Similarly, in trials involving patients with hepatic dysfunction, patients may enter the trial with grade 3 increases in liver enzymes, so the occurrence of this event during the trial would not be defined as a DLT.

A phase I trial must also define how the MTD will be identified. The definition of MTD is based on a targeted DLT rate and will depend on the dose escalation method. A 33% DLT rate is a common target rate in phase I oncology trials.

8. PHARMACOLOGIC EVALUATIONS

Pharmacologic evaluations are an important part of phase I oncology trials and are assuming increasing importance in the clinical development of compounds that are designed to target specific biomolecules. Most phase I trials include repetitive measurement of concentrations of the study drug in blood or plasma, in order to characterize human pharmacokinetics (e.g., volume of distribution, clearance) and the relationship between pharmacokinetic parameters and both dose and clinical outcomes. This information is often critical in selecting an optimal dose and schedule for a new compound. For example, analysis of plasma clearance of the epidermal growth factor receptor (EGFR) antibody C225 was used to identify a dose level associated with saturation of plasma clearance of this agent *(19)*. Since saturation of clearance may indicate saturation of antibody binding to its target, this dose level was recommended as the phase II dose for C225 *(19)*.

If a specific drug target is known, pharmacodynamic studies are often included to assess modulation of the target in the patient. In many cases these studies involve biochemical assays. Ideally these kinds of studies should be performed in tumor tissues, but this is impractical, with the exception of trials involving patients with hematologic malignancies, in which tumor cells may be obtained relatively easily by either venipuncture or bone marrow aspiration. Indeed, studies in peripheral blood leukemia cells of the protein CRKL, which is a substrate of the BCR-ABL tyrosine kinase, were useful in selecting the phase II dose for STI-571, an inhibitor of the BCR-ABL tyrosine kinase *(20)*.

Assessment of a drug target in nonmalignant tissues may also be helpful. For example, phase I trials of a proteasome inhibitor, PS-341, included a rapid and reliable assay of proteasome activity in whole blood that was used to define an optimal schedule of administration for this drug *(21,22)*.

The problem of assessing target modulation in tumor tissues in patients with nonhematologic malignancies may be solved by the use of imaging techniques, which allow noninvasive pharmacodynamic monitoring. This promising area of research has already proved useful in studies of antiangiogenic compounds. For example, dynamic contrast-enhanced magnetic resonance imaging was used to assess the effects of endostatin on tumor blood flow in phase I trials of this compound *(23,24)*.

With the availability of the human genome sequence, there is also increasing opportunity to identify and correlate patient genetic polymorphisms with pharmacokinetic parameters and clinical outcomes. For certain drugs, enzyme polymorphisms are known to predispose patients to either toxicity or lack of efficacy. For example, certain polymorphisms in the dihydropyrimidine dehydrogenase gene, which degrades fluoropyrimidines, and in the uridine diphosphate glucuronosyltransferase 1A1 gene, which when mutated results in Gilbert's syndrome, alter the metabolism of fluorouracil and irinotecan, respectively *(25,26)*. These polymorphisms result in increased toxicity in patients receiving these drugs. Other polymorphisms in the thymidylate synthase gene are associated with reduced survival in patients treated with methotrexate for leukemia *(27)*, or with 5-fluorouracil for colorectal cancer *(28)*. Conversely, a polymorphism in the glutathione *S*-transferase P1 gene is associated with improved survival in patients with colorectal cancer treated with a combination of 5-fluorouracil and oxaliplatin *(29)*. These findings have prompted banking of DNA from patients enrolled in phase I trials, in order to evaluate correlations between clinical outcomes and currently known or yet-to-be-discovered genetic polymorphisms that may be relevant to drug metabolism or drug-target interactions.

9. ETHICAL CONSIDERATIONS IN PHASE I ONCOLOGY TRIALS

Patients eligible for phase I oncology trials often have metastatic and refractory cancer with no options of proven therapeutic benefit. Thus, these patients may be viewed as particularly vulnerable to coercion for participation in phase I trials, in which the likelihood of benefit is unknown, and usually little is known regarding the likelihood of toxicity. Indeed, several studies suggest that many phase I trial patients do not understand the purpose of the trial, raising concerns over the informed consent process *(30–32)*. A recent study of written informed consent documents suggests that misunderstandings regarding the purpose of phase I trials do not arise from the written consent documents *(33)*. Additional results from a small survey suggest that patients enter a phase I trial for reasons of possible therapeutic benefit and are not strongly influenced in their decision making by physicians or family pressure *(30)*.

Although every effort should be made to ensure that patients understand the purpose of a phase I trial and are aware of alternatives to participation in such a trial, it is important to note that phase I oncology trials are performed with therapeutic intent. Specifically, these trials include repetitive assessments of disease status, and patients are removed from the study if there is evidence of disease progression. Although historical data indicate that the average response rate for phase I trials is low (about 5%) *(34)*, for a new compound that is being evaluated for the first time in humans, the response rate is not yet known. Indeed, it is possible that the response rate will be high, as evidenced by the nearly 100% hematologic response rate observed in phase I trials of the ABL tyrosine kinase inhibitor STI-571 in patients with chronic myelogenous leukemia *(20)*. Therefore, although it is not appropriate to suggest that a patient can expect direct benefit from participation in a phase I trial, it is possible that direct benefit will occur. Indeed, it could be argued that the generally low response rate in previous phase I oncology trials relates to a lack of knowledge regarding cancer biology (i.e., lack of good targets) and a lack of preclinical models that are predictive for efficacy in humans. Advances in both of these areas allow continued optimism regarding response rates in phase I trials of new anticancer compounds.

REFERENCES

1. Miller AB, Hoogstraten B, Staquet M, Winkler A. Reporting results of cancer treatment. *Cancer* 1981; 47:207–214.
2. Therasse P, Arbuck SG, Eisenhauer EA, et al. New guidelines to evaluate the response to treatment in solid tumors. European Organization for Research and Treatment of Cancer, National Cancer Institute of the United States, National Cancer Institute of Canada. *J Natl Cancer Inst* 2000; 92:205–216.
3. Boxenbaum H, DiLea C. First-time-in-human dose selection: allometric thoughts and perspectives. *J Clin Pharmacol* 1995; 35:957–966.
4. Storer BE. Design and analysis of phase I clinical trials. *Biometrics* 1989; 45:925–937.
5. O'Quigley J, Pepe M, Fisher L. Continual reassessment method: a practical design for phase 1 clinical trials in cancer. *Biometrics* 1990; 46:33–48.
6. Simon R, Freidlin B, Rubinstein L, Arbuck S G, Collins J, Christian MC. Accelerated titration designs for phase I clinical trials in oncology. *J Natl Cancer Inst* 1997; 89:1138–1147.
7. Stylianou M, Flournoy N. Dose finding using the biased coin up-and-down design and isotonic regression. *Biometrics* 2002; 58:171–177.
8. Babb J, Rogatko A, Zacks S. Cancer phase I clinical trials: efficient dose escalation with overdose control. *Stat Med* 1998; 17:1103–1120.
9. Cheung YK Chappell R. Sequential designs for phase I clinical trials with late-onset toxicities. *Biometrics* 2000; 56:1177–1182.
10. Mick R, Ratain MJ. Model-guided determination of maximum tolerated dose in phase I clinical trials: evidence for increased precision. *J Natl Cancer Inst* 1993; 85:217–223.
11. Collins JM, Grieshaber CK, Chabner BA. Pharmacologically guided phase I clinical trials based upon preclinical drug development. *J Natl Cancer Inst* 1990; 82:1321–1326.
12. Daugherty CK, Ratain MJ, Minami H, et al. Study of cohort-specific consent and patient control in phase I cancer trials. *J Clin Oncol* 1998; 16:2305–2312.
13. Yates JW, Chalmer B, McKegney FP. Evaluation of patients with advanced cancer using the Karnofsky performance status. *Cancer* 1980; 45:2220–2224.
14. Krikorian JG, Daniels JR, Brown BW Jr, Hu MS. Variables for predicting serious toxicity (vinblastine dose, performance status, and prior therapeutic experience): chemotherapy for metastatic testicular cancer with cis-dichlorodiammineplatinum(II), vinblastine, and bleomycin. *Cancer Treat Rep* 1978; 62:1455–1463.
15. Weitman S, Kamen BA. Cancer chemotherapy and pharmacology in children. In: Schilsky RL, Milano GA, Ratain MJ, eds. *Principles of Antineoplastic Drug Development and Pharmacology.* New York: Marcel Dekker, 1996:375–397.
16. Gronlund B, Hogdall C, Hansen HH, Engelholm SA. Performance status rather than age is the key prognostic factor in second-line treatment of elderly patients with epithelial ovarian carcinoma. *Cancer* 2002; 94:1961–1967.
17. Haak HL, Gerrits WB, Wijermans PW, Kerkhofs H. Mitoxantrone, teniposide, chlorambucil and prednisone (MVLP) for relapsed non-Hodgkin's lymphoma. The impact of advanced age and performance status. *Neth J Med* 1993; 42:122–127.
18. Tolcher AW, Takimoto CH, Rowinsky EK. The multifunctional, multi-institutional, and sometimes even global phase I study: a better life for phase I evaluations or just "living large"? [comment]. *J Clin Oncol* 2002; 20:4276–4278.
19. Baselga J, Pfister D, Cooper MR, et al. Phase I studies of anti-epidermal growth factor receptor chimeric antibody C225 alone and in combination with cisplatin. *J Clin Oncol* 2000; 18:904–914.
20. Druker BJ, Talpaz M, Resta DJ, et al. Efficacy and safety of a specific inhibitor of the BCR-ABL tyrosine kinase in chronic myeloid leukemia [comment]. *N Engl J Med* 2001; 344:1031–1037.
21. Orlowski RZ, Stinchcombe TE, Mitchell BS, et al. Phase I trial of the proteasome inhibitor PS-341 in patients with refractory hematologic malignancies. *J Clin Oncol* 2002; 20:4420–4427.
22. Lightcap ES, McCormack TA, Pien CS, Chau V, Adams J, Elliott PJ. Proteasome inhibition measurements: clinical application. *Clin Chem* 2000; 46:673–683.
23. Herbst RS, Mullani NA, Davis DW, et al. Development of biologic markers of response and assessment of antiangiogenic activity in a clinical trial of human recombinant endostatin. *J Clin Oncol* 2002; 20:3804–3814.
24. Eder JP Jr, Supko JG, Clark JW, et al. Phase I clinical trial of recombinant human endostatin administered as a short intravenous infusion repeated daily [comment]. *J Clin Oncol* 2002; 20:3772–3784.

25. Ridge SA, Sludden J, Wei X, et al. Dihydropyrimidine dehydrogenase pharmacogenetics in patients with colorectal cancer. *Br J Cancer* 1998; 77:497–500.
26. Wasserman E, Myara A, Lokiec F, et al. Severe CPT-11 toxicity in patients with Gilbert's syndrome: two case reports. *Ann Oncol* 1997; 8:1049–1051.
27. Krajinovic M, Costea I, Chiasson S. Polymorphism of the thymidylate synthase gene and outcome of acute lymphoblastic leukaemia. *Lancet* 2002; 359:1033–1034.
28. Iacopetta B, Grieu F, Joseph D, Elsaleh H. A polymorphism in the enhancer region of the thymidylate synthase promoter influences the survival of colorectal cancer patients treated with 5-fluorouracil [comment]. *Br J Cancer* 2001; 85:827–830.
29. Stoehlmacher J, Park DJ, Zhang W, et al. Association between glutathione S-transferase P1, T1, and M1 genetic polymorphism and survival of patients with metastatic colorectal cancer. *J Natl Cancer Inst* 2002; 94:936–942.
30. Daugherty C, Ratain MJ, Grochowski E, et al. Perceptions of cancer patients and their physicians involved in phase I trials [comment] [erratum appears in *J Clin Oncol* 1995; 13:2476]. *J Clin Oncol* 1995; 13:1062–1072.
31. Joffe S, Cook EF, Cleary PD, Clark JW, Weeks JC. Quality of informed consent in cancer clinical trials: a cross-sectional survey [comment]. *Lancet* 2001; 358:1772–1777.
32. Yoder LH, O'Rourke TJ, Etnyre A, Spears DT, Brown TD. Expectations and experiences of patients with cancer participating in phase I clinical trials. *Oncol Nurs Forum* 1997; 24:891–896.
33. Horng S, Emanuel EJ, Wilfond B, Rackoff J, Martz K, Grady C. Descriptions of benefits and risks in consent forms for phase 1 oncology trials. *N Engl J Med* 2002; 347:2134–2140.
34. Von Hoff DD, Turner J. Response rates, duration of response, and dose response effects in phase I studies of antineoplastics. *Invest New Drugs* 1991; 9:115–122.

18 Phase II Trials

Conventional Design and Novel Strategies in the Era of Targeted Therapies

Keith T. Flaherty, MD and Peter J. O'Dwyer, MD

CONTENTS

INTRODUCTION
PHASE II TRIAL BASICS
STANDARD PHASE II TRIAL DESIGN
NOVEL PHASE II TRIAL DESIGNS
INDIVIDUALIZING THERAPY IN PHASE II TRIALS

1. INTRODUCTION

Early clinical investigations in oncology are distinct from therapeutics evaluations in other medical disciplines. First, the risks associated with medicines for oncologic diseases dictate that they be evaluated in cancer patients only, and not in healthy volunteers. Second, dose-response relationships are essential to the understanding of potential therapeutic benefit and toxic side effects. Third, determining the specificity of therapeutic value for subsets of patients is essential to the development of effective therapies. For these reasons, a rational system of evaluation has been constructed to optimize the selection of tolerable and effective therapies for comparison with standard treatments in subsequent clinical trials.

Phase I trials are conducted to establish a recommended dose and schedule for phase II study. To determining the incidence, severity, and reversibility of adverse effects is the most essential function of phase I investigations. These outcomes are largely dependent on the disposition, metabolism, and clearance of the experimental drug amongst a heterogeneous patient population. Pharmacokinetic studies can quantify the variability in drug exposure among a genetically diverse population. The degree of variability is a determinant of a drug's suitability for further evaluation. Pharmacokinetics, in conjunction with toxicity, inform the selection of an administration schedule. These studies are typically carried out among a small number of patients with a varied treatment background. For

From: *Cancer Drug Discovery and Development:*
Anticancer Drug Development Guide: Preclinical Screening, Clinical Trials, and Approval, 2nd Ed.
Edited by: B. A. Teicher and P. A. Andrews © Humana Press Inc., Totowa, NJ

expediency, patients with all varieties of cancer are enrolled. Interindividual differences in drug metabolism and elimination will exist even among a population of patients with a uniform treatment history and baseline organ function. These variables introduce the risk that the appropriate phase II dose will not be identified. In such cases, phase II trials serve to further refine the dose to be investigated in subsequent studies.

The interaction between the drug and the host defines the pharmacokinetics of an agent. This must be considered apart from the interaction of the drug with its molecular targets and the subsequent effects, also referred to as the pharmacodynamic effect. The emphasis of phase I trials must be on pharmacokinetics, whereas in phase II trials, the focus shifts to pharmacodynamics. Put another way, the first goal in drug development is to establish that an investigational treatment is handled in a relatively uniform manner across a patient population and is associated with acceptable toxicity. However, phase I trials can explore the feasibility and reproducibility of a pharmacodynamic assay.

The primary endpoint of phase II clinical trials is the exploration of clinical or biologic activity in a predefined subset of patients. The definition of clinical activity and the methods used to assess it have undergone substantial revision in recent years. In the era of molecularly targeted therapy, biologic activity is ascertained in conjunction with clinical benefit. Phase I trials conducted with pharmacodynamic endpoints can identify the threshold dose for biologic activity. This can be substantially below the maximally tolerated dose, which has been the traditional stopping point for phase I trials. Phase II trials can be designed to simultaneously evaluate the relative clinical activity of a lower biologically effective dose and the maximally tolerated dose. Ultimately, the phase II study must provide compelling evidence to support the investment of many resources into phase III trials. A phase II trial with a uniquely active agent can lead to FDA approval if the treatment effect is unequivocally superior to standard therapies. The approval of STI571 for chronic myelogenous leukemia and gastrointestinal stromal tumors is a recent example.

2. PHASE II TRIAL BASICS

2.1. Selection of Agents

The typical costs of conducting phase I, II, and III clinical trials are US$200,000, $1 million, and $10 million, respectively. Usually, a novel anticancer agent is tested in one to four phase I trials to evaluate distinct schedules. Phase II trials will be conducted in five to ten tumor types. This step from phase I to phase II trials requires a 10-fold increment in investment. The limited public and private funding for clinical investigations mandates that agents be stringently selected for phase II development.

The criteria for selecting agents for phase II trials are evolving. Conventional cytotoxic agents are associated with strongly dose-dependent therapeutic effect and toxicity. A narrow therapeutic index is one reason for abandoning a drug after phase I trials. Furthermore, toxicity must be manageable and reversible to be considered acceptable for use as palliative therapy. The interindividual variability in drug clearance should minimal, generally less than threefold. And lastly, toxicity should be directly and predictably related to drug exposure. Molecularly targeted therapies appear to have a higher therapeutic index in animal models and are not restrained by the frequency of dose-limiting toxicities. The induction of the intended molecular effect in humans is the new standard for selecting molecularly targeted therapies for phase II development.

Table 1
Probabilities of Detecting True Rate
of Dose-Limiting Toxicity (DLT) in Cohorts of Three or Six Patients

No. of DLTs in a cohort of three patients	Probability of detecting true DLT rate				
True rate of DLT	0.10	0.20	0.30	0.40	0.50
0[a]	0.729	0.512	0.343	0.216	0.125
1[b]	0.243	0.384	0.441	.432	0.375
2 or more[c]	0.028	0.104	0.216	0.352	0.500
No. of DLTs in a cohort of six patients	Probability of detecting true DLT rate				
True rate of DLT	0.10	.20	0.30	0.40	0.50
0	—	—	—	—	—
1[b]	0.177	0.197	0.151	0.093	0.047
2 or more[c]	0.066	0.187	0.290	0.339	0.328

[a]Number of DLTs leads to advancing to the next cohort.
[b]Number of DLTs leading to enrolling an additional three patients in the cohort.
[c]Number of DLTs leading to stopping the study and defining the maximum tolerated dose (MTD).

2.2. Refining the Dose

While the primary function of phase I trials is to delineate a safe dose and schedule of administration, at times the recommended phase II dose cannot be generalized to a larger population. This can occur because of dissimilarities in treatment background, sample size limitations, and inability to detect cumulative toxicity. If the majority of patients enrolled on the phase I study have received multiple myelosuppressive chemotherapy regimens, then they may be more susceptible to the myelosuppressive effects of the investigational agent than patients who are receiving the drug as front-line therapy in a phase II study. This type of error can lead to under dosing of the investigational agent. The relatively small number of patients treated on a phase I study may not provide sufficient power to detect an infrequent but severe toxicity. In this case, the recommended phase II dose may be an overestimate of the tolerable dose. Lastly, patients selected for phase I evaluation typically have cancers that are refractory to standard therapy. They are unlikely to receive prolonged therapy on a phase I trial because of disease progression. If the majority of patients are discontinued from therapy within the first several weeks, data regarding cumulative toxicity will be unreliable owing to a small sample size.

Phase II trials can be designed to overcome these errors, adjusting the dose of investigational drug during the course of the study. A priori rules can be set to reduce the starting dose of the drug in the event of an unacceptably high rate of severe toxicity. For example, a 33% rate of grade 4 myelosuppression is generally deemed unacceptable. A stopping rule can be made so that the occurrence of grade 4 myelosuppression in a set number of an initial cohort of patients triggers the reduction in the starting dose for subsequent patients. This type of statistical calculation is routinely performed for efficacy but can apply equally to toxicity (Table 1).

Pharmacokinetic data from phase I trials can also be used to tailor the dose based on differences in drug clearance. This was accomplished in the development of carboplatin, a drug whose clearance is strongly correlated with creatinine clearance (1). A model was developed to determine the appropriate dose based on target area under the time-concentration curve, body surface area, and creatinine clearance. Using this method, the risk of renal failure and severe myelosuppression was significantly reduced compared to dosing based on body surface area alone.

2.3. Selecting the Treatment Group

2.3.1. PATIENT-SPECIFIC FACTORS

Several patient-specific factors have proven important in the accurate assessment of toxicity and clinical response in the context of phase II trials. Prior exposure to chemotherapeutic agents is an important predictor of certain side effects with subsequent treatment *(2)*. The mechanisms of resistance developed during exposure to previous treatments may contribute to overlapping resistance to an investigational agent. This may lead to an estimate of activity that is significantly lower than would be seen in a less heavily pretreated population. This was seen in the evaluation of mitoxantrone in women with breast cancer previously treated with doxorubicin *(3,4)*. Including only patients with normal organ function is required in the early investigation of drugs as clearance may be impacted, leading to increased drug exposure and excess toxicity.

The selection of patients with limited prior therapy raises important ethical questions regarding the place of experimental therapies in the treatment algorithm for cancer patients. It is agreed upon in situations where curative therapy exists that patients should receive the standard therapy as first-line treatment. Upon relapse, patients would then be eligible for participation in phase II trials of investigational agents. For diseases for which chemotherapy is palliative, there is debate regarding the appropriate sequencing of therapies. In the case of metastatic breast cancer, the median survival of patients, in the absence of treatment, from the time of diagnosis of metastatic disease is greater than 2-1/2 yr. Sequential therapy is capable of extending median survival to greater than 4 yr. While there are several active agents for treatment of breast cancer, it has not been shown that the introduction of an experimental agent early in the course of treatment negatively impacts overall survival. Furthermore, to assess the potential superiority of investigational agents to current front-line treatments, it is necessary to estimate activity in the front-line setting in the context of phase II trials. It is less clear how to order standard and investigational therapies in patients with disease whose natural history does not lend itself to multiple sequential therapies.

Performance status is a independent risk factor for increased toxicity and decreased clinical benefit from cytotoxic chemotherapy. Two validated scales have identified levels of performance status that are prohibitive to the administration of chemotherapy: Eastern Cooperative Oncology Group (ECOG) *(5)* and Karnofsky *(6)*. These tools are easily applied to general practice and are highly reproducible. They serve as an objective measure of disease progression and its physiological impact. In general, patients with an ECOG performance status of 0 or 1 are suitable for inclusion in phase II trials. For several novel agents, the side-effect profile is sufficiently tolerable to allow inclusion of performance status 2 patients.

Advanced age is not a mandatory restriction for inclusion in phase II trials. Many side effects from cytotoxic therapy have not shown age dependence. For those that do, careful assessment of organ function can often identify patients with predisposition to reduced drug clearance. There are examples of agents whose severe side effects were more prevalent among younger patients *(7)* and others for which the converse was seen *(8,9)*. The pharmacokinetics of several drugs are known to vary significantly in very young children compared to adults of all ages (10,11). For this reason, separate dose escalation, phase I trials are usually conducted among children. Gender is not typically seen as basis for differential sensitivity to nonhormonal therapies; however, some drugs can be metabolized differently owing to hormonal influences on the cytochrome P450 oxidoreductase system (12). Similarly, ethnic background has been associated with genotypic and phenotypic differences in P450 enzymes (13,14), although that is not felt to be grounds for restricting eligibility on the basis of ethnicity.

Single-agent activity seen in phase II trials can be compared to that reported with standard therapies evaluated in a similar patient population. The validity of such comparisons are limited by the possibility of confounding factors among the study populations, which may contribute to an underestimate or overestimate of clinical benefit. Although prone to error, the estimate of clinical activity in phase II trials remains the basis for undertaking a randomized phase III trial.

2.3.2. TUMOR-SPECIFIC FACTORS

The conventional strategy in choosing a target population for phase II trials selects patients whose cancers share histologic subtype and site of origin. There are two strengths to this inclusive method: ability to generalize results and the exploration of unanticipated mechanisms of action.

The appropriate selection of diseases to target in phase II trials is limited by the poor predictive value of in vitro systems and animal models. Traditionally, the most prevalent malignancies or diseases responsive to standard cytotoxic therapies were chosen as an initial screen for activity with an investigational agent (15). In the application of conventional cytotoxic or molecularly targeted therapy, this approach could fail to identify activity in unrepresented tumors and to invest excessive resources in the phase II trials with preclinical rationale. This was supplanted by the less empiric method of choosing tumor types based on activity in human tumors transplanted into mice. However, this also has been shown to have poor positive and negative predictive value (16). In vitro activity against a broad spectrum of human solid tumor cell lines emerged as more specific means of identifying target diseases. In isolation, these assays have also failed to accurately predict the activity of agents in phase II trials (17,18,19).

In retrospect, further work has elucidated some of the reasons why these systems are not representative of tumors in humans. Mouse xenografts models are possible only because of an immunocompromised host. Thus the induction of secondary immune responses is not possible in this system. This was a previously unknown mechanism of many effective cytotoxic therapies. Furthermore, the growth of xenografts in sites that are physiologically distinct contributes to the development of tumor stroma and microvasculature that are distinct from autochthonous human tumors. This has been shown to be particularly relevant for the activity of angiogenesis inhibitors. As antiangiogenic activity has also been described for many cytotoxic agents, this may also account for disparities between preclinical and clinical activity. In the early experience with therapies developed as specific agents against a pathogenetically important target, it appears that the combined assessment against molecular target, cell line with target dependence, and mouse xenografts of the corresponding human tumor cell lines are able to better identify active agents.

Including patients based on pathologic phenotype alone also allows for hypothesis testing of the proposed mechanism of action. For drugs with a known molecular target, it is commonly assumed that clinical activity will be limited to patients whose tumors overexpress or overutilize the molecular target. This hypothesis is based on the assumption that the drug is selective for a given target and that the function of that target is well understood. Preclinical studies of small-molecule inhibitors of the epidermal growth factor (EGF) receptor (erb-b1) suggested that antiproliferative activity was limited to tumor types where the receptor is overexpressed. However, separate studies in animal models revealed that tumor regression could be induced in tumor types where the receptor is not overexpressed. This activity correlates with inhibition of angiogenesis.

An alternative strategy in selecting patients for phase II study restricts eligibility based on a common molecular phenotype. There are several recent examples of successful identification of markers predictive of response to targeted therapy. Trastuzumab, a monoclonal antibody with affinity for the c-erb-2 receptor, has significant activity in the treatment of metastatic breast cancer. Overexpression of the c-erb-2 receptor is achieved through amplification of the wild-type gene in 30% of woman with breast cancer. The presence or absence of c-erb-2 gene amplification accurately predicts the subset of patients likely to receive clinical benefit from this therapy. This highlights the importance of the validity of the assay used to identify the molecular phenotype. In the case of c-erb-2 an immunohistochemical assay is available for the semiquantitative assessment of protein overexpression. In a head-to-head comparison of the two assays, the immunohistochemical assay is clearly less robust and, thus misclassifies patients who may or may not overexpress c-erb-2. With a focus on tailoring targeted therapy to individual patients, this type of error can lead to critical missteps in selecting appropriate therapies.

DNA mutation status and gene expression profiling offer another level of molecular definition for the selection of patients in phase II trials. Two-thirds of patients with metastatic melanoma were found to harbor somatic mutations in the kinase domain of *BRAF*. The expression of these mutant genes results in a constitutively active b-raf kinase, which appears to contribute to cell survival by signaling through the mitogen-activated protein (MAp) kinase pathway. A small-molecule inhibitor of raf kinase, BAY 43-9006, is being evaluated in phase II trials for patients with metastatic melanoma. Patients could be selected on the basis of *BRAF* mutation status; however, this would exclude patients who may respond to therapy. Misclassification of mutation status and alternative mechanisms of action could contribute to this error. In fact, antiangiogenesis appears to be an important mechanism for an inhibitor raf signaling. In this case, the appropriate selection strategy would be to include all patients with metastatic melanoma. Information regarding *BRAF* mutation status should be collected on all patients in order to make correlations with clinical benefit.

While gene expression profiling does not identify the presence or absence of a specific molecular target, it can create a molecular profile that meaningfully segregates patients with biologically distinct tumors. From this data, categorical variables can be derived to correlate phenotype with response to therapy. The identification of a predictive profile can be used to stratify patients in subsequent phase III trials. In patients with mantle cell lymphoma, two distinct expression profiles distinguish tumors with germinal center and follicular features. This categorization provides important prognostic information and may identify a subset of patients for whom standard treatments will prove ineffective.

This group can be spared the toxicity of ineffective treatment and selected for clinical trials of experimental therapies.

2.4. Defining the Endpoint

2.4.1. CLINICAL ENDPOINTS

Prolongation of survival is the benchmark of clinical benefit from anticancer treatment. However, it is not possible to accurately gauge survival benefits in the context of a small, single-arm clinical trial owing to confounding factors. Selection bias can result in the unintentional inclusion of patients with host or tumor characteristics that correspond to indolent or aggressive natural history of disease. These factors can outweigh the treatment effect and result in an erroneous estimate of efficacy. Relying on overall survival as the sole determinant of therapeutic benefit is further complicated by the impact of subsequent therapies on disease progression. This is especially important for relatively indolent tumors, where multiple courses of therapy may be administered prior to fatality. Time-to-disease-progression has been proposed as a better assessment of clinical benefit as it is not confounded by subsequent treatments. It is particularly endorsed for agents with a cytostatic or antiangiogenic mechanism of action. The interpretation of this endpoint in a single-arm clinical trial is also limited by selection bias.

Historically, objective response rate was the standard surrogate measure of the clinical activity of investigational agent. As tumors rarely undergo significant spontaneous regression, tumor shrinkage is considered to be a treatment-specific response. Improved and standardized guidelines have been developed to ascertain the reduction in the size of tumors in response to therapy. This system of evaluating clinical benefit is limited by the requirement that patients have visceral masses that are amenable to accurate measurement. Bone, lymph node, and subcutaneous metastases are sites where this method is of limited value. In diseases that preferentially manifest in these tissues, such as prostate cancer, relief of bone pain and reduction in serum tumor markers are introduced as surrogate markers of response. Although technically feasible, these measures correlate poorly with tumor burden or subsequent overall survival. Furthermore, the relevance of partial remission in predicting delayed tumor progression or prolonging survival is not established for several tumor types, particularly nonsmall lung and colorectal cancer. For these reasons, alternative surrogate endpoints have been proposed.

Quality of life has become an established component of phase II trials, as they can provide early quantification of the impact of qualitative side effects. Although the measurement of quality of life in a single-arm, phase II study is of limited value because of bias from patient selection, it can be a valuable point of comparison in a randomized phase II study. The development of standardized, operator-independent and facile instruments of assessment will strengthen the meaning of this endpoint in the development of investigational agents. Although the FDA will not approve an agent solely on the basis on an improvement in quality of life compared to standard therapy, a drug that is shown to be clearly inferior in this endpoint in the context of phase II trials may not warrant further investigation.

2.4.2. PHARMACOKINETIC ENDPOINTS

Though traditionally in the domain of phase I trials and preclinical studies, pharmacokinetics is now an established component of later stages of drug development *(20)*.

Since patient selection can profoundly influence clinical activity and tumor drug concentrations, it is advantageous to continue to examine the pharmacokinetic and pharmacodynamic properties of drugs in phase II trials. The goal is not only to expand the pharmacokinetic-pharmacodynamic database to support model development, but to determine those patient factors or covariates that influence drug disposition and response. The use of such models can not only improve patient response by aiding maintenance of a target plasma drug concentration or avoiding toxicity, but can also add insight into mechanisms of drug action. The models developed during phase I trials can be substantially refined with the data provided from phase II trials.

Motivating the emphasis on pharmacokinetics has been the ability to quantify patient variability through the application of pharmacokinetic and pharmacodynamic models, as well as the awareness that pharmacokinetic parameters such as AUC and steady-state concentration correlate better with tumor response and myelosuppression than does dose *(21)*. The development of limited sampling models, which allow for fewer samples to be taken to define the pharmacokinetics for given patient, provides a feasible mechanism for using pharmacokinetically based dosing under the data-sparse conditions of phase II trials.

Though computationally intense, population pharmacokinetic analysis allows incorporation of observational data collected in the course of phase II trials. These methods stand out in discriminating among interindividual, interoccasion, and intraindividual sources of pharmacokinetic and pharmacodynamic variability, while addressing study design problems, such as imbalance and confounding *(22,23)*. Patient attributes such as gender, age, and serum creatinine level, known to be important in drug action, pharmacokinetics, and patient response can be incorporated into the analysis. By use of the statistical technique of Bayesian individualization in conjunction with the output of population analysis, dosing adjustments for atypical patient subpopulations can be rationally made *(24)*.

The development of more tolerable targeted therapies allows for dosing strategies that were not feasible with more conventional cytotoxic agents. Many drugs in development are amenable to chronic administration without the development of cumulative toxicity. While the same pharmacokinetic parameters must be defined for these agents, dosing schedules are based more on serum half-life and less on the time to recovery from a dose-dependent side effect. The goal of schedule selection for these agents is either constant drug exposure above a threshold or constant suppression of the molecular target. In some cases the schedule for phase II study is based on the phase I schedule that results in a steady-state concentration that was associated pharmacodynamic effect in animal models. In others, the drug concentration may be undetectable, but the molecular target remains inhibited for a more prolonged time. In either case, the incorporation of pharmacokinetic analyses in phase II trials further explores the relationship and clinical activity. When correlated with pharmacodynamic endpoints, pharmacokinetic models can support the use of endpoints such as steady-state concentration as surrogates for pharmacodynamic response.

2.4.3. MOLECULAR ENDPOINTS

The emergence of molecularly targeted therapies and the availability of laboratory assays to quantify the activity of molecular targets provide a basis for validating the mechanism of action of experimental therapies in vivo (Fig. 1). There are several technical criteria that must be met for pharmacodynamic studies of this sort to provide mean-

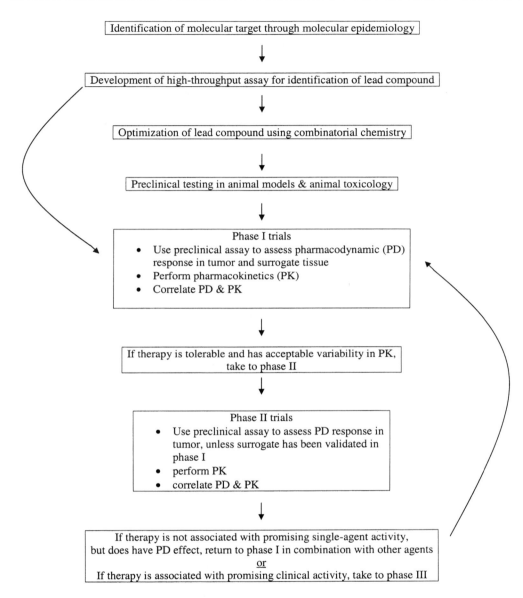

Fig. 1. Paradigm for evaluation of targeted therapy.

ingful predictive information. The molecular target must be reliably detectable. For agents that result in downregulation of the target or in molecules whose expression is regulated by the target, measurement of target expression alone suffices as an indicator of drug effect. However, for agents that inhibit or activate the molecular target, robust assays of activity must be available. Serial tumor biopsies performed before and during treatment generate paired tissue samples, which can be probed for target expression or activity. Alternatively, more easily accessed normal tissue can be obtained in a similar fashion to serve as a surrogate for tumor samples. Ideally, pharmacodynamic studies would be performed simultaneously in tumor and surrogate tissue. This would allow for an analysis of drug effect on molecular activity as well as validation of the surrogate tissue. The early identification of adequate surrogate tissue allows for the prospective assessment of pharmacodynamic effect in patients enrolled in subsequent, phase III trials.

Validation of target inhibition is lacking for the several therapies currently in development. In phase I trials of ZD1839, a small-molecule inhibitor of the epidermal growth factor receptor (EGFr) tyrosine kinase, serial skin biopsies were performed in a subset of patients to obtain surrogate tissue. EGFr tyrosine kinase activation results in autophosphorylation of the receptor. Monoclonal antibodies that recognize the phosphorylated intracellular domain of the receptor are available. Using antibodies that are not specific for the phosphorylated protein, the total amount of EGFr protein can be quantified. Skin is well suited for use as surrogate tissue for this drug as EGFr is highly expressed and active. At the recommended phase II doses, EGFr autophosphorylation was inhibited in all skin biopsy specimen obtained during treatment. In single-agent phase II trials, objective responses and prolonged disease stabilization were observed in a minority of patients. As tumor tissue was not assayed for EGFr expression or activity, it is not clear that EGFr activity was suppressed in tumors. This information is critical in the development of the entire class of EGFr targeted therapies. If responders and nonresponders can be distinguished by the residual activity of the EGFr tyrosine kinase, then EGFr is validated as a therapeutic target. Optimization of drugs against EGFr may overcome the resistance seen in nonresponders. If, on the contrary, EGFr tyrosine kinase activity is uniformly inhibited in tumors, then the target is invalidated. In that case, further investigation of agents whose sole mechanism of action is EGFr tyrosine kinase inhibition is not warranted.

3. STANDARD PHASE II TRIAL DESIGN

3.1. Single-Arm Studies in a Single Disease

The conventional strategy in phase II trials is to assess objective response rate in patients with histologically defined and organ-specific tumors. Clinical factors are typically utilized to select the study population and the rationale for targeting a given tumor type is typically empiric. A reference response rate is derived from historical data with standard therapies in similar patients. A target response rate is arbitrarily set to indicate a clinically significant difference from the standard. Probabilities of erroneously rejecting an active therapy or accepting an inactive therapy are set. The generally accepted chances of false positive or false negative results are 5% and 80–90%, respectively. These parameters dictate the sample size needed to detect the desired treatment effect. The consequence of a false positive result is that an ineffective therapy will be taken on to further clinical trials, which will presumably reveal the lack of activity. This puts patients at risk of receiving ineffective therapy, as opposed to the standard, when they are enrolled in a phase III trial. It also expends limited resources unnessarily. If a drug is evaluated in multiple phase II studies for different tumor types, the cumulative possibility of a false positive result increases. A falsely negative phase II trial results in the abandonment of that agent, which may have been added to the armamentarium of effective therapies.

In order to minimize the number of patients exposed to an ineffective agent, statistical strategies have been proposed to discontinue enrollment in a study before the total sample size has been accrued. The Simon two-stage design is the most widely employed early stopping rule of this type. Using the response rate to standard therapy as the lower limit, one can calculate the number of patients in an initial cohort that would need to respond to therapy in order to exclude, with 95% confidence, the possibility of inferior treatment. Provided that adequate data are available from trials of the standard therapy, a variety of clinical endpoints can be chosen as the primary focus of a phase II trial. Time-to-progression has been proposed a superior endpoint to objective response rate. One advantage is that patients may experience prolonged stabilization of disease with a new therapy and this benefit would be missed with traditional response criteria.

4. NOVEL PHASE II TRIAL DESIGNS

4.1. Compassionate Use or Expanded Access Phase II Trials

Although rare, it is possible for drugs to be approved on the basis of compelling data from phase II trials. The application of STI571 to primary chemotherapy-refractory gastrointestinal stromal tumors is an example. The current system of drug approval in oncology is founded on the demonstration of superior survival in the context of phase III clinical trials. The logistic limitation of the rapid completion of such a study results in delayed availability of very promising therapies to patients with refractory malignancies. For that reason, the FDA has created a provision for providing expanded access to investigational agents that are in the midst of phase III evaluation. For diseases that have proven survival prolongation with front-line therapy, but no survival benefit associated with subsequent therapy, promising experimental agents can be made available through such compassionate use phase II trials. These studies are preceded by more conventional phase II trials that demonstrate strong evidence of superiority to available therapies. The third-line treatment of metastatic breast cancer with docetaxel *(25)* and the third-line treatment of nonsmall lung cancer with ZD1839 were studied in this manner. Regimented toxicity monitoring is a requirement for such studies; however, rigorous correlative scientific study is typically not pursued. While awaiting the results of the pivotal registration trial, an expanded use phase II study can provide significantly more toxicity information and a more refined estimate of clinical activity.

4.2. Randomized Phase II Trials

Using pharmacodynamic methods described previously, it is possible to determine a minimum biologically effective dose (BED) for targeted therapies (Fig. 2). This may be substantially lower than the MTD. The clinical activity of the two doses may be different if the experimental agent has dose-dependent mechanisms of action that are not assessed with the assays used to determine the biologically effective dose. Furthermore, schedule dependent effects on pharmacodynamic response may not be appreciated among independent phase I trials. These hypotheses can be tested using a randomized phase II study. In this design, two or more doses or schedules can be compared in a head-to-head manner. With an adequate sample size, differences in efficacy can be detected.

Bevacizumab is an example of a drug shown to have superior clinical activity at the MTD compared to the minimum BED in a randomized phase II trial. Bevacizumab is a monoclonal antibody that binds circulating vascular endothelial growth factor-1 (VEGF-1) and results in degradation of the target protein. Single administration, dose escalation studies revealed that circulating VEGF could not be detected after administration of

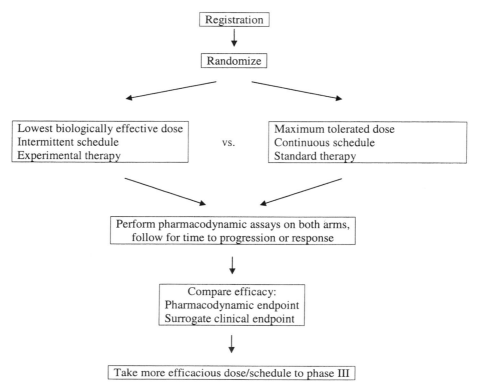

Fig. 2. Randomized phase II design.

doses of 3 mg/kg and higher. Although dose-limiting toxicities did not occur in a dose-dependent fashion, escalation was stopped at 10 mg/kg. The pharmacodynamic endpoint in the phase I study, serum VEGF concentration shortly after bevacizumab administration, does not necessarily reflect the impact on signaling through the VEGF receptor family. For that reason, a randomized phase II trial was conducted comparing the efficacy of 3 mg/kg, 10 mg/kg, and placebo in 110 patients with advanced renal cell carcinoma. Time-to-progression was significantly prolonged in the 10 mg/kg arm compared to 3 mg/kg or placebo arms. These results suggest that the pharmacodynamic endpoint used in the phase I trial is not an adequate predictor of clinical benefit. In this case the clinical activity of the minimum BED was significantly different than that associated with the MTD.

In addition to evaluating multiple doses, a randomized phase II trial can simultaneously evaluate multiple agents. In this setting, patient entry criteria are uniform across all treatment groups but the treatment is varied. The purpose of a phase II study is to explore activity, but not to make definitive comparisons between the investigational agent and the standard therapy, as the study is not adequately powered for direct comparison. These studies are typically not sufficiently large to infer relative superiority or inferiority based on an endpoint such as survival. However, this design can provide a basis for selecting which therapy looks most promising and for prioritizing agents to take on to phase III trials. A phase II trial can be powered to make inferences about the superiority of a given regimen with regard to pharmacodynamic endpoints. For this reason, phase II trials can include a standard therapy arm with the purpose of detecting differences in the surrogate endpoint.

The principle limitation of this design is the statistical power to detect clinically significant differences in efficacy. Traditionally, the sample size calculations performed in advance of a phase III trial depend on the time-to-progression and overall survival of patients treated in single-arm phase II trials. The event rate from the phase II trial and the desired magnitude of effect dictate the numbers of patients needed to have sufficient power to detect treatment benefit. Phase I studies cannot provide this type of data owing to small sample size and heterogeneity of the study population. Therefore, the sample size estimates for a randomized phase II trial are largely dependent on data from historical controls. This can result in an arbitrary and, at times, inappropriate estimation of sample size. An underpowered randomized phase II trial can result in the loss of considerable resources and a falsely negative result. An equivalent result in this design is generally assumed to support the further evaluation of the lowest dose. If an underestimation of sample size results in an erroneous inference of equivalence, subsequent phase III trials may be destined to fail because of under dosing.

4.3. Randomized Discontinuation Design

Several targeted therapies in development have shown a cytostatic effect in preclinical models. They are anticipated to confer clinical benefit through prolonged stabilization of disease as opposed to tumor regression. In the phase II evaluation of such drugs, time-to-progression is likely to be the most informative clinical endpoint. However, short-term disease stability can occur in untreated tumors. This limits the ability to extrapolate time-to-progression data in a single-arm trial. The randomized discontinuation design has been proposed as method to distinguish between treatment-related stability and natural history (Fig. 3). All patients are treated with investigational agent during the initial phase of the study. After a predetermined duration of treatment, patients are evaluated for objective response. Patients with complete or partial remissions are assumed to have treatment benefit and are continued on the investigational agent until the time of disease progression. Tumor progression at any time results in discontinuation of therapy. Patients with stable disease at the time of initial assessment are randomized to continue or discontinue the investigational agent. In order to avoid bias from the differential management of patients in the two groups, a placebo is administered to the patients on the discontinuation arm in a double-blinded fashion. The two cohorts are then followed until disease progression. A comparative increase in time-to-progression on the treatment arm implies that the disease stability was attributable to the experimental agent. This data can support the incorporation of cytostatic agents into phase III trials.

4.4. Pharmacodynamic Endpoints

Phase II trials powered according to objective response rate may underestimate the biologic activity of an experimental agent. For reasons discussed in Subheading 2.4.1., many targeted therapies may impact disease progression without inducing radiographic regression. In these cases it is especially important to assess the pharmacodynamic effect through correlative studies. In order to detect significant biologic activity that may co-exist with seemingly modest clinical measures of response, phase II trials must be powered according to pharmacodynamic endpoints. There are several hurdles to achieving

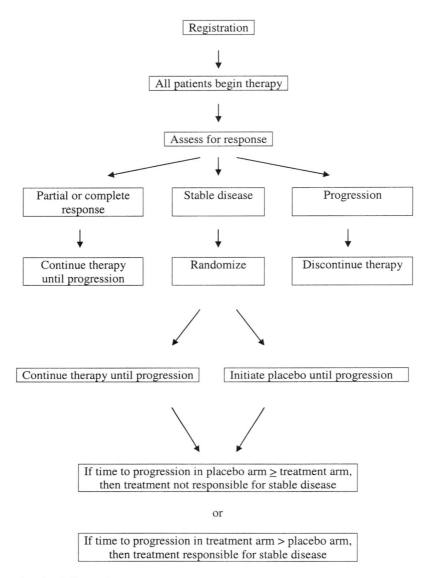

Fig. 3. Randomized discontinuation design.

this goal. The assay must be technically feasible in the vast majority of patients. In the case of serial tumor or surrogate tissue biopsies, patients must be selected based on the accessibility of the target tissue. This is the great advantage of peripheral blood mononuclear cells and other blood markers where feasibility is not an issue. Furthermore, the assay must be robust. This means that there must be limited intraindividual and interindividual variability. These operating characteristics must be worked out in phase I studies, if the assay is to be relied upon as the basis for choosing a sample size for phase II trials.

The principle limitation on tumor-tissue-based assays is the feasibility of obtaining samples from a meaningful number of patients in a safe manner. Surrogate tissues offer the advantage of greater accessibility, however, it cannot be assumed that the pharmacodynamic impact of a drug is the same in tissue that does not share the genotype and phenotype of the tumor. The field of molecular imaging is emerging as a method for assessing alterations in the tumor microenvironment. Positron emission tomography (PET) is being adapted to this purpose. PET is typically performed with ^{18}F-fluoro-2-deoxy-D-glucose (FDG) as the molecular tracer. A sample of a patient's blood is taken, mixed with FDG, and then reinfused into the patient. Cells take up FDG and unlabelled glucose proportionally to metabolic activity. The disproportionate uptake in tumor cells results in greater concentration of FDG. Positrons are emitted as the radionuclide decays and they can be detected with sensors placed around the patient.

FDG is capable of sensing metabolic alterations in response to therapy. If a treatment is capable of inducing cell death, then FDG-PET will detect this effect more quickly than conventional imaging modalities, such as computer tomography. This has been demonstrated in the phase II evaluation of STI571 in patients with gastrointestinal stromal tumors. The theoretical value of this finding is that nonresponders can be identified at an early point in their treatment and can be switched to another therapy. FDG-PET does not provide information regarding the impact of the therapeutic agent on the molecular target. Alternate tracers are being developed in order to assess the uptake of other compounds. ^{15}O-water is under evaluation as a marker of tumor perfusion and vascular permeability, a relevant endpoint for agents that inhibit angiogenesis.

More specific molecular alterations may be imaged with the labeling of a native and pharmacologic ligands. The ligand of the androgen receptor, 5α-dihydrotestosterone, is a recent example of the naturally occurring ligand that is amenable to this approach. The 16β-^{18}fluoro-5α-dihydrotestosterone species is taken up by androgen-independent prostate cancer cells, which are known to overexpress the androgen receptor, in vitro and in vivo. Imaging of patients with metastatic disease with this compound is capable of identifying active lesions. This imaging method is being tested as a means of assessing response to treatments that downregulate expression of the receptor. A similar strategy can be envisioned for the pharmacodynamic assessment of any drug that results in the downregulation of an receptor with a known ligand. The selective estrogen receptor modifying drugs, such as fulvestrant, are also ideal candidates for further investigation. While fulvestrant downregulates the estrogen receptor as a direct mechanism of action, there are many compounds that result in the decreased expression of cell surface, cytoplasmic, and nuclear receptors as a downstream event. These types of drugs are well suited for molecular imaging.

5. INDIVIDUALIZING THERAPY IN PHASE II TRIALS

The development of robust pharmacodynamic assays provides a basis for tailoring therapy to individual patients in the context of phase II trials. Variability in pharmacokinetics across a population will contribute to inappropriate dosing of some patients. In the case of patients with rapid clearance of the agent, the dose may be subtherapeutic or the schedule of administration may result in inadequate drug exposure. Tumor-specific factors can also introduce variability in pharmacodynamic response among patients with tumors of a common histologic subtype and molecular profile. This may or may not be reflected by pharmacodynamic effect on the same molecular target in surrogate tissue. In that sense, surrogate tissues are, at best, markers of response as opposed to predictors.

For molecularly targeted therapies the range of biologically effective doses may be very broad. Bevacizumab is an agent with at least a threefold difference between the minimum BED and the MTD. In the phase I trial, the dose was not escalated to the MTD, leaving the possibility that the difference is even greater. Dose escalation was discontinued largely because the data showed complete elimination of circulating VEGF levels at doses of 3 mg/kg and higher. The recovery of serum VEGF levels varied indirectly with dose such that higher doses were associated with a longer time to detectable VEGF levels. As measured by initial VEGF depletion, 3 mg/kg can be deemed the minimum BED. That dose and the highest dose evaluated in the phase I trial, 10 mg/kg, were both taken into phase II trials. In the randomized phase II trial in patients with renal cell carcinoma, the 10 mg/kg dose was superior to the 3 mg/kg in time-to-progression, which was the primary endpoint of the study. This result undermines the definition of the biologically effective dose and suggests that initial VEGF depletion is not the mechanistically relevant endpoint. It is possible that the depletion of VEGF over a threshold period of time is the predictive measure. This hypothesis can be tested in the phase II setting by prescribing dose adjustments according to the achievement of this endpoint.

The proposed dose modification method requires that the pharmacodynamic analysis can be performed in real time. The example of bevacizumab is instructive in that it is an assay that can performed on all patients and is not excessively labor intensive. Bevacizumab is administered every 2 wk in ongoing phase III trials. A randomized phase II trial could be designed in which patients are assigned to one of three arms: the minimum BED, the MTD, or a pharmacodynamically determined dose modification arm. In the third arm patients begin therapy at the minimum BED as the lower dose would be preferred if toxicity is dose-dependent but activity is not. The pharmacodynamic endpoint is assessed at regular intervals during the first cycle of therapy. Patients who achieve the threshold pharmacodynamic effect continue on therapy with no dose adjustment. For patients who do not demonstrate the target effect, the dose is escalated for subsequent cycles. An adequately powered study of this kind would be able to discern the superior treatment strategy with regard to reaching the pharmacodynamic goal. Equivalent pharmacodynamic efficacy between the MTD arm and the other two arms would suggest that the lower dose strategies should be pursued in phase III trials as this would minimize dose-related adverse effects.

A three arm, randomized phase II trial would require a larger sample size than the typical single arm phase II trial powered for comparison of objective response rate to historical controls. However, the investment of resources in phase II would optimize the selection of regimens for phase III evaluation. For drugs with clinical activity that is not obviously superior to standard therapies, only those with established pharmacodynamic effect would be attractive for further development. If the dose, schedule, and pharmacodynamic endpoints are not adequately studied in phase II trials, suboptimal regimens will be taken into phase III trials with a higher risk of failure. Alterations in these parameters are less likely to be undertaken after the completion of failed phase III trials.

The minority of human cancers is defined by single pathogenetic events. The ability of single-target therapy to substantially alter the natural history of a tumor is likely to be limited to these unusual cases. The sensitivity of chronic myelogenous leukemia and gastrointestinal stromal tumors to STI571 is, therefore, unlikely to generalize to the treatment of most tumor types. There is emerging evidence that the combination of targeted agents is associated with more profound anticancer effects. If the simultaneous targeting of multiple pathogenic pathways is required in order to improve upon standard therapy, there may be targeted agents, which have minimal activity as single agents, but are essential to the activity of the combination. It is critical, however, that drugs effectively impacting their target continue to be evaluated in phase II trials. Should they fail to demonstrate sufficient single-agent activity to warrant direct comparison with standard therapy in a phase III trial, they should continue to be evaluated in combination with other therapies based on preclinical evidence of complementary mechanism of action.

REFERENCES

1. Calvert AH, Newell DR, Gumbrell LA, et al. Carboplatin dosage: prospective evaluation of a simple formula based on renal function. *J Clin Oncol* 1989; 7:1748–1756.
2. Ettinger DS. Evaluation of new drugs in untreated patients with small cell lung cancer: Its time has come. *J Clin Oncol* 1990; 8:374–377.
3. Landys K. Mitoxantrone as a first-line treatment of advanced breast cancer. *Invest New Drugs* 1985; 3:133–137.
4. Henderson IC, Allegra JC, Woodcock T, et al. Randomized clinical trial comparing mitoxantrone with doxorubicin in previously treated patients with metastatic breast cancer. *J Clin Oncol* 1989; 7:560–571.
5. Moertel CG, Schmitt AJ, Hahn RG, et al. Effects of patient selection on results of phase II chemotherapy trials in gastrointestinal cancer. *Cancer Chemother Rep* 1974; 58:257–260.
6. Karnofsky DA, Burchenal JH. The clinical evaluation of chemotherapeutic agents in cancer. In: MacLeod CM, ed. *Evaluation of Chemotherapeutic Agents*. New York: Columbia University Press, 1949.
7. Alba E, Bastus R, de Andres L, et al. Anticipatory nausea and vomiting prevalence and predictors in chemotherapy patients. Oncology 1989; 46:26–30.
8. Robert J, Hoerni B. Age dependence of the early-phase pharmacokinetics of doxorubicin. *Cancer Res* 1983; 43:4467–4469.
9. Graves T, Hooks MA. Drug-induce toxicities associated with high-dose cytarabine arabinoside infusions. *Pharmacotherapy* 1989; 9:23–28.
10. Moore ES, Faix RG, Banagale RC, Grasela TH. The population pharmacokinetics of theophylline in neonates and young infants. *J Pharmacokinetics Biopharm* 1989; 17:47–66.
11. Grasela TH Jr, Donn SM. Neonatal population pharmacokinetics of phenobarbital derived from routine clinical data. *Dev Pharmacol Ther* 1985; 8:374–383.
12. Hunt CM, Westerkam WE, Stave GM. Effect of age and gender on the activity of human hepatic CYP3A. *Biochem Pharmacol* 1992; 44:275–283.
13. Kalow W. Ethnic differences in drug metabolism. *Clin Pharmacokinet* 1982; 7:373–400.
14. Liu HJ, Han CY, Liu BK, et al. Ethnic distribution of slow acetylator mutations in the polymorhphic N-acetyltransferase (NAT2) gene. *Pharmacogenetics* 1994; 4:125–134.
15. Marsoni S, Hoth D, Simon R, et al. Clinical drug development: an analysis of phase II trials, 1970-85. *Cancer Treatment Rep* 1987; 71:71–80.
16. Staquet MJ, Byar DP, Green SB, et al. Clinical predictivity of transplantable tumor systems in the selection of new drugs for solid tumors: rationale for a three-stage strategy. *Cancer Treatment Rep* 1983; 67:753–756.
17. Shoemaker RH, Wolpert-DeFilippes, Kern DH, et al. Application of a human tumor colony-forming assay to new drug screening. *Cancer Res* 1985; 45:2145–2153.
18. Shoemaker RH, Monks A, Alley MC, et al. Development of human tumor cell line panels for use in disease-oriented drug screening. *Prog Clin Biol Res* 1988; 276:265–286.
19. Alley MC, Soudiero DA, Monks et al. Feasibility of drug screening with panels of human tumor cell lines using a microculture tetrazoium assay. *Cancer Res* 1988; 48:589–601.
20. Peck CC, Barr WH, Benet LZ, et al. Opportunities for integration of pharmacokinetics, pharmacodynamics, and toxicokinetics in rational drug development. *Pharm Res* 1992; 9:826–833.
21. Workman P, Graham MA. Cancer Surveys 18 (Pharmacokinetics and Cancer Chemotherapy), 1993.
22. Sheiner LB, Ludden TM. Population pharmacokinetics/dynamics. *Annu Rev Pharmacol Toxicol* 1992; 32:185–209.
23. Whiting B, Kelman AW, Grevel J. Population pharmacokinetics: theory and clinical practice. *Clin Pharmacokinetics* 1986; 11:387–401.

24. Sheiner LB, Beal SL. Bayesian individualization of pharmacokinetics: simple implementation and comparison with non-Bayesian methods. *J Pharm Sci* 1982; 71:1344–1348.
25. Kruijtzer CMF, Verweij J, Schellens JH, et al. Docetaxel in 253 previously treated patients with progressive locally advanced or metastatic breast cancer: results of a compassionate use program in The Netherlands. *Anticancer Drugs* 2000; 11:249–55.

19 Drug Development in Europe

The Academic Perspective

Chris Twelves, BMedSci, MB ChB, MD, FRCP,
Mike Bibby, PhD, DSc, CBiol, FIBiol,
Denis Lacombe, MD, MSc,
and Sally Burtles, BSc, PhD

CONTENTS

INTRODUCTION
EUROPEAN ACADEMIC NETWORKS
PRECLINICAL COLLABORATION
EORTC EARLY CLINICAL TRIALS
CANCER RESEARCH UK EARLY CLINICAL TRIALS
HARMONIZING EUROPEAN REGULATORY REQUIREMENTS
CONCLUSIONS

1. INTRODUCTION

Europe has played a key role in the development of new anticancer drugs for many years and continues to make important contributions today. The historical importance of European drug development is perhaps best illustrated by endocrine therapy in breast cancer. Beatson in Scotland and Schinzinger in Germany demonstrated the hormonal dependency of breast cancer in animal models more than 100 yr ago *(1,2)*. This led to trials of synthetic estrogens, including diethylstilbestrol *(3)*, with the Royal Society of Medicine in the U.K. coordinating a trial that demonstrated the activity of diethylstilbestrol in breast cancer. Ultimately, this led to the development of tamoxifen, arguably the most important single anticancer drug currently in use, by the U.K.-based pharmaceutical company I.C.I. (now AstraZeneca). More recently, European centers played a leading role in the development of a novel class of antiestrogens, the aromatase inhibitors, that initially became standard second-line endocrine therapy but now appear as effective as

From: *Cancer Drug Discovery and Development:*
Anticancer Drug Development Guide: Preclinical Screening, Clinical Trials, and Approval, 2nd Ed.
Edited by: B. A. Teicher and P. A. Andrews © Humana Press Inc., Totowa, NJ

tamoxifen. Preliminary data from the recent ATAC (Arimidex, Tamoxifen Alone or in Combination) trial, which was carried out in collaboration with Cancer Research UK, show that anastazole (Arimidex®) is more effective than tamoxifen in reducing disease recurrence as adjuvant therapy in postmenopausal women with early breast cancer.

European academic networks have played an important and increasing role in drug development for many years. Temozolomide (Temodal®), which breaks down in vivo to the active moiety DTIC, was developed in a laboratory funded by the Cancer Research Campaign (now Cancer Research UK), then taken into trials by Cancer Research UK, and is now widely used in the treatment of glioma. One of the first specific aromatase inhibitors, 4-hydroxyandrostendione (Lentaron®), was also developed by Cancer Research UK. Likewise, results of studies by the European Organization for Research and Treatment of Cancer (EORTC) have been an important part of the registration dossier for several major new agents such as docetaxel, irinotecan, and topotecan.

This chapter focuses on the overlapping, but contrasting, roles of the two largest European academic drug development groups, the EORTC and Cancer Research UK (formed in the U.K. by the merger of the Cancer Research Campaign and the Imperial Cancer Research Fund). Links between the EORTC and Cancer Research UK are epitomized by the work of Tom Connors, who wrote this chapter for the previous edition but sadly died in 2002. Tom was very active in both organizations, founding and chairing the Cancer Research UK Phase I/II Committee and acting as Chairman of the Laboratory Research Division of the EORTC. Screening of new compounds and rodent-only toxicology, both important collaborative initiatives in European oncology drug development, are discussed. Important early clinical trials of the EORTC and Cancer Research UK are highlighted. Finally, some future challenges, especially in the regulatory area, are presented.

2. EUROPEAN ACADEMIC NETWORKS

National and international academic networks have played an important role in identifying novel targets and new agents, evaluating them in the laboratory, and testing them through all stages of their clinical development.

Early clinical trials now often incorporate relevant laboratory endpoints, not only pharmacokinetics but increasingly pharmacodynamic endpoints. Academic groups of clinical investigators, closely linked to a network of laboratories that have distinct areas of expertise, are well placed to promote rational drug development. This process extends from molecular pharmacology and biology into other areas such as functional imaging. Studies can also be implemented in phase III trials as well as additional objectives such as quality of life and health economics. A European perspective is important, as issues such as patients' attitude to their illness and its treatment as well as the costs of health care may well differ in the United States.

The EORTC was set up in 1962 by Professor Henri Tagnon, initially as the Groupe European de Chimiotherapie Anti-cancéreuse (GECA) and becoming the EORTC in 1968. The aim of the EORTC is to promote and coordinate high-quality laboratory research and clinical trials and to provide a central facility to support this network. The EORTC and its work in drug development were recently described in detail *(4)*.

In February 2002 the two main U.K. cancer charities, the Cancer Research Campaign and the Imperial Cancer Research Fund, merged to form the world's largest volunteer-supported cancer organization. Its stated objectives are "to protect and promote the health of the public by research into the nature, causes, prevention, treatment, and cure of all forms of cancer." As such, Cancer Research UK has a major commitment to new drug development, and the identification of new targets is a priority.

2.1. The European Drug Development Network (EDDN)

The EORTC and Cancer Research UK have a long history of involvement in drug development. More recently, the Southern European New Drug Organisation (SENDO) was established with the aim of coordinating preclinical and clinical studies specifically in Southern Europe. In 1999, the EORTC, Cancer Research UK, and SENDO formed the European Drug Development Network (EDDN) to optimize academic European drug development in phase I and II trials. The EDDN seeks to avoid competition between the groups and encourage collaboration. It also acts as a forum to address strategic issues, such as harmonization of regulatory procedures and methodological aspects of early drug development.

The ultimate aim of the EDDN is to share trials and facilities so that more scientifically and methodologically complex trials can be carried out based on a better understanding of cancer biology. The activities of the EDDN have recently been reviewed *(5)*.

3. PRECLINICAL COLLABORATION

3.1. The EORTC, Cancer Research UK, NCI Screening Program

An important early example of intragroup cooperation was the signing of agreements in the early 1970s among the EORTC, the CRC (Cancer Research UK), and the National Cancer Institute (NCI). The three organizations agreed to collaborate in the acquisition of compounds and in their screening, preclinical toxicity testing, and clinical evaluation. Initially, the NCI established a laboratory at the Institut Jules Bordet in Brussels that screened tens of thousands of compounds from Europe and selected some for clinical evaluation.

In 1993, the Laboratory Division of the EORTC, Cancer Research UK (then CRC), and NCI established a program to evaluate rationally in Europe new anticancer agents identified through the NCI screening program. First, members of EORTC and Cancer Research UK select promising compounds based on their COMPARE analysis, growth curve profiles, potency, and novelty of their molecular target and structure. Compounds of interest are then subjected to standardized preformulation, assay development, and stability studies to identify candidates for in vivo evaluation in mice. Those compounds in which a single intraperitoneal administration can achieve plasma levels approaching the median inhibitory concentration (IC_{50}) in vitro in the NCI cell line screen are selected for further in vitro and in vivo studies. Often hollow fiber data are available from the NCI indicating in vivo potential for a particular chemical structure or series.

In the 10 yr following the establishment of this joint venture, approx 1100 compounds have been reviewed by the EORTC/Cancer Research UK panel. Around 50 compounds have been selected for further evaluation, of which 26 have subsequently been dropped because of problems with solubility, impurity, stability, or bioavailability, 2 because there was insufficient activity in human xenografts in vivo, and 4 for other reasons. One compound did not exhibit these problems and showed significant preclinical activity so it has been moved on to further evaluation; the remaining compounds are currently undergoing preliminary evaluation (6).

Although this program has had limited success to date, it has been important in establishing a rational, collaborative structure for evaluating new compounds. With mechanism-based approaches increasingly being incorporated in this process, preclinical screening is becoming more sophisticated. The rational approach to preclinical testing has important implications in allowing phase I trials to be based around translational research with pharmacodynamic endpoints an integral part of the study. This has been a particularly useful component in the preclinical evaluation of Phortress® (7) and SJG 136 (8): specific mechanistic information has been collected to demonstrate in vivo proof of principle. These pharmacodynamic endpoints will be built into phase I studies of these compounds.

3.2. Rodent-Only Toxicology

Many regulatory authorities require preclinical toxicology studies in two species. This usually involves tests in a rodent and a nonrodent, in most cases the dog. European laboratory and clinical scientists have made a particular contribution to moves to stop unnecessary preclinical toxicology, especially in the dog, and to identify a scheme that is rapid but safe.

During the 1980s there was an appreciation that much animal toxicology was excessive and that the central requirement was a safe starting dose for phase I trials rather than a comprehensive picture of a drug's safety profile in different animal species. Short-term testing in rodents, avoiding tests on dogs, was seen as a means of expediting drug development and making the process more cost-effective. In 1980, the CRC defined the minimal requirements for toxicology prior to novel anticancer drugs entering phase I trials. These guidelines were soon adopted by the EORTC and subsequently published by a joint steering committee in 1990 (9). These guidelines were revised in 1995 (Table 1) to focus on clinically relevant schedules, doses, and routes of administration (10).

Rodent-only toxicology, carried out under these guidelines, allows starting doses to be chosen that are a satisfactory compromise between being very low and safe but homeopathic, and higher and potentially active but toxic. For small molecules, the starting dose is generally set at one-tenth of the maximum tolerated dose (MTD) in the most sensitive species, usually the mouse. Newell et al. (11) reviewed in detail the use of this approach with 25 drugs studied through Cancer Research UK. In 24 cases in which an MTD or lethal dose for 10% of subjects (LD_{10}) was defined in the mouse, this would have been safe in humans. Dose-limiting toxicities (DLTs) were seen in humans with two drugs at this dose, but these toxicities were emesis and asthenia/malaise, which cannot be evaluated in mice. For half of the compounds, the murine studies predicted the nature of the DLTs subsequently seen in humans. Caution is recommended with antimetabolites, in which interspecies variability in pharmacology and metabolic activation are well recognized, and with compounds that have mechanisms of action different from those of the 25 drugs that have been formally evaluated. Nevertheless, these data clearly demonstrate the adequacy of rodent-only toxicology prior to initiating phase I trials of new anticancer agents and have contributed to guidelines from the European Medicines Evaluation Committee on Proprietary Medicinal Products (EMEA CPMP) that include rodent-only toxicology for phase I trials of direct-acting anticancer drugs (12).

Table 1
Rodent-Only Toxicology Guidelines

Purpose

To provide a safe starting dose for clinical studies in humans

To define the most likely targets of toxicity

To determine whether cumulative toxicity occurs with repeated administration

To investigate the reversibility of toxicity

Procedure

Initial *single-dose* siting studies in mice to establish the maximum tolerated dose (MTD) or maximum administered dose (MAD) iv ± orally

The MTD/MAD can then be established in mice (one sex only), with *repeated dosing* reflecting proposed clinical schedule (e.g., orally or iv, daily or weekly)

Main study using above schedule and route in groups of 20 mice dosed at MTD/MAD, and control.

Necropsy 3 d (10 mice) and 28 d (10 mice) after last dose with hematology and histopathology of major organs, including bone marrow, as appropriate

Limited pharmacokinetic studies carried out in parallel.

In rats, MTD/MAD determined based on mice data and conducted as above to address need for studies in two species

Cancer Research UK has also contributed to the development of noncytotoxics with recommendations on the preclinical and early clinical testing of antibodies *(13)*, endocrine agents *(14)*, and products derived from recombinant DNA technology *(15)*. With greater emphasis on compounds with novel targets and modes of action, trial designs will continue to evolve. Preclinical testing will increasingly include the identification and validation of pharmacodynamic endpoints in addition to defining a safe starting dose.

4. EORTC EARLY CLINICAL TRIALS

In 1972 the U.S. NCI established a liaison office adjacent to the EORTC headquarters to coordinate transatlantic cancer research and 2 yr later supported the establishment of the EORTC data center. The data center now comprises more than 140 staff of 15 nationalities, including clinicians, statisticians, data managers, experts on quality of life and health economics, research fellows, and administrative staff. The EORTC has close links to the U.S. Food and Drug Administration (FDA). Since 1998, EORTC standard operating procedures (SOPs) have been filed at the FDA as a Drug Master File (number 13059). This can be used when seeking U.S. approval for drugs tested in Europe and puts EORTC trial data on an equal footing with that from the NCI and its collaborative groups. Also, in 1998 the EORTC was granted International Cooperative Project Assurance from the U.S. Office for Human Research Protection of the National Institutes of Health (NIH), enabling large phase III trials to be carried out jointly with U.S. cooperative groups in accordance with specific procedures.

Currently, the EORTC network comprises more than 2500 scientists and clinicians from 32 countries in about 30 multidisciplinary groups across Europe. These groups are based in hospitals and university laboratories across Europe and collaborate on a voluntary basis. The Functional Imaging, Pathology, Pharmacology, and Molecular Mechanisms, as well as the Receptors and Biomarkers Groups form the Laboratory Research

Division. Groups representing each tumor site, along with other modality-specific groups, quality of life, data management, nursing, and infection form the Clinical Research Division. Although the EORTC offers some grants through the Translational Research Fund and funds the data center, members of these groups do not receive core support from the EORTC.

Peer review of clinical trials is an important feature of the EORTC. The Protocol Review Committee brings together international expert opinion to guarantee high-quality protocols. This Committee is supported by the New Drug Advisory Committee (NDAC) and the Translational Research Advisory Committee (TRAC). The NDAC supports and makes recommendations to the clinical research groups including strategy and the prioritization of projects. The TRAC provides advice on all translational research conducted within the EORTC, from both a scientific and a practical perspective to ensure the relevance and validity of such work.

Each year more than 6500 patients with cancer are treated in phase I, II, and III trials for almost all tumor types, with around 100 EORTC protocols open at any one time. The EORTC has a database of over 100,000 patients, and over 27,000 patients are being followed up.

4.1. Background

EORTC trials have contributed to the registration of docetaxel, irinotecan, topotecan, ET-743, and STI571. Early work by the EORTC in phase I and II trials was reviewed by Schwartsmann et al. *(16)*. More recently, the EORTC NDDG has had the responsibility for conducting phase I and early phase II trials with logistical support from the New Drug Development Programme (NDDP). The EORTC does not fund its own drug discovery program so a drug acquisition consultant works with the NDDG, the NDDP, and the NDAC to identify targets and compounds of interest.

The NDDG conducts trials with small molecules (previously studied by the Early Clinical Studies Group [ECSG]) and trials using immunological approaches (previously studied by the Biological Therapies Development Group [BTDG]). The importance attached by the EORTC to new drug development was emphasized by the creation of the NDDP within the data center in 1999. The NDDP initially supported activities of the NDDG alone, but increasingly also supports other EORTC Clinical Groups in drug development studies in collaboration with the pharmaceutical industry and in the future will work more with the Laboratory Research Division.

4.1.1. THE NEW DRUG DEVELOPMENT PROGRAM

The NDDP is part of the data center and as such has adapted to new laws and directives in Europe as well as international standards of Good Clinical Practice (GCP) and the management of serious adverse events (SAEs). The Regulatory Affairs and Safety Desk was formed in 1997. The safety desk is responsible for managing SAEs according to both GCP and national guidelines and works with the Regulatory Affairs to expedite the reporting of SAEs to the competent authorities *(17)*. The Regulatory Affairs Desk is familiar with the legal requirements of more than 35 countries and has specific links with national health authorities. Since 1993, the data center has monitored clinical sites participating in EORTC trials, and in 1997 a specific Monitoring Unit was established. More than 1000 site visits have been performed, and summary reports are stored on a specific database. The Quality Assurance Unit was formed in 1994 to coordinate quality control

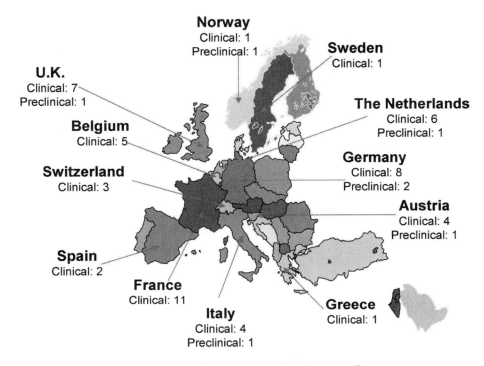

Fig. 1. Clinical and preclinical sites of the New Drug Development Group.

activities in line with policies filed at the FDA. Recently, the NDDP conducted a quality review of EORTC phase I trials that was fed back to the NDDG in order to maintain high standards and identify possible shortcomings.

The structures of the EORTC provide a unique framework for conducting high-quality clinical trials across many countries with differing legal, cultural, and practical characteristics. In addition, the EORTC performs these trials to GCP standards and has been subject to successful audits by both the FDA and the pharmaceutical industry. The U.S. NCI has also conducted regular site visits of the EORTC over the last 30 yr. These procedures guarantee rapid acceptance of such trials as compliant with U.S. requirements for the purpose of drug filing.

4.1.2. THE NEW DRUG DEVELOPMENT GROUP

The NDDG encourages a broad emphasis on target-based approaches. Together, the clinicians of the NDDG, and support structure of the NDDP, provide a single, comprehensive network for anticancer drug development.

The aims of the NDDG are (1) to conduct high-quality, rapid, independent early clinical trials; (2) to emphasize agents with novel targets or structures; (3) wherever possible, to incorporate translation research and strengthen links with the Laboratory Division Research; and (4) to facilitate phase II and III studies by forming networks with the disease-oriented groups.

The NDDG comprises around 50 centers across Europe (Fig. 1). All have expertise in early trials, with a core of 15 centers having particular experience in phase I trials. Between 1996 and 2002, the NDDG entered nearly 2000 patients into early clinical trials.

In the first 3 yr after formation of the NDDP alone, over 550 patients were entered into 22 studies. Like all EORTC trials, these studies are appraised by the Protocol Review Committee to confirm their scientific quality and relevance.

4.1.3. NDDG TRIALS

The NDDG seeks to have a portfolio of novel cytotoxic and "biological" agents that can be taken through phase I and early phase II testing and on to phase III trials by the disease-oriented groups.

Recent phase I trials of single-agent cytotoxics have included Men 10755 (third-generation anthracycline) given either weekly or three-weekly; E7070 (a novel sulfona-mide that blocks G[1]/S transition thus causing cell cycle arrest) given by three different infusion schedules, and CHS 828 (cyanoguanidine with an as yet unknown mechanism of action). Single-agent studies of biological agents include rViscumin (recombinant mistletoe lectin) given iv or sc, halofuginone (collagenase type inhibitor), SCH 66336 (oral farnesyl transferase inhibitor), and HuMV833 (a humanized monoclonal antibody against vascular endothelial growth factor [VEGF]). The combination of MS209 (a dihydroquinoline that inhibits drug efflux by binding to P-glycoprotein) and docetaxel has also been studied (18).

Phase II trials have recently been undertaken by the group in patients with a broad range of solid tumors. Many of these compounds, such as SCH66336 (19), E7070 (20), Men 10755, and ET743 (21,22), had previously been studied in EORTC phase I trials. Of the others, some are new cytotoxics including the combined topoisomerase I and II inhibitor XR5000 (23–25), the topoisomerase I inhibitor RFS 2000 (26), the glycosylated alkylating agent glufosfamide, a liposomal topoisomerase I inhibitor formulation, NX211 (27), and the oral fluoropyrmidine UFT (28) and S1. Others, such as the antisense mol-ecules ISIS5132 (directed at raf kinase) and 3512 (directed at protein kinase C) and STI571 (Glivec; directed at bcr/abl and platelet-derived growth factor receptor [PGDFR]) reflect more novel approaches.

Networks between EORTC groups will be increasingly important, with early trials placing greater emphasis on rational design coming from an understanding of the mecha-nism of action of drug action, with translational research at their core. Such research is facilitated by links with the Laboratory Research Division. Links with the other clinical groups allow early trials targeted at subpopulations of patients or less common tumors and also speed up the transition from early trials to large, randomized phase III trials. In this context, links with the Brain Tumour Group (BTG) have been especially successful, with selected BTG sites joining NDDG sites to conduct four early phase II trials of differing agents for recurrent glioma over the last 2 yr that accrued more than 160 patients.

4.2. EORTC Laboratory Division Research

The principal role of the Laboratory Division Research is to enhance translational research within EORTC clinical trials (6). This can be achieved (1) preclinically, through the identification and characterization of new therapies; (2) in mechanism-based early clinical trials that incorporate pharmacokinetics, pharmacodynamics, and functional imaging; and (3) through including molecular and cellular pathology studies in phase III trials.

The Laboratory Division Research comprises four research groups: Pharmacology and Molecular Mechanisms (PAMM), Receptor and Biomarker (RBG), Functional

Imaging (FIG), and Pathology Study (PSG). Each group has particular expertise, but they co-operate and work increasingly with the clinical groups through the TRAC. The former Screening and Pharmacology Group (SPG) was a mixture of chemists, biologists, and clinicians with an interest in drug development that met in closed session to maintain confidentiality. The SPG has merged with the PAMM. Among the compounds the SPG reviewed in detail are flavone acetic acid, EO9, AQ4N, C-1311, and NSC710305 (Phortress). Several of these compounds were generated by Cancer Research UK laboratories and subsequently went into clinical trials under the auspices of Cancer Research UK, further emphasizing the close links between the two organizations.

The PAMM Group was initially a subgroup of the then EORTC Early Clinical Trials Group and retains close links with the current NDDG. The Group led the implementation of pharmacokinetically guided dose escalation for phase I trials in Europe. More recently, an extensive evaluation of the pharmacokinetics of E7070 described in Subheading 4.3. below was carried out by members of the Group. Currently, the Group is co-ordinating the BIOMED project, funded by the European Union, to study the relationship between the population pharmacokinetics of cytotoxics and both therapeutic efficacy and toxicity in the first-line treatment of advanced breast or ovarian cancer. Links with the NDDG will be further strengthened by a project investigating correlations between genetic variability in drug-metabolizing enzymes and drug transporters and the pharmacokinetics of new anticancer drugs. In addition to molecular markers that the PAMM Group is evaluating as pharmacodynamic endpoints, other approaches including positron emission tomography (PET) and magnetic resonance imaging (MRI) are being studied by the FIG. This is a new area, with significant technical challenges, but the potential role of functional imaging was well illustrated by the phase I trial of the anti-VEGF antibody HuMV833 *(29)*.

Historically, the RBG was associated most closely with quality control for steroid receptor assays within EORTC centers but also at other laboratories in Europe and further afield. More recently, the Group has broadened its interests to evaluate other clinically relevant markers such as markers of proliferation and drug-metabolizing enzymes. The RBG has particular expertise in collecting and storing fresh and frozen tissues, which links closely with the PSG. The PSG is developing central support for histological review and banking of paraffin-embedded tissue. The central tumor bank will be based at the EORTC headquarters, with a virtual tumor bank of fresh tissue held at the clinical sites. The EORTC is addressing not only the practical aspects of tumor banking but also how to solve the legal and ethical issues. The PSG and RBG will be increasingly important in translational studies identifying potential therapeutic targets, their clinical validation, and the selection of patients for trials according to the cellular and molecular pathology of their tumors.

4.3. Translational Research

Members of the Laboratory Research Division Groups collaborate within academic networks and with the pharmaceutical industry in preclinical drug development. In 2001 the EORTC created a Translational Research Fund specifically to support work in relation to EORTC clinical trials and promote collaboration between the Laboratory Research Division and Clinical Research Groups. This support is intended to pump prime translational research with a view to subsequent external funding; five projects were funded in 2001, seven in 2002, and five in 2003. Another significant development in this area was the recent establishment of the TRAC that oversees translational research in the EORTC and provides a forum for contacts between the EORTC Laboratory and Clinical Research Divisions. Scientists and clinicians on the TRAC will advise EORTC Groups on translational aspects of clinical protocols and review Translational Research Fund applications.

Translational research has particular potential in trials of novel, noncytotoxic agents such as antiangiogenic drugs. This is illustrated by the recent EORTC study of HuMV833, a humanized version of an anti-VEGF monoclonal antibody with antitumor activity against several human tumor xenografts. Rather than seek a conventional MTD, patients received 0.3. 1, 3, or 10 mg/kg of HuMV833 with PET and MRI used in an attempt to define the optimum biologic dose (29). Distribution of the antibody into, and from, body tissues was measured by ^{124}I-HuMV833 PET and tumor vascular permeability by MRI. Vascular permeability fell 48 h following treatment, but this effect was not dose-dependent, and there was wide variability both between and within tumors. Likewise, although PET demonstrated antibody uptake in tumors, this was again highly heterogeneous. Importantly, there was no clear relationship between plasma pharmacokinetics and clearance of HuMV833 from tumors. This wide variability in tissue levels and biological activity of HuMV833 was only apparent because of the PET and MRI studies. Trials of biological therapies may require designs different from conventional cytotoxics such as intrapatient dose escalation or fewer but larger patient cohorts. Alternatively, these trials may need to be targeted at better defined patient populations.

The importance of translational research in trials of cytotoxics should not, however, be underestimated. The phase I program for E7070, a novel sulphonamide derivative with antiproliferative activity, evaluated four different infusion schedules. Neutropenia, thrombocytopenia, and fatigues were dose-limiting and there was evidence of clinical activity. These studies included extensive blood sampling, and E7070 pharmacokinetics appeared to be nonlinear, with disproportionately greater exposure to E7070 at higher doses in all studies, suggesting saturable processes. The reasons underlying this became clearer through a population pharmacokinetic analysis using data from all 143 patients (30). A three-compartment model was developed, with elimination from the central compartment by two processes, one linear and one saturable. E7070 is extensively metabolized (31), but a more likely explanation for these findings is that distribution of E7070 to red blood cells may be saturable. Bayesian analysis was used to generate a limited sampling for use in larger studies to define further the complex pharmacokinetics of E7070 and to investigate pharmacodynamic relationships (32).

5. CANCER RESEARCH UK EARLY CLINICAL TRIALS

During 2002 and 2003, Cancer Research UK spent £175 million (approx $280 or E245) on research. In contrast to the EORTC, Cancer Research UK directly supports scientists and clinicians. There is, therefore, a particular emphasis on evaluating new treatments that have been developed within Cancer Research UK. Indeed, in-house compounds account for 45% of new treatments, with 25% coming from other academic sources and 30% from industry. Preclinical testing is carried out by several Cancer Research UK groups. Rodent-only toxicology studies are performed to GLP standards in line with the Cancer Research UK/EORTC recommendations. The Cancer Research UK Formulation Unit it is specifically concerned with developing both iv and oral formulations, establishing stability of the final product, and manufacturing drug for clinical trials to Good Manufacturing Practice standards. Cancer Research UK also funds the Biotherapeutics Development Unit (BDU) for the development and production of biological agents. These are unique facilities in the academic sector in the U.K.

New compounds are brought to the New Agents Committee (NAC) for review of preclinical data. This should include a defined, validated target with information on the mechanism of action. A link should also be shown between the biological activity of the agent and the proposed mechanism of action. Pharmacokinetic data are required along with evidence that the drug is active in vivo at doses that can be tolerated. Wherever possible, preclinical testing should identify and validate laboratory parameters that can be incorporated in clinical trials to demonstrate proof of principle. When new agents meet these criteria and are approved, the NAC allocates resources for clinical trials to be undertaken. In 2001 the NAC considered 25 new anticancer agents.

5.1. History of the Phase I/II Committee

The work of the Phase I/II Committee has recently been reviewed in detail *(35)*. The Phase I/II Committee was established in 1980 by Tom Connors, along with Professor Laszlo Lajtha and Professor Brian Fox.

Within 3 yr the first compounds were in clinical trials, and to date 90 new agents have entered the clinic. Of these, 25 are cytotoxics, 5 endocrine agents, 26 antibody-targeted or immunological agents, 5 polymer-based therapies, and 28 others small molecules with novel or unknown mechanisms of action. Thirty-six compounds did not go beyond phase I trials, in most cases because of unacceptable toxicity. Thirty-one compounds have progressed into further trials, and 22 are currently in phase I trials. Of the 31 that went into phase II testing, trials have been completed with 19 compounds; 8 showed activity warranting further evaluation, and 4 were subsequently registered (4-hydroxy-androstenedione, temozolomide, biantrazole, and etoposide phosphate), with trials of others ongoing.

5.2. The Drug Development Office

Temozolomide is one of the most important compounds developed by the Phase I/II Committee. Initial trials were completed in 1992 *(33)*, and after activity had been demonstrated in patients with glioma, temozolomide was licensed to Schering Plough. Before undertaking phase III trials, the company performed a second phase I trial that identified the same recommended dose *(34)*, albeit some years later. Based on this experience, the Drug Development Office (DDO) was established in 1992 with the aim of ensuring that trials conducted by the Phase I/II Committee were conducted to the internationally accepted standards of GCP to the satisfaction of the pharmaceutical industry and ultimately the regulatory authorities.

The DDO is responsible for setting up, managing, monitoring, and analyzing the results of early trials with new agents for Cancer Research UK. Within the DDO, separate teams are responsible for preclinical and clinical development. Clinical studies by the DDO are conducted to ICH-GCP standards. There is also a dedicated Quality Assurance Manager for laboratories to ensure that laboratories conducting pharmacokinetic or other studies integral to the trial are working to GCP standards with SOPs for assay development, validation, and data handling. The DDO was inspected by the Medicine Controls Agency in 2000 and continues to update procedures in line with new regulatory requirements.

Like the EORTC, the DDO also has its SOPs filed at the FDA in a Drug Master File. This can be cross-referenced by companies using Cancer Research UK data for regulatory approval. Cancer Research UK was the first organization outside the United States to receive a Federal Wide Assurance (previously known as International Cooperative Project Assurance) from the U.S. Office of Human Research Protection.

5.3. Phase I/II Committee Trials

Phase I trials by Cancer Research UK over the last 20 yr were recently reviewed by Newell et al. *(35)*. The portfolio of small molecules includes signal transduction inhibitors, antivascular agents, repair inhibitors, platinum agents, bioreductives, antimetabolites, and polymer therapeutics. Other biological approaches include vaccines, immunotoxins, radioimmunotherapy, and antibody-directed enzyme prodrug therapy (ADEPT).

5.3.1. Targeted Therapy

Targeted, selective therapy has been a focus of many studies under the auspices of the Phase I/II Committee.

Selective activation of prodrugs is one way of targeting cancer therapy more effectively. One area that has been pursued by Cancer Research UK is ADEPT, first proposed by Bagshawe *(36)*. This involves a two-step approach, first administering an antibody-enzyme conjugate that binds to an antigen preferentially expressed by tumor cells, and then giving an inactive prodrug that is selectively converted to the active compound at the tumor site *(37)*. This approach has been refined through a series of laboratory and clinical studies using carboxypeptidase G2 (CPG2) as the activating enzyme and derivatives of alkylating agents as the cytotoxic *(38,39)*. Virus- and gene-directed enzyme prodrug therapy (VDEPT and GDEPT, respectively) are an extension of this approach. CB1954 is a monofunctional alkylating agent with striking antitumor activity in rat tumors. It is activated by the enzyme DT-diaphorase in rats, but the human enzyme has only limited ability to switch on CB1954. VDEPT has been used to deliver the enzyme nitroimidazole reductase, which is a potent activator of CB1954 *(40)*.

Monoclonal antibodies themselves have also been studied both as therapeutic agents and for imaging. Toxicities, in particular immunogenicity, have been an issue and lead to discontinuation of the chimeric B72.3 antibody. Studies of radioimmunotherapy with [67]Cu-C595-targeting MUC-1 expressed by many epithelial tumors, ^{131}I-CHT25 directed at the interleukin-2 (IL-2) receptor, and ^{131}I-A5B7 directed against carcinoembryonic antigen (CEA) are ongoing. In hematological malignancies, the anti-CD19 antibody BU 12-saporin and the anti-CD38 antibody OKT10-saporin for the treatment of childhood acute lymphoblastic leukemia and multiple myeloma, respectively, are in phase I trials. Several imaging agents have been studied, but ^{131}I-NY.3D11, SWA11, and ^{131}I-AFP161 A have not been successful.

Another immunological approach is vaccination, and studies with both antibody and plasmid vaccination have been undertaken *(41)*. In one ongoing trial for patients with

B-cell lymphoma, fragment C of tetanus toxin is fused with the lymphoma idiotype gene from individual tumors and the fusion gene administered repeatedly to achieve immunization. Other vaccines include 105AD7, an anti-idiotype CD55 vaccine, and 5T4, directed at epithelial tumors.

A different way to achieve selectivity is by exploiting the biology of the tumor itself. Hypoxia is characteristic of tumors, and bioreductive cytotoxics have been designed that are activated in hypoxic cells. Certain *N*-oxides can act as hypoxia-selective prodrugs, and the benzotriazine di-*N*-oxide, tirapazamine *(42)* and AQ4N, the di-*N*-oxide mitoxantrone analog *(43)*, are in clinical trials. The development of therapy targeted at hypoxia would be facilitated by a means to measure oxygen tension noninvasively in tumors. Magnetic resonance spectroscopy is being used in clinical trials to detect signal from SR4554 indicative of hypoxia *(44)*. Overexpression of reductive enzymes, in particular DT-diaphorase, is common in tumors and has been exploited to activate selectively drugs such as RH1, EO9, and CB1954 (*see* three paragraphs above).

By contrast, drug-polymer conjugates seek to exploit the combination of increased vascular permeability but reduced lymphatic drainage (the enhanced permeability and retention [EPR] effect) within tumors *(45)*. PK1 is an *N*-(2-hydroxypropyl)methacrylamide (HPMA) copolymer-doxorubicin conjugate that allowed the safe delivery of fourfold higher doses of the anthracycline than with conventional doxorubicin. ^{131}I-PK1 appeared to localize to tumor in at least some patients, and there was clinical evidence of antitumor activity *(46)*. A second polymeric agent, MAG-camptothecan, has also been studied but was less well tolerated and appeared not to accumulate selectively in tumor tissue. This approach has been refined by targeting the drug-polymer conjugate at tumor-specific antigens. PK2 is an HPMA copolymer-doxorubicin conjugate directed at the asialoglycoprotein receptor present on normal hepatocytes and hepatocellular carcinoma. Targeting of PK2 to the liver has been clearly demonstrated in patients by gamma camera imaging *(47)*. Other drug-polymer conjugates also being studied in the clinic.

5.3.2. NOVEL TARGETS AND MECHANISMS OF ACTION

Cancer Research UK has tested many agents directed at novel targets. One example is antivascular drugs, of which four have been taken into the clinic to date. The first of these was flavone acetic acid (FAA) ester (LM985), which emerged from the NCI screen and was active preclinically. In patients, however, LM985 caused hypotension. The free drug, FAA was identified as the active component and selected for further study. Differences emerged between the in vitro and in vivo activity of FAA, and the importance of vascular and immune effects was established, including the role of tumor necrosis factor-α (TNF-α) *(48)*. The striking preclinical activity of FAA was not reproduced in any of the phase II clinical trials *(49,50)*.

FAA analogs were synthesized in an attempt to identify an agent that would be as active in humans as in the laboratory. DMXAA achieved hemorrhagic necrosis similar to that seen with FAA but at much lower doses *(51)* and could also induce TNF-α *(52)*. A phase I trial has been completed incorporating dynamic contrast-enhanced (DCE)-MRI to measure blood flow in tumors and TNF-α levels, both as pharmacodynamic markers of activity. The final antivascular drug studied to date is combretastatin A4 phosphate (CA4P) *(53)*. This drug binds to tubulin and disrupts microtubule function, leading to massive hemorrhagic necrosis and antitumor activity in animals *(54)*. Again, a reduction in tumor blood flow has been shown using DCE-MRI and PET, although significant toxicities also emerged. Further studies, including combinations with cytotoxics, are planned with both DMXAA and CA4P.

Several small-molecule kinase inhibitors have been studied. Cancer Research UK has studied the protein kinase C modulator extensively and is working with the cyclin-dependent kinase inhibitor CYC202 *(55)*. Attempts to circumvent drug resistance continue, but PSC-833, an antagonist of P-glycoprotein, lacked efficacy *(56)*. One novel approach currently being evaluated is use of the demethylating agent decitabine to re-establish sensitivity to chemotherapy. With other agents such as elactocin, penclomidine, and SDZ 62-434, the precise mechanism of action was unknown.

5.3.3. Cytotoxics and Antiendocrine Agents

Although much of the current focus is on novel targets, three of the four Cancer Research UK compounds that came to be licensed are cytotoxics. The methylating agent temozolomide was one of a group of imidazotetrazine derivatives. The lead compound, mitozolomide, went into the clinic but caused severe and unpredictable myelosuppression *(57)*. Temozolomide did not have this limitation *(32)* and is now widely used in the treatment of gliomas. Etoposide phosphate was registered, as was the topoisomerase inhibitor biantrazole, although this drug was subsequently withdrawn.

In the search for agents with either a broader spectrum of activity or activity in tumors resistant to cisplatin and carboplatin, the novel platinums JM216, AMD473 (ZD0473), and BBR3464 were all studied in phase I and II trials, with JM216 and AMD473 remaining in development. Among the tubulin-binding agents, amphethinile and 1069-C85 ceased development after phase I because of unacceptable toxicity, whereas rhizoxin had insufficient activity. Of the antimetabolites that have been tested, MZPES, a nonclassical dihydrofolate reductase inhibitor, and AG2034 were discontinued, but nolatrexed (AG337) is still being evaluated.

Several antiendocrine agents have been evaluated through Cancer Research UK. Rogletimide is a pyridyl analog of aminoglutethimide, which acts by inhibiting aromatase, the final enzyme in estrogen synthesis. It was synthesized in an attempt to overcome metabolic inactivation, but, although it did reduce circulating estradiol levels, the potency of rogletimide was limited by induction of its own metabolism *(58)*. A much more potent aromatase inhibitor, 4-hydroxyandrostendione, was synthesized, tested, and then licensed to Novartis. As Lentaron®, 4-hydroxyandrostendione was available in many countries until it was superseded by more potent third-generation aromatase inhibitors.

Idoxifene was developed in an attempt to enhance the activity of tamoxifen by inhibiting its metabolism *(59)*. However, although active in women with breast cancer, idoxifene did not appear to have advantages over the parent compound. Other antiendocrine agents remain under evaluation including the sulfatase inhibitor coumate-667, for use in breast cancer, and abiraterone, which was developed for patients with prostate cancer and is an inhibitor of androgen synthesis in both the testis and adrenal gland.

5.3.4. Pharmacodynamic Endpoints

Several of the trials described above reflect the move toward targeted therapies with greater emphasis on identifying an optimal biological dose and pharmacodynamic endpoints rather than focusing solely on toxicity. Some of these require that tumor tissue be biopsied, whereas others are less invasive and use surrogate tissues. Least invasive of all are imaging studies.

Obtaining tumor biopsies is more difficult, but their value is well illustrated by work with 17-allylamino, 17-demethoxy geldanamycin (17AAG), an inhibitor of the heat shock protein 90 (HSP90) molecular chaperone. After treatment with 17AAG, clear effects on levels of the HSP client proteins Raf-1, HSP70, and CDK4 have been seen *(60)*. In the case of the thymidylate synthase inhibitor nolatrexed (AG337, Thymitaq®), plasma deoxyuridine levels were used as a surrogate marker for target inhibition. Although deoxyuridine levels fell after a 24-h infusion of nolatrexed *(61)*, they recovered rapidly, leading to the investigation of regimens achieving more prolonged exposure, of which the

5-d iv schedule was selected for further testing *(62)*. Measuring plasma deoxyuridine levels is not a burden for patients, but in some cases a surrogate tissue may not be feasible.

Noninvasive approaches are, however, preferable, and PET studies have been incorporated in several Cancer Research UK trials. XR5000 (DACA) is a combined inhibitor of topisomerase I and II. ^{11}C-XR5000 was synthesized, and PET studies were performed in both rats and humans ahead of phase I trials *(63)*. As part of the subsequent clinical trial ^{11}C-XR5000 PET scans were performed to follow drug distribution with ^{15}O PET used to relate tissue uptake to blood flow *(64)*. Although XR5000 did distribute into tumors, levels were lower than in adjacent tissues. PET has been used in other ways, with ^{18}F-fluorodeoxyglucose as an early marker of tumor response and ^{11}C-thymidine to measure thymidylate synthase inhibition with nolatrexed *(65)*.

6. HARMONIZING EUROPEAN REGULATORY REQUIREMENTS

Academic networks have played a major role in establishing a distinctive European perspective on drug development regarding all aspects of cancer clinical trial design. These groups have also been important in the implementation of European initiatives and directives to govern clinical research. The emergence of new compounds directed at novel targets is leading to a more scientific approach to clinical trials such as the incorporation of pharmacodynamic endpoints. In this setting academic networks will need to continue their work with European authorities and the FDA to ensure the prompt registration of new anticancer drugs.

Recently, the European Medicines Evaluation Agency (EMEA) met with representatives of academic groups, oncologists who advise the national regulatory authorities, and major pharmaceutical companies to review issues including dose-finding studies for noncytotoxics, the use of surrogate or pharmacodynamic endpoints, and mechanism-based approaches to clinical trials. The EMEA is also establishing Therapeutic Advisory Groups on oncology to advise the Committee for Proprietary Medicinal Products (CPMP) when reviewing oncology drugs.

6.1. The European Directive on Good Clinical Practice

Historically, European countries have each had their own regulatory systems, all of which are constantly being modified. One of the great strengths of the EORTC has been its knowledge of these differing regulatory requirements *(66)*. This has, however, been an unwieldy system, and in 2001 Europe started the process of harmonizing these regulations. The European Directive on GCP (Directive 2001/20/EC) applies not only to trials sponsored by the pharmaceutical industry with a view to registering new oncology drugs, but also to other therapeutic areas and noncommercial drug trials conducted independently in academic institutions.

The European Directive on GCP will affect many aspects of early trials. The aim of harmonizing and simplifying regulatory requirements has clear attractions if it does indeed facilitate the conduct of high-quality clinical trials. One positive aspect of the directive is the change to the process of ethical review so that approval from a single ethics committee will be valid throughout that country. Time should also be saved, as simultaneous submission to the ethical committee and to the competent regulatory authorities is permitted. Under the directive, all products have to be manufactured to Good Manufacturing Practice (GMP) standards, and procedures for the importation of new agents are specified. This will, however, carry additional costs that will be a further burden for academic research. The proposed database of clinical trials is also seen as a valuable resource to avoid duplication of trials, but it is unclear how this will work in practice.

The Directive takes effect from May 2004 and will be binding on all members of the EU. With the recent expansion of the EU, the GCP Directive will apply to the vast majority of Europe. There is, however, flexibility regarding both interpretation of the Directive and how it is incorporated into the legal statutes of each country. This may lead to contradictory interpretation of the Directive between countries. In some specific areas it is not clear to what extent the GCP Directive will resolve differences between European countries. The EORTC has, for example, drawn attention to wide variation in clinical trial insurance indemnity between countries (67). The requirements for insurance and indemnity are not, however, covered by the Directive, so sponsors will still need different policies for different countries.

There is also a concern that the new legislation will require more extensive preclinical toxicology testing than the rodent-only scheme advocated by Cancer Research UK and the EORTC. In other areas, the Directive may increase the bureaucracy and paper work and therefore the time and cost of initiating oncology trials. The new requirements may be particularly burdensome for smaller biotechnology companies and academic groups. This emphasizes again the importance of academic networks such as the EORTC and Cancer Research UK in new drug development. These groups already operate largely to GCP standards and have considerable resources and expertise, but incorporating the new requirements will be expensive. Although it is hoped that the European Directive will reduce red tape, there is concern that the reverse will be true and that it will increase the bureauocracy for initiating and conducting cancer clinical trials. The precise impact of the European Directive on cancer trials will only become apparent in the coming years.

7. CONCLUSIONS

Cancer Research UK and the EORTC are the two largest academic cancer research groups in Europe. Although their structures differ, both EORTC and Cancer Research UK have networks of preclinical scientists, oncologists, and offices to manage early drug development with due regard to regulatory affairs and quality control. Both Cancer Research UK and the EORTC are committed to incorporating translational research into early drug development through close links between clinical and preclinical scientists. Another important benefit for sponsors working with the EORTC or Cancer Research UK is the potential to move rapidly from phase I trials into phase II and III trials through their wider clinical trials networks. Cancer Research UK and EORTC work closely with the NCI, as epitomized by their collaboration in screening new drugs, and with U.S. regulatory bodies, so both organizations are well placed to participate in trials leading to international approval of agents tested in Europe. Significant challenges do, however, remain. In particular, the full implications of the European Directive for the conduct of cancer trials are not yet apparent. Academic researchers will be especially keen to ensure that the Directive does not impose unreasonable costs on early clinical trials in Europe.

REFERENCES

1. Beatson, G T. On the treatment of inoperable cases of the mamma. *Lancet* 1896; 2:104–107.
2. Schinziner, A. Uber carcinoma mammae. *Kongress Beilage Centralblat Chir* 1889; 29:55.
3. Dodds EC, Goldberg L, Lawson W, Robinson R. Oestrogenic activity of certain synthetic compounds. *Nature (Lond)* 1938; 141:247–248.

4. Lacombe D, Fumoleau P, Zwierzina H, et al., on behalf of the EORTC New Drug Development Group and New Drug Development Programme. *Eur J Cancer* 2002; 38(suppl 4):S19–S23

5. Lacombe D, Butler-Smith A, Therasse P, et al. Cancer drug development in Europe: A selection of new agents under development at the European Drug Development Network. *Cancer Invest* 2003; 21:137–147.

6. Brünner N, Double J, Fichtner I, et al. The EORTC Laboratory Research Division. *Eur J Cancer* 2002; 38(suppl 4):S14–S17.

7. Leong C-O, Gaskell M, Martin EA, et al. Antitumour 2-(4-aminophenyl)benzothiazoles generate DNA adducts in sensitive tumor cells in vitro and in vivo. *Br J Cancer* 2003; 88:470–477.

8. Hartley JA, Spanswick VJ, Pedley B, et al. In vitro antitumour activity and in vivo interstrand linking by the novel pyrrolobenzodiazepene dimer SJG-136 (NSC 694501). *Proc Am Assoc Cancer Res* 2002; 43:489.

9. Joint Steering Committee of the EORTC and CRC. General guidelines for the preclinical toxicology of new cytotoxic anticancer agents in Europe. *Eur J Cancer* 1990; 26:411–414.

10. Burtles SS, Newell DR, Henrar REC, Connors TA. Revisions of general guidelines for the preclinical toxicology of new cytotoxic anticancer agents in Europe. *Eur J Cancer* 1995; 31A:408–410.

11. Newell DR, Burtles SS, Fox BW, Jodrell DJ, Connors TA. Evaluation of rodent-only toxicology for early clinical trials with novel cancer therapeutics. *Br J Cancer* 1999; 81: 760–768.

12. European Agency for the Evaluation of Medicinal Products (1999). Committee for Proprietary Medicinal Products. Note for guidance on the pre-clinical evaluation of anticancer medicinal products. www.emea.eu.int. CPMP/SWP/997/96.

13. Joint Committee of the Cancer Research Campaign. Operation manual for control of production, preclinical toxicology and phase I trials of anti-tumour antibodies and rug antibody conjugates. *Br J Cancer* 1986; 54: 557–568.

14. Joint Committee of the Cancer Research Campaign, National Institute for Biological Standards and Control. Operation manual for control of selection, production, preclinical toxicology and phase I trials of endocrine agents for patients with cancer. *Br J Cancer* 1989; 60: 265–269.

15. Begent RHJ, Chester KA, Connors T, et al. Cancer Research Campaign Operation Manual for control recommendations for products derived from recombinant DNA technology prepared for investigational administration to patients with cancer in phase I trials. *Eur J Cancer* 1993; 29A:1970–1910.

16. Schwartsmann G, Wanders J, Koier IJ, et al. EORTC New Drug Development Office coordinating and monitoring programme for Phase I and II trials with new anticancer agents. *Eur J Cancer* 1991; 27: 1162–1168.

17. Dubois N, Lacombe D. SAE report handling in a multinational academic research environment. *Appl Clin Trials* 2000; April:38–45.

18. Dieras V, Degardin M, Benaoudia R, et al. An EORTC/ECSG phase I and pharmacokinetics (PK) study of MS209 in combination with docetaxel in patients with progressive solid tumors. *Clin Cancer Res* 2001; 7:437.

19. Eskens FALM, Awada A, Cutler DL, et al. Phase I and pharmacokinetic study of the oral farnesyl transferase inhibitor SCH 66336 given twice daily to patients with advanced solid tumors. *J Clin Oncol* 2001; 19:1167–1175.

20. Raymond E, Huinink WWT, Taieb J, et al. Phase I and pharmacokinetic study of E7070, a novel chloroindolyl sulfonamide cell-cycle inhibitor, administered as a one-hour infusion every three weeks in patients with advanced cancer. *J Clin Oncol* 2002a; 20:3508–3521.

21. Aune GJ, Furuta T, Pommier Y. Ecteinascidin 743: a novel anticancer drug with a unique mechanism of action. *Anticancer Drugs* 2002; 13:545–555.

22. Twelves C, Hoekman K, Bowman A, et al. Phase I and pharmacokinetic study of YondelisTM (Ecteinascidin-743;ET-743) administered as an infusion over 1 hour or 3 hours every 21 days in patients with solid tumors. *Eur J Cancer* 2003, in press.

23. Twelves C, Campone M, Coudert B, et al. Phase II study of XR5000(DACA) administered as a 120-h infusion in patients with recurrent glioblastoma multiforme. *Ann Oncol* 2002; 13:777–780.

24. Caponigro F, Dittrich C, Sorensen JB, et al. Phase II study of XR 5000, an inhibitor of topoisomerases I and II, in advanced colorectal cancer. *Eur J Can* 2002; 38:70–74

25. Dittrich C, Coudert B, Paz-Ares L, et al. Phase II study of XR 5000 (DACA), an inhibitor of topoisomerase I and II, administered as a 120-h infusion in patients with non-small cell lung cancer. *Eur J Cancer* 2003; 39:330–334.

26. Raymond E, Campone M, Stupp R, et al. Multicentre phase II and pharmacokinetic study of RFS2000 (9-nitro-camptothecin) administered orally 5 days a week in patients with glioblastoma multiforme. *Eur J Cancer* 2002b; 38:1348–1350.

27. Kehrer DFS, Bos AM, Verweij J, et al. Phase I and pharmacologic study of liposomal lurtotecan, NX 211: urinary excretion predicts hematologic toxicity. *J Clin Oncol* 2002; 20:1222–1231.

28. Borner MM, Schoffski P, de Wit R, et al. Patient preference and pharmacokinetics of oral modulated UFT versus intravenous fluorouracil and leucovorin: a randomised crossover trial in advanced colorectal cancer. *Eur J Cancer* 2002; 38:349–358

29. Jayson GC, Zweit J, Jackson A, et al. Molecular imaging and biological evaluation of HuMV833 anti-VEGF antibody: implications for trial design of anti-angiogenic antibodies. *J Natl Cancer Inst* 2002; 94:1484–1493.

30. van Kesteren C, Mathot RAA, Raymond E, et al. Population pharmacokinetics of the novel anticancer agent E7070 during four phase I studies: model building and validation. *J Clin Oncol* 2002a; 19: 4065–4073.

31. van den Bongard HJ, Pluim D, Rosing H, et al. An excretion balance and pharmacokinetic study of the novel anticancer agent E7070 in cancer patients. *Anticancer Drugs* 2002; 13:807–814.

32. van Kesteren C, Mathot RAA, Raymond E, et al. Development and validation of limited sampling strategies for prediction of the systemic exposure to the novel anticancer agent E7070 (N-(3-chloro-7-indolyl)-1, 4-benzenedisulphonamide). *Br J Clin Pharmacol* 2002b; 54:463–471.

33. Newlands ES, Blackledge GRP, Slack JA, et al. Phase I trial of temozolomide (CCRG 81045:M and B39831: NSC 362856). *Br J Cancer* 1992; 65:287–291.

34. Dhodapkar M, Rubin J, Reid JM, et al. Phase I trial of temozolomide (NSC 362856) in patients with advanced cancer. *Clin Cancer Res* 1997; 7:1093–1100.

35. Newell DR, Searle KM, Westwood NB, Burtles S. Professor Tom Connors and the development of novel cancer therapies by the Phase I/II committee of Cancer Research UK. *Br J Cancer* 2003; 89:437–454.

36. Bagshawe KD. Antibody directed enzymes revive anti-cancer prodrugs concept. *Br J Cancer* 1987; 56:531–532.

37. Bagshawe KD, Sharma SK, Springer CJ, Rogers GT. Antibody directed enzyme prodcrug therapy (ADEPT). A review of some theoretical, experimental and clinical aspects. *Ann Oncol* 1994; 5:879–891.

38. Senter PD, Springer CJ. Selective activation of anticancer prodrugs by monoclonal antibody-enzyme conjugates. *Adv Drug Delivery Rev* 2001; 53:247–264.

39. Francis RJ, Sharma SK, Springer C, et al. A phase I trial of antibody directed enzyme prodrug therapy (ADEPT) in patients with advanced colorectal carcinoma or other CEA producing tumors. *Br J Cancer* 2002; 87:600–607.

40. Chung-Faye G, Palmer D, Anderson D, et al. Virus-directed, enzyme prodrug therapy with nitroinidazole reductase: a phase I and pharmacokinetic study of its prodrug, CB1954. *Clin Cancer Res* 2001; 7: 2662–2668.

41. Hawkins RE, Russell SJ, Stevenson FK, Hamblin TJ. A pilot study of idiotypic vaccination for follicular B-cell lymphoma using a genetic approach. *Hum Gene Ther* 1997; 8:1287–1299.

42. Brown JM. SR-4233 (Tirapazamine)—a new anticancer drug exploiting hypoxia in solid tumors. *Br J Cancer* 1993; 67:1163–1170.

43. Patterson LH. Rationale for the use of aliphatic N-oxides of cytotoxic anthraquinones as prodrug DNA-binding agents—a new class of bioreductive agent. *Cancer Metastasis Rev* 1993; 12:119–134.

44. Seddon BM, Payne GS, Simmmons LM, et al. Phase I pharmacokinetics and magnetic resonance spectroscopic study of the non-invasive hypoxia probe SR-4554. *Proc Am Assoc Clin Oncol* 2002; 21:91b (abstract 2176).

45. Duncan R. Drug-polymer conjugates: potential for improved chemotherapy. *Anticancer Drugs* 1992; 3:175–210.

46. Vasey P, Twelves C, Kaye S, et al. Phase I clinical and pharmacokinetic study of PKI (HPMA copolymer doxorubicin) first member of a new class of chemotherapeutics agents: drug-polymer conjugates. *Clin Cancer Res* 1999; 5:83–94.

47. Seymour LW, Ferry DR, Anderson D, et al. Hepatic drug targeting: phase I evaluation of polymer bound doxorubicin. *J Clin Oncol* 2002; 20:1668–1676.

48. Bibby MC. Flavone acetic acid—an interesting novel therapeutic agent or just another disappointment? *Br J Cancer* 1991; 63:3–5.

49. Kerr DJ, Kaye SB, Cassidy J, et al. Phase I and pharmacokinetic study of flavone acetic acid. *Cancer Res* 1987; 47:6776–6781.

50. Kerr DJ, Maughan T, Newlands E, et al. Phase II trials of flavone acetic acid in advanced malignant melanoma and colorectal carcinoma. *Br J Cancer* 1989; 60:104–106

51. Rewcastle GW, Atwell GJ, Baguley BC, et al. Potential antitumour agents. 63. Structure-activity relationships for side-chain analogues of the colon 38 active agent 9-oxo-9*H*-xanthene-4-acetic acid. *J Med Chem* 1991; 34:2864–2870.

52. Ching LM, Joseph WR, Crosier KE, Baguley BC. Induction of tumour necrosis factor-alpha messenger RNA in human and murine cells by the flavone acetic acid analogue 5,6 dimethylxanthenone-4-acetic acid (NSC 640488). *Cancer Res* 1994; 54:870–872.

53. Pettit GR, Temple C, Narayanan VL, et al. Antineoplastic agents agents 322. Synthesis of combretastatin A4 prodrugs. *Anticancer Drug Des* 1995; 10:299–309.

54. Dark GG, Hill SA, Prise VE, Tozer GM, Pettit GR, Chaplin DJ. Combretastatin A4 an agent that displays potent and selective toxicity towards tumor vasculature. *Cancer Res* 1997; 45:1829–1834.

55. McClue SJ, Blake D, Clarke R, et al. In vitro and in vivo antitumor properties of the cyclin dependent kinase inhibitor CYC202 (R-roscovitine). *Int J Cancer* 2002; 102:463–468.

56. Gruber A, Bjorkholm M, Brinch L, et al. A phase I/II study of the MDR modulator Valspodar (PSC 833) combined with daunorubicin and cytarabine in patients with relapsed and primary refractory acute myeloid leukaemia. *Leuk Res* 2003; 27:323–328.

57. Newlands ES, Blackledge G, Slack JA, et al. Phase I clinical trial of mitozolomide. *Cancer Treat Rep* 1985; 69:801–805.

58. Dowsett M, MacNeill F, Mehta A, et al. Endocrine, pharmacokinetic and clinical studies of the aromatase inhibitor 3-ethyl-3-(4-pyridyl)piperidine-2,6-dione (pyridoglutethimide) in postmenopausal breast cancer patients. *Br J Cancer* 1991; 64:887–894.

59. Coombes RC, Haynes BP, Dowsett M, et al. idoxifene: report of a phase I study in patients with metastatic breast cancer. *Cancer Res* 1995; 55:1070–1074.

60. Banerji U, O'Donnell A, Scurr M, et al. A pharmacokinetically (PK)-pharmacodynamically (PD) driven phase I trial of the HSP90 molecular chaperone inhibitor 17-allylamino 17-demethoxygeldanamycin (17AAG). *Proc Am Assoc Cancer Res* 2002; 43:272(abstr 11352).

61. Rafi I, Taylor GA, Calvete JA, et al. Clinical pharmacokinetic and pharmacodynamic studies with the nonclassical antifoloate thymidylate synthase inhibitor 3,4-dihydro-2-amino-6-methyl-4-oxo-5-(4-pyridylthio)-quinazoline dihydrochloride (AG337) given by 24 hour intravenous infusion. *Clin Cancer Res* 1995; 1:1275–1284.

62. Rafi I, Boddy AV, Calvete JA, et al. Preclinical and phase I clinical studies with the non-classical antifolate thymidylate synthase inhibitor nolarexed dihydrochloride given by prolonged administration in patients with solid tumours. *J Clin Oncol* 1998; 16:1131–1141.

63. Osman S, Luthra SK, Brady F, et al. Studies on the metabolism of the novel antitumour agent [N-methyl-11C]N-2(dimethylamino)ethyl]acridine-4-carboxamide in rats and humans prior to phase I clinical trials. *Cancer Res* 1997; 57:2172–2180.

64. Propper DJ, deBono J, Saleem A, et al. Use of positron emission tomography in pharmacokinetic studies to investigate therapeutic advantage in a phase I study of 120-hour intravenous infusion XR5000. *J Clin Oncol* 2003; 21:203–210.

65. Wells P, Aboagye E, Gunn RN, et al. 2-[11C]thymidine positron emission tomography as an indicator of thymidylate synthase inhibition in patients treated with AG337. *J Natl Cancer Inst* 2003; 95:675–682.

66. Baeyens AJ, Lacombe D. Regulatory issues at EORTC: the way forward. *Eur J Cancer* 2002; 38(suppl 4):S142–S146.

67. Lacombe D. Insuring clinical trials, an academic viewpoint. *Appl Clin Trials* 1998; 7(March):24–29.

20 The Phase III Clinical Cancer Trial

Ramzi N. Dagher, MD and Richard Pazdur, MD

CONTENTS

INTRODUCTION
DEFINING THE POPULATION
RANDOMIZATION
TRIAL DESIGNS FOR PHASE III CANCER TRIALS
SAMPLE SIZE
PLACEBO AND BLINDING
ENDPOINTS
DATA MONITORING
CONCLUSIONS

The views expressed are the result of independent work and do not necessarily represent the views or findings of the United States Food and Drug Administration or the United States government.

1. INTRODUCTION

Phase III clinical trials in oncology represent the final step in a multistage process of evaluating the role of a new drug, combination regimen, or other treatment modality in the clinical cancer setting. In the United States, these trials are often conducted by large cooperative groups with support from the National Cancer Institute (NCI). Some cooperative groups were founded in the 1960s, and many now have world-wide clinical site affiliations. The major cooperative groups conducting phase III trials in adult and pediatric hematological malignancies and solid tumors in the United States are listed in Table 1. Phase III trials compare a new drug or combination to therapy regarded as standard of care in a specific cancer setting. Commercial sponsors often play an active role in the conduct of trials, either by assuming direct responsibility for clinical trial design and implementation or through agreements with cooperative groups. Input on the design of these trials is often sought from regulatory bodies such as the U.S. Food and Drug Administration (USFDA), the European Agency for the Evaluation of Medicinal Products (EMEA), or the Japanese regulatory authorities, owing to the potential regula-

From: *Cancer Drug Discovery and Development:*
Anticancer Drug Development Guide: Preclinical Screening, Clinical Trials, and Approval, 2nd Ed.
Edited by: B. A. Teicher and P. A. Andrews © Humana Press Inc., Totowa, NJ

Table 1
United States-Based Cooperative Groups

Cooperative group	Member institutions	Number of active clinical trials at any one time
Childrens Oncology Group (COG)	238 in the U.S., Canada, Europe, Australia	Approx 100
Southwest Oncology Group (SWOG)	283 in the U.S. and Canada	Approx 100
Eastern Cooperative Oncology Group (ECOG)	389 in the U.S., Canada, Australia, Peru, Israel, South Africa	90 or more
Radiation Therapy Oncology Group (RTOG)	250 in the U.S. and Canada	Approx 40
National Surgical Adjuvant Breast and Bowel Project (NSABP)	Approx 200	Approx 10 (treatment and prevention)
Cancer and Leukemia Group B (CALGB)	29 University Centers and 185 Community Hospitals in the U.S.	Approx 90
North Central Cancer Treatment Group (NCCTG)	20 in the U.S.	Approx 60
American College of Surgeons Oncology Group	13 Organ Committees	Approx 15–20
Gynecologic Oncology Group (GOG)	84 in the U.S., Canada, U.K., and Japan	Approx 45

tory impact of some phase III trials. The design, conduct, and outcome analysis of phase III cancer trials is a complex interaction among academic institutions, cooperative groups, commercial sponsors, and regulatory bodies.

Although phase III trials conducted in the oncology setting seek to compare a new drug or regimen with standard therapy, there are instances in which standard therapy does not exist and supportive care alone would be an appropriate comparator. Although the primary objective of such trials is often to determine whether a new approach is superior to standard therapy, there are instances in which a new treatment may be equally effective and associated with less toxicity or a more convenient form of administration (e.g., oral vs intravenous). These studies must demonstrate preservation of efficacy (noninferiority analysis). Well-designed and properly conducted phase III trials share basic elements, which are outlined in a study protocol. These elements include a clear definition of the objectives, endpoints, study population, treatment plan including clinical and laboratory assessments, statistical considerations including sample size and randomization process, data monitoring, and informed consent. Special considerations relevant to these elements are outlined below. For a discussion of regulatory considerations relevant to clinical trials design, *see* Chapter 23, " FDA Role in Cancer Drug Development and Requirements for Approval."

2. DEFINING THE POPULATION

The patient population is defined by outlining eligibility criteria, consisting of inclusion and exclusion criteria. Documentation of the histological diagnosis is usually required. Rare exceptions arise when obtaining a sample for pathological examination poses great risk to the patient, and the diagnosis can be made with relative certainty based on a compendium of clinical, radiological, and/or laboratory considerations (e.g., brainstem gliomas). Pathological evaluation may take into account factors other than histology alone. Cytogenetic evaluation and examination of cell surface markers by immunohistochemistry or flow cytometry can aid in the proper diagnosis and classification of disease in hematological and select pediatric malignancies (1,2). Recently, agents with a putative molecular target have been introduced into clinical development (3–5). In many cases, there is uncertainty regarding the relative contribution of the target of interest to the disease process. Whether or not (and by what methods) the molecular target should be included in the definition of the study population remains a challenge for the academic community, commercial sponsors, and regulatory bodies.

Aside from pathological considerations, eligibility criteria should address clinical concerns relevant to defining the population. Although many phase III cancer trials focus on newly diagnosed patients, other trials enroll patients with some prior therapy. The extent of prior therapy (surgery, radiotherapy, or chemotherapy) should be recorded in a precise fashion. Another major consideration is defining thresholds for adequate organ function, especially given the cytotoxic nature of many cancer chemotherapy agents and their impact on hematopoietic, gastrointestinal, and in some cases, hepatic or renal function. Since pediatric cancer patients are usually treated on separate trials from adults, phase III trials enrolling adults usually have a minimum age requirement of 18 or 21 yr. A number of clinical trials in oncology have historically excluded elderly patients. Even when elderly patients are not excluded, economic issues and the frequency of concomitant serious comorbid conditions contribute to under-representation of the elderly population in clinical cancer trials (6,7). In response, some oncology cooperative groups such as the Cancer and Leukemia Group B (CALGB) have developed protocols that specifically target older patients (7,8). Although a desire to define eligibility criteria rather narrowly exists, this approach must be balanced against the need to maintain the generalizibility of the study results to the population for whom the intervention is intended (9).

3. RANDOMIZATION

Attempts to compare results of single-arm trials with historical controls may be misleading owing to potential differences in baseline patient characteristics (e.g., performance status, prior therapy), diagnostic criteria, staging, supportive care, evaluation, and follow-up between the current trial and historical data. Even when matched historical or concurrent controls can be selected, matching for known factors does not guarantee that unknown factors are evenly distributed between two groups. Randomization in a large well-controlled trial will usually accomplish this task (10).

After a patient has been screened for eligibility and has given consent to participate, randomization should be performed through a central office that allocates treatment through an independent process. To ensure that at any time point in the conduct of the study a relatively equal number of patients is being enrolled to each of the treatment arms, a process of "blocked randomization" can be used: in a "block," or sequence of a fixed number of patients, the treatment arms are allocated an equal number of times *(11)*.

When prognostic factors are known for patients participating in a randomized phase III trial, these must be taken into consideration when interpreting differences in outcome between study arms. This can be done by distributing prognostic factors evenly between treatment arms at the time of randomization through a process of stratification *(12)*. The categories used in defining a particular stratification factor must be mutually exclusive (e.g., stage IIIB vs stage IV nonsmall-cell lung cancer or age less than 60 yr vs 60 yr old or older), and the stratification factors must be known for each patient at the time of randomization. Examples of stratification factors used in cancer trials include stage of disease, performance status, age, and geographic region.

4. TRIAL DESIGNS FOR PHASE III CANCER TRIALS

Phase III clinical cancer trials involve randomization to two or more parallel treatment arms with a uniform treatment approach in each arm for a finite treatment duration. In some cases, alternative approaches are utilized such as a crossover or factorial design. Figure 1 illustrates designs for phase III trials utilized in oncology. In a crossover design, each patient serves as his or her own control with respect to each of the treatments being investigated. When two treatments A and B are being evaluated, half the patients are randomly assigned to initially receive A followed by B and the other half B followed by A *(13)*.

For a valid comparison between the two treatments, a number of assumptions are made. First, the effect observed in the first period of treatment should not carry over into the second period. In addition, the patient should be in the same overall clinical state at the beginning of the second period as in the beginning of the first period. In cancer patients, crossover designs are often problematic. The important endpoint of survival benefit associated with a specific therapy may be obscured by crossover. In addition, patient performance status and tolerance to toxicities may decrease after the initial treatment. Settings in which a crossover design may be applicable include those evaluating supportive care modalities, such as in the evaluation of growth factor support, antiemetic therapy, or pain control *(14)*. Factorial designs are employed when two (or more) different treatment modalities are being tested simultaneously *(15)*. In the example of a 2×2 factorial design, one could test two local control methods (e.g., surgery or radiotherapy) and simultaneously test two different systemic chemotherapy regimens. In such a 2×2 factorial design, patients are randomized to four treatment groups. Hence, two efficacy questions can be answered simultaneously by this approach. However, a factorial design is not ideal when a negative interaction or overlapping toxicity profiles between the individual treatment modalities being tested may exist.

5. SAMPLE SIZE

5.1. Superiority Trials

The number of patients to be enrolled in a phase III trial should be specified in the relevant protocol. Methods of sample size determination are based on the assumption that at the conclusion of the follow-up period, a test for statistical significance will be conducted. A one-sided significance level represents the probability of obtaining a difference

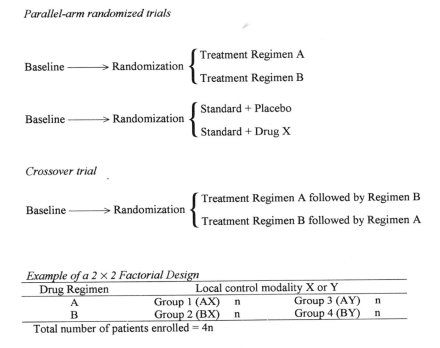

Fig. 1. Phase III clinical trial designs used in oncology.

as large and in the same direction as that actually observed. In contrast, a two-sided significance level represents the probability of obtaining, by chance, a difference *in either direction* as large in magnitude as that actually observed. A two-sided significance level of 0.05 has become widely accepted as a standard level of evidence *(10)*.

The probability of obtaining a statistically significant result when the treatments differ in effectiveness is called the power of the trial. In general, the power of a trial increases as the sample size and extent of follow-up increase. However, the power of a trial also depends on the size of the true difference in effectiveness between two treatment regimens. Trials are usually sized so that the power is 0.8 or 0.9 when the true difference in effectiveness between two treatments is the smallest size that is considered clinically meaningful.

5.2. Noninferiority Trials

A noninferiority analysis ensures that a survival advantage, the "control effect" associated with a standard drug or regimen, will not be lost with a new agent or treatment approach. Noninferiority trials require that the treatment effect is no less than the control effect by a clinically acceptable margin in a randomized setting. To determine the control effect, external information (e.g., drug effect in a historical control vs placebo) is required, and a certain portion of the control effect should be preserved. Noninferiority designs should be applied when the benefit of standard treatment is of substantial magnitude, is precisely estimated, and is considered clinically meaningful. The control effect to be preserved and the margins to be utilized in the analysis of results should be prospectively defined.

6. PLACEBO AND BLINDING

Biases inherent in the evaluation of clinical endpoints can be minimized with the use of a placebo control and blinding in the context of a randomized trial. Cancer clinical trials have not often utilized blinding and/or placebos. The toxicity profile of most oncology drugs and the different schedules and routes of administration utilized (oral vs bolus intravenous or continuous infusion) make blinding difficult. With the advent of oral dosing forms of oncology drugs with limited toxicity profiles, randomized placebo controlled trials are being implemented. The new oral treatment is tested against placebo or in an add-on setting; the drug is added to a chemotherapy regimen and compared with chemotherapy plus placebo.

7. ENDPOINTS

Protocols for phase III cancer trials usually delineate one primary endpoint to be evaluated as evidence of clinical benefit and one or more secondary endpoints related to biological activity and safety. In the following sections, a discussion of endpoints commonly examined in the context of phase III cancer trials is provided.

7.1. Time to Event Endpoints

7.1.1. SURVIVAL

Overall survival (OR), defined as time from randomization to time of death from any cause, is often considered an optimal efficacy endpoint in phase III cancer trials. Small improvements in survival may be considered evidence of meaningful clinical benefit. As an endpoint, survival is assessed daily and is relatively easily documented through direct patient contact during hospitalizations, office visits, or verbal contact by phone. Date of death is usually confirmed with little difficulty and is independent of causality. For patients who are lost to follow-up prior to documentation of death, censoring is usually undertaken at the time of last documented contact.

Disease-free survival (DFS), defined as time from randomization to disease recurrence or death owing to disease progression, is also frequently examined as a primary endpoint in phase III clinical cancer trials. In some instances, DFS is more difficult to document as an endpoint compared with OS since it requires careful follow-up to detect disease recurrence, and the cause of death can be difficult to ascertain in cancer patients *(16)*. Cancer patients often have comorbid conditions (e.g., cardiovascular disease) that may confound the interpretation of DFS. Furthermore, cancer patients often die outside of a hospital setting, and autopsies are not routinely performed.

7.1.2. TIME TO PROGRESSION

Time to progression (TTP) is defined as the time from randomization to time of progressive disease or death. Potential advantages associated with the use of TTP include a smaller sample size and shorter follow-up than is necessary when a survival endpoint is utilized. In addition, differences in TTP will not be obscured by secondary therapies if a crossover effect exists. There is interest in enhancing this endpoint by correlating radiographical changes with a delay of onset of new symptoms or delay of symptomatic worsening.

There are a number of difficulties associated with the use of TTP as an endpoint in the oncology setting. First, most oncology trials are not blinded, potentially introducing bias into the decision-making process regarding TTP. Second, patients must be evaluated on a regular basis with complete ascertainment of all sites of disease at baseline and follow-up visits. The same assessment technique and evaluation schedule should be used in all patients in order for TTP findings to be interpretable. Third, determination of a magnitude of difference that would be considered clinically meaningful can be problematic since most measurements are performed every 2–3 mo and the differences in TTP may be of a similar magnitude. Finally, handling of missing data and censoring decisions can be difficult.

7.1.3. TIME TO TREATMENT FAILURE

Time to treatment failure (TTF) is defined as time from randomization to documentation of progressive disease, death, withdrawal owing to adverse events, patient refusal to continue on the study, or introduction of a new therapy. The composite nature of TTF allows for a potential tradeoff of efficacy for toxicity reduction, and hence TTF is not usually utilized as a primary endpoint of phase III clinical cancer trials.

7.2. Palliation, Patient-Reported Outcomes, and Health-Related Quality of Life

Aside from survival, endpoints relevant to patient benefit include those related to palliation or symptom control, such as a reduction in pain or decreased analgesic use. These endpoints are usually reported as patient-reported outcomes. The credibility of such endpoints can be enhanced by blinding and an association with a biological effect of the drug (e.g., response rate). Instruments used to measure these endpoints should be relatively simple, prospectively designed, and tailored around an expected outcome.

Health-related quality of life measures are included in many clinical trials and may provide the patient's perspective on treatment effects. However, a number of limitations are associated with their use. They may be associated with significant reporting bias on the part of investigators and patients, especially in the setting of a nonblinded trial. Cultural factors such as lack of availability of measures used in multiple languages may limit the ability to apply such endpoints consistently in the setting of multicenter, multinational phase III trials, which are becoming more global in nature. In addition, interpretation of results of such measures can be difficult owing to the problems of missing data, multiple endpoints, and multiple comparisons with baseline that must be adjusted for in the statistical analysis plan, and lack of prior validation of many of these measures in the cancer setting.

7.3. Objective Tumor Response

Objective tumor response, defined in the case of solid tumors as a reduction in tumor size over baseline, is an endpoint usually evaluated in the phase II setting. This endpoint provides initial evidence of a treatment's biologic activity, providing credence for further clinical development in the phase III setting. Tumor response is often a secondary endpoint of many phase III trials. In this setting, response data can provide insight into a treatment's activity in a more homogeneous, often less refractory patient population than that typically evaluated in phase II cancer trials. In contrast to endpoints such as survival and TTP, in which both a treatment effect and the natural history of the disease affect the duration of the endpoint, tumor size reduction can usually be attributed entirely to treatment.

In evaluating response, the response duration must be taken into account. Response rates are a compilation of complete and partial responses. Stable disease and minor

Table 2
Commonly Used Response Criteria in Clinical Cancer Trials

Disease setting	Response criteria
Solid tumors	SWOG (Southwest Oncology Group), WHO (World Health Organization) RECIST (WHO, NCI, EORTC)
Chronic lymphocytic leukemia	International Workshop on CLLNCI
Multiple myeloma	European Group for Bone Marrow Transplantation, SWOG, Chronic Leukemia-Myeloma Task Force

response are excluded from the determination of response rate. One of the limitations of assessing response data is the variation in criteria used for response determination in clinical trials. Another is the subjectivity introduced by use of individual readers of varying skill and experience. Finally, methodological issues related to the evaluation and interpretation of response data include the need to prospectively identify lesions to be measured and the potential variability in imaging techniques used (e.g., nature of imaging scan, types of cuts used). Recently, the World Health Organization (WHO), U.S. NCI, and the European Organization for Research and Treatment of Cancer (EORTC) have jointly adopted a new set of tumor response criteria that define evaluable lesions and enable the use of newer imaging modalities, such as spiral computed tomography (CT) and magnetic resonance imaging (MRI) *(17)*. These criteria are being widely adopted in cancer trials for solid tumors *(18)*. Response criteria commonly used in clinical cancer trials of solid tumors and some hematological malignancies are listed in Table 2 *(17,19–21)*.

8. DATA MONITORING

During the conduct of a phase III trial, the integrity and credibility of the clinical study must be maintained in order for the final results to be interpretable and applicable to clinical practice. To achieve this goal, a data monitoring committee (DMC) or data monitoring safety board (DMSB) is often charged with the task of reviewing safety and efficacy data from a phase III trial on a continuing basis. This is usually the only group reviewing data by treatment assignment. Sponsors, investigators, and regulatory bodies are unaware of treatment allocation during the trial conduct *(22)*. The membership of a DMC or DMSB for a clinical cancer trial should include representatives from medical oncology, biostatistics, and ethics. To provide objective recommendations, membership should be limited to individuals who maintain independence from the sponsor and investigators *(23)*. If interim data demonstrate that a treatment benefit is emerging, or that the treatment under evaluation is associated with undue harm, a monitoring board may recommend early termination of a trial or protocol modification. A decision to terminate a trial prior to completion or to modify the design must be made with careful consideration, as early/interim results may be misleading. This decision could have irreversible consequences *(24)*.

Statistical monitoring procedures can assist monitoring boards in the review of safety and efficacy data. Although there can be wide variations in the statistical methodologies and stopping rules utilized by monitoring boards, these methodologies are intended only as guidelines. A common approach is the group sequential design. This method requires more extreme results for early termination than conventional stopping criteria. This approach requires very strong early evidence of a treatment difference and "slackens" that criterion as the trial progresses. Such an approach relies on the p value for a difference in effect between study groups.

A less conventional approach uses bayesian methods *(25)*. With this approach, participating clinicians are asked their opinions on the expected difference between the conventional and study treatments. These opinions are used to form an "enthusiastic" and a "skeptical" prior distribution. These prior distributions are combined with trial data at each of the annual DMC meetings. The DMC decides whether the information may convert skeptics or enthusiasts. DMCs and DSMBs must ensure the confidentiality of interim data. Maintenance of the confidentiality of interim results minimizes the risk of widespread prejudgment of early information *(22)*. Confidentiality allows the continuation of timely accrual of study participants to ensure adherence to the study regimen and to maintain objective and complete assessment of outcome measures. Although arguments have been made in support of making interim results available to the public, enabling patients to make individual decisions on the basis of data that might rationally provoke different choices from different people *(26)*, this practice has been largely avoided.

9. CONCLUSIONS

Phase III clinical cancer trials are often the product of multiple interactions among commercial sponsors, cooperative groups, local institutions, and regulatory bodies. DMCs or DMRBs also play an important role in the conduct of phase III clinical cancer trials. Their role enables the safe and ethical conduct of such trials. Prospective, randomized designs employing survival as the primary endpoint are usually the preferred methods of evaluating the benefit of a new drug or treatment regimen. Efforts to minimize subjectivity and bias in endpoint selection and analysis should be encouraged. Randomization allows time to event endpoints to be utilized. It allows an informative comparison of toxicities associated with new treatments compared with standard regimens and also permits known and potentially unrecognized factors to be adequately distributed between treatment arms. Finally, it provides statistical confidence regarding the selection of new therapies.

REFERENCES

1. Pagnucco G, Vanelli L, Gervasi F. Mlutidimensional flow cytometry immunophenotyping of hematologic malignancy. *Ann NY Acad Sci* 2002; 963:313–321.
2. Wang NP, Marx J, McNutt MA, et al. Expression of myogenic regulatory proteins (myogenin and MyoD1) in small round blue cell tumors of childhood. *Am J Pathol* 1995; 147:1799–1810.
3. Fox B, Curt GA, Balis FM. Clinical trial design for target-based therapy. *Oncologist* 2002; 7:401–409.
4. Korn EL, Arbuck SG, Pluda JM, et al. Clinical trial design for cytostatic agents: are new approaches needed? *J Clin Oncol* 2002; 19:265–272.
5. Chabner BA. Cytotoxic Agents in the era of molecular targets and genomics. *Oncologist* 2002; 7(s):34–41.
6. Balducci L. Geriatric oncology: challenges for the new century. *Eur J Cancer* 2000; 36:1741–1754.
7. Wymenga ANM, Slaets JPJ, Sleijfer DT. Treatment of cancer in old age, shortcomings and challenges. *Netherlands J Med* 2001; 59:259–266.
8. Muss HB, Cohen HJ, Lichtman SM. Clinical research in the older cancer patient. *Hematol/Oncol Clin North Am* 2000; 14:283–291.

9. Furberg CD. To whom do the research findings apply? *Heart* 2002; 87:570–574.

10. Simon R. Clinical trials in cancer. In: DeVita VT, Hellman S, Rosenberg SA, eds. *Principles and Practice of Oncology*, 5th ed. Philadelphia: Lippincott-Raven. 1997:513–542.

11. Staquet M, Otilia Dalesio. Designs for phase III trials. In: ME Buyse, MJ Staquet, Sylvester RJ, eds. *Cancer Clinical Trials—Methods and Practice*. Oxford, United Kingdom: Oxford University Press. 1990:261–275.

12. Friedman LM, Furberg CD, DeMets DL. The randomization process. In: *Fundamentals of Clinical Trials*, 2nd ed. Littleton, MA: PSG Publishing. 1985:51–69.

13. Senn S. *Cross-over Trials in Clinical Research*. Chichester, UK: John Wiley & Sons. 1993.

14. Ellison N, Loprinzi CL, Kugler J. Phase III placebo-controlled trial of capsaicin cream in the management of surgical neuropathic pain in cancer patients. *J Clin Oncol* 1997; 15:2974–2980.

15. Byar DP, Piantadosi S. Factorial designs for randomized clinical trials. *Cancer Treat Rep* 1985; 69: 1055–1063.

16. Machtay M, Glatstein E. Just another statistic. *Oncologist* 1998;3:III–IV.

17. Therasse P, Arbuck SG, Eisenhauer EA, et al. New guidelines to evaluate the response to treatment in solid tumors. *J Natl Cancer Inst* 2000;92:205–216.

18. Padhani AR, Ollivier L. The RECIST criteria: implications for diagnostic radiologists. *Br J Radiol* 2001;74:983–986.

19. Gahrton G, Tura S, Ljunman P, et al. Prognostic factors in allogeneic bone marrow transplantation for multiple myeloma. *J Clin Oncol* 1995; 13:1312–1322.

20. Gahrton G, Svensson H, Cavo M, et al. Progress in allogeneic bone marrow and peripheral blood stem cell transplantation for multiple myeloma; a comparison between transplants performed 1983–93 and 1994–98 at European Group for Blood and Marrow Transplantation centres. *Br J Haematol* 2001;113:209–216.

21. Cortes JE, et al. Chronic lymphocytic leukemia. In: Pazdur R, Coia LR, Hoskins WJ, Wagman LD, eds. *Cancer Management: A Multidisciplinary Approach*, 6th ed. Melville, NY: PRR. 2002:721–734.

22. Fleming TR, Ellenberg S, DeMets DL. Monitoring clinical trials: issues and controversies regarding confidentiality. *Stat Med* 2002; 21:2843–2851.

23. DeMets DL, Pocock SJ, Julian DG. The agonising negative trend in monitoring of clinical trials. *Lancet* 1999; 354:1983–1988.

24. Green SJ, Fleming TR, O'Fallon JR. Policies for study monitoring and interim reporting of results. *J Clin Oncol* 1987; 5:1477–1484.

25. Parmar MK, Griffiths GO, Spiegelhalter DJ, et al. Monitoring of large randomised clinical trials: a new approach with Bayesian methods. *Lancet* 2001; 358:375–381.

26. Lilford RJ, Braunholtz D, Edwards S, et al. Monitoring clinical trials-interim data should be publicly available. *BMJ* 2001; 323:441–442.

21

Assessing Tumor-Related Symptoms and Health-Related Quality of Life in Cancer Clinical Trials

A Regulatory Perspective

Judy H. Chiao, MD, Grant Williams, MD, and Donna Griebel, MD

CONTENTS

INTRODUCTION
DEFINITIONS
TUMOR-RELATED SYMPTOMS AND HRQL AS EFFICACY ENDPOINTS
INSTRUMENT
STUDY DESIGN
DATA ANALYSIS
CLINICAL INTERPRETATION
CONCLUSIONS

This chapter reflects independent work of the authors and does not necessarily represent the view of the Food and Drug Administration.

1. INTRODUCTION

Improving survival has traditionally been the goal of anticancer therapy. Although great strides have been made in cancer therapeutics, it is relatively uncommon that new drugs or biological agents provide substantial improvement in survival. Most of these agents have side effects, some of which are severe, resulting in discomfort and disability. For patients with incurable cancers, overall quality of their remaining life is particularly important. Adequate palliation of cancer-related symptoms, especially pain, may ease suffering and fear, allowing the final journey to be taken with peace and dignity.

In 1985, the Oncologic Drugs Advisory Committee recommended that beneficial effects on quality of life (QOL) endpoints could serve as the basis for approval of new oncology drugs. Therefore, from a regulatory standpoint, for drugs that do not have an

From: *Cancer Drug Discovery and Development:*
Anticancer Drug Development Guide: Preclinical Screening, Clinical Trials, and Approval, 2nd Ed.
Edited by: B. A. Teicher and P. A. Andrews © Humana Press Inc., Totowa, NJ

impact on survival, demonstration of a favorable effect on QOL would be considered more compelling than improvements in other measures, such as objective tumor response rate *(1)*. From January 1, 1990 to October 1, 2001, the Food and Drug Administration (FDA) granted marketing approval to 62 oncology drug applications *(2)*. Relief or improvement of tumor-related symptoms provided critical support for approval in 11 of these approvals (Table 1). It should be noted that a favorable effect on QOL scores alone on a QOL instrument has not been used as the basis for granting marketing approval.

Health-related quality of life (HRQOL) endpoints are increasingly being incorporated into randomized, controlled clinical trials in oncology. Pharmaceutical companies are seeking novel approaches to establish the benefits of drug treatment and to differentiate their products from other marketed products. Health care providers and cancer patients need definitive information when choosing among potentially toxic therapies *(1)*. The challenges in designing the QOL component of a cancer clinical trial include identifying and measuring tumor-related symptoms, treatment-related symptoms, and other factors that may significantly affect a patient's perception of health. Although assessing tumor-related symptoms may seem intuitive, it is not straightforward. The most relevant symptoms for many cancer settings have not been well defined. Furthermore, methodology issues related to the timing of assessments, "placebo effect," and missing data present additional difficulties. Given these complexities, it is unlikely that a single, one-size-fits-all approach will be adequate for assessing tumor-related symptoms and HRQL in cancer clinical trials.

2. DEFINITIONS

The World Health Organization (WHO) defines health as "complete physical, psychological, and social well-being and not merely the absence of infirmity and disease" *(3)*. This inclusive definition goes well beyond the cure of the disease to address the multidimensional aspect of health. The term *health-related quality of life* refers to the physical, psychological, and social domains of health that are influenced by a person's experiences, beliefs, expectations, and perceptions *(4)*. Most experts agree that HRQL is a multidimensional construct that represents the patient's perspective on valued aspects of health and functioning. Consequently, the expert for assessing HRQL is the patient. Proxy ratings given by family members or health care providers may not provide reliable information because assessment of HRQL by an observer is likely to be biased by the observer's own internal standard of what is a desirable HRQL state, which may be different from that of the patient's *(5)*.

Symptom status is defined as "a patient's perception of an abnormal physical, emotional, or cognitive state" *(6)*. In cancer patients, there is a high prevalence of somatic and psychological symptoms such as pain, dyspnea, dysphagia, cough, weight loss, nausea, anorexia, fatigue, and depression. It is not always possible to attribute a symptom exclusively to tumor or to differentiate tumor-related symptoms from treatment-related side effects. Most experts agree that symptoms alone do not encompass HRQL because there are other influences that may affect the patient's perspective on valued aspects of health and functioning.

Table 1
Regular Marketing Approvals Based on or Supported
by Relief or Improvement of Tumor-Related Symptoms (1990–2001)

Drug (yr of approval)	Study design	Treatment indication
Alitretinoin gel (1999)	Double-blind, vehicle-controlled, RCT	Cutaneous lesions in patients with AIDS-related Kaposi's sarcoma
Bexarotene capsules (1999)	Open-label, phase II	Cutaneous manifestations of CTCL in patients who are refractory to at least one prior systemic therapy
Bexarotene gel (2000)	Open-label, phase II	Cutaneous manifestations of CTCL (IA and IB) in patients who have refractory or persistent disease after other therapies or are intolerant of other therapies
Gemcitabine (1996)	Single-blinded, RCT	Locally advanced or metastatic pancreatic cancer
Liposomal daunorubicin (1994)	Open-label, RCT	Advanced HIV-associated Kaposi's sarcoma (first-line treatment)
Liposomal doxorubicin (1999)	Open-label, phase II	AIDS-related Kaposi's sarcoma in patients with disease progression on prior combination chemotherapy or intolerant of such treatment
Mitoxantrone/prednisone (1996)	Open-label, RCT	Palliation of pain related to advanced hormone-refractory prostate cancer.
Pamidronate (1998)	Double-blind, placebo-controlled RCT	Treatment of osteolytic bone metastases (breast/myeloma)
Methoxsalen (1999)	Open-label, phase II	For use in combination with photopheresis in the palliative treatment of the skin manifestations of CTCL that is unresponsive to other forms of treatment
Paclitaxel (1997)	Open-label, phase II	AIDS related Kaposi's sarcoma (second-line treatment)
Porfimer sodium (1995, 1998)	Open-label, phase II (esophageal cancer); open-label, RCT (NSCLC)	Obstructive esophageal cancer or obstructive endobronchial NSCLC

ABBREVIATIONS: RCT, Randomized controlled trial; NSCLC, nonsmall-cell lung cancer; CTCL, cutaneous T-cell lymphoma.

3. TUMOR-RELATED SYMPTOMS AND HRQL AS EFFICACY ENDPOINTS

In the drug regulatory setting, primary endpoints are those that describe the major perceived efficacy of a new drug; secondary endpoints describe important though not central findings. Primary efficacy endpoints generally serve as the primary basis for new drug approval. Prominent findings from secondary endpoints are sometimes described in the drug's package insert. In general, it is not feasible to measure all influences on health and functioning in cancer clinical trials. Measures directed at tumor-related symptoms are preferable to measures of "larger" psychosocial consequences, as the former are likely to be more sensitive to medical interventions *(7)*. Improvement in tumor-related symptoms and delay of onset or worsening of tumor related symptoms is clinically meaningful to patients and represents clinical benefit of a drug therapy. Described below are several representative examples in which tumor-related symptoms played a critical role as primary or secondary efficacy endpoints supporting new oncology drug approval.

Relieving or preventing tumor-related symptoms was the primary efficacy endpoint in the registration trials of three New Drug Applications (NDAs). Pain relief was the basis for the approval of mitoxantrone in combination with corticosteroids for treatment of pain related to hormone-refractory prostate cancer. The efficacy endpoint was a 2-point decrease in pain intensity on a 6-point pain scale (McGill-Melzack Pain Questionnaire) lasting at least 6 wk and not accompanied by an increase in analgesic use. In an open-label, randomized controlled trial of 161 patients with hormone-refractory prostate cancer suffering from pain, 29% of patients who received mitoxantrone and prednisone met the prospectively defined pain response criteria, compared with 12% of patients who received prednisone alone ($p = 0.011$). Median duration of pain response and median time to progression (defined as an increase in pain intensity and/or analgesic use, disease progression on radiographical studies, or requirement for radiotherapy) were also prolonged in patients treated with mitoxantrone and prednisone. Survival was similar in both arms.

A composite endpoint may be appropriate when the benefit of a drug is multifaceted. The components of the endpoint should be related and generally of equal clinical importance. Pamidronate was the first bisphosphonate drug approved for treatment of skeletal metastases, initially approved for myeloma, and subsequently for breast cancer. The goal of treatment with pamidronate is to decrease the morbidity of bone metastases. The approval was based on a composite benefit endpoint consisting of one or more skeletal-related events (SREs) that would be anticipated to be associated with pain and other distress. SREs are defined as pathological fractures, radiation therapy to bone, surgery to bone, and spinal cord compression. In the myeloma and breast cancer trials, treatment with pamidronate resulted in both a decrease in the proportion of patients with at least one SRE and an increase in time to first SRE. In addition, decreases in pain scores from baseline were observed in multiple myeloma patients who had pain at baseline and were randomized to the pamidronate arm. Clinical Benefit Response, a composite endpoint of pain and analgesic consumption reported by the patient and performance status assessed by a physician, was supportive of regular approval of gemcitabine for treatment of pancreatic cancer. Patients who were randomized to the gemcitabine arm had a small, statistically significant survival improvement compared with those randomized to the control arm of 5-flurouracil.

Objective measurement of response to a new drug therapy, e.g., tumor response, is indicative of the biological activity of the new drug, which may or may not be associated with prolongation of survival or symptom palliation. Measures of symptom relief in patients or evidence of relief of distress caused by lesions in patients who have achieved tumor response or stable disease may establish the clinical benefit associated with achieving a tumor response or stable disease.

The approval of alitretinoin gel for treatment of cutaneous Kaposi's sarcoma (KS) was based on cutaneous tumor responses supported by photographs documenting cosmetic improvement of disfiguring lesions. Paclitaxel was approved for second-line treatment of KS based on response rate and retrospective collection of information that reflected relief of distress caused by lesions, e.g., improved ambulation in patients with KS that involved the feet, healing of cutaneous ulcers, and resolution of disfiguring facial lesions. Bexarotene capsules and bexarotene gel received regular approval for treatment of cutaneous manifestations of cutaneous T-cell lymphoma (CTCL) based on a Composite Assessment of Index Lesion Severity that assessed erythema, scaling, elevation, and pigmentation of lesions. Luminal tumor responses supported by patient report of relief of symptoms of obstruction were the basis for regular approval of porfimer sodium for photodynamic therapy (PDT) in patients with completely obstructing esophageal cancer and completely or partially obstructing endobronchial nonsmall-cell lung cancer. Palliation of obstructing esophageal cancer was defined as a 2-point change on a 5-point dysphagia scale. In endobronchial cancer, palliation was defined as a 2-point change on 5-point pulmonary symptom severity scales for dyspnea, cough, or hemoptysis.

There is continuing debate over whether HRQL outcomes should be analyzed using group measurements (e.g., median, mean scores across the treatment arm) or by individual scores (e.g., response rate). Clinicians generally find effects described in individuals to be more intuitive and relevant. Regardless of the analysis method used, the study protocol should prospectively define the magnitude of change constituting meaningful clinical benefit. The relationship between changes in tumor-related symptoms and changes in other domains of HRQL, especially general functioning, should be evaluated. Given the toxicity profile of many cancer drugs, it is quite possible that while tumor-related symptoms are improved, other aspects of HRQL, e.g., emotional functioning or physical functioning, are adversely affected by the treatment. By collecting data on different domains of HRQL, a more thorough evaluation of treatment can be accomplished.

4. INSTRUMENT

A spectrum of instruments has been developed for the evaluation of patients with cancer, ranging from global QOL scales, to disease- or symptom-specific scales, to *ad hoc* instruments that are specific to a single study *(8)*. Detailed discussion of the relative strengths and weaknesses of each type of scale is beyond the scope of this chapter. Two widely used instruments designed for cancer patients are the FACT and EORTC-QLQ-

30. These cancer-specific core instruments can be supplemented with disease-specific assessment modules. For example, the EORTC-QLQ-30 and the FACT have lung cancer-specific modules, the QLQ-LC13 and FACT-lung, respectively. Even with disease-specific assessment modules, one may need to supplement these modules with study-specific questions for specific stages of tumors, specific symptom subsets within tumors, or specific treatment side effects. Strictly speaking, a validated instrument supplemented with study-specific questions should be considered an unvalidated instrument. Ideally, substantive validation of a new instrument should be performed prior to its use in the principal trials, but this is not always possible owing to the vast amount of time and effort required. It remains to be determined what constitutes the appropriate level of validation when items from one validated instrument are extracted to supplement another validated instrument.

5. STUDY DESIGN

QOL research should be hypothesis-driven and subject to the same rigor as all other elements of clinical research. The study design should be optimized to provide informative, reliable, and consistent results to allow determination of whether a new drug or a new therapeutic regimen provides clinical benefit to patients. In general, the sample size in a randomized controlled cancer trial is based on the efficacy endpoint of survival or time to progression. Frequently, HRQL data collection and descriptive analyses are added without a formal hypothesis. As a result, the HRQL analyses are usually underpowered because the sample size is not adequate to detect relevant changes in the HRQL parameters. To optimize the ability of a study to provide reliable and interpretable HRQL information, the clinical investigator and the QOL investigator should work together during the trial design stage to identify the clinically important HRQL question or objective. With a clear and specific objective, the investigators can prospectively identify the appropriate HRQL parameters to evaluate and the best strategy to measure and analyze them. If these studies intend to demonstrate improvement of tumor-related symptoms, a sufficient number of symptomatic patients should be enrolled.

Ideally, a pilot study should be performed to identify the relevant tumor-related symptoms or aspects of HRQL that are likely to be improved by a new drug therapy and the major toxicity(ies) expected to impact negatively on patient well-being. An estimate of the magnitude of symptom improvement or change in HRQL scores allows a preliminary assessment of the clinical significance of the drug effect and can provide a realistic estimate of sample size for the confirmatory studies. In general, confirmatory studies should be randomized and double-blinded to remove or reduce the bias that is attendant on knowledge of one's treatment (9). Although it is well recognized that a patient's perception of health and functioning or symptoms can be influenced by taking a promising new drug or new treatment regimen (placebo effect), it is less well appreciated that an investigator's preference toward a new drug or new treatment regimen may exert a subtle but potentially important influence on the patient's perceptions. The timing of measurement should be prior to a patient's discussion with health care providers, especially prior to a patient's knowledge of tumor response. Procedures should be implemented to ensure patient compliance so that missing data or incomplete data are minimized.

6. DATA ANALYSIS

The statistical analysis of HRQL data should be prospectively defined. Because HRQL has multiple domains and repeated measurements over time, the strategy for dealing with a multiplicity of endpoints should be prespecified. There is a major concern about the false-positive error inflation owing to the multiplicity of endpoints and/or statistical tests performed. If large numbers of endpoints and analyses are performed, it is difficult to determine whether the observed positive outcomes are truly positive or just random associations arising within a large number of analyses.

Primary hypotheses should be prespecified and limited to a small number, if possible. Appropriate adjustment for multiplicity should be prospectively specified in the protocol. Strategies for adjustment include, but are not limited to, alpha-level adjustments, closed testing procedures, and the use of summary measures. The choice of the right summary measure depends on the research question and the expected pattern of change in the patient population exposed to the new drug. Detailed discussions on these strategies are beyond the scope of this chapter, and interested readers should consult the relevant statistical literature.

To collect HRQL data, HRQL instruments are administered repeatedly to subjects for the duration of their time on a given trial. Perhaps with the exception of short-term studies, a longitudinal analysis should be an essential component of the statistical evaluation of the HRQL measures. Longitudinal analyses are needed to characterize temporal patterns, investigate the effects of dropouts, study the influence of baseline covariates on time trends, and place univariate comparisons in context (9).

In cancer clinical trials, data are frequently missing because patients drop out of the study for progression of disease, and/or intolerable drug toxicities. Missing data is a significant problem in HRQL assessment. The reason that the assessment is missing is often related to the actual value of the HRQL parameter at the scheduled time of assessment. For example, patients who are not feeling well on the day of assessment because of disease progression or toxicity will be less likely to fill out the questionnaire. Because patients who did poorly dropped out of the study, there is a tendency for the study population to become skewed over time toward those who are doing better. Statistically, this phenomenon is called "missing not at random" (MNAR) and will introduce bias in statistical inferences unless appropriate analyses are performed. There is no definitive rule on the amount of missing data that is considered unacceptable for a clinical study. It depends on the objective of the study and the intended use of the inference.

There is also no gold standard analytical method for dealing with MNAR data because the relationship of the missing data to outcome or even the assumption that it is "missing not at random" is untestable because data are missing. Acceptable methods include repeated measures ANCOVA (analysis of covariance), if the proper assumptions are met, or the GEE (general estimating equations) approach if ANCOVA is not justified (10). Sensitivity analyses using various models under different assumptions should be performed to determine whether results from different models are consistent and robust.

7. CLINICAL INTERPRETATION

Small numerical differences in mean scores derived from HRQL assessment instruments may give statistically significant results when large samples of subjects are involved, but the clinical interpretation of the meaning of small numerical differences is uncertain *(11)*. Many experts would agree that statistically significant changes are not equivalent to clinically significant changes. Jaeschke et al. *(12)* defined "minimal clinically important difference" as the smallest difference in score, in a domain of interest that patients perceive as beneficial and that would mandate, in the absence of troublesome side effects and excessive cost, a change in the patient's management. Although this definition is conceptually attractive, there is no best method for determining the magnitude of changes in scores that will achieve the "minimal clinically important difference." Proposed methods include "anchoring" changes seen in QOL measures to other clinical changes or results, or using statistical distributions of the results for distribution-based interpretation. The most commonly cited of the distributional-based measures is the effect size in which the importance of the change is scaled by comparing the magnitude of the change with the variability in stable subjects, for example, on baseline or among untreated individuals *(13)*.

Regardless of the methods used, clinically meaningful changes in scores should be defined and justified *a priori*. Patients enrolled into the trial should have a level of symptom intensity at baseline that would allow demonstration of the prospectively defined clinically relevant change in scores. Furthermore, the clinical significance of a change in scores should also be interpreted in the context of available palliative approaches using standard techniques. For example, if improvement in pain palliation is the primary therapeutic goal of a new cancer drug treatment, the clinical significance of the pain relief achieved by the new drug will be evident if only patients who have been receiving optimal pain management are entered, and the side effects from the new drug treatment are comparable to or less than those from other available palliative approaches.

8. CONCLUSIONS

Interest in HRQL outcomes in oncology drug trials continues to grow. HRQL endpoints will probably be included in many future randomized cancer trials. Careful planning during the protocol design stage is essential to allow valid and meaningful analysis of HRQL data. Continued attention should be directed to ensuring: (1) the HRQL objective of the study is clinically relevant; (2) appropriate measures from validated instruments are used; (3) enough patients in a given disease setting (e.g., symptomatic patients) are enrolled in the trial to address the study objective; and (4) the HRQL data are accurately recorded and analyzed without bias by appropriate statistical methods that have been prospectively described. Improvement in tumor-related symptoms (or prolongation in time to symptomatic progression) represents evidence of clinical benefit for cancer patients and will continue to be used for decision making in granting marketing approval to new oncology drugs.

ACKNOWLEDGMENT

The authors thank Dr. Clare Gnecco from the Food and Drug Administration for helpful discussion of statistical issues during the preparation of this manuscript.

REFERENCES

1. Transcript of the Quality of Life Subcommittee of the Oncologic Drug Advisory Committee to the Food and Drug Administration, February 10, 2000.
2. Johnson JR, Williams G, Pazdun R. Endpoints for FDA approval of Oncology Drugs. ASCO abstract #1018, 2002.

3. World Health Organization. *The First Ten Years of the World Health Organization.* Geneva: WHO. 1958.

4. Testa MA, Simonson DC. Assessment of quality-of- life outcomes. *N Engl J Med* 1996; 334:835–840.

5. Osoba D. Lessons learned from measuring health-related quality of life in oncology. *J Clin Oncol* 1994; 12:608–616.

6. Wilson IB, Cleary PD. Linking clinical variables with health-related quality of life-a conceptual model of patient outcomes. JAMA 1995; 273:59–65.

7. Beitz J. Quality-of-life endpoints in oncology drug trials. Oncology 1999; 13:1439–1445.

8. Aaronson NK. Methodologic issues in assessing the quality of life of cancer patients. Cancer 1991; 67(3 suppl):844–850.

9. Gnecco C, Lachenbruch PA. Regulatory aspects of quality of life. In: Mesbah M, et al., eds. *Statistical Methods for Quality of Life Studies, Design, Measurement and Analysis.* Dordrecht: Kluwer Academic. 2002.

10. Beitz J, Gneco C, Justice R. Quality-of-life endpoints in cancer clinical trials: The U.S. Food and Drug Administration Perspective. *J Natl Cancer Inst Monogr* 1996; 20.

11. Osoba D, Rodrigues G, Myles J, Zee B, Pater J. Interpreting the significance of changes in health-related quality-of-life scores. *J Clin Oncol* 1998; 16:139–144.

12. Jaeschke R, Singer J, Guyatt GH. Measurement of health status: ascertaining the minimal clinically important difference. *Control Clin Trial* 1989; 10:407–415.

13. Lydick E, Epstein RS. Interpretation of quality of life changes. *Quality Life Res* 1993; 2:221–226.

22

The Role of the Oncology Drug Advisory Committee in the FDA Review Process for Oncologic Products

Leslie A. Vaccari, BSN, RAC

CONTENTS

INTRODUCTION
ODAC FUNCTION
ODAC STRUCTURE AND MEMBERSHIP
PREPARATION FOR THE ODAC MEETING
ODAC MEETING CONDUCT
CONCLUSION

1. INTRODUCTION

Whether or not the topic of the Oncology Drug Advisory Committee (ODAC) sounds interesting or not, no one can afford not to read every word written on the subject, because the role of the ODAC in the review process for oncological products is often misunderstood. The role of the ODAC is simple, but the expectations for the committee's performance range from the misconception that the ODAC approves drugs to the lack of confidence that ODAC impacts Food and Drug Administration (FDA) decisions.

In reality, the ODAC falls in the middle of the spectrum of these expectations. When there are close-call situations in the review process during which the safety and efficacy of the product is not clearly substantiated by the data, the FDA requests ODAC's advice on applications to supplement and balance their expertise. This is the typical and most common type of ODAC meeting. The scheduling of an application for presentation before ODAC is made during the review of an application only when the FDA review division determines that ODAC's advice would be beneficial to the FDA's review.

Oncological products presented to ODAC may be drugs, biologics, or combination drug- or biological-device products. Biological products may be presented before either the ODAC or the Biological Response Modifier Advisory Committee. The presentation of an oncologic product to ODAC is a milestone for both the product development

From: *Cancer Drug Discovery and Development:*
Anticancer Drug Development Guide: Preclinical Screening, Clinical Trials, and Approval, 2nd Ed.
Edited by: B. A. Teicher and P. A. Andrews © Humana Press Inc., Totowa, NJ

timeline and also for the FDA's application review timeline. Therefore, it is essential, even as early as phase I, to become an astute observer of this process. By observing ODAC meetings regularly, attendees can not only learn how the committee functions but can take advantage of the opportunity to look through this unique FDA window. Observers at ODAC meetings gain knowledge of the FDA review process for oncology products and of the regulatory strategies to use or avoid in the oncological product development process. No matter where a product is on the development continuum, it is never too early to develop a thorough understanding of the purpose and function of the ODAC, because meetings at which similar products are presented may not occur frequently. The development of a clear understanding of the ODAC's role and function will result in a realistic approach to the overwhelming task of preparation for and participation in the ODAC meeting process.

The ODAC affects the FDA drug review process both directly and indirectly. The ODAC affects the review process directly for the specific product presented because ODAC's recommendations are taken into consideration by the FDA during the subsequent review process. Indirectly, the ODAC meetings influence the current cancer products in development. At open, public ODAC meetings, all drug developers benefit by having access to the applicant's and FDA's meeting materials for the pending applications. By observing the FDA's presentation of their concerns and questions before ODAC and the resulting interactions and deliberations, an appreciation is gained of ODAC's role in the FDA review process. As a result, the product development process also becomes much clearer.

In the following discussion, the overall function of ODAC is described. A comprehensive understanding of the ODAC and its purpose is critical in order to develop realistic expectations about the Committee's performance.

2. ODAC FUNCTION

The function of ODAC is consistent with other FDA advisory committees that meet to provide independent expert medical and scientific advice to the FDA regarding the safety, effectiveness, and appropriate use of products that are under its jurisdiction. In the last decade, the performance and availability of the resources afforded by advisory committee meetings has enhanced the FDA review of all drug and biological products for the treatment of cancer. In addition, the advisory committee process affords cancer patients and cancer advocate groups the opportunity to impact on the cancer therapy review and approval process. It is the goal of the FDA to make the advisory committee process as transparent as possible while complying with the requirements of the law.

As established in the Committee's Charter, the ODAC advises the Commissioner of the FDA or designee in discharging responsibilities to ensure safe and effective drugs and other products for human use for which the FDA has regulatory responsibility. The Sunshine Act of 1977 ensures that all drug advisory committee meetings are public meetings except when an open discussion of the agenda item would be an invasion of privacy or when confidential, commercial, or trade secret information is presented and discussed. All advisory committee recommendations are offered as advice and are not binding on the FDA decisions for the applications under review. The ODAC, like all advisory committees, functions under a charter that must be renewed every 2 yr. The renewal must be approved by both the Secretary of Health and Human Services and the Administrator of the General Services Administration. The charter is available on the FDA website at www.fda.gov/cder/audiences/acspage/acslist.htm.

3. ODAC STRUCTURE AND MEMBERSHIP

The ODAC is composed of a core group consisting of the chairperson and 12 members that includes clinical scientists, one consumer representative, one patient representative, and one industry representative. To ensure the independence and diversity of the committee, clinical scientists are selected with extensive experience in clinical research from a broad and diverse range of backgrounds and expertise. Usually three to four new clinical scientists are named to the committee yearly, because members generally serve a 4-yr term. The nonscientific representative role on the committee was created in recent years and expands the ODAC's diversity by including consumers, patients with cancer, and an industry constituent.

The consumer representative is a voting member of the committee who serves a 4-yr term and ensures representation of the consumer perspective on issues and actions before the committee. The consumer representative must be able to analyze data, understand research design, discuss benefits and risks, and evaluate the safety and effectiveness of products under review. A patient representative is selected from a standing panel of patient representatives who serve 2-yr terms.

There is a patient representative for each session of the ODAC meeting with a background based on the treatment of the disease being discussed. The patient representative may or may not be a voting member but is always expected to represent the particular interests of a patient with the disease being treated by the product under evaluation. Patient representatives only serve on ODAC and other committees that review products and therapies relating to serious and life-threatening diseases.

The industry representative is a relatively new addition to the membership complement as stipulated in the Food and Drug Administration Modernization Act passed by Congress in 1997. As a nonvoting member, the industry representative serves a 4-yr term to act on behalf of regulated industry at ODAC meetings. The representative evaluates and discusses issues before ODAC from the perspective of the affected industry and not as an individual from a specific pharmaceutical company.

4. PREPARATION FOR THE ODAC MEETING

4.1. Notification of Meetings

Meetings are tentatively scheduled a year in advance in order to provide the appropriate times for the reviewing division to present applications and to accommodate application review goal dates. Additional meetings may be scheduled as needed, and tentatively scheduled meetings may be cancelled if input from the committee is not needed. The tentative meeting schedule is published yearly in the *Federal Register*. Specific meeting announcements including agendas also appear in the *Federal Register*. Pending applications are scheduled for presentation to the ODAC very shortly after submission to the FDA. During the Investigational New Drug (IND) stage of development, it is in a sponsor's best interest to pose the question of the possibility of presentation of the application before the ODAC. As a result, a timely dialogue regarding the timelines and requirements for the background package can occur. At the time of submission of the application to the FDA, contact with the ODAC Executive Secretary at the Advisory and Consultant Staff of the Center for Drug Evaluation and Research (CDER) may be helpful, especially when special scheduling considerations will be needed. The staff contacts are available on the website www.fda.gov/cder/audiences/acspage.

4.2. Configuration of the ODAC for a Meeting

An ODAC meeting can only be convened with a minimum quorum. The ODAC Charter states that the FDA may, in connection with a particular committee meeting, specify a quorum that is less than a majority of the current-voting members owing to the size of the Committee and the variety in the types of issues that it will consider. The membership of the core Committee may be expanded to include recognized expert consultants who will provide unique scientific expertise regarding issues being addressed for specific oncology products. These consultants perform as Special Government Employees with voting privileges.

4.3. Conflict of Interest

In advance of a scheduled meeting and before any confidential information is provided for review, all ODAC members and consultants must undergo evaluation for any conflicts of interest with regard to the product or application. If there is a conflict of interest, the member is either excluded or granted a waiver. If the FDA's need for the member's participation outweighs the conflict of interest, a waiver is granted after careful evaluation. The FDA Waiver Criteria 2000 provides the information on the FDA's management of conflict of interest issues. The criteria within the document do not translate to rigid decisions, and each situation is evaluated within the context and consideration of all factors involved. On average, every meeting has several members who have received waivers that are disclosed at the opening of the meeting. It is important for industry staff to remain alert to these disclosures. The disclosure statement my reveal important information about the member who may be considered for involvement in a future product's development. The waiver criteria are available on the website www.fda.gov/oc/advisory.

4.4. Preparation Materials Provided to Advisory Committee Members

In order to prepare for an ODAC meeting, members are provided with both the FDA's and sponsor's preparation materials before the meeting. In collaboration with the ODAC Chairperson, the FDA finalizes the questions to be posed to the Committee. It is expected that all members will come to the meeting prepared to comment on the basis of their review of the materials provided. The applicant and FDA presentations before the ODAC provide clarification of the meeting materials that have been reviewed by the members.

4.5. Public Access to Materials for ODAC Meetings

Before January 1, 2000, preparation materials provided to any FDA advisory committee for open meetings were not available to the public in written form prior to or after the meetings. As a result of the final court agreement among the Public Citizen, the FDA, and the Pharmaceutical Research and Manufacturers of America, CDER now makes all materials available either 24 h before the meeting or at the meeting when it is practical. This procedure complies with the disclosure requirements of the Federal Advisory Committee Act (the FACA; 5 U.S.C. App. 2) agreement and FDA's regulation governing disclosure of information concerning new drug applications in 21 CFR 314.430. This requirement does not apply to a Biologic Licensing Applications (BLA) or Premarket Approval Application (PMA) unless the product is used in combination with a drug.

In order for the CDER Advisors and Consultant Staff to accomplish this required disclosure process, submission of a sponsor's briefing package must be made as recommended in the CDER guidance document entitled Guidance for Industry, Disclosure of Materials Provided to Advisory Committee Meeting Convened by the Center for Drug Evaluation and Research Beginning on January 1, 2000. The restrictive deadlines that are imposed to meet the requirements for disclosure of the ODAC meeting preparation materials can impact on the timelines of the 6-mo priority reviews. The ODAC meeting is normally scheduled within 4–5 mo of receipt of an application targeted for a priority review. When the applicant designates the background package to be exempt from the disclosure requirements, the FDA will consider this designation to be the applicant's agreement to extend the review time by 2 mo for the review cycle in which the meeting will be held. No adjustment to the review timeline is made for standard review applications of 10 mo. Guidance for industry for disclosure of information provided to advisory committees is available on the FDA website at www.fda.gov/cder/guidance/index.htm.

5. ODAC MEETING CONDUCT

5.1. Overview of ODAC Meeting

The conduct of ODAC meetings is consistent with the requirements for all FDA advisory committee meetings. The conflict of interest statement is read by the Executive Secretary and is usually followed by a period of time for the required open public hearing (although this may occur at any designated time during the course of the meeting). Because both the FDA and the applicant provide summary reviews of the safety and efficacy data before the meeting, the applicant's and the FDA's presentation enhance the clarity of the data for the ODAC members. Historically, the presentations have been restricted to approx 1 h to allow for the maximum amount of time for the ODAC deliberations. After the applicant's presentation and the ODAC's subsequent questions to the applicant, the FDA reviewer(s) summarizes findings from the review of the application. The interpretations of the data by the applicant and the FDA often appear divergent, dissimilar, or contradictory, but this should be expected. When the ODAC members finish questioning the FDA reviewers, further discussion of issues among the members continues in order to achieve clarity and focus. Then the ODAC members discuss and respond to the FDA questions. The Committee remains cognizant that the questions have been carefully crafted by the FDA to target the major issues that are critical to the FDA review of the application. When all questions have been voted on or addressed satisfactorily, the meeting is concluded.

5.2. Source of Available ODAC Meeting Materials

The meeting agenda, the FDA questions, and the preparation materials are made available at www.fda.gov/ohrms/dockets/as/acmenu.htm at least 24 h before the meeting in compliance with the FDA's responsibility under FACA and 21 CFR 314.340. In addition, copies of the agenda and the questions are available at the meeting. Following the meeting, the transcript of the proceedings is placed on the FDA dockets website as soon as it becomes available at www.fda.gov/ohrms/dockets/ac/acmenu.htm.

5.3. Applicant's Presentation Before ODAC

The applicant's presentation is a summary of the safety and efficacy results from the studies supporting the application. The applicant's demeanor should convey professionalism and respect for the ODAC and the FDA. No new data should be presented to the ODAC that has not been submitted in the application to the FDA. The precision and clarity of an applicant's presentation and the subsequent responses to the ODAC's questions on the data may affect the ODACs recommendations, which in turn may affect the FDA's decision on the application.

Usually, the FDA's presentation is made after the applicant's presentation and this may be the first time the applicant discovers the details of the application's deficiencies. The FDA's critique of the data will provide insight into deficiencies of the application that will have to be addressed for approval. The FDA's review of the data often provokes an adversarial atmosphere between the FDA and the applicant. Thorough premeeting preparation of all staff is imperative in order to desensitize all attendees and prevent any inappropriate response to the less than optimal findings. In addition, the applicant must be prepared to respond in a nonconfrontational manner to questions from the Committee after the FDA presentation.

5.4. ODAC's Discussion and Vote on FDA Questions

The focal point of the meeting is ODAC's final recommendations on an application or other topic presented for comment. It is crucial to have a thorough appreciation of the deliberation process to understand the final ODAC recommendations and their ramifications. Topics for presentation may include a New Drug Application (NDA), a BLA, a supplemental application for a new indication for either a drug or biologic, a discussion of the single-patient use of nonapproved oncology drugs and biologics, or a discussion of a new regulatory policies. When the topic of an ODAC meeting is an issue not specific to an application, the comments and recommendations have ramifications for development for all oncological products. The questions posed to the ODAC directly relate to the review issues of the application or global scientific or regulatory issues of interest to the FDA. The following list provides a sampling of questions with varying themes that have been posed to the ODAC:

- Do the results of the phase II trials in patients with relapsed glioblastoma multiforme provide confirmatory evidence that the product is effective in this indication?
- Is time-to-progression a surrogate for a patient benefit other than survival?
- The FDA believes the relevance of the symptom improvement data discussed above cannot be adequately evaluated without a randomized, blinded study with an adequate control arm. Does ODAC agree?

- Given the lack of clinical benefit in two large studies of the product in combination with standard first-list nonsmall-cell lung cancer (NSCLC) chemotherapy, is the Study 0039 response rate of 10% in 139 patients with resistant or refractory NSCLC reasonably likely to predict the product's clinical benefit in NSCLC?
- More that 12,000 NSCLC patients have received this product under an expanded access protocol. Please discuss what position the FDA should take on the expanded access if marketing approval of the product is not granted at this time.
- Regardless of whether this product is granted accelerated approval for treating NSCLC, additional trials may be needed. Please discuss potential study designs to demonstrate that the product provides clinical benefit to NSCLC patients.

It is the role of the ODAC to maintain flexibility to accommodate the changing agenda and needs of the FDA. The question repeatedly arises in some form of whether a positive recommendation by the ODAC will be indicative of FDA approval of the product. It is often reiterated that the FDA accepts the ODAC recommendations as advice only and must make a decision in compliance with the regulations.

6. CONCLUSION

The objective of this chapter has been to describe the role of the ODAC. When requested by the FDA, the ODAC provides independent expert medical and scientific advice regarding the safety, effectiveness, and appropriate use of products that are under its jurisdiction. The ODAC recommendations are advice and are not binding on the FDA decisions for the applications under review. Even though the recommendations are only advice, the FDA generally accepts the recommendations made by the ODAC unless there are scientific and regulatory obstructions that preclude certain FDA decisions. In addition to the advice to the FDA, there is the immediate benefit from the ODAC's deliberations on oncology drug development as well as benefit to cancer patients. The ODAC process also confirms the integrity and quality of the FDA review process.

It is essential to remember that it is never too early to develop a keen awareness of the function of the ODAC. Many sponsors of INDs with development issues do not start to prepare for their ODAC presentation until immediately prior to submission of the application, and this is a critical strategic error in planning. Oncology drug development is detailed at the ODAC meetings in the applicant's presentations. Everyone can learn from this. It should not be assumed that a product will not be presented to ODAC unless the review division specifically conveys this decision. Attend as many meetings as possible. The ODAC is a meeting of scientists who make recommendations impartially on the issues and questions posed by the FDA. Develop a thorough understanding of the ODAC and how it functions over a number of years. On the basis of a sound understanding of the ODAC, preparation for an ODAC meeting has a high probability of a reasonable expectation for success.

23

FDA Role in Cancer Drug Development and Requirements for Approval

Susan Flamm Honig, MD

CONTENTS

INTRODUCTION
SUMMARY OF FOOD AND DRUG LAW: THE STATUTORY BASIS
    FOR REGULATION
IND APPLICATIONS AND REVIEW
MEETINGS
ENDPOINTS AND TRIAL DESIGNS FOR ONCOLOGY PRODUCTS
NDA SUBMISSIONS AND REVIEW
SPECIAL REGULATORY TOPICS IN ONCOLOGY DRUG DEVELOPMENT
CONCLUSIONS

1. INTRODUCTION

The preceding chapters in this book have described screening and in vivo testing techniques to identify potential anticancer agents, animal studies needed to support a safe starting dose in humans, and fundamental aspects of clinical trial design. This chapter details the regulatory aspects of oncology drug development, review, and approval. The basis of approval, acceptable endpoints and clinical trial designs for oncology drugs, and mechanisms to decrease oncology drug development and review times are discussed. These issues are critically important to ensure good communication between the Food and Drug Administration (FDA) and industry, so that safe and effective new treatments for cancer patients can be developed carefully and efficiently.

2. SUMMARY OF FOOD AND DRUG LAW: THE STATUTORY BASIS FOR REGULATION

The Food and Drug Administration regulates drugs and biologic agents on a statutory basis enacted in the Pure Food and Drug Act of 1906, which prohibited interstate commerce of misbranded food and drugs *(1)*. The Federal Food, Drug, and Cosmetic Act was

From: *Cancer Drug Discovery and Development:*
Anticancer Drug Development Guide: Preclinical Screening, Clinical Trials, and Approval, 2nd Ed.
Edited by: B. A. Teicher and P. A. Andrews © Humana Press Inc., Totowa, NJ

passed in 1938 after the sulfanilimide-related deaths of more than 100 people and required demonstration of product safety prior to marketing *(2)*. Proof of efficacy was not required until 1962, when the Kefauver-Harris Drug Amendments were passed after thalidomide-related birth defects were identified in Europe. The amendments mandated submission of Investigational New Drug (IND) applications with supportive primary data to the FDA prior to human testing and established the requirement for informed consent prior to study participation. Comparable legislation was passed for biologic products, including the 1902 Biologics Control Act (safety and manufacturing oversight of serum, antitoxins, and vaccines), the 1944 Public Health Service Act (blood safety), the establishment of the Bureau of Biologics in 1972, and the 1973 provisions for biologic agents in the Public Health Service Act *(3)*. As reflected in the parallel legislation, drugs and biologic products were initially regulated separately in the Bureau of Drugs and the Bureau of Biologics. The Bureaus merged into the National Center for Drugs and Biologics in 1982 and then separated into the Center for Drug Evaluation and Research (CDER) and the Center for Biologics Evaluation and Research (CBER) in 1988 *(3)*. In 2002, the Office of the Commissioner announced that that review of biologic products (except for vaccines, blood cells, tissues, and gene therapy) would be transferred to CDER *(4)*. Despite these changes, it has been the practice in CDER and CBER to work closely together and to use similar standards for review and approval of oncology products.

The Code of Federal Regulations (CFR) contains specific requirements for IND applications, New Drug Applications (NDAs), and Biologic Licensing Applications (BLAs). New laws shortened product development and review times. The following sections discuss the scope of these regulations. It is important to remember that whereas scientific interchange with industry and investigators is critical to drug development and that expert knowledge and clinical judgement are required for review, these processes arise from the legislative requirements that govern the FDA.

3. IND APPLICATIONS AND REVIEW

The CFR describes the requirements for use of an investigational new drug in clinical investigations and the content and format of the IND submission *(5)*. Figure 1 illustrates the IND and drug development timelines. The IND is held by a sponsor, defined as a pharmaceutical company, an individual investigator, or an academic institution. The application must contain all available information on the chemistry and manufacturing controls (CMCs) of the drug substance, the pharmacology and drug disposition, prior human experience with the product, and the proposed clinical trial protocol. The proposed study may be designed as a phase I, II, or III trial, depending on whether the IND is for the first trial in humans or whether initial development was performed outside the United States. A phase I trial is reviewed to verify the selection of a safe starting dose. A phase II or III trial is reviewed for safety, the scientific quality of the study, and the likelihood that it will yield data permitting evaluation of drug efficacy. The sponsor may begin the proposed study 30 d after the FDA receives the IND unless the FDA notifies the sponsor that the investigation is subject to Clinical Hold *(6)*. Grounds for a Clinical Hold include

- Unreasonable and significant risk of injury or illness to the human subject
- Lack of qualified investigators

Drug Development Timeline

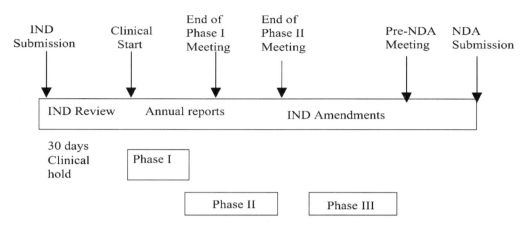

Fig. 1. Drug development timeline. IND, Investigational New Drug: NDA, New Drug Application.

- Misleading, erroneous, or incomplete Investigator's Brochure
- Insufficient data submitted to evaluate risk.

Phase II or III trials may be placed on Hold if the protocol is clearly deficient in design to meet the stated objectives. The Division Director must inform the sponsor of the Clinical Hold in a teleconference, followed by a written deficiency list. Clinical Holds are uncommon in the Division of Oncology Drug Products (DODP) and usually result from insufficient data to support the starting dose or schedule.

Once the IND has been approved, the sponsor may proceed with the requested protocol and may continue to conduct clinical trials with the investigational agent. The sponsor must submit new protocols and protocol amendments to the FDA, but no additional waiting period is required. Additional reporting requirements include changes in investigators, Information Amendments (changes in CMC, new toxicology information, trial analyses), IND safety reports, and Annual Reports.

4. MEETINGS

The Division encourages a series of meetings with the sponsor in order to understand the drug development plan and reach consensus on study designs used to support a marketing application. Regular communication with the FDA ensures that regulatory requirements and precedents are met so that well-designed and well-executed trials can efficiently determine the safety and efficacy of new products. This series of meetings can begin prior to IND submission and continue until the NDA submission.

To ensure a timely start to the clinical investigation, the sponsor may request a *pre-IND meeting (7)*. Issues for discussion include adequacy of completed animal studies to support the requested dose and schedule, problems with the drug substance or formulation, pharmacokinetic issues related to dosing schedule or active metabolites, proposed novel phase I dose-escalation schemes, or proposals for clinical monitoring of an anticipated organ toxicity.

Once clinical investigations begin, the next meeting is the *end of phase II (EOP2) meeting (8)*. The designs of the randomized controlled trials planned to support approval are reviewed. This meeting is considered critical to drug development by the Agency. The meeting usually includes a discussion of the patient population to be studied, the primary and secondary efficacy endpoints, sample size considerations, preliminary statistical plans, specific safety concerns raised in earlier studies, and the appropriate comparator. The FDA Guidance on Available Therapy cites the best comparator as a treatment labeled for the indication to be studied *(9)*. However, in oncology, many products were initially approved in the 1970s and early 1980s with broadly written indications; off-label use of oncology drugs is common. Thus, labeled indications frequently are not consistent with the clinical standard of care. The Division usually recommends a comparator that represents the current standard of care and has a quantitative assessment of efficacy derived from well-controlled clinical trials documented in the medical literature. In the DODP, an Advisory Committee member participates in the EOP2 meeting as does a patient who has personal experience with the type of cancer to be studied. These representatives provide important perspectives.

After the EOP2 meeting, sponsors are encouraged to submit the pivotal study protocols for a *Special Protocol Assessment (SPA) (10,11)*. The SPA, enacted in FDAMA, states that the FDA will review special protocols (carcinogenicity, stability, and pivotal phase III trials) within 45 d of receipt. If the FDA approves the protocol, the FDA will not change its mind unless public health concerns unrecognized at the time of the agreement emerge. Approval of the protocol by the FDA is limited to specific questions regarding trial design, sample size, and the proposed data analysis methods. Approval does not imply a commitment to general regulatory issues, such as the number of trials required for approval, a specific p-value needed to define statistical significance, or the degree of improvement in an endpoint such as time to progression or survival required to demonstrate clinical benefit.

The final meeting is the *pre-NDA meeting*, in which the sponsor presents a brief summary of the trial results *(8)*. The purpose of this meeting is to identify the appropriate studies for NDA submission, address unresolved outstanding problems, discuss data formatting, and discuss (but not rewrite) the statistical analysis plan. It is important to emphasize that prospective planning should be performed during the EOP2 meeting and SPA discussions. The pre-NDA meeting is not a venue in which to adjust the study results retrospectively for previously unappreciated critical aspects of trial design.

5. ENDPOINTS AND TRIAL DESIGNS FOR ONCOLOGY PRODUCTS

Sponsors may develop products for full, or traditional, approval or for Accelerated Approval *(10,12,13)*. Full approval is based on demonstration of clinical benefit, whereas Accelerated Approval (refractory disease only) is based on a surrogate endpoint reasonably likely to demonstrate clinical benefit. Endpoints traditionally used to demonstrate clinical benefit include survival, disease-free survival in the adjuvant setting, durable complete response (applicable in some hematologic malignancies), and palliation of tumor-related symptoms in combination with a meaningful clinical response. To date, the endpoint most commonly used to support Accelerated Approval is response rate. Response rate reflects the biologic activity of the drug product, since tumors rarely shrink spontaneously. However, because response rate has not been shown to correlate with survival and because many oncology patients in clinical trials are asymptomatic, response rate is considered a surrogate endpoint. Response rate is used for full approval only for hormonal therapies: the decreased toxicity of these agents has been traditionally considered by the FDA to outweigh the uncertainty of the magnitude of the benefit. Time to progression has been used as the basis of full approval in the second-line treatment of metastatic cancer and in combination with response rate for hormonal therapy.

In considering trial designs, it is important to define the patient population. The type of cancer, the stage of cancer, and whether the product will be developed for first-line, second-line, or refractory metastatic cancer must be determined. The sponsor must decide whether to design a superiority or a noninferiority trial based on review of phase I and phase II data, select the number of trials, and consider the design of the confirmatory study, if Accelerated Approval will be sought. It is important to consider regulatory precedents, as the Agency strives for consistency in its approach to product approval.

6. NDA SUBMISSIONS AND REVIEW

The CFR describes the New Drug Application for marketing (14). The application must contain all relevant information about CMC, preclinical pharmacology and toxicology, human pharmacokinetics and bioavailability, clinical data, and statistical analyses so that the applicant's claims of safety and efficacy can be independently verified by FDA reviewers. Case report forms (CRFs) and case report tabulations (CRTs) must be submitted to provide confirmation of individual patient results. Electronic submission of data is common, with increasing use of entirely electronic NDAs. Figure 2 illustrates the drug review and marketing timelines.

Applicants must submit Financial Disclosure information (15). The purpose of Financial Disclosure is to ensure that the applicant identifies financial interests of or arrangements with principal investigators that could affect the reliability of the data submitted to the FDA in support of a marketing application. FDA reviewers must consider whether the financial interests had an effect on the submitted data. Disclosure is required for applications for drugs, biologics, and devices and must be made for any study that demonstrates effectiveness, including bioequivalence studies that link a clinical trial formulation to a to-be-marketed formulation. The Rule took effect on February 2, 1999 and applies to all applications submitted after that date, even if the studies contained in the application were conducted prior to the effective date. Failure to provide Financial Disclosure may constitute a Refuse to File issue.

Once the NDA is submitted, the division meets (45-d Filing Meeting) to determine the filing status and the review classification of the application (16). Reasons for Refuse to File decisions are delineated in 314. 101. A Refuse to File decision is uncommon; when it occurs, it frequently results from primary data that are insufficient to permit verification of the primary endpoint. During the Filing meeting, the application is classified as a standard (10-mo) or a priority (6-mo) review. The criteria for priority review are listed in Table 1.

A multidisciplinary team, which includes a chemist, a pharmacologist, a biopharmaceutical reviewer, a physician, and a statistician, reviews the application. Communication with the applicant and processing of the application is coordinated by a

Drug Review Timeline

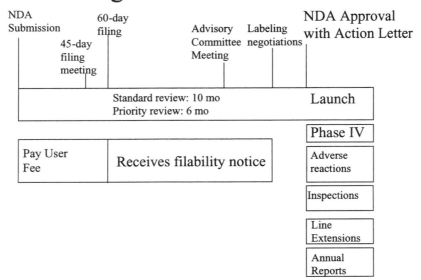

Fig. 2. Drug review timeline. NDA, New Drug Application.

Table 1
Criteria for Priority review (6 Months)

Demonstrates increased effectiveness over existing therapy
Provides therapy where none exists
Eliminates or reduces treatment-limiting adverse events
Enhances patient compliance
Demonstrates safety and efficacy in a new subpopulation

project manager. Once the reviewers agree that efficacy has been demonstrated, the relative risks and benefits are considered in determining whether the application is approved. The application may be discussed at the Oncologic Drugs Advisory Committee (ODAC) meeting in order to obtain the input of qualified oncologists on review issues.

Based on the review, the NDA may be approved, may be deemed Approvable with a list of correctable deficiencies sent to the applicant, or may be Not Approved with communication of the noncorrectable deficiencies sent to the applicant. The Division may require postmarketing (phase IV) studies to evaluate safety or efficacy in subpopulations. Also, drugs given Accelerated Approval are required to demonstrate clinical benefit in a postmarketing trial *(10,12)*. All phase IV studies must be reported to Congress on an annual basis as legislated in FDAMA *(10)*. Due diligence of the sponsor in completing the studies and due diligence of the FDA in reviewing the results of the study will be made public.

After approval, reporting requirements continue. The applicant must submit postmarketing reports of adverse events and Annual Reports containing significant new information about the drug identified in the past year. All labeling changes must be reported to and approved by the FDA.

7. SPECIAL REGULATORY TOPICS IN ONCOLOGY DRUG DEVELOPMENT

7.1. Reinventing the Regulation of Cancer Drugs (REGO)

As part of the Clinton-Gore "Reinventing Government" program in the National Performance Review, four initiatives for oncology drug review were published in March, 1996 *(13)*. These initiatives included access to cancer therapies approved in other countries, Accelerated Approval, voting patient representatives on ODAC, and exemption of some INDS for marketed products.

The first initiative evaluated access to cancer therapies approved in other countries. A survey of worldwide regulatory authorities demonstrated that most products approved in other countries but not in the United States represented first-generation therapies, whereas the United States had already approved the second- or third-generation product. Thus, this initiative led to the recognition that Americans had access to new and promising medicines for cancer and that the United States did not lag behind Europe in oncology drug approvals, as previously perceived.

The second initiative formalized the Accelerated Approval mechanism, which is discussed in detail in the next section.

The third initiative provided for a voting patient representative on ODAC. Patients participate in a series of lectures on regulatory requirements for drug approval. As mentioned in Subheading 4. (Meetings), these patients also participate in EOP2 meetings and have the opportunity to provide input for pivotal trial design.

The fourth initiative permitted exemption of INDs for marketed products when the product is used in generally the same patient population and dose/schedule for which it was approved. Exemption is permitted, therefore, when the use of the approved agent will not substantially increase patient risk. In addition, the study should not be intended to support approval of the new use or a significant change in labeling or advertising. Guidance is available on the FDA website *(17)*.

7.2. Accelerated Approval

Accelerated Approved was first legislated under Subpart E in 1988 *(18)*. This law outlined procedures to expedite the development and approval of new therapies to treat patients with life-threatening and severely debilitating illnesses for which no satisfactory alternative treatments exist. It provided the potential for NDA approval on the basis of phase II trials and was intended to expedite the development of drugs for HIV-related disease in particular. Subsequently, the Clinton-Gore REGO initiatives included Accelerated Approval and emphasized its applicability to cancer therapies (1996) *(13)*. The initiative stated that marketing approval for drugs for serious and life-threatening illnesses could be granted based on a surrogate endpoint "reasonably likely to predict clinical benefit." Additional studies confirming clinical benefit must be completed after approval. Accelerated Approval was restated in FDAMA to emphasize its applicability to any serious and life-threatening illness (including diseases other than HIV-related or cancer) without available therapy *(10)*.

Table 2
Drugs Approved Under Accelerated Approval

Dexrazoxane (Zinecard®)
Docetaxel (Taxotere®)
Irinotecan (Camptosar®)
Liposomal doxorubicin (Doxil®—two indications)
Capecitabine (Xeloda®)
Cytarabine liposomal injection (Depocyt®)
Temozolomide (Temodar®)
Celecoxib (Celebrex®)
Gemtuzumab (Mylotarg™)
Imatinib mesylate/STI-571 (Gleevec™, two indications)
Oxaliplatin (Eloxatin™)
Amifostine (Ethyol®)
Anastrozole (Arimidex®)
Gefitinib (Iressa®)

To date, 14 oncology drugs have been granted 12 indications under Accelerated Approval (Table 2). Response rate has been the most commonly used surrogate endpoint. Several drugs completed postmarketing studies in order to convert to Full Approval. Studies are ongoing for the remaining products. Although this process does not decrease the amount or quality of data required to support approval, it can expedite the availability of an effective drug to a refractory population.

7.3. Fast Track

FDAMA included a new provision for Fast Track designation designed to facilitate development and expedite review of drugs and biologics for serious or life-threatening disease that demonstrate the potential to address unmet medical needs *(10)*. Fast Track applies to products used for the diagnosis, prevention, or treatment of a serious and life-threatening disease, or of a serious side effect or complication of the disease. Both the disease itself and the specific aspect of the disease to be treated must be serious and life-threatening. Thus, a therapy designed to improve survival in a cancer patient has the potential to qualify for Fast Track. In contrast, a product that prevents alopecia, despite its potential to improve quality of life significantly in cancer patients, does not treat a life-threatening aspect of cancer and would not qualify that product for Fast Track consideration. In addition, the product must have the potential to address an "unmet medical need," defined in the Guidance *(19)*. The product must treat a disease without available therapy, must be anticipated to have efficacy superior to available therapy, must provide benefit comparable to available therapy but with less toxicity or different toxicity or better compliance, or affect a serious aspect of the disease not treated by available therapy. If granted, the Fast Track designation refers to the overall development plan for the drug and describes a collaborative series of meetings between the sponsor and the Agency. It should be noted that this meeting schedule is available to any sponsor developing products for any indication and is not limited to Fast Track designees.

The unique advantage to Fast Track is Submission of Portions of an Application (SoPA). At present, in CDER but not in CBER, sponsors may presubmit completed CMC and preclinical pharmacology sections prior to submission of the complete NDA. Fast

Track designation permits rolling submissions. Sponsors must submit reviewable, complete sections of the NDA, but broader definitions of "reviewable unit" can be used. The reader is referred to the draft guidances for Continuous Marketing Applications on the FDA website *(20,21)*.

It is expected that the NDA application will be complete within 12 months of the first submission. The sponsor must negotiate the timeline for submission of the NDA with the review division. User fees must be paid at the time of the first submission.

Fast Track status can be requested as early as the time of IND submission and as late as the pre-NDA meeting. The type of data used to support the Fast Track request must be consistent with the stage of development at the time Fast Track is requested. Thus, at the IND stage, preclinical and animal data are acceptable. Requests made during phase II must be supported by phase II human data.

Because Fast Track refers to the combination of the product and the specific treatment, Fast Track designation is conferred on the indication, not the product itself. Separate applications must be made for each indication, and each will be considered independently. Thus, a sponsor who develops a product for lung cancer, colon cancer, and breast cancer must submit three Fast Track applications if the data warrant such an expectation; one application will not cover all proposed uses of the drug.

It is important to note that although this book describes oncology drug development, the Fast Track mechanism applies to products developed for any serious and life-threatening disease. Products for diseases such as Alzheimer's disease, stroke, advanced debilitating rheumatoid arthritis, coronary syndrome, diabetic vascular compromise, and many others are appropriate for Fast Track applications.

Although the criteria for Fast Track are similar to those used for other programs, there are important differences between Fast Track and other legislation, as follows:

1. *Fast Track is not the same as priority review*. Priority review means that a submitted NDA has been determined to demonstrate a significant improvement in safety or effectiveness compared with standard therapy (Table 1) and has been assigned to a 6-month review clock. Fast Track refers to the entire development process; Priority review refers to the length of time needed to review an application, after development is complete. Fast Track drugs will usually fulfill the criteria for Priority review, but such a designation can only be made after preliminary review of the efficacy findings from the completed NDA. Drugs without Fast Track designation may also be granted Priority review status.
2. *Fast Track is not the same as Treatment Use of a new drug*. Treatment Use (also called Expanded Access or Compassionate Use) refers to drugs provided to patients with serious or life-threatening illnesses without available therapy while the NDA is prepared or reviewed. It describes availability of the new drug at the end of the drug development timeline, whereas Fast Track refers to the drug development process. Fast Track products are often good candidates for Treatment Use protocols, but non-Fast Track drugs may qualify as well.
3. *Fast Track is not the same as Accelerated Approval*. Both Accelerated Approval and Fast Track apply to drugs developed for serious and life-threatening diseases, and the definition of "serious and life-threatening" is the same for both. Accelerated Approval refers to the use of a surrogate endpoint as the basis of approval, with subsequent confirmation of clinical benefit. Fast Track products are frequently good candidates for Accelerated Approval but may be developed for full or traditional approval. Products without Fast Track designation may use the Accelerated Approval mechanism.

Table 3
Supplemental Indications Potentially Supported by One Efficacy Trial

For approval in a second cancer biologically similar to the approved cancer
For approval in children with the same type of cancer as that approved in adults (if the cancer and
    drug have similar biologic behavior in children and adults)
For approval in a second cancer of an agent that reduces adverse treatment effects but does not
    interfere with treatment efficacy in the approved cancer
For approval of a new dosing regimen
For approval in an earlier stage of the approved refractory cancer
For approval of monotherapy when the product is approved for combination therapy

Table 4
Characteristics of a Convincing Single Trial to Support Efficacy

Large sample size
Randomized trial
Prospective design and statistical plan
Multicenter study
Statistically powerful findings
Statistically significant results for multiple endpoints
Results consistent across strata
Results consistent across subsets
Results consistent between centers

7.4. Use of One Trial to Support Safety and Efficacy

The regulations state that the basis of approval rests on the demonstration of efficacy with acceptable safety in adequate and well-controlled trials. The use of the plural form in the regulations has been interpreted as a requirement for at least two trials. Two guidances, Clinical Evidence of Effectiveness for Human Drug and Biologic Products and FDA Approval of New Cancer Treatment Uses for Marketed Drug and Biologic Products, were published and subsequently legislated in FDAMA *(22,23)*. These guidances describe the circumstances under which a single trial can be used as the basis of approval for marketed products (Table 3). Characteristics of a single study that provide convincing evidence of efficacy are summarized in Table 4. Submission of one trial leaves little room for problems with the trial design or inconsistencies in the data. The use of one trial is preferred when where the results of the first trial make it unethical to perform a second study.

The guidances and FDAMA reiterate that alternate sources of study data, such as data from cooperative group trials or from foreign centers, can be used to support approval *(10,22,24)*. The DODP has approved many drugs using cooperative (Table 5) and foreign data.

7.5. Clinical Trials Databank

The Clinical Trials Databank was established as mandated in FDAMA and requires submission of information about all efficacy trials (phase II, III, and IV studies, treatment IND protocols, and group C studies) for serious and life-threatening diseases, whether

Table 5
Drugs Approved Using Cooperative Group Data

Cooperative group	Drug	Indication
RTOG	Ethyol	Xerostomia after radiotherapy, head/neck
SWOG	Carboplatin	Ovarian cancer
NCCTG	Leucovorin and 5-FU	Metastatic colorectal cancer
NCIC	Mitoxantrone	Prostate cancer
GOG	Taxol	First-line ovarian cancer
ECOG	Taxol	Nonsmall-cell lung cancer
NSABP	Tamoxifen	1. To reduce the risk of breast cancer in women at high risk of breast cancer 2. Ductal carcinoma *in situ*
Intergroup	Taxol	Node-positive adjuvant breast cancer
Intergroup	Temozolomide	Anaplastic astrocytoma

federally or privately funded *(10,25)*. Information about the trial design, eligibility criteria, trial sites, and contact information must be entered in language readily understood by the public. Submission of information for other trials, including Treatment Use studies, is encouraged. It is hoped that establishment of a comprehensive database will increase patients' ability to access information about clinical trials for which they are eligible and to improve accrual to studies designed to support marketing of important medicines for serious and life-threatening illnesses.

7.6. Pediatric Initiatives

In an effort to obtain needed pediatric studies, Congress enacted the Pediatric Rule, Pediatric Exclusivity, and, most recently, the Best Pharmaceuticals for Children Act. Each of these important pieces of legislation will be discussed in turn.

The Pediatric Rule (1998) required pediatric studies for new drugs when the requested indication in adults also exists in children *(26–28)*. The Rule was invalidated in Federal District Court in October 2002.

Because many drugs are developed for adult indications that do not exist in children, Section 111 of FDAMA (1997) created Pediatric Exclusivity *(10,29)*. Pediatric Exclusivity encourages voluntary submission of pediatric studies for any disease for products with existing patent protection. The FDA issues a Written Request to the sponsor, which contains specific information about the type, number, and design of the requested studies and a deadline for submitting the completed study reports. If the results provide important pediatric information, whether positive or negative, the sponsor may receive an additional 6 months of exclusivity for all approved indications for the studied drug. The review may result in labeling changes important for safe and effective use of the product in children.

The Best Pharmaceuticals for Children Act (2002) established a research fund to encourage pediatric studies for drugs without exclusivity or patent protection *(30)*. The sponsor of the approved application has the right of first refusal. If the sponsor refuses the Written Request, the Request is open to any sponsor or to the National Institutes of Health (NIH). The resulting exclusivity attaches to the sponsor who actually performs the study. The Act also states that if sponsors of drugs with patent protection decline the Written Request, FDA may refer the Request to the Foundation for NIH for further study.

This legislation, as well as the establishment of the Office of Pediatric Therapeutics at the FDA and of two pediatric advisory committees, will help to ensure that the best possible treatments can be safely provided to children *(31)*.

8. CONCLUSIONS

The responsibility for the regulation of cancer treatments lies with the FDA. Although development and review of products is based in legislation, the Agency can adapt to changing scientific and clinical considerations. Oncology products are developed and reviewed in close cooperation with the pharmaceutical industry, oncology experts in academic and private practice, patients and their advocacy groups, and other parts of the federal government including the National Cancer Institute. Together, our efforts provide safe and effective cancer products to the American public.

REFERENCES

1. Federal Food and Drugs Act of 1906 (the "Wiley Act"), public law number 59-384, 34 STAT. 768 (1906), 21 U.S.C. Sec 1-15 (1934).
2. Federal Food, Drug, and Cosmetic Act, title 21, as amended by the FDA Modernization Act of 1997. Washington, DC: U.S. Government Printing Office.
3. Science and the regulation of biological products, CBER Centennial Committee, www.fda.gov/cber/inside/cberbkp.1.pdf, September, 2002.
4. http://www.fda.gov/bbs/topics/NEWS/2002/NEW00834.html.
5. 21CFR 312.
6. 21 CFR 312.42.
7. 21 CFR 312.82.
8. 21 CFR 312.47.
9. Draft Guidance for Industry: Available Therapy, www.fda.gov/cder/guidance/3057dft.htm, posted 2/6/2002.
10. Food and Drug Modernization Act of 1997, Public law 105-115, 111 STAT. 2296 (1997), 21 U.S. C. 301.
11. Guidance for Industry: Special Protocol Assessment, http://www.fda.gov/cder/guidance/3764fnl.htm, May, 2002.
12. 21 CFR part 314.500.
13. Reinventing the Regulation of Cancer Drugs, National Performance Review, Clinton and Gore, March 1996. Washington, DC: U.S. Government Printing Office.
14. 21 CFR part 314.
15. 21 CFR 54 2/2/98 and 12/31/98.
16. 21 CFR 314.101.
17. Draft Guidance for Industry: IND Exemptions for Studies of Lawfully Marketed Cancer Drug or Biological Products, http://www.fda.gov/cder/guidance/3760dft.pdf, posted 4/9/2002.
18. 21 CFR 312.80.
19. Guidance for Industry: Fast Track Drug Development Programs—Designation, Development, and Application Review, http://www.fda.gov/cder/guidance/2112fnl.pdf, posted 11/17/1998.
20. Guidance for Industry: Continuous Marketing Applications: Pilot 1—Reviewable Units for Fast Track Products Under PDUFA. http://www.fda.gov/cder/guidance/5739-fnl.doc. October 2003.
21. Guidance for Industry: Continuous Marketing Applications: Pilot 2—Scientific Feedback and Interactions During Development of Fast Track Products Under PDUFA. http://www.fda.gov/cder/guidance/5740-fnl.doc. October 2003.
22. Guidance for Industry: FDA Approval of New Cancer Treatment Uses for Marketed Drug and Biological Products, http://www.fda.gov/cder/guidance/1484fnl.htm, posted 2/2/1999.

23. Guidance for Industry: Providing Clinical Evidence of Effectiveness for Human Drug and Biological Products, http://www.fda.gov/cder/guidance/1397fnl.pdf, posted 5/14/1998.

24. Guidance for Industry: Acceptance of Foreign Clinical Studies, http://www.fda.gov/cder/guidance/fstud.htm, posted 3/12/2001.

25. Guidance for Industry: Information Program on Clinical Trials for Serious or Life-Threatening Diseases: Establishment of a Data Bank, http://www.fda.gov/cder/graveyard/guidance/3585dft.htm, posted 3/28/2000.

26. 21 CFR 314.55 (a).

27. 21 CFR 601.27 (a).

28. Guidance for Industry: Recommendations for Complying with the Pediatric Rule, http://www.fda.gov/cder/guidance/3578dft.htm, posted November, 2000.

29. Guidance for Industry: Qualifying for Pediatric Exclusivity under Section 505A of the Federal Food, Drug, and Cosmetic Act, http://www.fda.gov/cder/guidance/2414fnl.htm, June, 1998.

30. Best Pharmaceuticals for Children Act, amendment to the Federal Food, Drug, and Cosmetic Act.

31. Pediatric Medicine page, http://www.fda.gov/cder/pediatric/index.htm.

Index

Accelerated Approval, new oncology drugs, 435, 436

Acute myelocytic leukemia in Brown Norway rat (BNML), minimal residual tumor biomarker model, 246–248

ADME-Tox assays, high-throughput screening, 33, 34

Adriamycin, orthotopic metastatic mouse model studies, 204

Alamar Blue, vital staining for drug screening in vitro, 14–17

Angiogenesis,
    drug screening utility, 180
    in vitro assays,
        aortic ring assays, 162
        applications, 162, 164
        chemotaxis assay, 160, 161
        cord formation assay, 159, 160
        growth inhibition assay, 158, 159
        overview, 157, 158
    in vivo assays,
        Matrigel plug assay, 164
        syngeneic tumor models, 165
        TNP-470 activity in xenograft models, 166–168

B

Batimastat (BB-94), orthotopic metastatic mouse model studies, 201

BB-94, see Batimastat

B-cell leukemia/lymphoma murine model (BCL1), minimal residual tumor biomarker model, 248, 249

BCL1, see B-cell leukemia/lymphoma murine model

Bevacizumab, phase II trials, 373, 374

Bladder cancer,
    dog model, 274, 275
    orthotopic metastatic mouse models, 191

BNML, see Acute myelocytic leukemia in Brown Norway rat

Breast cancer,
    cat mammary tumors, 272, 273
    dog mammary tumors,
        clinical features, 272
        relevance to human disease, 272
        treatment, 272
    orthotopic metastatic mouse models, 198

Brown Norway rat, see Acute myelocytic leukemia in Brown Norway rat

C

Cancer,
    animal kingdom distribution, 101
    mortality, 63
    prevalence, 63

Cancer Research UK,
    Drug Development Office, 391, 392
    drug development examples, 382, 391–395
    grants, 390, 391
    Phase I/II Committee,
        historical perspective, 391
        trials,
            cytotoxics and antiendocrine agents, 394
            novel targets and mechanisms of action, 393, 394
            pharmacodynamic endpoints, 394, 395
            targeted therapy, 392, 393
    preclinical collaborations, 383–385

Cancer vaccines, nonclinical testing, 333, 334

Carboplatin, scheduling and sequencing of high-dose therapy, 234

Cat models,
    advantages of companion animal models, 260, 261
    cancer epidemiology, 261
    cell lines, 261, 262
    hemangiosarcoma,
        clinical features, 268
        treatment, 268, 269
    in vivo assessments, 262
    mammary tumors, 272, 273
    non-Hodgkin's lymphoma,
        classification, 266
        etiology, 265, 266
        incidence, 265
        relevance to human disease, 266
        treatment, 266
    pathogenesis of tumors, 262, 263
    soft tissue sarcoma,
        classification, 266–268
        etiology, 266
        incidence, 266
        relevance to human disease, 268
        treatment, 268

Cisplatin,
    combination therapy preclinical model analysis, 219, 220
    drug delivery systems in dog model of osteosarcoma, 271

Clonogenic assays, see also Human tumor cloning assay,

drug screening in vitro, 5, 6
principles, 64, 65
Colon cancer, orthotopic metastatic mouse
models, 190, 191
Combination therapy nonclinical testing, *see*
Oncology drug product nonclinical
testing
Combination therapy preclinical models,
endpoints, 213, 214
high-dose therapy scheduling and sequencing,
231, 232, 234, 235
isobologram method, 218, 221–223, 225, 226
median effect/combination index method,
218–221
stem cell support model, 226–229
tumor excision assay, 214–218
Contract research organization (CRO),
common problems in toxicology testing, 310,
311
toxicology study outsourcing,
criteria for selection, 307–309
monitoring toxicology studies, 309, 310
quotation request, 309
CRO, *see* Contract research organization
CT1746, orthotopic metastatic mouse model
studies, 201, 202
CS-682, metastatic mouse model study, 204
Cyclophosphamide,
combination therapy preclinical model
analysis, 222, 223
scheduling and sequencing of high-dose
therapy, 231, 232, 234
Cytotoxic drugs, categorization by drug
administration schedule for animal
tumor models, 110, 111

D

DDG, *see* Drug Development Group
Developmental Therapeutics Program (DTP),
functions, 339–341
grants and contracts programs, 347
repositories, 347
Web site, 41, 348
Dog models,
advantages of companion animal models, 260,
261
bladder carcinoma, 274, 275
cancer epidemiology, 261
cell lines, 261, 262
hemangiosarcoma,
clinical features, 268
treatment, 268, 269
in vivo assessments, 262
mammary tumors,
clinical features, 272
relevance to human disease, 272
treatment, 272
non-Hodgkin's lymphoma,
classification, 263, 264
incidence, 263

prognostic factors, 265
relevance to human disease, 265
treatment, 265
oral melanoma,
clinical features, 273, 274
prognosis, 274
treatment, 274
osteosarcoma,
cisplatin drug delivery systems, 271
clinical features, 269, 270
L-MTP-PE immunotherapy, 269, 271
pathogenesis of tumors, 262, 263
soft tissue sarcoma,
classification, 266–268
etiology, 266
incidence, 266
relevance to human disease, 268
treatment, 268
Doxorubicin, in mouse model study, 204, 205
Drug Development Group (DDG),
collaboration, 34
functions, 341–343, 345
DTP, *see* Developmental Therapeutics Program
DX-895, orthotopic metastatic mouse model
studies, 203

E

Eastern Cooperative Oncology Group (ECOG)
performance status scale, clinical
trial patient selection, 357, 366
ECOG performance status scale, *see* Eastern
Cooperative Oncology Group
performance status scale
EMT-6/CTX cells, tumor excision assay, 217,
218
EMT-6/Parent tumors, tumor excision assay,
214–218
Endpoints, *see also* Health-related quality of life;
Tumor-related symptoms,
combination therapy preclinical models, 213,
214
phase II clinical trials,
clinical endpoints, 369
molecular endpoints, 370–372
pharmacokinetic endpoints, 369, 370
phase III clinical trials,
health-related quality of life, 407, 412,
415, 416, 419
objective tumor response, 407, 408
palliation, 407
survival, 406
time to progression, 406, 407
time to treatment failure, 407
tumor-related symptoms, 407
toxicology studies,
body weight, 301
clinical pathology, 303
clinical signs, 300–303
food consumption, 301
histopathology, 304–307

sampling volumes and good practices, 303, 304

tumor characterization in rodent tumor models, 115, 116

EORTC, *see* European Organization for Research and Treatment of Cancer

Etoposide, combination therapy preclinical model analysis, 220, 221

European drug development, *see also* Cancer Research UK; European Organization for Research and Treatment of Cancer,

academic networks, 382, 383

European Drug Development Network, 383

harmonization of European regulatory trials, 395, 396

preclinical collaborations, 383–385

European Organization for Research and Treatment of Cancer (EORTC),

drug development examples, 386, 388

Laboratory Division Research, 388, 389

New Drug Advisory Committee, 386

New Drug Development Group goals and trials, 387, 388

New Drug Development Program, 386, 387

preclinical collaborations, 383–385

structure, 385, 386

Translational Research Advisory Committee, 386

translational research, 389, 390

F

Fast Track designation, new oncology drugs, 436–438

FCS, *see* Fluorescence correlation spectroscopy

FDA, *see* Food and Drug Administration

FISH, *see* Fluorescence *in situ* hybridization

Fluorescence correlation spectroscopy (FCS), high-throughput screening, 30

Fluorescence *in situ* hybridization (FISH), minimal residual disease detection, 249, 250, 253, 254

Fluorescence polarization (FP), high-throughput screening, 28, 29

Fluorescence resonance energy transfer (FRET), high-throughput screening, 28, 29

5-Fluorouracil, orthotopic metastatic mouse model studies, 192

Food and Drug Administration (FDA),

end of phase II meeting, 432

endpoints and trial designs for oncology products, 432, 433

Investigational New Drug applications and review, 430, 431

New Drug Application submissions and review, 433–435

Oncology Drug Advisory Committee, *see* Oncology Drug Advisory Committee

pre-IND meeting, 431

pre-NDA meeting, 432

regulatory reform,

Accelerated Approval, 435, 436

Clinical Trials Databank, 438, 439

Fast Track designation, 436–438

pediatric initiatives, 439, 440

single trial support of safety and efficacy, 438

Special Protocol Assessment, 432

statutory basis for regulation, 429, 430

FP, *see* Fluorescence polarization

FR-118487, orthotopic metastatic mouse model studies, 205

FRET, *see* Fluorescence resonance energy transfer

G

G-CSF, *see* Granulocyte colony-stimulating factor

Gemcitabine,

combination therapy preclinical model analysis, 219, 220, 225, 226

orthotopic metastatic mouse model studies, 202

Gene therapy, nonclinical testing, 330–332

GFP, *see* Green fluorescent protein

GI_{50}, calculation, 18, 19

Granulocyte colony-stimulating factor (G-CSF), cell protection from chemotoxicity, 228, 229

Green fluorescent protein (GFP), orthotopic metastatic mouse models,

dual-color imaging of tumor–host interaction, 207

imaging of tumors, 192, 193, 197–199

H

Halichondrin B, pharmacological characterization, 175, 176

Head and neck cancer, orthotopic metastatic mouse models, 193, 194

Health-related quality of life (HRQL),

data analysis, 418, 419

definition, 413

endpoint in phase III trials, 407, 412, 415, 416, 419

instruments, 416, 417

study design, 417

Hemangiosarcoma, dog and cat models,

clinical features, 268

treatment, 268, 269

High-throughput screening (HTS),

ADME-Tox assays, 33, 34

automation technology, 30–32

cell-based screening, 30

compound library management, 33

data management, 34–36

high-content screening, 30

historical perspective, 23, 24

homogeneous and heterogeneous assay technologies, 28, 29

lead compound discovery, 27, 28
mechanism-based anticancer drug
    discovery, 24–27
miniaturization, 32
prospects, 37
protein kinase inhibitor assays, 29
Hollow fiber assays,
    luciferin-based technologies, 156
    molecular target screening, 156
    pharmacological characterization of agents,
        ex vivo pharmacology bioassay,
            operational steps, 171
            phenylurea thiocarbamate
                characterization, 176, 178, 179
            strategy, 170, 171
        in vitro concentration ⌈ time drug exposure
            assay,
            NSC 652287 characterization, 171,
                173–175
            principles, 169, 170
        in vitro concentration ⌈ time drug stability
            assay,
            halichondrin B characterization, 175,
                176
            principles, 170
    overview, 167, 169, 180
    principles, 154
    routine screening, 154–156, 180
HRQL, *see* Health-related quality of life
HTCA, *see* Human tumor cloning assay
HTCFA, *see* Human tumor colony formation
    assay
HTS, *see* High-throughput screening
Human tumor cloning assay (HTCA),
    applications, 66
    chemosensitivity versus chemoresistance
        assays, 66
    clinical applications, 68, 70
    comparison with other chemosensitivity tests,
        72, 73
    drug development, 70–72
    overview, 66
    statistical analysis, 67, 68
Human tumor colony formation assay (HTCFA),
    historical perspective, 127
Human tumor xenograft models, *see also specific*
    models,
    advanced-stage xenograft models,
        anti-tumor activity calculations, 134, 135
        overview, 133, 134
        toxicity parameters, 134
    alternative models, 145–149
    challenge survival models, 136
    detailed drug evaluation strategy, 143–145
    development of models, 128, 129, 133
    drug sensitivity profiles, 136–142
    early-stage xenograft models, 135, 136
    historical perspective, 186–189
    initial compound evaluation strategy, 141–143

tumor growth characteristics by tumor origin,
    130–132

I

IC50, calculation, 18, 19
IIP, *see* Inter-Institute Program
IL-1, *see* Interleukin-1
ILS, *see* Increase in life span
Immunodeficient mice,
    athymic nude mice,
        orthotopic implants, *see* Orthotopic
            metastatic mouse models
        subcutaneous implant tumor models, *see*
            Human tumor xenograft models
    history of development, 185, 186
Immunogenicity, indications in transplantable
    tumor models, 104, 105
Immunostaining, minimal residual disease
    detection, 250, 251, 253
Increase in life span (ILS), calculation, 136
IND, *see* Investigational New Drug
Inter-Institute Program (IIP), collaborations, 347
Interferon-γ, orthotopic metastatic mouse model
    studies, 203, 204
Interleukin-1 (IL-1), cell protection from
    chemotoxicity, 227, 228
Investigational New Drug (IND), applications
    and review, 430, 431
In vitro screening, *see* Screening, in vitro
Irinotecan, combination therapy preclinical model
    analysis, 220, 226
Isobologram method, combination therapy
    preclinical model analysis, 218,
    221–223, 225, 226

K

Karnofsky performance status scale, clinical trial
    patient selection, 357, 358, 366
KDR/Flk-1 antisense oligonucleotide, orthotopic
    metastatic mouse model studies,
    204, 205

L

L1210 leukemia model,
    characteristics of leukemia, 80, 81
    drug screening, 79, 80
    drug-resistant models,
        alkylating agent resistance, 89, 92
        antimetabolite resistance, 92
        DNA- and tubulin-binding agent
            resistance, 92, 93
        types, 88, 89
    historical perspective, 126
    minimal residual tumor biomarker models, 244,
        245
    predictive value, 86–88
    prospects, 93, 96
    sensitivity to clinical agents, 81–84, 86
Luciferin, hollow fiber assay utilization, 156
Lung cancer, orthotopic metastatic mouse
    models, 195–197

M

MDR, *see* Multiple drug resistance
Median effect/combination index method,
      combination therapy preclinical
      model analysis, 218–221
Melanoma, dog model of oral melanoma,
   clinical features, 273, 274
   prognosis, 274
   treatment, 274
Melphalan, scheduling and sequencing of high-
      dose therapy, 231, 232, 234
Metastasis, *see* Orthotopic metastatic mouse
      models
Minimal residual tumor biomarker models,
   acute myelocytic leukemia in Brown Norway
      rat, 246–248
   B-cell leukemia/lymphoma murine model,
      248, 249
   detection of minimal residual disease,
      colony formation assay, 252
      fluorescence *in situ* hybridization, 249,
         250, 253, 254
      immunostaining, 250, 251, 253
      polymerase chain reaction, 251–254
      sensitivity of techniques, 252–254
   historical perspective, 243–246
Mitomycin C, orthotopic metastatic mouse model
      studies, 192
MMI-166, orthotopic metastatic mouse model
      studies, 202
Monoclonal antibody products, nonclinical
      testing, 328, 329
Monolayer cultures, drug screening in vitro, 5,
      7
MTT, vital staining for drug screening in vitro, 8–
      11, 44–46
Multiple drug resistance (MDR), resistant cell
      lines in drug screening, 17, 18
Murine leukemia models, *see* L1210 leukemia
      model; P388 leukemia model

N

National Cancer Institute (NCI),
   Cancer Therapy Evaluation Program, 339,
      340, 345, 346, 348
   Developmental Therapeutics Program, 41,
      339–341, 348
   Drug Development Group,
      collaboration, 346
      functions, 341–343, 345
   grants and contracts programs, 347
   history of drug development program, 340,
      341
   Inter-Institute Program, 347
   Rapid Access to Intervention Development,
      346
   Rapid Access to NCI Discovery program, 236,
      347

   repositories, 347
   stages of drug development,
      advanced screening and preclinical
         development, 344
      clinical development, 344–346
      drug discovery and screening, 343, 344
      overview, 341–343
   Web resources, 41, 348
National Cancer Institute 60-cell screen,
   Developmental Therapeutics Program Web
      site, 41
   implementation,
      assay selection, 44–46
      cell line panel, 46
      information technology, 47
      oversight, 43
      review and recommendation to operational
         status, 47
      standardization and reproducibility, 47
   operation,
      research applications, 50, 52–54
      service screening operations, 48, 49
   origins, 42, 43
   preclinical collaborations with European
      groups, 383–385
   prospects, 54, 56
National Cooperative Drug Discovery Group
      (NCDDG) program, grants, 347
NCDDG program, *see* National Cooperative Drug
      Discovery Group program
NCI, *see* National Cancer Institute
NDA, *see* New Drug Application
Neutral red, vital staining for drug screening
      in vitro, 8
New Drug Application (NDA), submissions and
      review, 433–435
NHL, *see* Non-Hodgkin's lymphoma
Non-Hodgkin's lymphoma (NHL),
   cat model,
      classification, 266
      etiology, 265, 266
      incidence, 265
      relevance to human disease, 266
      treatment, 266
   dog model,
      classification, 263, 264
      incidence, 263
      prognostic factors, 265
      relevance to human disease, 265
      treatment, 265
Nonclinical safety development program,
   biologic product testing, *see* Oncology
         biologic product nonclinical testing
   common problems in toxicology testing, 310,
      311
   contract research organization outsourcing,
      criteria for selection, 307–309
      monitoring toxicology studies, 309, 310
      quotation request, 309

design,
    balance among sound science, regulatory
        expectations, and corporate
        objectives, 288, 289
    cost estimates and timelines, 291–295
    toxicology program for oncology products,
        289–291
drug testing, *see* Oncology drug product
        nonclinical testing
toxicology study design,
    administration routes, 295, 296
    dose level selection, 299
dose volumes and good practices, 296, 297
    endpoints,
        body weight, 301
        clinical pathology, 303
        clinical signs, 300–303
        food consumption, 301
        histopathology, 304–307
        sampling volumes and good practices,
            303, 304
    number of animals, 299
    species selection considerations, 296, 298,
        299
NSC 652287, pharmacological characterization,
    171, 173–175

O

ODAC, *see* Oncology Drug Advisory Committee
Oncology biologic product nonclinical testing,
    ancillary products, 332, 333
    cancer vaccines, 333, 334
    design of studies, *see* Nonclinical safety
        development program
    gene therapy, 330–332
    general safety principles, 326–328
    goals, 334, 335
    monoclonal antibody products, 328, 329
    recombinant proteins, 333
    regulatory oversight, 325, 326
    somatic cell therapy, 329, 330
Oncology Drug Advisory Committee (ODAC),
    functions, 421–423
    importance of functional understanding, 421,
        427
    meetings,
        applicant presentation, 426
        conflict of interest evaluation, 424
        discussion and vote on questions, 426, 427
        format, 425
        notifications, 423, 424
        preparation materials and public access,
            424–426
        quorum, 424
    product types for review, 421
    structure and membership, 423
Oncology drug product nonclinical testing,
    chronically administered, molecularly targeted
        drugs,

phase I trial support, 315–317
        phase II trial support, 315–317
        phase III trial support, 316
    combination therapy,
        cytotoxic drug combinations, 318
        cytotoxic drug combinations with
            molecularly targeted drugs, 318, 319
        molecularly targeted drug combinations,
            319
    design of studies, *see* Nonclinical safety
        development program
    expanded acute studies, 314, 322
    immunotoxicology requirements, 321
    interspecies dose conversions, 321, 322
    marketing applications nonclinical program,
        carcinogenicity, 317, 318
        developmental and reproductive toxicology
            screens, 318
        genetic toxicity, 317
        targeted toxicity studies, 318
    normal volunteer trials, 319, 320
    overview, 313–315
    phototoxicology requirements, 321
    safety pharmacology requirements, 320, 321
    starting dose selection, 321
Organ culture, drug screening in vitro, 4
Orthotopic metastatic mouse models,
    bladder cancer, 191
    breast cancer, 198
    colon cancer, 190, 191
    drug discovery studies, 201–207
    green fluorescent protein,
        dual-color imaging of tumor–host
            interaction, 207
        imaging of tumors, 192, 193, 197–199
    head and neck cancer, 193, 194
    historical perspective, 184, 185, 189
    lung cancer, 195–197
    mechanisms of enhanced metastasis, 199, 200
    ovarian cancer, 198
    Paget's *see*d and soil hypothesis, 184, 200,
        201
    pancreas cancer, 191–193
    prostate cancer, 197, 198
    stomach cancer, 194, 195
Osteosarcoma, dog model,
    cisplatin drug delivery systems, 271
    clinical features, 269, 270
    L-MTP-PE immunotherapy, 269, 271
Ovarian cancer, orthotopic metastatic mouse
        models, 198

P

P388 leukemia model,
    characteristics of leukemia, 80, 81
    drug screening, 3, 42, 79, 80
    drug-resistant models,
        alkylating agent resistance, 89, 92
        antimetabolite resistance, 92

DNA- and tubulin-binding agent
    resistance, 92, 93
  types, 88, 89
historical perspective, 126
minimal residual tumor biomarker models, 244,
    245
predictive value, 86–88
prospects, 93, 96
sensitivity to clinical agents, 81–84, 86
supersensitive model limitations, 100, 101
Paclitaxel, combination therapy preclinical model
    analysis, 220, 221
Paget's seed and soil hypothesis, 184, 200, 201
Pancreas cancer, orthotopic metastatic mouse
    models, 191–193
Parathyroid hormone-related protein (PTHrP),
    orthotopic metastatic mouse model
    studies, 193
PCR, *see* Polymerase chain reaction
Pharmacological characterization of agents,
  ex vivo pharmacology bioassay,
    operational steps, 171
    phenylurea thiocarbamate characterization,
        176, 178, 179
    strategy, 170, 171
  in vitro concentration ⌈ time drug exposure
    assay,
      NSC 652287 characterization, 171, 173–
          175
      principles, 169, 170
  in vitro concentration ⌈ time drug stability
    assay,
      halichondrin B characterization, 175, 176
      principles, 170
  overview, 167, 169, 180
Phase I clinical trials,
  costs, 364
  dose escalation strategies, 354–356
  drug schedules, 352, 353
  ethics in oncology trials, 360
  initial dose level determination, 353, 354
  nonclinical testing support, 315–317
  objectives, 351, 352
  patient selection, 356–358
  pharmacologic evaluations, 359, 360
routes of administration, 353
  toxicity assessment, 358, 359
Phase II clinical trials,
  agent selection, 364
  costs, 364
  designs,
    expanded access trials, 373
    pharmacodynamic endpoints, 375–377
    randomized discontinuation design, 375
    randomized trials, 373–375
    single-arm studies of a single disease, 372,
        373
  dose refinement, 365, 366

endpoint selection,
  clinical endpoints, 369
  molecular endpoints, 370–372
  pharmacokinetic endpoints, 369, 370
individualization of therapy, 377–379
nonclinical testing support, 315–317
objectives, 363, 364
patient selection factors,
  patient-specific factors, 366, 367
  tumor-specific factors, 367–369
Phase III clinical trials,
  cooperative groups in United States, 401, 402
  costs, 364
  data monitoring, 408, 409
  designs, 404
  endpoints,
    health-related quality of life, 407, 412,
        415, 416, 419
    objective tumor response, 407, 408
    palliation, 407
    survival, 406
    time to progression, 406, 407
    time to treatment failure, 407
    tumor-related symptoms, 407
  nonclinical testing support, 316
  objectives, 401, 402
  patient selection, 403
  placebo and blinding, 406
  randomization, 403, 404
  regulatory oversight, 401, 402, 409
  sample size,
    noninferiority trials, 405
    superiority trials, 404, 405
Phenylurea thiocarbamate (PTC),
    pharmacological characterization,
        176, 178, 179
Polymerase chain reaction (PCR), minimal
    residual disease detection, 251–254
Prostate cancer, orthotopic metastatic mouse
    models, 197, 198
PTC, *see* Phenylurea thiocarbamate
PTHrP, *see* Parathyroid hormone-related protein

R
R*A*N*D, *see* Rapid Access to NCI Discovery
RAID, *see* Rapid Access to Intervention
    Development
Rapid Access to Intervention Development
    (RAID), collaborations, 346
Rapid Access to NCI Discovery (R*A*N*D),
    collaborations, 346, 347
Recombinant therapeutic proteins, nonclinical
    testing, 333
Rodent tumor models, *see also specific models*,
  discovery goal of primary screening, 116, 117
  drug development and secondary evaluation,
    criteria, 118–120
    overestimation of drug potential, 117
    protocol design considerations, 118

underestimation of drug potential, 117
history of development, 101–104
immunogenicity indications, 104, 105
prescreening importance, 105
protocol design considerations for screening,
controls, 115
drug administration,
dosing, 111, 112
formulations, 113, 114
routes, 112, 113
schedules, 110, 111
implantation sites for tumors, 109
mouse weighing, 114
toxicity assessment, 114, 115
tumor stage, 108, 109
selection for primary screening, 106–108
tumor characterization,
cell kill calculation, 116
endpoints, 115, 116
tumor growth delay, 116

S

S-1, orthotopic metastatic mouse model studies,
205
SBIR, *see* Small Business Innovation Research
Scintillation proximity assay (SPA), high-
throughput screening, 29
Screening, in vitro,
clonogenic assays, 5, 6, 64–66
historical perspective, 4
human tumor screening, *see* Human tumor
cloning assay
large-scale screening, *see also* High-
throughput screening,
criteria, 6
dye exclusion assays, 7
monolayer cultures, 7
resistant cell lines in screening, 17, 18
vital staining,
Alamar Blue, 14–17
MTT, 8–11
neutral red, 8
XTT, 12–14
monolayer culture, 5
organ culture, 4
rationale, 3, 4, 105
60-cell screen, *see* National Cancer Institute
60-cell screen
spheroids, 5
toxicity reporting, 18, 19
60-cell screen, *see* National Cancer Institute 60-
cell screen
Small Business Innovation Research (SBIR),
grants, 347

Small Business Technology Transfer (STTR)
program, grants, 347
Soft tissue sarcoma, dog and cat models,
classification, 266–268
etiology, 266
incidence, 266
relevance to human disease, 268
treatment, 268
Somatic cell therapy, nonclinical testing, 329, 330
SPA, *see* Scintillation proximity assay
Spheroids, drug screening in vitro, 5
SRB, *see* Sulforhodamine B
Stem cell support model, combination therapy
preclinical model, 226–229
Stomach cancer, orthotopic metastatic mouse
models, 194, 195
STTR program, *see* Small Business Technology
Transfer program
Sulforhodamine B (SRB), drug screening in vitro,
45, 46

T

Thiotepa,
combination therapy preclinical model
analysis, 222, 223
scheduling and sequencing of high-dose
therapy, 231
TNP-470,
activity in xenograft models, 166–168
orthotopic metastatic mouse model studies,
206, 207
Toxicology studies, *see* Nonclinical safety
development program; Oncology
biologic product nonclinical testing;
Oncology drug product nonclinical
testing
Tumor cell kill, calculation, 116, 134, 135
Tumor growth delay, calculation, 116, 134
Tumor-related symptoms,
definition, 413
endpoint in phase III trials, 407, 415, 416
instruments, 416, 417
regular marketing approvals, 413–416

V

Vascular endothelial growth factor neutralizing
antibodies, orthotopic metastatic
mouse model studies, 205, 206
Vinblastine, combination therapy preclinical
model analysis, 221
Vinorelbine, combination therapy preclinical
model analysis, 225

X

XTT, vital staining for drug screening in vitro,
12–14, 44, 46

ABOUT THE EDITORS

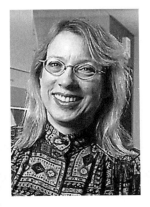

Dr. Beverly A. Teicher is Vice President and Director of the Oncology Portfolio at Genzyme Molecular Oncology and Genzyme Corporation, Framingham, MA. Upon completion of her PhD in Bioorganic Chemistry at the Johns Hopkins University, Dr. Teicher accepted a postdoctoral position in the laboratory of Dr. Alan C. Sartorelli in the Department of Pharmacology at Yale University School of Medicine, where she studied the response of hypoxic cells to anticancer therapies and the synthesis of potential hypoxic cell-selective cytotoxic agents. Dr. Teicher joined the staff of the Dana-Farber Cancer Institute as an assistant professor of pathology in July 1981 and over 16 years there rose to the rank of associate professor of medicine and radiation therapy, Harvard Medical School at the Dana-Farber Cancer Institute and Joint Center for Radiation Therapy. She pioneered the application of perfluorochemical and hemoglobin oxygen delivery agents in cancer therapy and tumor imaging. Dr. Teicher also elucidated mechanisms by which solid tumors are resistant to antitumor agents, especially antitumor alkylating agents, developing 25 alkylating agent-resistant human tumor cell lines and exploring the mechanisms of their drug resistance. Dr. Teicher established a model system where drug resistance in a solid tumor was developed in vivo and went on to incorporate antiangiogenic agents into solid tumor treatment paradigms. In July 1997, Dr. Teicher was appointed Research Advisor in Cancer Drug Discovery at Lilly Research Laboratories. Dr. Teicher joined Genzyme Corporation in January 2002, where she is heading the antiangiogenesis effort and leading the oncology application effort in the transforming growth factor-β program. Dr. Teicher is a very active member of the international scientific community. She has written or coauthored more than 400 scientific publications, has edited five books, is senior editor for the journal *Clinical Cancer Research,* and is series editor of the Cancer Drug Discovery and Development book series.

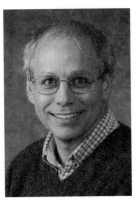

Dr. Paul Andrews is Senior Director, Preclinical Sciences, at Aton Pharma Inc., where he develops, implements, and manages nonclinical safety assessment programs to support clinical development of oncology drugs. He received a BA in Chemistry from Johns Hopkins University and his PhD in Medicinal Chemistry from the University of Maryland at Baltimore. Dr. Andrews has more than 25 years of experience in preclinical drug development, as well as extensive background in academia, where he has directed a research laboratory investigating various aspects of the cellular pharmacology of anticancer agents. He is an expert in nonclinical regulatory issues and oncology drug development strategies from both governmental and industry perspectives. Prior to joining Aton, Dr. Andrews was a consultant at Cato Research Ltd and had previously worked at the Food and Drug Administration, ultimately as the Pharmacology Team Leader in the Division of Oncology Drug Products. He also served a term as the Associate Director for Pharmacology and Toxicology at the Office of Drug Evaluation I.